CT and MRI in Oncology

Springer

Paris
Berlin
Heidelberg
New York
Barcelona
Budapest
Hong Kong
London
Milan
Santa Clara
Singapore
Tokyo

Didier Buthiau, David Khayat (eds)

CT and MRI in Oncology

Preface by James F. Holland

Springer

Didier Buthiau
Radiologue. Ancien Chef de Clinique-Assistant
des Hôpitaux de Paris
Centre d'Imagerie Scanner Paris 14
119 avenue du Général Leclerc, 75014 Paris
et Centre RMX, 80 avenue Félix Faure, 75015 Paris

David Khayat
Cancérologue. Professeur des Universités, Praticien
Hospitalier. Chef du Service d'Oncologie Médicale
Hôpital de La Salpêtrière
47 boulevard de l'Hôpital, 75013 Paris

Drawings and diagrams: S. Buthiau

Original French edition
Scanner et IRM en Cancérologie

ISBN-13: 978-3-642-46844-5 e-ISBN-13: 978-3-642-46842-1
DOI: 10.1007/978-3-642-46842-1

Library of Congress Cataloging-in-Publication Data
Scanner et IRM en Cancérologie. English.
CT scan and MRI in Oncology/D. Buthiau, D. Khayat, (eds) ;
Foreword by J.F. Holland
p. cm.
Includes bibliographical references and index.
ISBN-13: 978-3-642-46844-5
1. Cancer- -Tomography. 2. Cancer- -Magnetic resonance imaging.
I. Buthiau, D (Didier) II. Khayat, David. III Title.
[DNLM: 1. Neoplasms- - diagnosis. 2. Tomography, X-Ray Computed- -methods. 3. Diagnosis Imaging- -methods QZ 241 S283c 1998a]
RC270.3.T65S28 1998
616.99'20757- -dc21
DNLM/DLC
for Library of Congress 97-45146
CIP

Softcover reprint of the hardcover 1st edition 1998

SPIN: 1055722 Printed on acid-free paper

To Sylvie, Norman and Candice

D. Buthiau

To Jocelyne, Julie, Barbara and Cécile

D. Khayat

Contents

Contributors

C. Aboulker
Radiologue. Ancien Chef de Clinique-Assistant des Hôpitaux de Paris
Centre Chirurgical de Boulogne-Billancourt
105 avenue Victor Hugo, 92100 Boulogne

E.-Ch. Antoine
Cancérologue. Chef de Clinique-Assistant des Hôpitaux de Paris
Service d'Oncologie Médicale
Hôpital de La Salpêtrière
47 boulevard de l'Hôpital, 75013 Paris

L. Arrivé
Radiologue. Praticien Hospitalier
Service de Radiologie, Hôpital St-Antoine
184 rue de Fbg St-Antoine, 75012 Paris

F. Assadian
Chirurgien Cervico-Facial et Oto-Rhino-Laryngologiste. Board de l'État de Californie
Service d'ORL, Centre Hospitalier Privé du Montgardé
78410 Aubergenville

T. Bach-Gansmo
Nycomed Imaging As. Oslo

P. Baldeyrou
Pneumologue
Centre Médico-Chirurgical de la Porte de Choisy
6 place Port au Prince, 75013 Paris

P. Banzet
Professeur des Universités, Praticien Hospitalier
Chef de Service de Chirurgie Plastique et Reconstructrice. Hôpital St-Louis
1, avenue Claude Vellefaux, 75010 Paris

A. Benhammouda
Cancérologue. Attaché des Hôpitaux de Paris
Service d'Oncologie Médicale, Hôpital de la Salpêtrière
47 boulevard de l'Hôpital, 75013 Paris

J.-L. Bensimon
Radiologue. Oto-Rhino-Laryngologiste
91 boulevard Haussmann, 75008 Paris

J. Berge
Neuroradiologue. Praticien Hospitalier
Service de Neuroradiologie Diagnostique et Thérapeutique. Hôpital Pellegrin
33076 Bordeaux Cedex

O. Bernard
Assistant-Chef de Clinique
Service de Radiothérapie Oncologique
Hôpital du Val de Grâce
74 boulevard du Port Royal, 75005 Paris

Ch. Billote
Ophtalmologiste. Praticien Hospitalier
Service d'Ophtalmologie
CHU Côte de Nacre. 14033 Caen

A. Biondi
Neuroradiologue. Attachée des Hôpitaux de Paris
Service de Neuroradiologie
Hôpital de La Pitié-Salpêtrière
83 boulevard de l'Hôpital, 75013 Paris

J. Biserte
Urologue. Professeur des Universités
Praticien Hospitalier. Service d'Urologie
Hôpital C. Huriez, CHRU de Lille
1 place de Verdun, 59037 Lille Cedex

O. Blétry
Médecin Interniste. Professeur des Universités
Praticien Hospitalier
Chef de Service de Médecine Interne
Hôpital Foch, 40 rue Worth, 92151 Suresnes

S. Bobin
Oto-Rhino-Laryngologiste et Chirurgien Cervico-Facial. Professeur des Universités, Praticien Hospitalier Chef de Service d'ORL et de Chirurgie Cervico-Faciale
Hôpital de Bicêtre, 78 avenue du Général Leclerc
94270 Le Kremlin Bicêtre

L. Boiteau
Radiologue. Chef de Clinique-Assistant des Hôpitaux
Département de Radiologie
CHU Côte de Nacre, 14033 Caen

F. Bolgert
Neurologue. Praticien Hospitalier
Service de Neurologie. Unité de Réanimation
Hôpital de La Salpêtrière
47 boulevard de l'Hôpital, 75013 Paris

C. Borel
Cancérologue. Attaché des Hôpitaux de Paris
Service d'Oncologie Médicale.
Hôpital de La Salpêtrière
47 boulevard de l'Hôpital, 75013 Paris

M. Bouaziz
Cancérologue. Service d'Oncologie Médicale
Hôpital de La Salpêtrière
47 boulevard de l'Hôpital, 75013 Paris

D. Brasnu
Oto-Rhino-Laryngologiste et Chirurgien Cervico-Facial. Professeur des Universités, Praticien hospitalier
Chef de Service d'ORL et de Chirurgie Cervico-Faciale
Hôpital Laennec, 42 rue de Sèvres, 75007 Paris

J.-L. Breau
Cancérologue. Professeur des Universités
Praticien Hospitalier. Chef du Service d'Oncologie
Hôpital Avicenne
125 route de Stalingrad, 93000 Bobigny

P. Brunet
Neurologue. Professeur des Universités
Praticien Hospitalier. Chef de Service de Neurologie
Hôpital de La Salpêtrière
47 boulevard de l'Hôpital, 75013 Paris

D. Buthiau
Radiologue. Ancien Chef de Clinique-Assistant des Hôpitaux de Paris. Centre d'Imagerie Scanner Paris 14
119 avenue du Général Leclerc, 75014 Paris
et Centre RMX, 80 avenue Félix Faure, 75015 Paris

J.-M. Caillé
Neuroradiologue. Professeur des Universités
Praticien Hospitalier. Chef du Service de Neuroradiologie Diagnostique et Thérapeutique
Hôpital Pellegrin, 33076 Bordeaux Cedex

J.V. Chantelard
Cancérologue. Ancien Chef de Clinique-Assistant des Hôpitaux de Paris. Clinique Oncologique et Radiothérapique de la Croix de Chavaux
42 boulevard de Chanzy, 93100 Montreuil

C. Chapelon-Abric
Médecin Interniste. Praticien Hospitalier
Service de Médecine Interne. Hôpital de la Pitié
83 boulevard de l'Hôpital, 75013 Paris

B. Charbonnel
Endocrinologue. Professeur des Universités, Praticien Hospitalier. Chef du Service d'Endocrinologie
Hôtel-Dieu, BP 1005, 44035 CHU Nantes

H. Charreyre
Attaché des Hôpitaux de Paris
Service de Gynécologie-Obstétrique. Hôpital de La Pitié
83 boulevard de l'Hôpital, 75013 Paris

P. Chaumier
Médecin Interniste et Pneumologue. Ancien Chef de Clinique-Assistant des Hôpitaux de Paris
Service de Médecine Interne et Pneumologie. Centre Hospitalier Privé du Montgardé, 78410 Aubergenville

B. Chiche
Chirurgien Viscéral. Professeur Associé au Collège de Médecine des Hôpitaux de Paris.
Chef du Service de Chirurgie.
Centre Raymond-Garcin
2 bis rue d'Alésia, 75014 Paris

D. Coeffic
Cancérologue. Chef de Clinique-Assistant des Hôpitaux de Paris. Service d'Oncologie Médicale.
Hôpital de La Salpêtrière
47 boulevard de l'Hôpital, 75013 Paris

G. Cohen-Aloro
Chirurgien Viscéral. Ancien Chef de Clinique-Assistant des Hôpitaux de Paris. Clinique du Mont-Louis
8-10 rue de la Folie Régnault, 75011 Paris

J.-M. Cosset
Radiothérapeute. Professeur des Universités
Praticien Hospitalier
Chef du Département d'Oncologie Radiothérapique
Institut Curie, 26 rue d'Ulm, 75005 Paris

P. Courtheoux
Radiologue. Professeur des Universités, Praticien Hospitalier. Chef du Département de Radiologie
CHU Côte de Nacre, 14033 Caen

C. Courtieu
Gynécologue-Obstétricien. Praticien Hospitalier
Service de Gynécologie-Obstétrique
CHT Carremeau, 30900 Nîmes

Y. Darbois
Gynécologue-Obstétricien. Professeur des Universités
Praticien Hospitalier
Chef du Service de Gynécologie-Obstétrique
Hôpital de la Pitié
83 boulevard de l'Hôpital, 75013 Paris

D. Dargent
Gynécologue-Obstétricien. Professeur des Universités Praticien Hospitalier. Chef du Service de Gynécologie-Obstétrique. Hôpital Édouard Herriot
5 place d'Arsonval, 69437 Lyon Cedex 03

J. Dauplat
Gynécologue-Obstétricien. Professeur des Universités Praticien Hospitalier. Chef du Service de Gynécologie-Obstétrique. Centre Jean Perrin
58 rue Montalembert, BP 392, 63011 Clermont-Ferrand

G. Delépine
Chirurgien Orthopédiste. Cancérologue. Ancien Chef de Clinique-Assistant des Hôpitaux de Paris
Service d'Orthopédie (Pr Goutallier)
Hôpital Henri Mondor
51 avenue de Lattre de Tassigny, 94000 Créteil

N. Delépine
Pédiatre. Cancérologue. Médecin des Hôpitaux de Paris Ancien Chef de Clinique-Assistant
Service d'Oncologie Pédiatrique. Hôpital Robert Debré
48 boulevard Serurier, 75019 Paris

R. Dendale
Cancérologue. Interne des Hôpitaux de Paris. Service d'Oncologie Médicale. Hôpital de La Salpêtrière
47 boulevard de l'Hôpital, 75013 Paris

J.C. Desbois
Pédiatre. Cancérologue. Professeur des Universités Praticien Hospitalier. Chef de Service d'Oncologie Pédiatrique. Hôpital Robert Debré
48 boulevard Serurier, 75019 Paris

E. Dieu
Psychiatre. Clinique Villa Montsouris
115 rue de la Santé, 75013 Paris

R.F. Dondelinger
Radiologue. Professeur de Radiologie. Université de Liège. Chef du Service d'Imagerie Médicale. CHU Sart Tilman, Domaine Universitaire du Sart Tilman
BP 35, 4000 Liège, 1

D. Dormont
Neuroradiologue. Praticien Hospitalier. Service de Neuroradiologie. Hôpital de La Pitié-Salpêtrière
83 boulevard de l'Hôpital, 75013 Paris

M. Dousset
Radiologue. Ancien Assistant en Radiologie
Harvard Medical School, Massachusetts General Hospital, Boston
Centre d'Imagerie Médicale
17 rue de Milan, 75009 Paris

V. Dousset
Neuroradiologue. Chef de Clinique-Assistant. Service de Neuroradiologie Diagnostique et Thérapeutique
Hôpital Pellegrin, 33076 Bordeaux Cedex

J.P. Droz
Cancérologue. Professeur des Universités, Praticien Hospitalier. Chef de Service d'Oncologie. Centre Léon Bérard, 28 rue Laennec, 69373 Lyon Cedex 08

B. Dupas
Radiologue. Praticien Hospitalier. Chef du Service Central de Radiologie et d'Imagerie Médicale
Hôtel-Dieu, BP 1005, 44035 CHU Nantes

C. Durier
Université Necker-Enfants Malades (René Descartes)
156 rue de Vaugirard 75015 Paris

A. Eche
Cancérologue. Interne des Hôpitaux de Paris
Service d'Oncologie Médicale
Hôpital de La Salpêtrière
47 boulevard de l'Hôpital, 75013 Paris

J.M. Faintuch
Radiologue. Ancien Chef de Clinique-Assistant des Hôpitaux de Paris. Service de Radiologie
Hôpital Tenon, 4 rue de la Chine, 75020 Paris

L. Feuvret
Cancérologue. Interne des Hôpitaux de Paris
Service de Radiothérapie Oncologique
Institut Curie, 26 rue d'Ulm, 75005 Paris

A. Foulet
Anatomo-Pathologiste. Ancien Chef de Clinique
Laboratoire d'Anatomo-Pathologie
CH du Mans, 72037 Le Mans Cedex

M. Gayet-Delacroix
Radiologue. Praticien Hospitalier
Service Central de Radiologie et d'Imagerie Médicale
Hôtel Dieu, BP 1005, 44035 CHU Nantes

F. Gelbert
Radiologue. Praticien Hospitalier
Service de Neuroradiologie et Angiographie Thérapeutique. Hôpital Lariboisière
2 rue Ambroise Paré, 75010 Paris

S. Gerber
Neuroradiologue. Attachée des Hôpitaux de Paris
Service de Neuroradiologie. Hôpital Pitié-Salpêtrière
47 boulevard de l'Hôpital, 75013 Paris

M. Gil-Delgado
Cancérologue. Praticien Hospitalier. SOMPS
47 boulevard de l'Hôpital, 75013 Paris

B. Gosselin
Anatomo-Pathologiste. Professeur des Universités
Praticien Hospitalier. Chef de Service d'Anatomo-Pathologie. Hôpital A. Calmette, CHRU Lille
boulevard du Professeur Leclercq, 59037 Lille Cedex

M. Gozy
Cancérologue. Chef de Clinique-Assistant
Service d'Oncologie Médicale. Hôpital de la Salpêtrière
47 boulevard de l'Hôpital, 75013 Paris

R. Grob
Neurochirurgien. Ancien Chef de Clinique-Assistant des Hôpitaux de Paris. Clinique Bachaumont
18 rue de Bachaumont, 75002 Paris

D. Grosskopf
Neurochirurgien. Ancien Chef de Clinique-Assistant des Hôpitaux de Paris. Clinique Geoffroy St-Hilaire
59 rue Geoffroy St-Hilaire, 75005 Paris

F. Guinet
Cancérologue. Centre Médico-Chirurgical Léonard de Vinci, 95 avenue Parmentier, 75011 Paris

A.C. Hardy
Cancérologue. Attachée des Hôpitaux de Paris. Service d'Oncologie Médicale. Hôpital de La Salpêtrière
47 boulevard de l'Hôpital, 75013 Paris

F. Hecht
Cancérologue, Radiothérapeute. Unité d'Oncologie Chirurgicale. Service de Chirurgie
Hôpital Bichat, 46 rue Henri-Huchard, 75018 Paris

D. Herbreteau
Radiologue. Chef de Clinique-Assistant des Hôpitaux de Paris. Service de Neuroradiologie et Angiographie Thérapeutique. Hôpital Lariboisière
2 rue Ambroise Paré, 75010 Paris

M. Housset
Cancérologue, Radiothérapeute. Professeur des Universités, Praticien Hospitalier, Service de Radiothérapie. Hôpital Saint-Louis
1 avenue Claude Vellefaux, 75010 Paris

D. Khayat
Cancérologue. Professeur des Universités, Praticien Hospitalier. Chef du Service d'Oncologie Médicale
Hôpital de La Salpêtrière
47 boulevard de l'Hôpital, 75013 Paris

H. Laccourreye
Oto-Rhino-Laryngologiste et Chirurgien Cervico-Facial
Professeur des Universités, Praticien Hospitalier
Ancien Chef de Service d'ORL et de Chirurgie Cervico-Faciale
Hôpital Laennec, 42 rue de Sèvres, 75007 Paris

O. Laccourreye
Oto-Rhino-Laryngologiste et Chirurgien Cervico-Facial
Professeur des Universités, Praticien Hospitalier
Service d'ORL et de Chirurgie Cervico-Faciale
Hôpital Laennec, 42 rue de Sèvres, 75007 Paris

J.P. Laissy
Radiologue. Professeur des Universités
Praticien Hospitalier. Service de Radiologie Viscérale
Hôpital Bichat, 46 rue Henri Huchard, 75018 Paris

P. Lapresle
Chirurgien Orthopédiste. Ancien Chef de Clinique-Assistant des Hôpitaux de Paris
Clinique Arago, 95 boulevard Arago, 75014 Paris

D. Lardé
Radiologue. Ancien Chef de Clinique-Assistant des Hôpitaux de Paris. Centre de Radiologie
34 rue des Mèches, 94000 Créteil

J.-P. Le Bourgeois
Cancérologue. Professeur des Universités
Praticien Hospitalier. Chef du Service de Radiothérapie-Oncologie. CHU Henri Mondor
51 av. du Maréchal de Lattre de Tassigny, 94010 Créteil

T. Le Chevalier
Cancérologue. Professeur des Universités, Praticien Hospitalier. Assistant des Centres Anti-Cancéreux
Chef de Service de Médecine Oncologique
Institut Gustave Roussy
39-53 rue Camille Desmoulins, 94800 Villejuif

G. Lefebvre
Gynécologue-Obstétricien. Praticien Hospitalier
Service de Gynécologie-Obstétrique
Hôpital de la Pitié
83 boulevard de l'Hôpital, 75013 Paris

J.-P. Lefranc
Gynécologue-Obstétricien. Professeur des Universités
Praticien Hospitalier. Service de Chirurgie Gynécologique. Hôpital de La Salpêtrière
47 boulevard de l'Hôpital, 75013 Paris

H. Lemaignen
Assistant Directeur Médical. Laboratoires Nycomed
25 quai Panhard et Levassor, 75013 Paris

L. Lemaître
Radiologue. Professeur des Universités. Praticien Hospitalier. Chef de Service de Radiologie Ouest
Hôpital C. Huriez, CHRU Lille
1 place de Verdun 59037 Lille Cedex

E. Malaurie
Cancérologue. Praticien Hospitalier. Service de Cancérologie. Hôpital Intercommunal de Créteil
40 avenue de Verdun, 94000 Créteil

B. Marro
Radiologue. Ancien Chef de Clinique-Assistante des Hôpitaux de Paris. Service de Neuroradiologie
Hôpital de la Pitié-Salpêtrière
47 boulevard de l'Hôpital, 75013 Paris

C. Marsault
Neuroradiologue. Professeur des Universités
Praticien Hospitalier. Chef de Service
de Neuroradiologie
Hôpital de La Pitié-Salpêtrière
47 boulevard de l'Hôpital, 75013 Paris

P. Martinat
Radiologue. Interne. Service de Radiologie Ouest
Hôpital C. Huriez, CHRU Lille
1 place de Verdun, 59037 Lille Cedex

M. Marty
Cancérologue. Professeur des Universités
Praticien Hospitalier. Chef de Service
Policlinique d'Oncologie Médicale
Hôpital Saint-Louis
1 avenue Claude Vellefaux, 75010 Paris

A. Maubon
Radiologue. Ancien Chef de Clinique-Assistant
CMC Beausoleil
119 avenue de Lodève, 34000 Montpellier

E. Mazeman
Urologue, Professeur des Universités, Praticien Hospitalier. Chef de Service d'Urologie
Hôpital C. Huriez, CHRU Lille
1 place de Verdun, 59037 Lille Cedex

B. Mégarbane
Cancérologue, Interne des Hôpitaux de Paris
Service d'Oncologie Médicale
Hôpital de La Salpêtrière
47 boulevard de l'Hôpital, 75013 Paris

G. Michaux
Docteur en Chirurgie Dentaire
Docteur en Sciences Odontologiques
90 rue du Bac, 75007 Paris

G. Missenard
Chirurgien Orthopédiste. Ancien Chef de Clinique-Assistant des Hôpitaux de Paris
Clinique Arago, 95 boulevard Arago, 75014 Paris

J.L. Misset
Cancérologue. Professeur des Universités
Praticien Hospitalier. Chef de Service
d'Oncologie Médicale. Hôpital Paul Brousse
14, avenue Paul-Vaillant-Couturier
94804 Villejuif Cedex

J.M Mussini
Neurologue, Attaché au Service de Médecine Interne
Hôtel Dieu. BP 1005, 44035 CHU Nantes

D. Nizri
Cancérologue Radiothérapeute
Professeur Associé de Cancérologie
Attaché du Service d'Oncologie Médicale
Hôpital de La Salpêtrière
47 boulevard de l'Hôpital, 75013 Paris

P.Y. Pagan
Physicien d'Hôpital. Service de Radiothérapie Oncologique. Hôpital du Val de Grâce
74 boulevard du Port-Royal, 75005 Paris

D. Paraiso
Cancérologue. Attaché des Hôpitaux de Paris
Service d'Oncologie Médicale
Hôpital de La Salpêtrière
47 boulevard de l'Hôpital, 75013 Paris

N. Perrot
Radiologue. Attaché-Consultant des Hôpitaux de Paris
Service de Radiologie et de Gynécologie
Hôpital Tenon
4 rue de la Chine, 75020 Paris

T. Petit
Cancérologue. Ancien Chef de Clinique-Assistant des Hôpitaux de Paris
Service d'Oncologie Médicale
Hôpital de La Salpêtrière
47 boulevard de l'Hôpital, 75013

C. Petitjean
Chirurgien Vasculaire. Ancien Chef de Clinique-Assistant des Hôpitaux de Paris. Clinique Labrouste
64 rue Labrouste, 75015 Paris

J.D. Picard
Radiologue. Membre de l'Académie Nationale de Médecine. Ancien Chef de Service de Radiologie
Hôpital Foch, 40 rue Worth, 92150 Suresnes

P. Piedbois
Cancérologue. Professeur des Universités, Praticien Hospitalier. Service de Radiothérapie-Oncologie
CHU Henri Mondor
51 av. du Maréchal de Lattre de Tassigny
94010 Créteil

J.C. Piette
Médecin Interniste. Professeur des Universités
Praticien Hospitalier. Chef du Service de Médecine Interne. Hôpital de La Pitié
83 boulevard de l'Hôpital, 75013 Paris

M. Poisson
Neurologue. Professeur des Universités
Praticien Hospitalier. Chef de Service de Neurologie
Hôpital de La Salpêtrière
47 boulevard de l'Hôpital, 75013 Paris

P. Pouillart
Cancérologue. Professeur des Universités, Praticien Hospitalier. Chef de Service de Médecine Oncologique
Institut Curie, 26 rue d'Ulm, 75005 Paris

P. Priollet
Médecin Interniste. Chef du Service d'Hypertension Artérielle, Médecine Vasculaire et Médecine Interne
Hôpital Saint-Joseph,
7 rue Pierre Larousse, 75014 Paris

M. Raynaud
Neuroradiologue. Praticien Hospitalier. Service de Neuroradiologie Diagnostique et Thérapeutique
Hôpital Pellegrin, 33076 Bordeaux Cedex

J. de Recondo
Neurologue. Professeur des Universités
Praticien Hospitalier. Chef du Service de Neurologie
Centre Raymond Garcin, 2 bis rue d'Alésia, 75014 Paris

D. Régent
Radiologue. Professeur des Universités, Praticien Hospitalier. Chef de Service de Radiologie Adultes
CHU Nancy-Brabois, allée du Morvan
54511 Vandoeuvre Cedex

N. Renody
Cancérologue. Médecin Spécialiste des Centres Anti-Cancéreux
Centre Pleyel, 223 rue du Fg St-Honoré, 75008 Paris

O. Rixe
Cancérologue. Ancien Chef de Clinique-Assistant des Hôpitaux de Paris
Service d'Oncologie Médicale
Hôpital de La Salpêtrière
47 boulevard de l'Hôpital, 75013 Paris

Y. Robert
Radiologue. Praticien Hospitalier
Service de Radiologie Ouest
Hôpital C. Huriez, CHRU Lille
1 place de Verdun, 59037 Lille Cedex

M.A. Rocher
Cancérologue. Attachée du Service d'Oncologie Médicale. Hôpital de la Salpêtrière
47 boulevard de l'Hôpital, 75013 Paris

J.-P. Rouanet
Radiologue. Professeur des Universités
Praticien Hospitalier
Chef du Service d'Imagerie Médicale
Centre Médico-Chirurgical Beausoleil
119 avenue de Lodève, 34000 Montpellier

M. Sahel
Neuroradiologue. Attaché des Hôpitaux de Paris
Service de Neuroradiologie
Hôpital de la Pitié-Salpêtrière
83 boulevard de l'Hôpital, 75013 Paris

D. Salandre
Médecin Interniste et Gastro-Entérologue
Ancien Chef de Clinique-Assistant des Hôpitaux de Paris. Service de Médecine Interne et de Gastro-Entérologie
Centre Hospitalier Privé du Montgardé
78410 Aubergenville

M. Schlumberger
Chef d'Unité d'Hospitalisation
Service de Médecine Nucléaire
Institut Gustave Roussy
39-53, rue Camille Desmoulins
94805 Villejuif Cedex

P. Schmit
Radiologue. Ancien Chef de Clinique
Assistant des Hôpitaux de Paris
Centre Chirurgical de Boulogne-Billancourt
105 avenue Victor Hugo, 92100 Boulogne

C. Soubrane
Immunologiste. Docteur en Médecine
Docteur Ès Sciences. Chargée de Recherche INSERM
Laboratoire du Service d'Oncologie Médicale
Hôpital de La Salpêtrière
47 boulevard de l'Hôpital, 75013 Paris

J.-P. Spano
Cancérologue. Ancien Interne des Hôpitaux de Paris
Service d'Oncologie Médicale
Hôpital de La Salpêtrière
47 boulevard de l'Hôpital, 75013 Paris

H. Szpirglas
Stomatologiste-Oncologue. Médecin des Hôpitaux
Service de Stomatologie. Hôpital de La Salpêtrière
47 boulevard de l'Hôpital. 75013 Paris

P. Tassan
Neurologue. Praticien Hospitalier. Centre Hospitalier
Poissy-St-Germain-en-Laye
20 rue Armagis, 78105 St-Germain Cedex

A. Thomas
Stomatologiste-Oncologue. Service de Stomatologie
Hôpital de La Salpêtrière
47 boulevard de l'Hôpital, 75013 Paris

J. Traversat
Médecin-Interniste et Cardiologue. Ancien Chef de
Clinique-Assistant des Hôpitaux de Paris. Service de
Médecine Interne et de Cardiologie. Centre Hospitalier
Privé du Montgardé, 78410 Aubergenville

A. Vacheron
Cardiologue. Professeur des Universités
Praticien Hospitalier, Chef du Service de Cardiologie
Hôpital Necker, 149 rue de Sèvres, 75015 Paris

D. Vadrot
Radiologue. Professeur des Universités
Praticien Hospitalier. Chef du Service de Radiologie
Hôtel Dieu de Paris
1 place du Parvis de Notre-Dame, 75004 Paris

E. Vuillemin
Cancérologue. Ancien Chef de Clinique-Assistant des
Hôpitaux de Paris. Service d'Oncologie Médicale
Centre Saint-Yves, 56000 Vannes

A. Wacrenier
Gynécologue-Obstétricien. Attaché des Hôpitaux de
Paris. Service de Gynécologie-Obstétrique
Hôpital de La Pitié
83 boulevard de l'Hôpital. 75013 Paris

B. Wechsler
Médecin Interniste. Médecin des Hôpitaux
Professeur au Collège Hospitalier
Service de Médecine Interne. Hôpital de La Pitié
83 boulevard de l'Hôpital, 75013 Paris

M. Weil
Hématologue-Cancérologue. Maître de Conférences
des Universités. Praticien Hospitalier
Service d'Oncologie Médicale
Hôpital de la Salpêtrière
47 boulevard de l'Hôpital, 75013 Paris

C. Yana
Radiologue. Ancien Chef de Clinique des Hôpitaux
de Paris. Clinique Bachaumont
18 rue de Bachaumont, 75002 Paris

A. Zamora
Chirurgien, Gynécologue-Obstétricien. Ancien Chef de
Clinique-Assistant des Hôpitaux de Paris
Centre Médico-Chirurgical Galien
15 Clos des Cascades, 93160 Noisy le Grand

L. Zelek
Cancérologue. Interne des Hôpitaux de Paris. Service
d'Oncologie Médicale, Hôpital de La Salpêtrière
47 boulevard de l'Hôpital, 75013 Paris

J. Zerbib
Oto-Rhino-Laryngologiste et Chirurgien Cervico-
Facial. Attaché-Consultant des Hôpitaux de Paris
Service d'ORL et de Chirurgie Cervico-Faciale
Hôpital de Bicêtre, Centre d'ORL
95 avenue du Général Leclerc, 75014 Paris

J.M. Ziza
Rhumatologue. Ancien Chef de Clinique-Assistant des
Hôpitaux de Paris. Chef du Service de Médecine
Interne et de Rhumatologie
Hôpital de la Croix St-Simon
125 rue d'Avron, 75020 Paris

Preface

Despite a relatively young discipline of only a hundred years of age, imaging has seen remarkable advances over the past 25 years due largely to the development of CT and, more recently, MRI. CT and MRI have made extraordinary progress in body imaging and moreover MRI has opened the way for studying the specific composition of tissues.

Imaging is routinely used in oncology, playing an essential role in tumor diagnosis, accurately defining spread to different organs and detecting recurrent disease. It is also vital both in research and clinical practice, providing a way of objectively measuring tumor responses to treatment. Nowadays it is impossible to specify the therapeutic indications for a cancer patient and monitor the response to the chosen treatment without comparing the clinical and imaging findings. This textbook by Didier Buthiau and David Khayat and their co-authors studies the relative roles of CT and MRI for all tumors: by constant comparison with clinical results, essential for evaluating these new technologies, the respective indications for these techniques are clarified, possible pitfalls highlighted and any difficulties encountered are analyzed.

This work is indispensable because oncologists, although still requiring expert image interpretation by competent radiologists, should themselves be able to understand the images they encounter in order to improve their clinical examination.

In this field, the technology is improving all the time: the future prospects for these new techniques are presented in this book (MR angiography, helical CT, multiplanar and 3-dimensional reconstructions). Digital image storage and transmission onto high definition computers opens up multiple possibilities for comparing images in different planes.

The further education of oncologists necessitated by the advances in imaging will be greatly enhanced by this book by Didier Buthiau and David Khayat and their co-authors who have combined a clarity of text and superb illustrations with their incomparable experience in clinical oncology. However, it will also be invaluable to hospital doctors and general practitioners alike.

Professor James F. Holland
Chief of the Department of Neoplasic Disease
Mount Sinai Hospital, New York
Ex-President of the ASCO and AACR
Ex-President of the CALGB

Acknowledgments

To General Electric Medical Systems Europe for their scientific collaboration.

To Nycomed Laboratories for their help in the development of this book.

To Sterling for their help in collecting iconography.

To Dr. A. Wacrenier, Dr. F. Gelbert, Dr. L. Zelek, Dr. D. Herbreteau and to Ms B. Cedreau for their support in this project.

Cancer, internal medicine and new imaging

Clinician
J.-C. Piette

The true revolution in medical practice as a result of modern imaging over the last 20 years has primarily been concerned with the diagnosis and management of cancers, imaging playing a major role in the detection of a tumor and often raising the suspicion of its malignant nature. The combination of ultrasound, CT and more recently MRI in clinical practice has occurred so quickly and impressively that these investigations have become part of our daily routine and seem to have always existed. The best way of measuring the major impact of these techniques on our practice is to take a quick look into the past with the help of a few examples. Is a first epileptic fit the presenting feature of a cerebral tumor? In situations such as this, only the neurologist could even attempt to consult the oracle in order to unravel the secrets hidden within the skull vault which was opaque to x-rays. Although the investigation of pulmonary or mediastinal masses was aided by tomography, the abdominal contents and retroperitoneal space remained areas where the clinician was at a loss. Morphological assessment of the pancreas also depended on indirect tests, radiological investigation of the kidney was essentially reduced to visualization of the renal tracts, and the performance of lymphography was too selective for visualizing the retroperitoneal space. Certainly arteriography, performed secondarily, was contributive for large tumor masses, but had definite limitations. The creation of an artificial air contrast (air encephalogram, pneumoretroperitoneogram) could resolve some diagnostic problems but the painful experience of these examinations is certainly more deeply ingrained in the memories of patients than of the medical profession. Younger doctors might say that this is a walk into a medical museum from an other age: a museum certainly, but a contemporary one

For the internist, the visualization of tumor masses by modern imaging has shown itself to be particularly important in two circumstances: the investigation of prolonged fever of unknown origin (FUO) and paraneoplastic syndromes. The causes of the former are extremely diverse, neoplastic diseases being responsible for 15-30 % of cases. Pelvic and abdominal ultrasound, being simple, repeatable and inexpensive, has become the initial examination of choice. The bile ducts, liver, kidneys, sometimes the pancreas and retroperitoneum are well demonstrated. However, ultrasound does not detect small lesions and meticulous patient preparation is necessary. The clinician, who is rarely capable of personally analyzing the images, must consult a trained ultrasonographer, and the reliability of the examination is highly operator and equipment dependent. In addition, ultrasound is dependent on certain characteristics of the patient, particularly obesity. Abdominal and pelvic CT with the injection of contrast having previously excluded any contraindications is able to simultaneously demonstrate viscera (liver, spleen, pancreas, kidneys, uterus, ovaries) and the retroperitoneum (vessels and particularly lymph nodes). CT must be performed early to reduce diagnostic delays and provides an answer in a quarter of cases as demonstrated in a coordinated study by our team, and all this is achieved with minimal risk or discomfort to the patient. It also has the advantage of providing hard copies which can be subsequently reviewed. Thoracic CT is of less value in the investigation of persistent fever but sometimes demonstrates lesions missed by the chest x-ray, particularly mediastinal lymphadenopathy and thymic pathology. Magnetic Resonance Imaging (MRI), which can be performed if there is a contraindication to iodinated contrast, has the added advantage of sagittal and coronal images. However, its role in the investigation of persistent fever remains less well evaluated than CT. Overall, these new imaging techniques, combined where indicated with endoscopic or endoscopic-ultrasound findings, have replaced the need for the exploratory laparotomy which was sometimes performed in the investigation of a FUO. The reasons for this are two fold. Certainly an exploratory laparotomy may still sometimes be indicated but today, far from being performed blind, it is guided by the imaging findings to suspicious areas within specific organs from which a histological diagnosis can be obtained. However, surgical intervention is often unnecessary to obtain a biopsy due to the advances in the performance of CT or ultrasound guided percutaneous biopsies. Undeniable improvements have so far been achieved using this technique in terms of peri-operative morbidity, patient comfort, cost, and healing delay before commencing chemotherapy. Nonetheless, these should not hide the limitations of this technique. These include inaccessible lesions (due to their small size and/or perivascular position), particularly inadequate specimen or specimens for precise histological typing of a non-Hodgkin's lymphoma, and missing the true nature of a retroperitoneal fibrosis due to a paucity of neoplastic cells.

The problem of paraneoplastic syndromes for the internists similar to that of a FUO with two important differences: on the one hand, the search for a tumor is the principle or even the exclusive goal; on the other hand, certain conditions are only inconsistently associated with a cancer (only a quarter of adult cases of dermatomyositis) so that even a systematic approach is often negative, thus questioning its justification in terms of cost benefit. Sometimes the presenting symptoms strongly guide the search for a tumor towards a specific organ: the Schwartz-Barter or Eaton-Lambert syndrome/anaplastic small cell cancer, myasthenia/thymoma, to quote just two examples. Investigation by CT and/or MRI of the incriminated organ or region often gives the diagnostic answer. In certain situations, endoscopic ultrasound is the examination of choice: assessment of the prostate, systematic assessment of an ovarian carcinoma in a woman with dermatomyositis, visualization of a small pancreatic endocrine tumor. Moreover, the problems are even more complex. The presenting symptoms may be associated with a variety of cancers or the search for the tumor at statistically the most likely site is negative. The performance of a systematic multi-organ assessment is then guided by the levels of tumor markers and can justifiably be repeated several weeks or months after the initial targeted investigation because the first examination may miss a very small tumor. Since the prognosis following treatment is strongly dependent on the size of the lesion, repeating the scan to monitor size, which in the eyes of the manager may seem a complete waste of resources, is clearly totally justifiable. Apart from the clearly dramatic contribution to the initial diagnosis of the tumor, modern imaging has an equally important role in pre-therapeutic oncological staging. MRI is particularly useful in the staging of locoregional disease due to its ability to distinguish healthy from pathological tissue (fig. I.1) and to perform coronal and sagittal images which gives a representation of the tumor in three dimensions. All this is extremely important both for the choice of treatment strategies and for the calculation of the optimal dose. In a rather more anecdotal fashion, the non-surgeon can appreciate finally the rewards for all the time spent studying anatomy in his youth. CT has also a central role in the assessment of distant spread, not only reducing the indications for lymphography in malignant lymphoma to Hodgkin's disease but also in certain diseases where the investigation of the brain or lungs has become indispensable in the initial evaluation.

MRI and CT also have an important role in the follow-up of patients after treatment. In the early stages, these are used to confirm the expected response to chemotherapy, sometimes allowing deferred surgical excision to be performed which was initially impossible, or conversely to identify treatment failure leading to a rapid change in therapy. In many sites, these constitute the only objective ways of assessing the efficacy of treatment. At a later stage, in association with monitoring tumor markers, modern imaging plays an important role in confirming complete remission or persistent disease. The diagnosis of recurrent disease can also be made, either local recurrence (sometimes very subtle in an area highly altered by the treatment) or distant metastases. The internist is often confronted with the difficult problem of a fever occurring in a known cancer patient in whom the answer is not always recurrent tumor or associated infection. Other causes, such as drugs, endocrine problems induced by interferon, as well as any other pathology which is independent of the initial disease must be excluded.

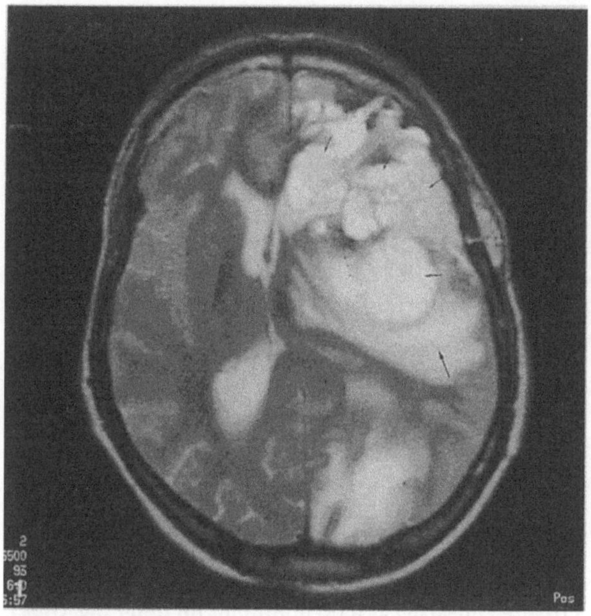

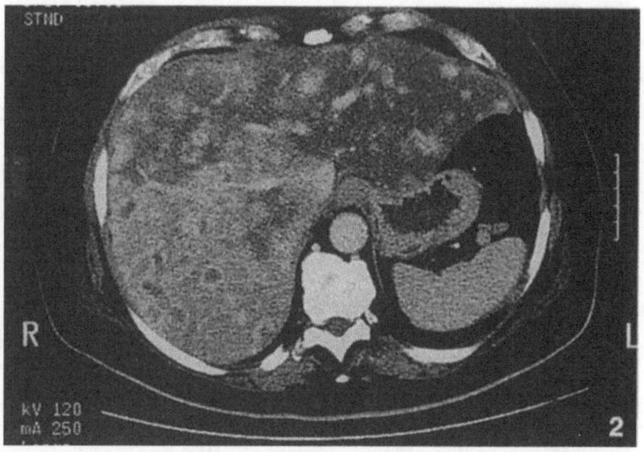

Fig. I.1. Diffuse metastases of the left hemisphere from a facial carcinoma (intermaxillary commissure) on axial SE T2: small arrows), edema, perilesional gliosis (large arrow) and normal tissue are well demonstrated on the MRI. Note the extrinsic compression of the midline ventricular structures and the subfalcine herniation

Fig. I.2. Contrast enhanced helical CT: diffuse form of hepatic epithelioid hemangio-endothelioma, demonstrating a combination of infiltrative zones of low density pseudosteatosis, and diffuse multiple micronodular lesions, as well as extrinsic compression of the hepatic veins and inferior vena cava. The short delay time and rapid acquisition result in good quality images despite difficulties with cooperation in this 64 year old patient presenting with a significant general deterioration in health

The role of CT and MRI in these circumstances is often conclusive.

In reviewing the evidence and the major contribution to oncology made by these modern imaging techniques, one must not forget the limitations of these techniques and meticulous skills required for image interpretation. Let us look at a few examples which are by no means exhaustive. CT, although extremely sensitive in the assessment of parenchymal disease and the detection of small effusions, does not pick up, on the other hand, some peritoneal metastases and intraperitoneal lymphadenopathies. In addition, it is less sensitive than ultrasound in the detection of hepatic metastases and in the study of the biliary system. Despite considerable improvements in the image resolution since the first generation scanners, the risk of a false negative remains for subcentimetre lesions, even using contiguous sections. The latest scanners with continuous rotation should, at least partially overcome this problem. Conversely, in the presence of large tumor, it is sometimes difficult to determine with certainty its site of origin. Moreover, the proliferation in the number of imaging examinations performed has produced a new phenomenon, namely the incidentaloma, particularly in the adrenal glands. Despite the value of MRI in distinguishing between benign and malignant lesions, the clinician is often still faced with difficult decisions. The individual treatment of the patient cannot be reliably based on statistics alone and a histological diagnosis is often considered essential. In addition, the pre-treatment assessment of the degree of tumor extension into adjacent tissues and the determination of the nature of residual masses following treatment of large tumors, particularly lymphomas, remain extremely difficult, even with MRI.

The situation is fortunately not static. CT, which had appeared to have reached its peak, has experienced a revival with the production of high resolution thin sections and the arrival of continuous rotation and helical mode scanners (fig. I.2), software for image reconstruction and the ability to perform ultrafast real time acquisitions, particularly for the evaluation of cardiac tumors. MRI is in a state of constant change: MR angiography (fig. I.3) and techniques of signal

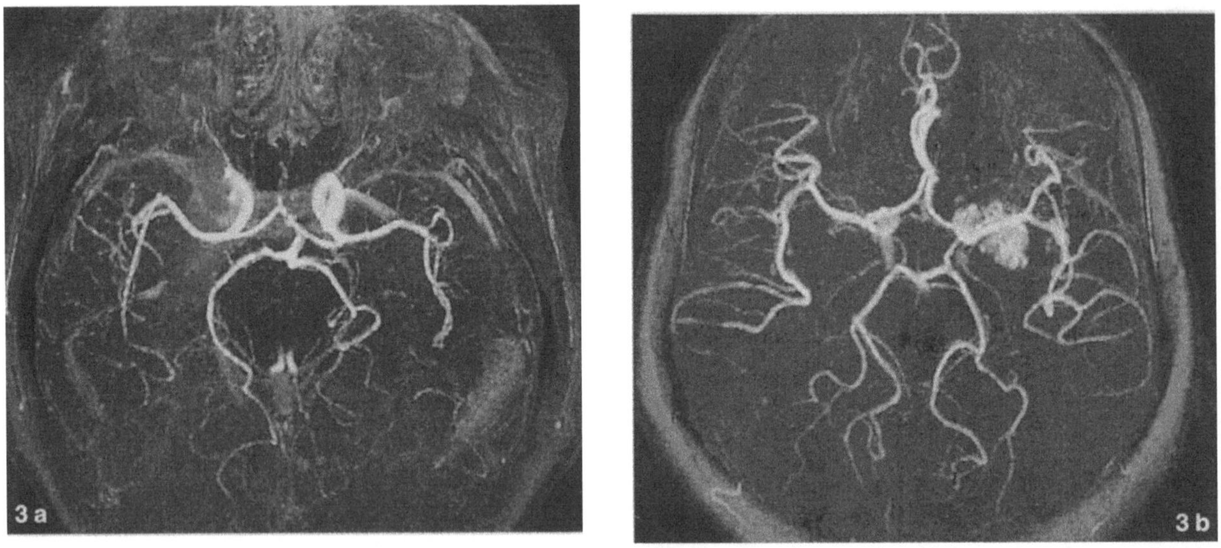

Fig. I.3. Cerebral MR angiography. **a** Normal appearances of the cerebral vasculature on MR angiography. **b** Axial MR angiogram showing an arteriovenous malformation in the left Sylvian fissure appearing as a pseudotumor on other investigations (CT and standard MRI). (Images courtesy of Dr D. Buthiau, Centre RMX)

suppression are some of the most important advances in imaging; new contrast agents are under evaluation; MR spectroscopy, which may be able to measure the local concentration of certain drugs and their metabolites, is opening important avenues of therapeutic research.

Nonetheless, patients will only fully benefit from these technical developments, either now or in the future, if practitioners learn to preserve two fundamental values, ancestral but not obsolete, which are so important to modern medicine: namely good sense and modesty. The former is well illustrated by three aphorisms coming from a daily experience:

- imaging complements but does not replace clinical examination;
- a normal abdominal CT does not exclude an abnormality in the pelvis, a combined examination of both regions should be routine in the situations mentioned in this chapter;
- in the investigation of fever of unknown origin, the detection of a heterogeneous mass almost certainly indicates a neoplastic process, but could also indicate necrosis of a benign tumor or an inflammatory lesion (particularly tuberculosis).

Finally, the clinician must be modest and acknowledge his own shortcomings, especially in image interpretation: if it is his wish to attempt to understand the new semiology arising from CT and MRI, only an experienced radiologist can avoid pitfalls such as the partial volume effect or a rare anatomical variant, and particularly assess the new MRI sequences. A comprehensive knowledge of the patient's previous medical history is also extremely important for the correct interpretation of scans and requires regular multidisciplinary collaboration between radiologists and clinicians (internists, oncologists and system-specific specialists). This has been the approach of our own team for a long time and has proved to be invaluable for optimizing the management of cancer patients.

References

1. Edelman RR, Warach S (1993) Magnetic resonance imaging. N Engl J Med 308: 708-716 & 785-791
2. Hatron PY, Gosset D, Savinel P, Devulder B (1991) Manifestations systémiques des cancers. In: MF Kahn, A Peltier, O Meyer, JC Piette (eds) Les maladies systémiques. Flammarion Médecine-Sciences, Paris, pp 1081-1114
3. Lebas J, Pariente D, Blétry O, et al (1985) Fièvres prolongées et syndromes inflammatoires inexpliqués. Intérêt diagnostique de la tomodensitométrie abdominale. Etude prospective randomisée de 36 observations. Presse Med 14 : 577-581
4. Wechsler B. Piette JC (3-1990) Fièvres au long cours de l'adulte. Encycl Med Chir Paris, Maladies infectieuses, 80003, P 10

CHAPTER 1

Principles and performance of CT and MRI

Radiologists
M. Dousset, D. Buthiau

CT: performance and techniques

CT image is formed by obtaining a measurement of the x-ray absorption coefficient of each volume element which characterizes the anatomical structure.

Performance of a CT examination

Patient explanation and details

It is important to explain to the patient the non-invasive nature of the examination which, at most, usually requires only an intravenous injection of a contrast agent.

Before proceeding any further, the type of examination required is determined by studying the patient's notes and taking into account previous biochemical and radiological results.

Contraindications

Any contraindications to the injection of contrast agent must be recognized. The patient must be fasted for 5 - 6 hours.

The only absolute contraindication is an allergy to the iodine in patients who have not received prophylactic premedication.

The other contraindications are relative; miscellaneous allergic conditions, renal failure, diabetes, multiple myeloma, thyroid disease treated with iodine.

Patient preparation

All cases require adequate preparation:
- an combination of tranexamic acid, betamethasone, and oxazepam given 2 days prior to the examination;
- in diabetics on biguanides, the treatment should be stopped 48 hours before the contrast examination and recommenced 2 days after the injection to avoid occurring of lactic acidosis;
- more than 100 mg of hydrocortisone should be injected immediately before the examination for a high risk patient in the knowledge that it is essential that a person adequately trained in resuscitation techniques is present for the injection;
- in patients with signs of dehydration, multiple myeloma, severe renal failure or if the patient is elderly, adequate hydration is necessary.

Additional preparation is necessary in cases where whole body CT is being performed:
- the bladder should be half empty;
- bowel opacification is achieved by the ingestion of a diluted water soluble contrast agent,
  • for the level proximal to the mesocolon, a moderate quantity of 500-800 ml should be administered approximately 30 minutes before the examination;
  • for the peritoneal and upper pelvic levels, a volume of a 1000-1500 ml is taken in fractionated doses,
  • for the pelvis, 1000 ml is given orally the day before the examination:
  • in certain cases (specific study of the liver and biliary system), the examination can be performed without bowel opacification.

Performance of the examination

The patient is usually asked to lie supine, rarely prone with the head in maximum extension (for coronal slices for example), or in lateral decubitus position.

Viewing of the images

The x-ray absorption coefficients calculated by computer are converted into Hounsfield units according to a scale with 200 levels covering a range of -1000 to +1000.

The window is the range of densities represented by the whole of the grey scale on the monitor.

The window width can be altered and its level should always be adjusted to the value of the average density of the structure being studied.

The absorption coefficients in Hounsfield units of the most important tissues are (0 arbitrarily being the density of water):

Cortical	+ 300 to + 100
Medullary bone	+ 180 to + 250
Muscles	+ 55 to + 60
White matter	+ 30 to + 55
Grey matter	+ 45 to + 60
Recent hematoma and clot	+ 50 to + 70
Liquid, simple cyst	+ 5 to + 25
Fat	- 20 to - 100
Air	- 1000

Acquisition techniques and parameters

Scanogram or scout view

From a lateral or frontal digital image, the centering point and orientation can be selected and the slices covering the regions of interest can be defined.

Thickness and spacing of the slices

The majority of machines currently can obtain slice thickness of between 1 mm and 10 mm, the interspace between the sections is determined by the localization and extent of the lesion under investigation. Optimal results are achieved by using contiguous sections which have less chance of missing small lesions.

Interslice delays

Previously of the order of 2-15 seconds per image, these are now very short on the latest generation rapid CT scanners (spiral and electron beam CT), and are down to 50 ms per image.

Contiguous sections with single breath hold through an anatomical region of interest with dynamic contrast enhancement can be performed.

Improved detection and characterization of lesions is achievable, particularly in the thorax and abdomen.

Small lesions, which may be missed due to respiratory movement on conventional scanners, are well visualized. The study of very tired patients is greatly facilitated.

Field of view

The size of the field of view varies with the dimensions of the organ being studied.

Matrix

The higher the number of pixels, the better the image quality obtained, at the expense of a longer acquisition time.

Filters

These enable the examination to be adapted to the type of structure under study (notably the bone filter for the examination of bony structures).

Continuous rotation and helical mode

(see fig. 1.3)

Continuous rotation is a technique in which the tube and detector rotate at constant velocity. In helical mode, several rotations are performed while the table top moves at a constant velocity. The images are reconstructed differently. This technique enables very rapid performance of an examination covering a large volume on a single breath hold, reduces the injected contrast load and produces contiguous sections.

Image reconstructions

From a series of sections of the order of a millimeter thickness performed in one plane, notably in helical mode (see above), thin slices can be obtained in orthogonal planes (for example coronal and sagittal reconstructions from slices obtained in the axial

Table 1.1. MRI terminology [3]

A: MRI terminology and signal intensities as a function of T1, proton density and T2-weighted sequences. This table simplifies any influence on the relaxation times (T1, T2) by the acquisition of parameters (TR, TE) and the resultant contrast observed on the images. The short TR and long TE sequences are difficult to interpret due to the opposing T1 and T2 effects.

	Sequences	T1-weighted sequence	Proton density weighted sequence (P)	T2-weighted sequence
	Acquisition parameters	Short TR (500 ms) Short TE (20 ms)	Long TR (1.5 s) Short TE (< 50 ms)	Long TR (1.5 s) Long TE (> 50 ms)
Contrast	Hyperintense	Short T1 (fat, blood)	Increased (minimal soft tissue contrast)	Long T2 (liquid, edema)
	Hypointense	Long T1 (liquid, edema)	Minimal signal (cortical bone and air)	Short T2*

(*) Short T2 is not a distinctive criterion.

B: Other terminology used includes:

- T1-weighted sequence corresponds to the short TR sequence;
- proton density weighted sequence for the long TR and short TE sequence;
- T2-weighted sequence for the long TR and long TE sequence.

For simplification remember:
- that the T1-weighted sequence gives high contrast but poor tissue discrimination (fairly similar to the axial CT image);
- that the proton density weighted sequence produces pleasing images but little tissue detail;
- that the T2-weighted sequence is less pleasing to the eye but highly informative for the composition of tissue (principally the degree of hydration) which aids tissue characterization.

plane). As a result of recent advances and rapid data processing (particularly on the latest generation rapid CT scanners, spiral and electron beam CT), these techniques are now used in current practice and even 3D reconstructions are possible giving a 3-dimensional representation of the lesion.

MRI: performance and techniques

Magnetic resonance imaging (MRI) has greater inherent soft tissue contrast in many areas compared to the other imaging modalities. The tissue contrast depends on the choice of the imaging sequences which highlight the influence of certain tissue characteristics, essentially the T1 and T2 relaxation times.

Basically, these are responsible for the fall off in signal following excitation. The majority of pathological processes, neoplastic or otherwise, are associated with an alteration in these two parameters to variable degrees.

The terminology used in MRI is summarized in table 1.1 (see also table 6.2, chapter 6 "Sellar, parasellar and skull base tumors").

Performance of MRI

There are a limited number of **contraindications** to the performance of MRI.

Absolute contraindications:
- cardiac pacemaker,
- surgical and vascular clips,
- small ferromagnetic foreign bodies (cardiac valves, intraocular foreign bodies, cochlear implants).

In doubtful cases, it is the responsibility of the referring clinician to seek the advice of a radiologist to determine whether it is safe to perform the examination.

Relative contraindications :
- claustrophobia primarily: prior to the examination, the doctor should explain to the patient the non-invasive nature of the examination, the well ventilated and open nature of the two ends of the magnet, the normally expected noise levels produced by the echo gradients, and the constant patient contact with the MR technician (video, intercom and alarm button);
- the first trimester of pregnancy, as a precaution, although MRI has not been shown to be teratogenic.

Types of magnet

Resistive

The magnetic field is produced by the passage of current through a coil made from materials based on copper and aluminum. This causes a quite marked heating effect requiring significant cooling which, in practice, limits the field strength to a maximum of 0.5 Tesla (T).

Superconducting

The coils, in this case, are constructed with material having the property of superconductivity. This removes the problem of resistance and hence heating, which is such a drawback in resistive magnets, but necessitates the immersion of the coils in liquid helium to maintain their superconductive properties. The liquid helium itself is cooled by liquid nitrogen in order to reduce evaporation. The superconducting magnets are used in the high field systems, up to 4 Tesla.

Permanent

In practice, these are rarely used due to their great weight which limits the field strength.

Field strength

This is categorized as:
- low and ultralow field, up to 0.35 T,
- mid field, from 0.35 to 0.6 T,
- high field, from 1 T to 4 T.

Although increasing field strength results in an improved signal to noise ratio (SNR), the picture is not as simple as this.

The T1 relaxation (longitudinal) time, which increases with the field strength, is one factor which reduces the SNR for a given TR (repetition time). In addition, the inhomogeneity of the radiofrequency increases with field strength, and the movement and chemical shift artefacts are accentuated at high field system.

Comparative studies between low, mid and high field systems have tended to show that the selection of sequence parameters and available sequences rather than the field strength per se determine the optimal contrast between the lesion and healthy tissue (CNR).

However, it should be noted that more research and the development of new sequences are currently undertaken on high field systems.

Coils

These can be divided into:
- body coil (thorax, abdomen, thigh),
- head coil,
- surface coil (spine, extremities, shoulders).

The surface area of the coil should correspond to that of the anatomical region under study. It should be noted that for the small surface coils, the SNR is excellent in the region immediately adjacent to the coil but falls off dramatically with increasing distance from the coil. The SNR is better with large coils for the lesion which is away from the coil itself.

Having selected the receiver coil and positioned the patient, the examination consists of several successive multi-image sequences. The type of sequence, impulse and a number of other acquisition parameters must be selected for each imaging sequence.

Types of sequence

(See table 1.1 and also table 6.2, chapter 6 «Sellar, parasellar and skull base tumors»)

Spin echo (SE) (fig. 1.1)

This sequence, the most frequently used in current practice, can produce different contrasts depending on the values of the two main essential parameters: the repetition time (TR) and the echotime (TE).

Predominantly T1-weighted contrast is obtained by selecting a short TR, usually around 300 ms to allow a sufficient number of slices, and more importantly the lowest TE possible allowed by the machine (e.g. 10 ms). This reduction in TE has also the advantage of reducing respiratory artefacts by signal averaging and increasing the number of possible slices without altering the TR.

T2-weighted contrast is obtained by using a TR (e.g. 2000 ms) and a long TE (> 50 ms). Different contrast can be simultaneously acquired using several echoes which become increasingly T2-weighted with longer TE. However, excessive prolongation of the TE results in signal loss and is responsible for very noisy images. The acquisition time is directly proportional to the TR, thus a T2-weighted image (WI) requires a longer imaging time.

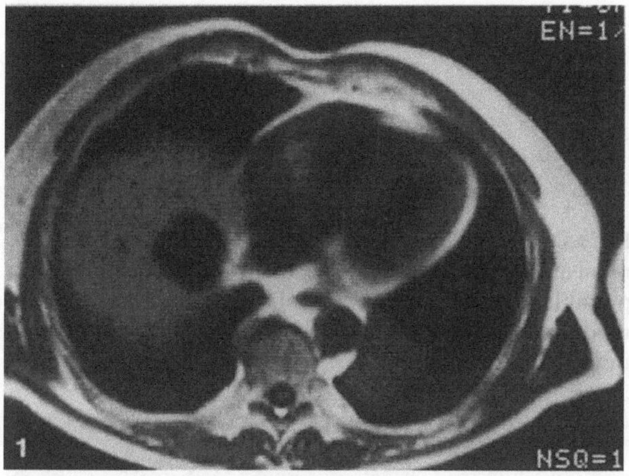

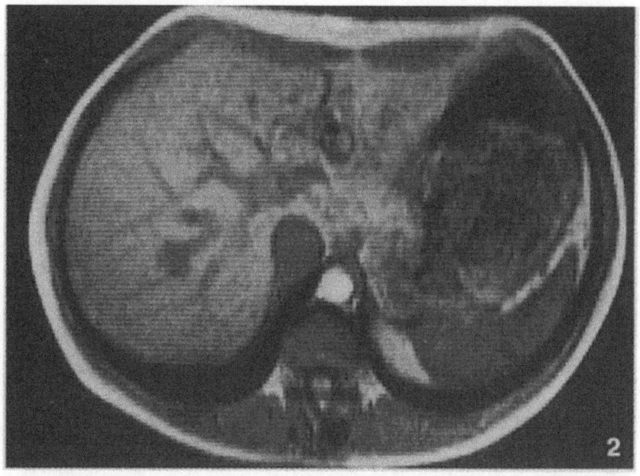

Fig. 1.1. SE sequence 275/14 (TR/TE) demonstrating a cyst in the dome of the liver; note the excellent CNR (contrast to noise ratio) between the lesion and normal liver (courtesy of DD Stark)

Fig. 1.2. SE sequence 130/11 with flip angle of 60° performed with a 16 second breath hold, demonstrating a secondary deposit in the right lobe of the liver adjacent to the portal vessel (courtesy of DD Stark)

Proton density contrast is obtained using a long TR and a very short TE.

Inversion recovery (IR)

A third parameter must be introduced for this sequence in addition to the TR and the TE: the inversion time (TI).

A classical inversion recovery sequence (TR/TE/TI) optimizes T_1 contrast at the expense of a long acquisition time.

The use of a short TI (STIR sequences) nulls the fat signal. The optimal value of TI is around 100 ms but may vary slightly depending on the machine. This sequence, which has a relatively short acquisition time, gives images with a combination of both T_1- and T_2-weighting. The suppression of the fat signal reduces respiratory motion artefacts of the fat and increases the CNR between the lesion and healthy tissue. In addition, the fatty nature of a high signal intensity structure is confirmed by its suppression on the STIR sequence (see figs 1.4 & 1.5)

Gradient echo (GE) (fig. 1.2)

By varying the flip angle (= a) and values of TR (around 10 ms), imaging times of the order of 1 second are possible. This technique has numerous applications such as GRASS (gradient recalled acquisition at the steady state), FLASH (fast low angle shot), FISP (fast imaging with steady state precession) and FAST (Fourier acquired steady state technique).

In these sequences, the weighting of the image is determined not only by the choice or TR and TE but also by the value of the flip angle.

Essentially, for angles > 45° and a short TE, the images tend to be T_1-weighted, and for angles < 25°, the images tend to be proton density or T_2-weighted depending on the value of TE.

Opposed phase sequence (Dixon method or chemical shift)

This type of sequence is used equally well in SE and IR sequences. It opposes the magnetic moments of fat and water at the time of the spin echo resulting in a clear differentiation of fat within tissues with a high water content. This sequence also increases the CNR between the lesion and healthy tissue (particularly on T_2-weighted images).

Echoplanar imaging (EPI)

This technique of the future is obtained by forming as many echoes as lines required in k space (the frequency domain within which the data processing and sampling is performed) by the application of a rapid train of gradient echoes.

Each image is obtained in < 40 ms.

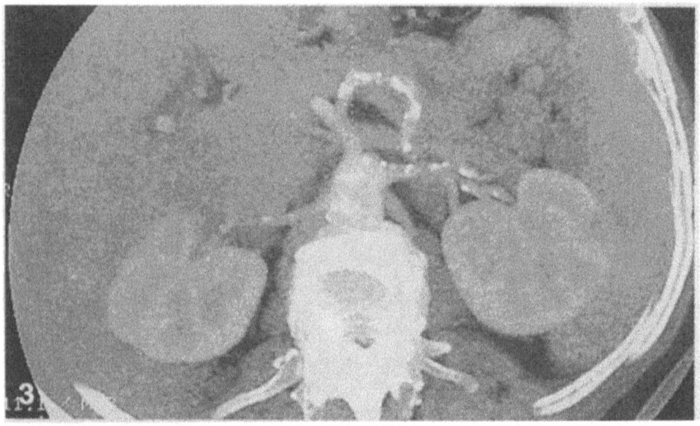

Fig. 1.3. Helical CT, performed at the level of the celiac trunk, renal arteries and kidneys. Note that with this technique it is possible to achieve a good vascular resolution and cortico-medullary differentiation in the kidney using a small volume of contrast (35 ml)

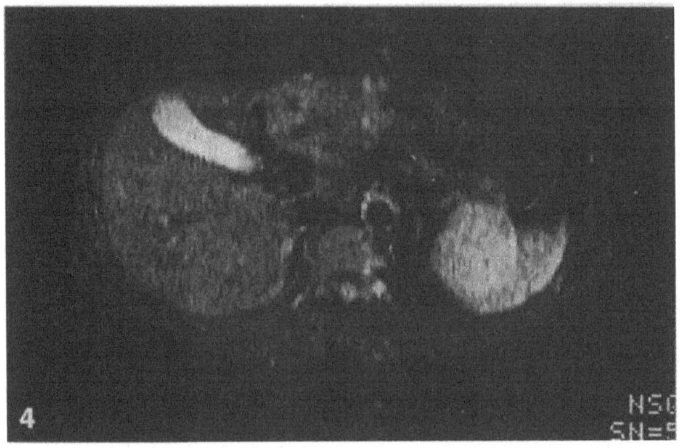

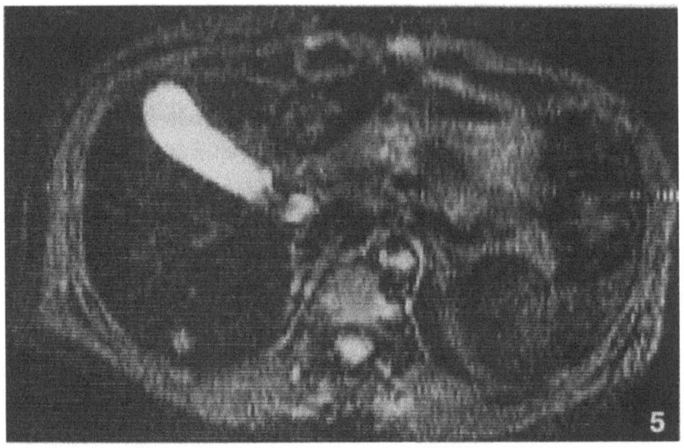

Fig. 1.4. STIR sequence 1500/80/30 (TR/TI/TE) before injection of paramagnetic ferrous oxide in a patient presenting with a known primary malignant lesion: no hepatic, metastatic lesion is demonstrated. The value of STIR sequences, despite the poor SNR (signal to noise ratio) and therefore relatively poor anatomical definition, is to improve the CNR (contrast to noise) between a lesion and normal liver as demonstrated by the excellent CNR between the spleen and liver (courtesy of D.D. Stark)

Fig. 1.5. STIR sequence 1500/80/30 (TR/TI/TE) following the injection of paramagnetic ferrous oxide, in the same patient, demonstrating a secondary lesion in the inferior portion of the right lobe of the liver (courtesy of D.D. Stark)

The different types of contrast (proton density, T1 and T2) can be obtained:
- T2 contrast is achieved by increasing the TE,
- T1 contrast is improved by applying a 180 ° inversion pulse as in the inversion recovery sequences.

So, in little less than 17 seconds, a series of 16 snapshot images (at 1 second intervals) with simultaneous dynamic bolus contrast studies can be performed. This also makes artefacts with abdominal respiratory movement.

Other acquisition parameters

Orientation of the scan plane

It is often useful to start with a very rapid coronal, sagittal or axial localizing sequence, depending on the region of study, in order to obtain a centering point and select subsequent slices to cover the anatomical region of interest.

Number of acquisitions

The number of acquisitions (or excitations) considerably influences the degree of background noise. An increase in the number of acquisitions (NA) results in a reduction in artefacts by signal averaging [noise = f(NA-1/2)]. The increase in scan time is therefore proportional to NA. Although it is possible to use 4 to 8 acquisitions when the TR is short, a long TR is more limiting.

Field of view (FOV)

This varies between 10 and 50 cm and should be tailored to the anatomical region of interest.

Acquisition matrix (NX × NY)

It may be useful to use an asymmetrical acquisition matrix (NX × NY) of 128 by 256, which halves the acquisition time compared to a 256 by 256 matrix. The volume element is larger with a slightly inferior spatial resolution.

Slice thickness

This varies between 1.5 and 20 mm; the spacing between slices can be zero thus giving contiguous slices, but this may result in interference of the signal between two adjacent slices. A minimum interspace of 10 to 15% is therefore advisable.

Number of slices

The maximum allowed depends on the selected parameters and is increased by prolonging the TR and shortening the TE.

Acquisition time

This can be calculated by the formula TR × NA × NY (acquisition matrix)

Gating

Electrocardiogram gating is not routinely used. Respiratory gating, if necessary, reduces motion artefacts but is associated with increased imaging times.

The influence of the different tissue parameters (proton density, T1 T2, flow) on the signal intensity, and the fact that the contrast between the lesion and healthy tissue depends on various parameters (TE, TR, TI, Flip angle) explains why certain lesions may be well demonstrated and characterized within normal tissues whereas others may be missed by using an inappropriate imaging sequence. MRI is, therefore, highly operator dependent.

References

1. Boulin A, Korach G (1988) Les techniques. In: Vignaud J, Boulin A (eds) Tomodensitométrie crânio-encéphalique. Vigot, Paris, pp 11-20
2. Brasch RC, Drayer BP, Weissleder R (1992) Contrast agents for MR imaging (RC), 81, RSNA 992
3. Buthiau D (1991) TDM et IRM Notions générales. In: D. Buthiau (ed) TDM et IRM Cliniques. Frison Roche, Paris
4. Bydder GM (1988) Clinical application of Gadolinium DTPA. In: Stark DD, Bradley WG Jr (eds) Magnetic Resonance Imaging. Mosby, St Louis, pp 182-200
5. Dousset M, Weissleder R, Hendrick RE, et al (1989) Short Tl inversion recovery imaging of the liver: pulse sequence optimization and comparison to spin echo imaging. Radiology 171: 327-333
6. Dousset M, Weissleder R, Stark DD, et al (1988) Comparison of image quality in abdominal MR imaging at Low, Mid and High Field. RSNA 843: 275
7. Ferrucci JT (1990) Liver tumor Imaging : currents concepts. AJR 155: 473-484
8. Gerstman BB (1991) Epidemiologic critic of the report on adverse reactions and non ionic contrast media by Japanese committee on the safety of contrast media. Radiology 17
9. Hendrick RE. Osborn AG (1988) Introduction to MR imaging, Il, pulse sequences and image contrast. In: Stark DD, Bradley WG Jr (eds) Diagnostic categorical course in MR Imaging. Chicago RSNA: 15-25
10. Katayama H, Yamaguchi K, Kozura T, Takashima T, Seez P, Matsuura K (1990) Adverse reactions and non ionic contrast media: a report from the Japanese committee on the safety of contrast media. Radiology 75: 621 -626
11. Kneeland JB (1988) Instrumentation. In: Stark DD, Bradley WG Jr (eds) Magnetic Resonance Imaging. Mosby, St Louis, pp 3-23
12. Korach G, Boulin A (1988) Principes de la tomodensitométrie. In: Vignaud J, Boulin A (eds) Tomodensitométrie crânio-encéphalique. Vigot, Paris, pp 3-10
13. Low RN, Francis IR Herkens RJ, et al (1993) Fast Multiplanar Spoiled Gradient Recalled Imaging of the liver: pulse sequence Optimization and comparison with spin echo imaging. AJR: 501-509
14. Sagel SS, Fishman EK, Sheedy PF II (1992) Fast scanning: clinical application of spiral and electron beam CT (RC), RSNA :69
15. Stark DD (1990) Contrast agents for abdominal MR imaging. In: Kressel HY, Modic MT, Murphy WA (eds) Syllabus: "Special course in MR Imaging", Chicago. RSNA: 147- 152
16. Stark DD (1988) Liver. In: Stark DD, Bradley WG Jr (eds) Magnetic Resonance Imaging. Mosby, St Louis, pp 934-1029
17. Wehrli FW (1990) Fast MR Imaging. In: Kressel HY, Modic MT, Murphy WA (eds) Syllabus: "Special course in MR Imaging", Chicago. RSNA 31-46

CHAPTER 2

Contrast agents

Radiologists
H. Lemaignen, T. Bach-Gansmo

Iodinated contrast agents in CT

Current data and applications in imaging

Introduction

CT is a technique with a higher contrast resolution than conventional radiology.

At the time of the introduction of this technique it was thought that intravenous contrast agents would not be necessary. However, it soon became apparent that these were indispensable for the visualization of many pathological processes, and today one would not perform a CT examination without considering iodinated contrast enhancement, particularly in the field of oncology.

Iodinated urographic contrast agents currently available are all derivatives of iodinated benzoic acid. The contrast agents are classified as highly hyperosmolar ionic monomers (iotalamate, ioxitalamate, metrizoate), slightly hyperosmolar ionic dimers (ioxaglate), and slightly hyperosmolar non-ionic monomers (iohexol, iopamidol, iopentol, iopromide, ioversol). The highly hyperosmolar agents have an osmolality of the order of 2100 mOsm/kg H_2O per 370 mg of iodine per ml plasma: 300 mOsm/kg H_2O and as a result the tolerance is far from ideal: pain, sensation of burning at the injection site, osmotic overload, higher incidence of pseudo-allergic reactions, etc. [2]. As a result, the use of these contrast agents has been reduced to a minimum in a number of countries. The use of minimally hyperosmolar non-ionic agents (600-800 mOsm/kg H_2O per 300-350 mg of iodine/ml) is today widespread in most developed countries due to the better local and systemic tolerance which has been confirmed by the numerous comparative and clinical epidemiological studies [3, 11-13, 16, 18, 21]. Nonetheless, economic constraints prevent their universal usage due to their highly cost.

General pharmacokinetics of uro-angiographic contrast agents

Whatever their chemical nature, all the uro-angiographic iodinated contrast agents have the same pharmacokinetics following intravascular injection. These small molecules, not (or very weakly) bound to plasma proteins, are rapidly distributed throughout the plasma and, more slowly, to the extracellular interstitial space following a compartmental model. Their kinetic is therefore biphasic: the initial phase corresponds to the equilibration of the concentrations between the two compartments (approximately 3 minutes duration). The second phase corresponds to the retrodiffusion from the interstitial space into the plasma which is parallel to the renal excretion by glomerular filtration, without either reabsorption or tubular secretion. The mean biological half life is 90 minutes.

Certain features must be highlighted:

– the important role of the blood brain barrier (BBB), the impermeable histo-physiological interface between

the plasma and the neurological tissue which prevents diffusion of iodinated contrast media into the interstitial space of the brain;
- the absence of any metabolism of these agents which are excreted unchanged;
- the impact on the thyroid gland due to traces of free iodine contained within the contrast solution which are sufficient to block the uptake of iodides for several weeks thus preventing the performance of scintigraphy or the treatment of thyroid cancer or its metastases by radioactive iodine.

These general principles of pharmacokinetics may vary from patient to patient and depend to some extent on the injection protocols used in CT. These inter- and intra-patient variations explain the impossibility of quantitatively characterizing a lesion by its degree of enhancement.

Pharmacokinetics applicable to CT

Bolus injection

Intravenous bolus injection of uro-angiographic contrast agent gives a curve of contrast concentration as a function of time (time-concentration curve) defined as the following: peak concentration within the aorta (and therefore of enhancement) at 15 seconds followed by a rapid fall in concentration. The geometry of the bolus following injection as a function of time (time-concentration curve) is shown in figure 2.1 [19]:

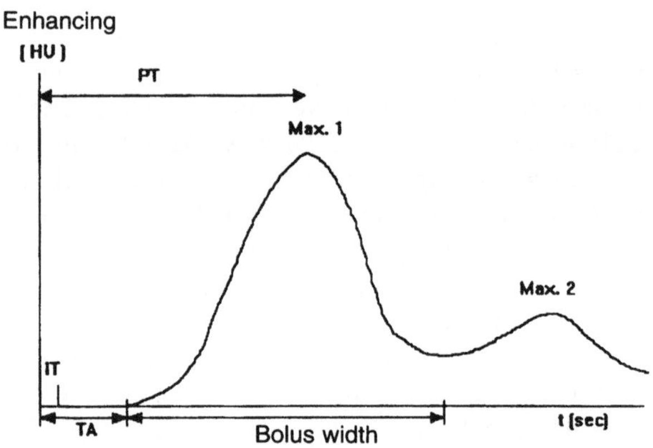

Fig. 2.1. Time-concentration graph following peripheral intravenous injection. IT length of injection (seconds); TA time to appearance (seconds): max 1, maximal peak concentration (Hounsfield units); max 2, second concentration peak, corresponding to the first recirculation; PT, time to peak (seconds); HU degree of enhancement (Hounsfield units)

Importance of the time to peak

This parameter is a function of the transit time of the contrast bolus from the intravenous injection site to the target organ. A value can be calculated by applying Schad's equation:

$$PT = n \times 60/FC$$

PT: time to peak in seconds; FC: heart rate per minute; n: number of heart beats between the brachial artery and target organ.

Values of n for different organs: right ventricle = 4; left ventricle = 11; thoracic aorta = 12; brain = 13; iliac artery =15.

For the brain, the PT will on average, for a heart rate of 60 per minute, be equal to:

$$13 \times 60/60 = 13 \text{ seconds.}$$

This theoretical data should only serve as an indicator to help synchronize the injection parameters with the acquisition sequences as a function of the target organ or heart rate of the patient. The commencement of data acquisition will be a function of the time to peak and the scan time of the machine. The total acquisition time for an arterial enhancement (scan time) will be related to the duration of the bolus injection, the scan time above all must be at least as long as the duration of the bolus. A bolus injection produces a high contrast peak resulting in a better opacification of blood vessels and the vascular component of tumors by increasing their contrast relative to adjacent tissues. Another advantage of a high contrast peak is that more contrast crosses the blood brain barrier, disrupted by a tumor if this peak is important. This constitutes the mechanism for contrast enhancement of a lesion within the brain. An automatic injection device should be used if all the injection parameters are to be controlled.

Injection by slow infusion

With this technique a constant concentration of iodine is maintained but without a concentration peak, the dynamic information of the bolus technique is lost. It has a very limited role except in otorhinolaryngology where it clearly highlights the vessels with contrast. In other cases it may be dangerous because tumors as hepatic metastases may be missed [4].

Bolus infusion

The benefits of the dynamic features of the bolus and the maintenance of adequate opacification for a longer time can be achieved by combining the two techniques. This also allows for an increase of the acquisition time [4].

Intra-arterial injection

This technique may be employed in liver imaging; CT portography consists in injecting the contrast agent via a selective catheter in the superior mesenteric artery. The contrast agent reaches the liver via the portal system in a high concentration, as there is in first passage through the heart and lungs. This is being performed more and more frequently to complement intravenous techniques in cases where nature of the lesion is uncertain [4, 19].

Other applications

Gastrointestinal tract (GIT)

In cases where barium is contraindicated (intestinal obstruction or perforation), it is possible to opacify the lumen of the GIT with a dilute water soluble iodinated contrast agent (approximately 5 g iodine per 100 ml) administered orally or rectally. This procedure helps differentiate the GIT from adjacent abdominal organs.

Spinal canal

A CT scan performed after myelography has the advantage of contrast within the cerebrospinal fluid (CT myelography). The use of a non-ionic iodinated contrast agent is absolutely obligatory in these cases

Future prospects

Safety and tolerance

The non-ionic contrast agents available today represent a significant medical advance in terms of improved patient tolerance compared to the ionic contrast agents used previously. Nonetheless, the non-ionic agents are by no means perfect: their osmolality varies from 2-3 times that of plasma and a small but significant degree of chemotoxicity persists [2]. The pharmaceutical industry has directed its research towards two principal and related aims: to reduce the osmolality for a given concentration of iodine and to reduce the chemotoxicity [2, 7]

Reduction in osmolality

The currently available non-ionic contrast agents are monomers containing three iodine atoms per molecule (ratio 3:1). The chemical structure of the latest agents -iodixanol, iotrolan- is a non-ionic dimer containing of 6 iodine atoms per molecule (ratio 6:1). The osmolality is therefore halved to equal that of plasma.

Intravascular injection of iodixanol (Nycomed Imaging AS) has been shown to be extremely well tolerated in several phase III clinical trials [17] and is in daily use in the countries where it is marketed (Sweden, Great Britain, Switzerland). Iotrolan (Schering AG) was specifically developed for myelography and for the visualization of body cavities.

Reduction in chemotoxicity

Generally the chemotoxicity of contrast agents is related to their hydrophylism: increased hydrophylism can reduced chemotoxicity [2]. For the non-ionic monomers, the best tolerated are the most hydrophilic. The non-ionic dimers are also extremely hydrophilic, proportionally to the number of hydroxyl radicals.

Iodine concentration imaging

Enhancement on CT is directly proportional to the concentration of iodine. However, it is possible that the newer techniques, such as spinal CT, particularly of the thorax, will result in lower concentrations of iodine being used, of the order of 100-150 mg of iodine per ml [5, 14, 15]. Spinal CT is such a recent technique that the precise injection protocols (volume, delivery, iodine concentration), have yet to be strictly defined (see fig 1.3)

Product aims

The intravascular injection of a contrast agent is non-specific. The contrast is distributed throughout the organism by the blood stream. It is therefore tempting to anticipate the production of organ specific agents. Several directions of research are possible:

Intravascular liposomes consisting of microspheres containing a classical iodinated contrast agent can be injected intravenously. These are actively taken up by the reticulo-endothelial system and persist for a sufficient time to obtain quality images. These compounds appear to be most promising in hepatic imaging [7].

The lymphographic contrast agents currently available (oil-based contrast agents) are certainly efficacious but are associated with numerous inconveniences and contraindications, particularly the very slow excretion rate and undesirable cardio-pulmonary side effects. Water soluble iodinated contrast agents encapsulated within liposomes could be a satisfactory alternative and provide CT images of the lymphatic system and the lymph nodes [7].

Contrast agents using an alternative to iodine

There have been several attempts to replace the iodine by another metal. Unfortunately, so far it has not been possible to replace iodine due to excessive toxicity or insufficient efficacy. The use of gadolinium chelates in MRI, which are extremely well tolerated, may soon change this. In fact, gadolinium is perfectly capable of having a physical effect on the x-ray due to its high atomic number (Z), with an attenuation slightly greater than for iodine. This would allow for the use of higher energy x-rays with less biological interference [7].

Contrast agents in MRI

Current data and applications in imaging

Introduction

The inherent contrast between different tissues and between normal and neoplastic tissues is excellent in many cases. However, the ability to appreciate breakdown of the blood brain barrier (BBB) has very rapidly opened the way for the paramagnetic contrast agents which are now equally important in neuro-MRI as iodinated contrast agent.

Classification of MRI contrast agents

These agents can be divided in three different categories.

Paramagnetic agents

Based on gadolinium, manganese or iron, these agents shorten T1 and T2. The effect on T1 predominates at the usual clinical concentrations. At a higher concentration the T2 effect becomes more important. The result of the T1 shortening is a marked increase in the signal intensity in areas with high contrast uptake, on T1-weighted sequences.

Mechanism of action: within the primary magnetic field of the MRscanner, the protons, which behave as tiny magnets, are preferentially aligned in the direction of the magnetic field and are consequently in a low energy state. The initial effect of all imaging sequences is to excite a proportion of these protons to a higher energy state. T1 is the time taken for 63% of these protons to relax back to their original low energy state. Paramagnetic materials are magnets capable of destabilizing the protons and shortening the relaxation time of these protons back to the low energy state, i.e. the T1.

Superparamagnetic agents or magnetic susceptibility agents

These also shorten T1 and T2 but the T2 shortening is the dominant factor. T2 shortening has opposite effect of T1 shortening; it results in a reduction in the signal from tissues effected by these contrast agents.

Mechanism of action: superparamagnetic agents are magnetic ferrous oxide particles with a combined magnetization from all the ferrous oxide molecules within each «grain». A collection of these grains forms a particle of the contrast agent. By definition each grain of the superparamagnetic contrast agent must be sufficiently small (< 40 nm). That thermal agitation prevents the alignment of the inherent magnetic fields of each of the grains. However, when the external magnetic field becomes stronger, these grains align themselves more and more with the external field. In the strong collective magnetic field of an MRscanner, all the grains align with the external field resulting in a strong magnetization, and a significant magnetic gradient is created in their vicinity. The diffusion of protons within this gradient is responsible for the reduction in signal.

Thus, the mode of action of these T2 agents is based on their capacity to create local inhomogeneity within the primary magnetic field. In addition, these agents act by shortening T1 and T2, analogous to the paramagnetic agents [20].

Products containing few or no protons, such as perfluorooctylbromide

The proton is the source of the common MR signal. The replacement of a tissue or the contents of a body cavity by these agents results in a reduction in signal. These products will not be described in detail here; suffice to say that perfluorooctylbromide (PFOB) is still in the process of development as a gastrointestinal marker and perfusion agent.

Products currently available for diagnostic clinical use

The chelates of gadolinium, markers of the extracellular space

Based on our knowledge of scintigraphy which has the same requirement of administering a toxic insoluble metal, these metals must be bound to a ligand (chelating agent) to give a chelate. The ligands are the distinctive elements of this class of contrast agents. They primarily have the effect of reducing toxicity and increasing solubility, which are the only requirements for markers of the extracellular space. The ligands can also have a role in targeting. There are two groups of ligands for the extracellular space agents which are either linear or macrocyclic. This distinction is only based on the visualization of the molecule in one dimension because, in the three-dimensional space, both types form a pocket around the gadolinium.

More recently, non-ionic contrast agents have been developed. Their non-ionic nature reduces the osmolality and toxicity, and alters the affinity of the ligand for gadolinium. There are four classes of extracellular agents (table 2.1). Initially, discussions between the manufacturers of these various agents was dominated by the thermodynamic dissociation constant and the acute toxicity. In general, the macrocyclic agents have a greater affinity for gadolinium with a higher «log K» (thermodynamic stability constant). However, macrocyclic agents have a greater inherent chemotoxicity than the linear agents. This becomes apparent by comparing the LD50 of the various agents.

More rigorous studies have shown that the selectivity constant (which represents the stability of the ligand-metal complex in the presence of endogenous metals such as zinc) is a better indicator of the stability in vivo than the thermodynamic stability constant (which represents the general stability in vitro). There are still arguments over the relative importance of either of these properties. However, it is important to underline that all these agents are well tolerated at the usual dosage of 0.1 mmol/kg.

Primary or metastatic cerebral tumors were the first indications of these agents, demonstrating a breakdown of the BBB. Today, the demonstration of enhancement is the method of choice for proving the presence of cerebral metastases [10]. Moreover, the BBB may be involved to a variable extent. In particular, the degree of enhancement of astrocytomas is proportional to their malignant potential so that the absence of enhancement of an astrocytoma would classify it as a low grade tumor [10]. On the other hand, other tumors enhance so intensely that a lower dose can be used, such is the case for neurinomas of the VIII cranial nerve where a dose a 0.05 mmol/kg is sufficient. However, in cases of suspected small cerebral metastases a dose of 0.3 mmol/kg may demonstrate lesions which otherwise would not be detected [7].

The indications outside the CNS are numerous, and specific protocols are often necessary. In addition, the dose of gadolinium may need to be doubled or tripled. Dynamic imaging is becoming an increasingly utilized technique: following injection of a bolus of contrast, the slope of the enhancement curve rather than the enhancement itself gives an indication of the pathology. In this context of rapid and high dose injection, the better tolerated non-ionic contrast agents would seem to be advantageous. The dynamic enhancement technique may mask pathology in certain tissues such as on the pituitary gland and liver, therefore strict examination protocols are imperative.

Table 2.1. LD50 in mice after intravenous injection, thermodynamic stability (log Ktherm) and selectivity (log Ksel). Comparison of MR contrast agents (UD: unpublished data)

Chelates	Log Ktherm	Log Ksel	DL50
Gd-DTPA-BMA/Omniscan	16.85	9.04	34
Gd-DTPA/Magnevist	22.46	7.04	5.6
Gd-DOTA/Dotarem	25.4	UD	11.4
Gd-DOTA/Pro-Hance	22.8	UD	12

Superparamagnetic agents

The superparamagnetic agents currently available are bowel markers in a similar fashion to barium or Gastrografin used in CT; opacification of the stomach and small bowel facilitates the recognition of normal or pathological structures outside the digestive tract. Abdoscan (Oral Magnetic Particles, Nycomed Imaging AS) and Lumirem (Advanced Magnetics) both seem to facilitate examinations. The iron particles are in suspension in 600 to 1000 ml of liquid, either with a viscous substance or an osmotic agent to give optimal distribution of the contrast.

Future prospects

Tissue specific agents

Several agents in which the ligand has a specific hepatic affinity are under development of which Mn-DPDP is the most advanced. The dipyridamol-diphosphate ligand allows delivery of manganese in a non-toxic form although some of the manganese is liberated [9]. Mn-DPDP is also used as a pancreatic parenchymal contrast agent.

Sufficiently the lipophilic Gd-BOPTA is captured by normal hepatocytes to obtain enhancement of the normal liver [8]. These two agents enter into the normal hepatocytes and are partially excreted in the bile. Hepatic metastases, and primary tumors depending on their differentiation, do not take up these agents. Tumors appear as areas of reduced signal intensity within the normal liver parenchyma which exhibits marked T1 shortening [8].

Specific agents for the examination of the reticuloendothelial system may also be developed (see figs 1.4 & 1.5 in previous chapter). The Kupffer cells of the liver are the principle targets but the spleen and bone marrow may also become targets for these agents. Liver tumors, neither primary nor metastatic, do not contain any functioning Kupffer cells. Superparamagnetic and paramagnetic particles in the form of liposomes have been suggested and tested. The only contrast currently in the process of being marketed is AMI-25 (Advanced Magnetics), composed of superparamagnetic particles [20]. The use of particles based on gadolinium is possible but the gadolinium must gain access to the hepatocytes or remain within the liver sinusoids in order to be of any value [6].

Fast bolus tracking

For a long time there has been a desire to study perfusion. By injecting a gadolinium based contrast agent, it is possible to follow the effect of magnetic susceptibility within tissues during the first passage which is proportional to the blood supply. This technique (fast bolus tracking) depends on ultrarapid imaging, such as echo planar imaging, to obtain several simultaneous sections. Research has centered on the heart and brain in order to demonstrate ischemia. The superparamagnetic particles and macromolecules containing gadolinium derivatives can also be useful as perfusion agents, having the advantage of remaining intravascular.

Notes

Omniscan and Abdoscan are trade marks of Nycomed Imaging AS, Oslo, Norway.

Magnevist and Gastrografin are trade marks of Schering AG, Berlin, Germany.

Lumirem and Dotarem are trade marks of Guerbet Laboratories, Aulnay-sous-Bois, France

Pro-Hance is a trade mark of Squibb, Princeton, NJ, USA

References

1. Akeson P, Larsson EM, Kristofferssen DT, Johnson E, Holtas S (1993) Comparison of contrast enhanced MRI at standard and high dose, using gadodiamide injection in patients with brain metastasis (Abst) ESMRMB, Rome, p 23
2. Almen T (1989) Relation between chemical structure, animal toxicity and clinical adverse effects of contrast media. In: Enge I and Edgren J (eds) Patients safety and adverse events in contrast media examination. Excerpta Medica, Amsterdam, p 25
3. Brismar JB, et al (1991) Miscellancous adverse effects of low- versus high-osmolality contrast media: a study revised. Radiology 179: 19-23
4. Buthiau D, Gardeur D (1986) Produits de contraste en tomodensitométrie. In: Protocoles d'examen en tomodensitométrie. Schering, p 4
5. Costello P, et al (1992) Spiral CT of the thorax with reduced volume of contrast material: a comparative study. Radiology 183: 663-666
6. Fahlvik AK, Holtz E. Klaveness J (1990) Relaxation efficacy of paramagnetic and superparamagnetic microspheres in liver and spleen. Magn Reson Imaging 8: 363-369
7. Fritzsch T, et al (1992) Status of contrast media research in MRI, ultrasound and X-ray. Eur Radiol 2, 2- 13: 1 - 13
8. Giovannoni A, Bourne MW, Paci E. Terilli F, Pirovano G, Whitehouse GH (1993) The value of GdBOPTA/ dimeg for focal lesions in MRI of the liver (Abst) SMRMB. Rome, p 104
9. Grant D, Holtz E, Zech K (1993) Biodistribution and excretion of ^{54}Mn and ^{14}C labelled MnDPDP in rats and dogs (Abst) ESMRMB, Rome, p 251
10. Hasso AN, Kortmann KE, Bradley WG (1988) Supratentorial neoplasms. In: DD Stark and WG Bradley Jr (eds) Magnetic Resonance Imaging. Mosby, St Louis, p 770
11. Jacobsson BF, et al (1988) Non-ionic versus ionic media in intravenous urography: clinical trial in 1000 consecutive patients. Radiology 167: 601-605
12. Katayama H, et al (1990) Adverse reactions to iodinated contrast media. A report from the Japanese Committee on the Safety of Contrast Media. Radiology 175: 601 -605
13. Palmer FJ (1988) The RACR survey of intravenous contrast media reactions. Final report. Australas Radiol 32: 426-428
14. Rémy J (1993) Chest-CT (spiral). 8th European Congress of Radiology, Vienne (Autriche), 12- 17 Septembre
15. Rémy-Jardin M, et al (1992) Central pulmonary thromboembolism: diagnosis with spiral volumetric CT with the single breath-hold technique. Comparison with pulmonary angiography. Radiology 185: 381 -587
16. Thomsen HS, Dorph S (1993) Review article: High-osmolar and low-osmolar contrast media. An update on frequency of adverse drug reactions. Acta Radiol 34: 205-209
17. Thornbury JR (1992) Phase III clinical trial of iodixanol (non-ionic, isotonic) as a body CT contrast agent: genitourinary and general results. Am J Roentgenol 158: 1400
18. Vacek JL, et al (1990) Frequencies of reactions to iohexol versus ioxaglate. Am J Cardiol 66: 1277-1278
19. Wegener OH (1992) Contrast media. In: Whole body computed tomography, 2nd edn. Blackwell Scientific Publications, Oxford, p 97
20. Weissleder R, Papisov M (1992) Pharmaceutical iron oxides for MR Imaging. Rev Magn Reson Med 4: 1-20
21. Wolf GL (1991) Comparison of the rates of adverse drug reactions - Ionic contrast agents, ionic agents combined with steroids, and non-ionic agents. Invest Radiol 26: 404-410

CHAPTER 3

Malignant intracerebral tumors

Clinicians
F. Bolgert, M. Poisson, E. Dieu, J.-V. Chantelard, R. Grob, P. Tassan, O. Rixe

Radiologists
J.-M. Caillé, M. Raynaud, D. Buthiau, F. Gelbert, V. Dousset, J. Berge

Currently there are many indications for a CT or MR examination. A scan should be performed in the presence of a clinical suspicion not just for advanced disease. In this chapter dedicated to malignant cerebral tumors (primary and secondary), the most characteristic CT and MRI appearances of these neoplasms are summarized. The pretreatment evaluation and role of imaging in follow-up of these malignant tumors are discussed.

Classification of intracranial tumors

(tables 3.1a & 3.1b)

Presenting signs

The commonest presenting sign is epilepsy. Other signs include:

- headaches, the nature of which suggests organic disease (daily, often early morning, atypical, sometimes ipsilateral to the tumor);
- intracranial hypertension is common in the posterior fossa tumors in children. In adults, a rapidly developing intracranial hypertension is suggestive of a tumor;
- functional deficit syndromes. These are usually progressive and the symptomatology depends on the localization, size of tumor and associated edema;
- sudden onset of a deficit which more or less recovers and suggests a vascular origin must be routinely investigated by CT. About 10-15% of metastases may present in this fashion. Hemorrhage is generally the rule in glioblastoma multiform or metastasis (kidney, melanoma, choriocarcinoma);
- more rarely, the presenting signs may be:
  - problems with thought process or memory,
  - meningeal hemorrhage,
  - alteration in general state,
  - vomiting in a young child.

In fact, any neurological signs suggesting an organic etiology must be radiologically investigated by CT which may subsequently be complemented by MRI.

The psychological problems of cerebral tumors are strongly associated with the symptoms of superior functional deficit, neurologic disorders (epilepsy), confusion and endocrine diseases. However, these disorders are still isolated, and the diagnosis of cerebral tumors is difficult for

- midline tumors (frontal, rhinencephalic, hypothalamic),
- difficult disease (frontal indifference, tumoral Korsakoff) or manifestation of indistinct symptom of psychotherapy (equilibrium problem of posterior fossa tumor).

Psychiatric symptomatology is very diverse:

- changes of mood (euphoria of frontal tumor, depression syndrome of psychotherapy),
- akinetic mutism (3rd ventricule),
- changes of character (agressiveness of diencephalic and temporal tumors),
- hallucinations (comitative symptom)

Table 3.1a. Classification of tumor type (OMS)

	GRADES			
Origin	I	II (Survival > 3 years)	III (Survival 1-3 years)	IV (Survival < 1 year)
I. Neuroepithelial				
Astrocytoma (A)	A. of cerebellum Juvenile pilocytic Glioma of optic nerve	A. differentiated	A. anaplastic	
T. oligodendroglial		Oligodendrogliomas	Anaplastic oligodendrogliomas	
T. of the ependyma		Ependymomas	Anaplastic ependymomas	
T. pineal				Pinealblastoma
T. poorly differentiated			Glioblastoma	Medulloblastoma
II. Nerve sheath	Neurinomas (Schwannomas)		Anaplastic neurinoma	
III. T. Anaplastic meningeal	Meningioma		Meningioma	
IV. Lymphomas		Primary cerebral lymphoma		
	Teratoma	Germinoma (pineal gl.)		Choriocarcinoma
V. T. malformations	Craniopharyngioma, Lipoma, Epidermoid and dermoid cyst Colloid cyst of the third ventricle			
VI. Metastases				

Table 3.1b. Characteristics of primary cerebral tumors [from D. Balériaux and J. Hildebrand (1991) In: D. Buthiau (ed) Clinical CT and MRI. Frison-Roche, Paris, pp 173-210]

Type of tumor	Grade	Peak incidence (age)	Commonest localization	Incidence (%) all ages	Before 15
Pilocytic astrocytoma	I	Before 20 years	Cerebellum		12
			Cerebral hemisphere	10	
			Optic nerve	< 5	
Differentiated astrocytoma	II	Young adults or middle age	Cerebral hemisphere	5-10	15
Anaplastic astrocytoma	III	Peak 46 years	Cerebral hemisphere	10-15	10
Glioblastoma	IV	Peak 56 years	Cerebral hemisphere	20-30	
Ependymoma	II	Before 20 years	Fourth ventricle	5	10
Oligodendroglioma	II	Peak 40 years	Hemisphere (frontal lobe 60%)	< 5	1
Medulloblastoma	IV	60% before 10 years	Cerebellum	< 8	20
Neurinoma	I	Middle age	VIII nerve, V (rare)	< 8	< 1
Meningioma	I	Middle age		15	1
Primary lymphoma	III, IV	Peak 55 years	Periventricular hemisphere	< 2	–
Germinoma					
Teratoma	I to III	Before 20 years	Pineal region	< 1	2

- modification of libido (related to hypophysis adenoma, exuberant sexual component of temporal tumor),
- changes of alimentary tract (boulimia or anorexia, behavior of diencephalic tumor),
- hypersomnia (di- and mesencephalic tumor),
- false «Attention Deficit Disorder and Hyperactivity» of infant (posterior fossa tumor).

Imaging of intracranial tumors: general points [1, 12, 19, 22] (table 3.2)

There are three stages in the imaging of intracranial tumors:
- detection of the abnormality;
- identifying the abnormality as a tumor and determining its benign, malignant, intra-, extra-axial nature, etc.;
- establishing a pretreatment strategy as precisely as possible by defining the nature, volume, localization and relationship of the tumor with the different anatomical structures at risk.

The first two stages are often linked, and a combination of the clinical examination and scan findings can provide the answer in the majority of cases. Usually the pretherapeutic assessment is performed and subsequently requires several examinations.

The patients are selected on a clinical basis and referred for the most appropriate initial examination, namely CT. A combination of the clinical findings and CT appearances will diagnose a tumor in 95% of cases and give an indication of its nature in more than 80% of cases.

CT [4, 20, 22] (table 3.2)

This should be the initial examination of choice. The performance of the CT examination must obey certain rules when looking for an intracranial tumor:
- routine lateral «scout view» from which the different scan planes can be visualized and accurately defined;
- routine performance of sections from the foramen magnum to the vertex;
- contiguous axial sections of 5 mm thickness through the posterior fossa and 10 mm thickness supratentorially. Supplementary coronal sections are necessary for the examination of certain areas (hypophysis, optic chiasma, orbit, vertex). These greatly assist in defining the relationships of the tumor with different anatomical structures (tentor-

Table 3.2. MR and CT appearances of cerebral tumors [from D. Balériaux and J. Hildebrand (1991) In: D. Buthiau (ed) Clinical CT and MRI Frison-Roche, Paris, pp 173-210]

Cerebral tumor	CT		IRM							
	– C	+ C	T1	T2	Gd	E	Cy	Ca	H	M
Pilocytic astr.	Iso/hypo	++	Hypo	Hyper	++	+	+++	+/–	–	+/–
Cerebellar astr.	Iso/hypo	+	Hypo	Hyper	+	+/–	+++	+/–	–	+/–
Grade I hemispheric astr.	Hypo	– (+)	Hypo	Hyper	– (+)	+/–	– (+)	–	–	+/–
Subependymal astr.	Iso/hyper	+++	Hypo/iso	Hypo/hyper	+++	+	–	+++	–	+
Grade II astr.	Hypo	+/–	Hypo	Hyper	+/–	+/–	+/–	–	–	+/-
Grade III astr.	Hypo/iso	++	Hypo	Hyper	++	+	+	–	+/–	+
Glioblastoma	Hypo/iso/hyper	++/+++	Hypo/iso	Hyper	++	+++	+	–	++	++
Oligodendroglioma I and II	Hypo/iso/hyper	–/+	Hypo	Hyper	–/+	+/–	+	+++	++	+/–
Oligodendroglioma III and IV	Hypo/iso/hyper	++	Hypo/iso	Hyper	++	++	+++	+/–	+++	++
Ependymoma	Iso/hyper	+	Iso/hypo	Hyper	+/++	++	+/–	++	+/–	++
Medulloblastoma	Hyper	++	Iso/hypo	Iso/hyper	++	+	+/–	+/–	++	+
Metastasis	Hypo/iso/hyper	+/++	Hypo	Hyper	+/++	++/+++	+	+/–	+	+/++
Neurinoma	Iso/hypo	+++	Iso/hypo	Hyper	+++	+/–	+/–	–	–	+/-
Meningiona	Hyper	+++	Iso/hypo	Iso/hypo	+++	+/++	–	++	–	+/++
Primary lymphoma	Hyper	+++	Hypo	Hyper	++	+++	+/–	–	–	++
Pineal T.	Iso/hyper	+++	Iso	Hyper	+++	+/–	–	+/–	+/–	+/–

C: contrast media; Ca: calcification; Cy: cyst; E: edema; H: hemorrhage; M: mass effect

ium cerebelli, skull base, etc.). However, in other areas coronal sections must be performed with care due to the risk of decompensating a cerebral edema or even coning following extension of the head. Multiplanar examination of space occupying lesions should nowadays be reserved for MRI;
- sections obtained before and after the intravenous injection of a contrast agent. Potentially, post-contrast scans can be performed straight-away. Unenhanced scans can be performed at a later date since only contrast scans may misdiagnose blood as tumor enhancement;
- apart from a few specific cases (investigation of hypophyseal tumors), a rapid infusion technique (2 ml per kg body weight) is employed using a contrast agent with an iodine concentration of approximately 30%;
- scans must be obtained immediately or within half an hour of the infusion;
- the sections through the skull base must be imaged both with the bony and soft tissue windows (e.g. windows: 100, 500);
- other techniques are sometimes used: density measurement to confirm the lipid nature of a tumor and 3D reconstruction.

Findings

This is based on changes in density and in morphology. There is no characteristic density measurement apart from fat (negative density) and hence the density measurement will only give a degree of guidance: liquid density if the measurement is around 10 Hounsfield units, probable calcification if the density is greater than 300 Hounsfield units, etc.

Indirect signs

These are variable depending on the origin and length of onset, but are useful for determining the intra- or extra-axial localization of the lesion.

Bony signs

- Signs of intracranial hypertension,
- enlargement of a skull base foramen,
- changes in the skull vault: thinning, hyperostosis, deformity.

Signs involving the cisterns

A compression or conversely an enlargement of a cistern.

Mass effect

This is a function of tumor size, degree of edema, the localization of the tumor and the rapidity of growth. It is assessed by analyzing the cerebrospinal fluid spaces and midline structures and should routinely be looked for.

Early mass effect

This does not affect the midline structures and may be seen as localized effacement of the convexity gyri or slight deformity of the ventricular wall.

Marked mass effect

A very significant deformity of the cerebrospinal fluid spaces and displacement of the reference anatomical structures:
- effacement of the gyri of a whole region or hemisphere,
- ipsilateral ventricular compression,
- corresponding compression of the cisterns.

Herniation

- Subfalcine herniation of the corpus callosum is relatively easy to appreciate on axial sections: midline shift, compression of the lateral ventricle and/or inferior displacement of the roof of the involved lateral ventricle;
- transtentorial temporal herniation into the foramen ovale is characterized by effacement of the ipsilateral peripeduncular and suprasellar cisterns with displacement of the brainstem. This may result in infarction due to ischemia in the territory of the ipsilateral posterior cerebral artery;
- transtentorial infero-superior herniation is characterized by elevation of the cerebellar vermis and therefore deformity of the quadrigeminal cisterns and anterior displacement of the brainstem;
- herniation of the cerebellar tonsils is quite difficult to appreciate on CT. It requires very caudal sections through the long axis of the foramen magnum at which level the spino-medullary junction may be recognized as being compressed anteriorly by the paired tonsils well visualized in the cervical part of the cisterna magna;

Hydrocephalus

Ventricular dilatation is easy to recognize. Formal measurements are of little value. The diagnosis of hydrocephalus can be made on the basis of rounding of the lateral and third ventricles, the presence or absence of a periventricular hypodensity around the frontal and occipital horns. This parenchymal hypodensity corresponds to transependymal resorption of the cerebrospinal fluid.

Direct signs

These must be assessed both on the pre- and post-contrast scans.

Pre-contrast

The finding of intracranial tumors is in fact quite poor. The density of the tumors should be compared to the adjacent tissues and may be described as hypodense, hyperdense, heterogeneous, calcified or cystic.

Post-contrast

Tumors may or may not be enhanced following injection of an intravenous iodinated contrast agent depending on the histology. Tumor enhancement depends on two factors, the vascular pool and the diffusion of the contrast from the intravascular space into the extracellular space via the intervening capillary fenestrations.

Any tumor developing from structures which normally possess capillary are impermeable, therefore enhanced following the injection of the contrast agent. This is the case for all lesions affecting the extra-axial structures: bone, meninges, cranial nerves and hypophysis will be all enhanced after the contrast injection.

Intra-axial structures, however, possess a blood brain barrier: the capillaries are impermeable and prevent the diffusion of certain molecules including iodinated contrast. In the normal state, the iodine injected intravenously remains strictly within the intravascular space. This space represents only 5% of the total cerebral blood volume and is too small to produce a significant change in density following the intravenous injection. There is, therefore, no detectable enhancement of the cerebral parenchyma following the intravenous contrast injection. In certain pathological circumstances, the brain capillaries lose their impermeability and the iodine can be diffused into the extracellular space of the lesion. As an oversimplification, all primary or metastatic tumors will be enhanced following the contrast injection as will all inflammatory or acute infectious processes: encephalitis, brain abscess, brain softening, etc.

It is vital to understand that this enhancement does not necessarily represent the whole tumor volume, particularly in the case of astrocytic gliomas. Non-enhancement of the center of a tumor does not necessarily indicate central necrosis or cystic change.

Differences between intra-axial and extra-axial tumors

Theoretically it should be easy to differentiate an intra-axial from extra-axial tumor. However, in certain cases it is not easy to determine the exact localization of a tumor, and supplementary CT examinations are necessary, notably coronal sections, although these have progressively been superseded by MRI (risks previously discussed).

Extra-axial tumor (fig. 3.1)

- May affect bone;
- may cause dilatation of the cistern within which it has developed;
- compression of the parenchyma;
- in general, these tumors elicit less edema. A hypodensity in the periphery of the lesion is likely to be «liquid» if it remains very limited and does not extend into the white matter;
- extra-axial tumors always enhanced after intravenous injection.

Intra-axial tumors (fig. 3.2)

- Usually these develop in the white matter and are therefore surrounded by brain parenchyma;
- these lesions elicit the rapid development of vasogenic edema which spreads along the affected white matter fibers, a very characteristic appearance;
- effacement of the gyri and compression of the ipsilateral cisterns;
- variable enhancement;
- the adjacent bone is not affected.

The *distinction* between intra- and extra-axial tumor is not always easy.

Certain extra-axial tumors invade or are closely adherent to the cortex. Conversely, some glioblastomas or metastasis may invade the dura.

Nodular extensions of some intra-axial tumors may invade the cisterns and appear as extra-axial tumors (brainstem tumor, tumor of the fourth ventricle lodged in the cerebello-pontine angle, etc.).

Some intra-axial tumors extend along the skull vault or falx and resemble a meningioma.

Finally and most importantly no pattern of enhancement is really characteristic.

Overall in the majority of cases, the CT appearances with the help of the clinical details allow one to make the diagnosis of a tumor, to differentiate an intra-axial from extra-axial tumor, to give some idea of the exact diagnosis for the commonest tumors: glioma, metastasis, meningioma, neurinoma, etc.

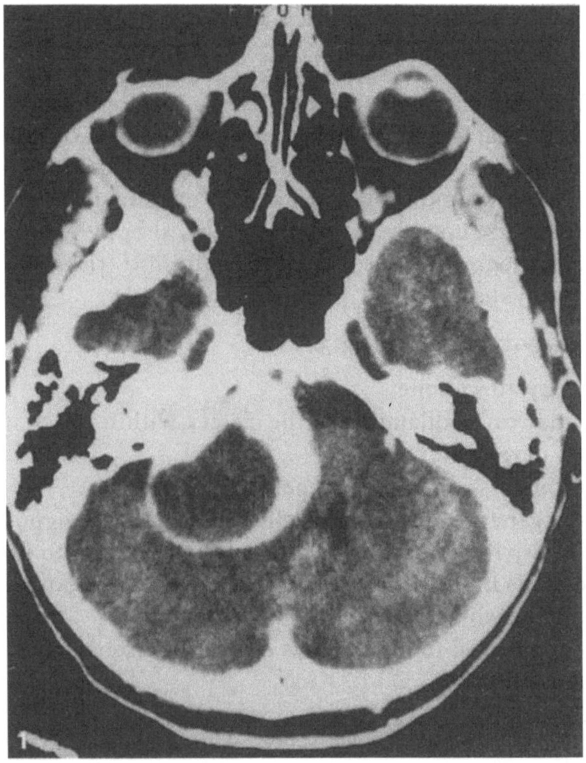

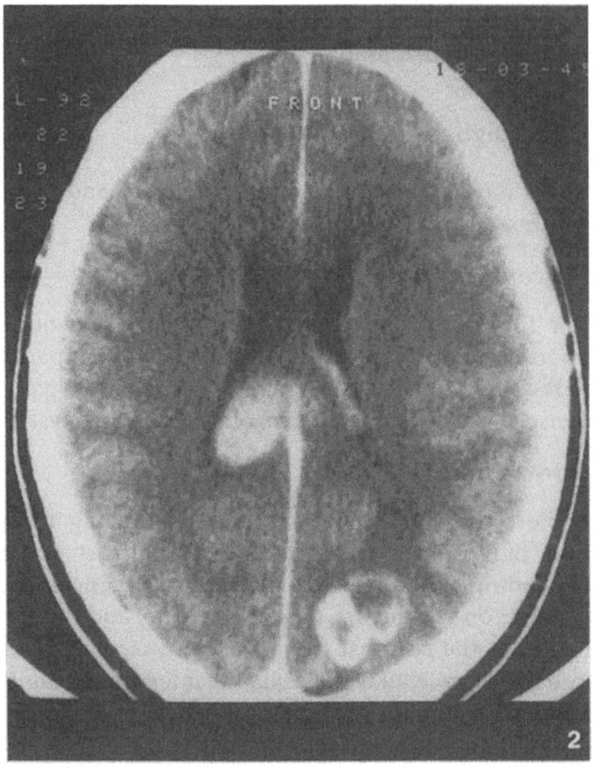

Fig. 3.1. Neurinoma of the right VIII nerve. Typical appearances of an extra-axial tumor: bony changes (enlargement of the internal auditory canal), enlargement of adjacent subarachnoid spaces, displacement of the brainstem, peripheral enhancement following contrast on CT

Fig. 3.2. Intra-axial tumor. CT shows that the tumor is completely surrounded by interdigitating edema of the white matter which is effacing the gyri. No apparent bone change

MRI [1, 2, 12, 21] (table 3.2)

Essentially the image produced is a function of intrinsic and extrinsic factors.

The intrinsic factors are characteristics of the tissue or organ under investigation: proton density, T1- and, T2 relaxation times, flow.

The extrinsic factors depend on the type of scanner and sequences used:
- the finding may change with field strength,
- proton density, T1- and T2-weighted sequences. These different weightings are achieved by varying the repetition time (TR), echo time (TE), and less frequently the inversion time (TI).

Normal appearances

On T1-weighted sequences, the cerebrospinal fluid (CSF) appears hypointense, the grey/white matter differentiation is variable depending on the sequence used but the signal of the white matter is always more intense than that of the grey matter. These are the so-called anatomical sequences.

The T2-weighted sequences are less «anatomical» but are much more sensitive to differences in the chemical composition of tissues. The CSF signal intensity increases with lengthening of the echo time and therefore appears more and more white. The signal intensity of the white matter changes in the other direction: the later the echo, the more hypointense signal. The signal intensity of the white matter changes with prolongation of the TE.

The T2-weighted sequences are the most sensitive to pathology: very minor alterations in water content show up as signal changes.

MRI contrast agents [5, 11, 21, 24]

It is possible to use contrast agents which are complexes of gadolinium (Gd) which is a paramagnetic ion. These gadolinium compounds are used essentially with T1-weighted sequences.

These MR contrast agents are not dissimilar to the uro-angiographic iodinated contrast agents, possessing comparable general and local pharmacokinetic properties. They diffuse across all capillary walls except for those within normal brain (blood brain barrier). However, MRI appears to be more sensitive than CT. The equivalent diffusion of iodine and gadolinium into the same extracellular space would be more readily detected by MR than CT due to the more marked signal change.

Performance of MRI for intracranial tumors

By modifying the acquisition parameters it is possible to obtain images with variable appearance (T1- or T2-weighting by varying the TE) in three orthogonal planes: axial, coronal and sagittal.

The examination usually comprises of images acquired in the three orthogonal planes with at least two types of sequence (T1- and T2-weighted). Typically, the sagittal sections are T1-weighted in order to best define the anatomical relationships. Coronal and axial sections are more often T2-weighted and may be performed with reference to landmarks which can subsequently be used for stereotactic surgery and radiotherapy.

Small and clinically silent areas of high signal intensity may be apparent in the white matter in normal adults over 50 years of age:

- high signal intensity in the region of the frontal horns of the lateral ventricles: stage I of Zimmerman;
- linear periventricular high signal intensity: stage II of Zimmerman;
- multiple patchy high signal changes within the white matter.

Findings specific to MRI

(figs 3.3-3.6)

This is more elementary than CT. Essentially, for the great majority of tumors:

- the appearances are similar with very small differences: hypointense on T1-weighted imaging, hyperintense on T2-weighted imaging,

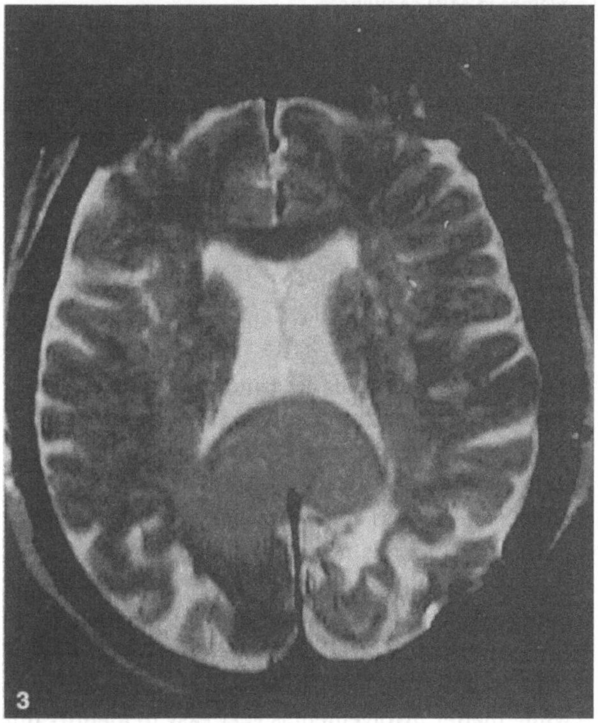

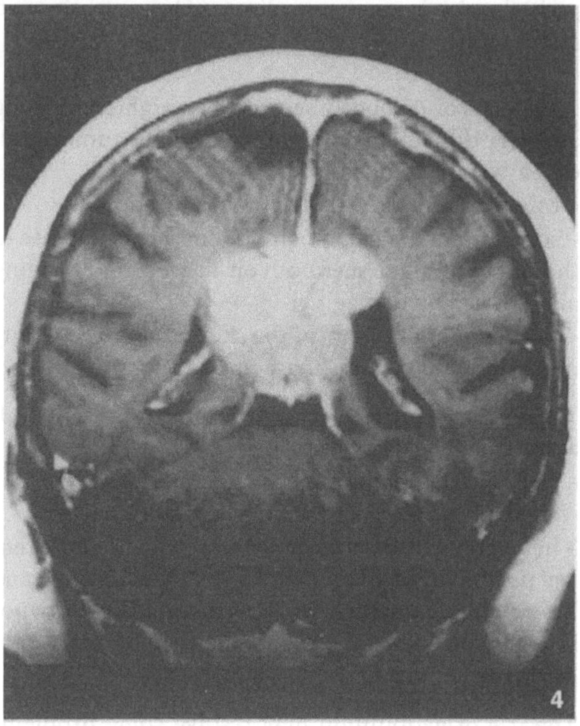

Figs 3.3 & 3.4. Meningioma. MRI, T2-weighted (fig. 3.3) and post-gadolinium T1-weighted images (fig. 3.4). The lesion appears isointense to the cerebral parenchyma on the T2-weighted images, fairly characteristic of meningiomas with marked enhancement following gadolinium. The contrast injection demonstrates the characteristic enhancement of the meninges in contact with the tumor

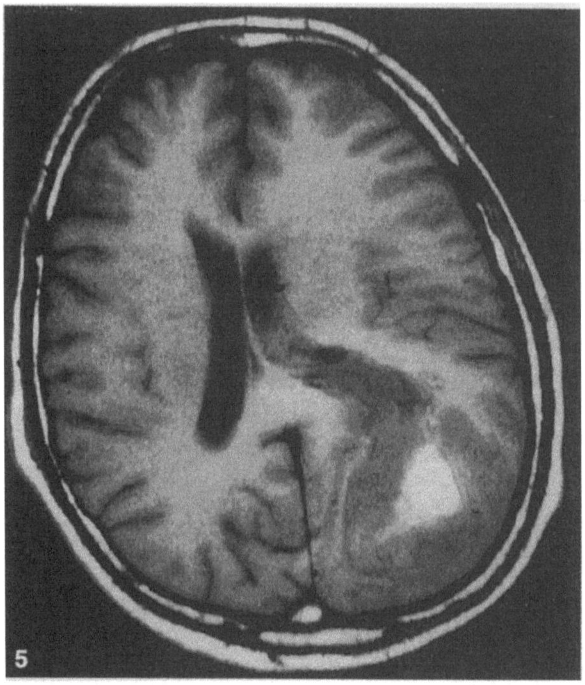

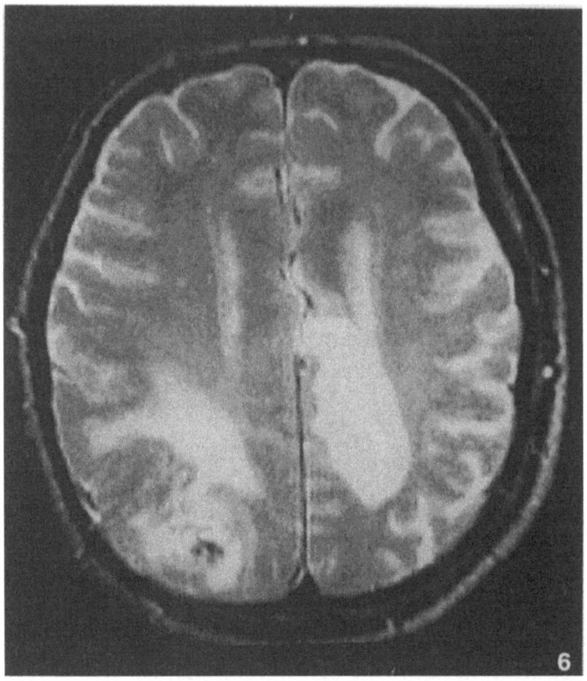

Fig. 3.5. Glioblastoma: post-gadolinium T1-weighted MRI section. Mass compressing and displacing the lateral ventricle and effacing the cortical sulcal pattern. The central enhancement is not an indicator of the true extent of the tumor

Fig. 3.6. Multiple lesions in cerebral lymphoma: intratumoral hemorrhage within the lesion located in the right posterior parietal region is seen as a small area of hypointensity on the T2-weighted MRI sequences

- edema is often poorly seen on T1-weighted imaging and very difficult to differentiate from the tumor itself on T2-weighted imaging;
- calcifications are usually not visualized;
- some tumors, such as meningioma, are isointense to the surrounding tissues both on T1-weighted imaging and T2-weighted imaging;
- the bones and tumors of the skull base are generally more difficult to assess than on CT.

There is no truly characteristic appearance on MRI, apart from a few exceptions:
- fatty or fat containing tumors: hyperintense on T1-weighted and T2-weighted imaging fat signal on;
- hemorrhagic tumor or cavernous hemangioma: central portion hyperintense on T1-weighted imaging and T2-weighted imaging with a peripheral ring of hypointensity on T2-weighted imaging (hemosiderin deposition).

The use of gadolinium may resolve some problems but the same limitations exist as for iodinated contrast:
- good definition of tumors which take up the contrast. Simplistically, enhancement is seen in all extra-axial tumors, malignant intra-axial tumors and metastases, as well as a number of non-neoplastic lesions;
- excellent visualization of extra-axial tumors, particularly those in the posterior fossa and skull base.

Indirect signs

Apart from the bony changes, indirect signs are easier to appreciate when compared to CT:
- effects on the cisterns (compression or enlargement);
- effects on the gyri and ventricles;
- mass effect is extremely well shown by MRI.

A detailed description of the MRI appearances would require a whole day on its own, particularly in relation to the temporal lobe. Very small lesions may be detected despite a negative CT:
- white matter involvement is very easy to identify due to the three orthogonal scan planes;
- hydrocephalus: MRI is the examination of choice, particularly for assessing the region of the mesencephalon and posterior fossa.

In summary, very small tumors can be demonstrated by MRI due to its high sensitivity and exquisite anatomical detail. Precise diagnosis of extra-axial tumors can be made with the use of gadolinium which seems to be superior to CT. The acquisition of images in three orthogonal planes precisely defines the tumor localization, volume and anatomical relationships .

In summary

Currently, the diagnosis of an intracranial tumor is made by CT in the majority of cases. MRI is clearly more sensitive than CT in certain areas: midline, posterior fossa, temporal lobe. The identification of a tumor is usually independent of its intrinsic characteristics either on CT or MRI but highly dependent on the clinical findings and the location of the tumor. Pretherapeutic assessment is obtained by a combination of CT and MRI, complemented in certain cases by angiography.

We describe the imaging of a variety of tumors encountered in the two classically described areas, namely the supratentorial and infratentorial levels.

Tumor localization

The principal aim is to define whether a tumor is intra- or extra-axial. CT and particularly MRI are able to make this distinction in the majority of cases. This distinction is essential in order to determine the correct treatment. In effect, the majority extra-axial tumors are benign.

Supratentorial tumors

The three commonest types of tumors encountered in the adult are gliomas, metastases and meningiomas.

Whatever the nature of the lesion, the diagnosis of a tumor is made from the clinical details, localization (intra- or extra-axial tumor), age of the patient (the specific features of childhood tumors will be highlighted), and imaging appearances.

Intra-axial tumors

In making the diagnosis of an intra-axial mass, imaging is unable to determine the histological nature of the tumor but certain signs are suggestive of malignancy:

- absence of calcification,
- necrosis,
- contrast enhancement,
- edema,
- multiple lesions.

Other pathologies can give identical appearances on CT or MRI:
- brain-softening conditions,
- old hematomas,
- abscesses.

The combination of the imaging findings and clinical history will suggest the diagnosis of the tumor in the majority of cases. The two most important types of intra-axial tumor are astrocytic gliomas and metastases.

Gliomas [1, 4, 10, 12, 25]

Arising from the glial cells, gliomas are the commonest primary intracranial tumors. Their incidence varies between 30-60% of all primary tumors depending on the series quoted.

Astrocytic gliomas

These represent 30-35% of gliomas. In the vast majority of cases, the diagnosis poses no problem and the CT examination is all that is required.

• Low grade astrocytomas (fig. 3.7)

There is no evidence histologically of malignancy in these tumors but they are susceptible to malignant transformation. They tend to evolve slowly and may recur after treatment with or without malignant transformation. The tumors may contain micro- or macrocysts and sometimes areas of calcification. It is extremely important to make the diagnosis of a low grade astrocytoma localized in a functionally silent zone of the brain in a young patient from the imaging findings. MRI, due to its very high sensitivity, is at least partially able to achieve this.

CT

Usually these tumors appear as a poorly defined hypodense area on the pre-contrast scan. The majority do not enhance after the injection of contrast. However, some studies have demonstrated that enhancement may occur, particularly at the periphery of the lesion. The exact boundaries of the tumor are impossible to define because it is an infiltrative lesion.

The indirect signs of a low grade astrocytoma are not very obvious: reactive edema is generally absent or only minimal; often there is no mass effect until late in the disease process.

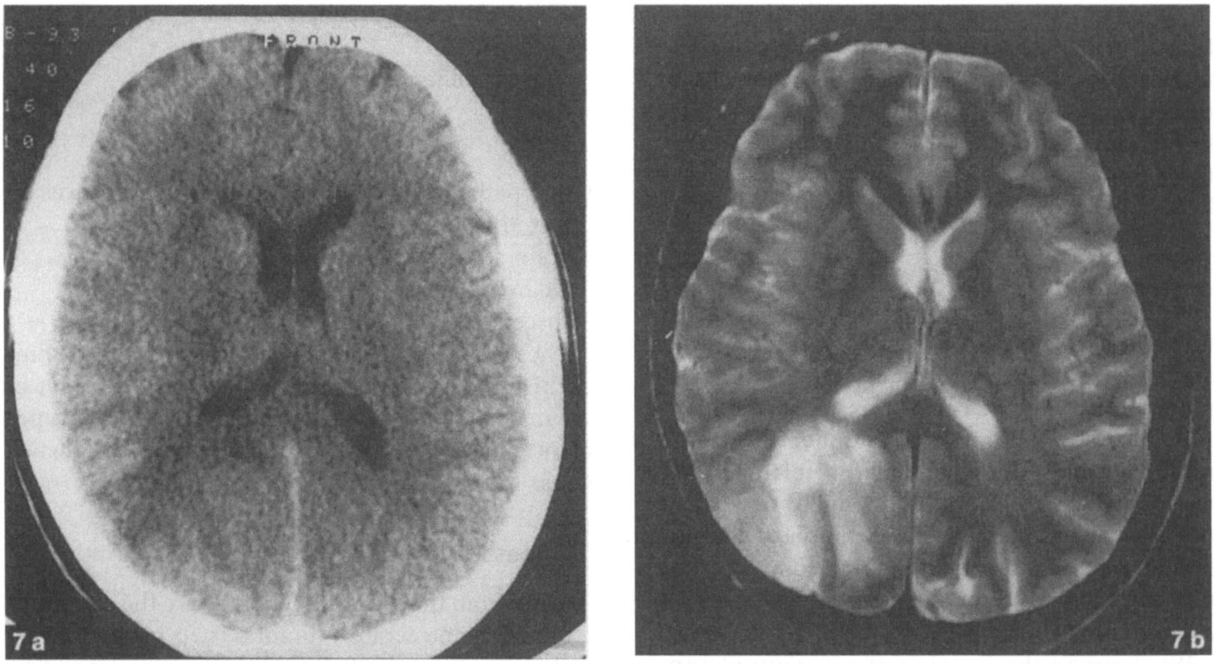

Fig. 3.7 a, b. Low grade astrocytoma. **a** CT: poorly defined hypodense area which is difficult to appreciate and located in the right parietal region causing slight mass effect on the right lateral ventricle. **b** MRI: T2-weighted image: large area of hyperintensity making the diagnosis much easier than CT

MRI

Low grade astrocytomas appear hypointense on T1-weighted imaging and hyperintense on T2-weighted imaging which does not differentiate them in any way from other lesions. However, the high sensitivity of MRI is particularly valuable in two circumstances:
- there is clinical suspicion of a tumor despite a negative CT. MRI may detect an abnormality (hyperintense on T2) particularly within the temporal lobe. The MR examination should always include in these cases sagittal T1-weighted images and axial and coronal T2-weighted images;
- the diagnosis of a low grade astrocytoma has been made on the CT examination. When surgical treatment and/or radiotherapy are planned, a complementary MRI should be performed before deciding on the correct treatment strategy. In fact, these astrocytomas are often highly infiltrative and MRI will demonstrate (hyperintense on T2) a considerable degree of extension not appreciated on the CT examination.

• Anaplastic astrocytomas and glioblastomas

These occur generally in older adults(fig. 3.8)

CT

The appearances are often highly suggestive even on pre-contrast scan: areas of hypodensity extending to a variable extent into the white matter (an appearance suggestive of an intra-axial lesion), heterogeneous hypodensity, sometimes slightly hyperdense without hemorrhage (grade 3). Occasionally there is a hyperdensity surrounded by hypodensity due to hemorrhage. Following contrast injection, there is a thin irregular ring of enhancement or poorly defined nodular enhancement alternating with non-enhancing areas.

The indirect signs depend on the size and site of the lesion: usually a mass effect, herniation or rarely hydrocephalus. The tumor is often large and already extensive at the time of the initial CT examination: temporo-frontal glioma, glioma involving the grey matter nuclei, «butterfly» glioma; extension bilaterally across the corpus callosum.

The combination of clinical examination and CT is sufficient to confirm the diagnosis in 98% of cases. In very rare cases, some CT appearances could theoretically be confused with extra-axial lesions.

It is therefore important to understand the limitations of CT:
- the enhancing tissue does not necessarily represent the whole tumor volume. Infiltrative tumor tissue may actually extend beyond the outer limit of the enhancing tissue;

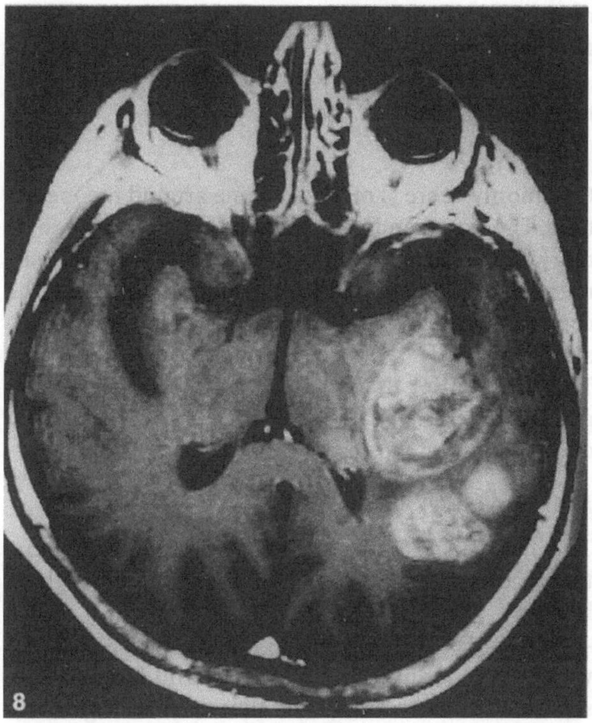

Fig. 3.8. Glioblastoma on post-gadolinium T1-weighted MRI: multilobulated heterogeneous mass demonstrating enhancement

- the enhancement pattern does not grade the tumor; it simply confirms the presence of abnormal capillary permeability suggestive of a malignant lesion;
- the unenhanced hypodense center is not necessarily synonymous with necrosis. It may represent a cystic area or even tumor tissue which exhibits delayed enhancement.

MRI

MRI is not indispensable for making the diagnosis but its multiplanar capability may be necessary for pretreatment assessment to define the tumor volume, extent and anatomical relationships.

The appearances on MRI are:

- hypointense on T1; edema and tumor are of similar signal intensity,
- hyperintense on T2 which confuses edema and tumor extension. However, it is possible on the late echo images to differentiate edema form the tumor.

MRI is only really valuable when combined with the use of contrast agents. The high signal intensity caused by the diffusion of gadolinium on T1-weighted images and the three imaging planes improve the assessment of tumor volume, extension and anatomical relationships. The same reservations exist for the gadolinium compounds as do for the iodinated agents since they possess the same properties.

The diffusion of gadolinium does not necessarily represent the border and hence the extent of tumor. The diffusion of gadolinium gives no indication of the grade of malignancy. The absence of diffusion into the center of the tumor does not always indicate necrosis.

• Oligodendroglioma

These represent 9-10% of glial tumors, occur in adults and develop particularly in the frontal lobes. Calcification is present in approximately 9% of cases. CT appearances are very typical:

- hyperdense area without mass effect with associated calcification. The peripheral calcifications may have a linear or eggshell appearance but the nodular pattern of calcification is the commonest. The association of these two types of calcification is characteristic;
- inhomogeneous enhancement following contrast injection;
- occasionally cystic center containing a fluid/fluid level.

The only value of MRI is the improved assessment of tumor volume and its relationships. The calcifications may be indeed missed on MRI, and CT remains the examination of choice.

• Ependymoma [1, 12, 31]

These glial tumors usually develop in the ventricular system close to the foramina of Monro, the aqueduct

or at the level of the fourth ventricle. CT appearances are fairly characteristic:
- hyperdense on the pre-contrast scan with associated micro- and occasionally macrocalcifications. The tumor is adherent to or projects into the ventricular lumen or causes ventricular collapse;
- intense, well defined, and homogeneous enhancement following contrast.

MRI gives no further information concerning the exact nature of the tumor.

• Papilloma of the choroid plexus

These are rare tumors (0.5 - 0.6% of all intracranial tumors). They effect particularly the young but may also occur in adults, particularly within the fourth ventricle. Their CT appearances are described with the infratentorial tumors.

• Tuberous sclerosis of Bourneville [30]

See following chapter

Cerebral metastases [1, 2, 12, 22]

Usually there is a known primary tumor, carcinoma is commoner than sarcoma or lymphoma. The diagnosis is evident from the multiple nature of the lesions which occur both infra- and supratentorially. More rarely, there is no known primary tumor but the multiplicity of the lesions is highly suggestive. However, the diagnosis is more difficult in cases of a solitary lesion without a known primary tumor. It should be remembered that 20% of patients presenting with disseminated cancer develop cerebral metastasis (e.g. lung).

CT

Direct signs

Metastases are characterized by a hypo- or isodensity and are one to several cm in diameter. They almost invariably enhance, usually in a thin, regular ring pattern. Enhancement takes the form of a homogeneous nodule when the metastasis is small: usually the lesions are multiple. CT examination should also always be viewed on a bone window. The association of a bony lesion with a parenchymal lesion is a strong indicator of metastatic disease.

Metastases may be intrinsically hyperdense, in other words hemorrhagic, and are most commonly from a malignant melanoma or rarely from a gastro-intestinal carcinoma.

Exceptionally, metastases are calcified (melanoma, colonic carcinoma, osteogenic sarcoma) or less rarely, necrotic or cystic (causing possible confusion with a glioblastoma).

Lesions are frequently localized at the grey/white matter interface.

Indirect signs

Commonly, there is marked edema around the metastasis. The extent and degree of this hypodensity can be markedly reduced by the effect of anti-edema treatment. The CT diagnosis is usually obvious and the combination of a known primary tumor with multiple supra- and infratentorial lesions is very suggestive. The differential diagnosis of a solitary metastasis poses problems: glioma, abscess, cerebrovascular accident, meningioma, etc.

MRI (fig. 3.9)

The majority of metastases are hypointense relative to the normal parenchyma on the T1-weighted images:
- the signal difference on the delayed echo T2-weighted sequences using long TE and long TR, can separate the metastasis from the surrounding edema (hyperintense edema, hypointense metastasis);
- the MR appearances following gadolinium injection on the T1-weighted sequences is comparable to the post-contrast CT but smaller lesions are demonstrated on the MRI.

The differential diagnostic problems are different to those encountered in CT. In older subjects, focal areas of abnormal signal are often seen (hypointense on T1- and hyperintense on T2-weighted sequences). These localized hyperintense areas in the white matter which may correspond to ischemic lesions or gliosis but also can simulate multiple metastasis. The clinical context is usually sufficient to exclude this diagnosis. In particular, these anomalies do not enhance following gadolinium injection.

Lymphoma [1, 2, 9, 12] (fig. 3.10)

Intracranial lymphoma may be primary or secondary and is encountered with increasing frequency in cases of AIDS. The radiological appearances are not characteristic.

CT

The lesions may be solitary or multiple and appear hypo-, iso- or hyperdense on the pre-contrast scans, with or without perilesional edema. They are usually located in the periventricular region and central grey nuclei. The infiltrative type of lesions, diffuse subependymal or bifrontal, are particularly suggestive.

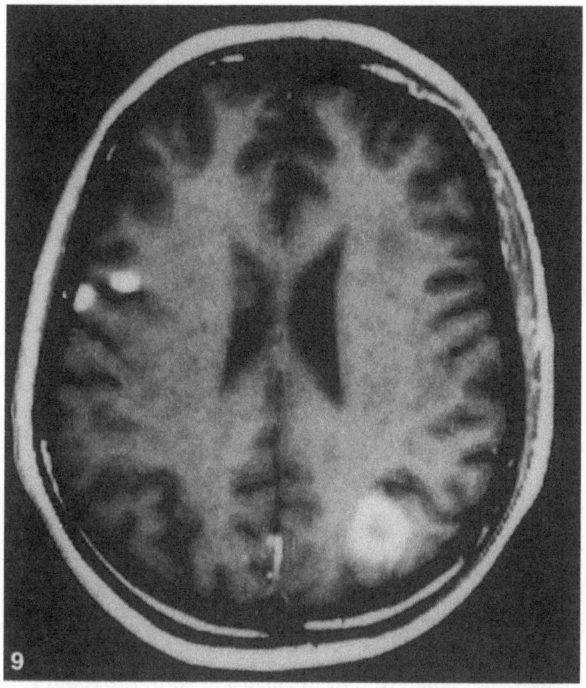

Fig. 3.9. Metastasis on post-gadolinium T1-weighted MRI section: only the lesion in the left parietal region was demonstrated on CT. MRI shows the unexpected contralateral lesions indicating cerebral metastasis. Large metastasis have a regular thin ring enhancement pattern whereas small lesions demonstrate a homogeneous nodular enhancement pattern

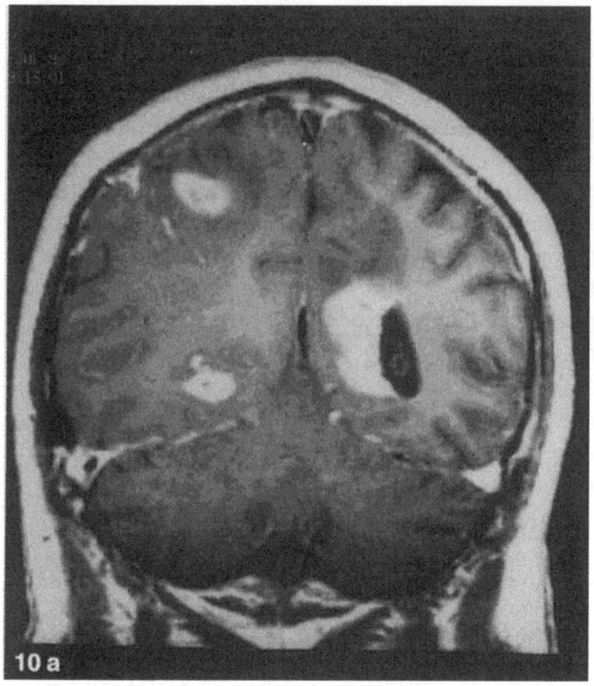

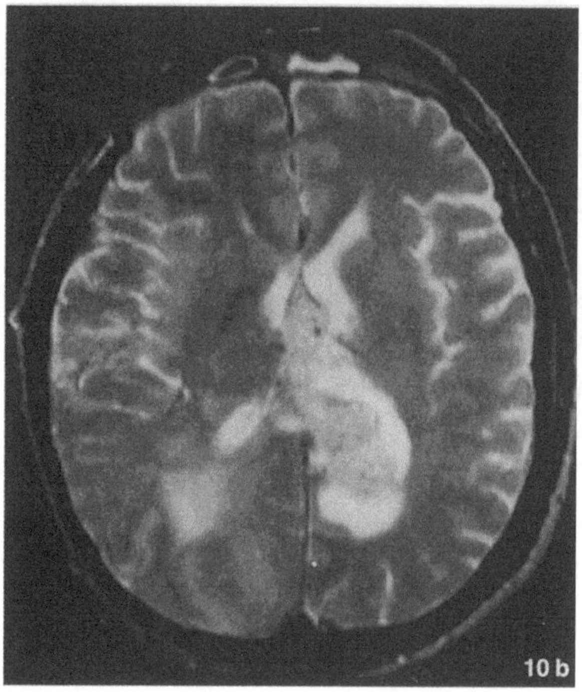

Fig. 3.10 a, b. Lymphoma on MRI. **a** Post-gadolinium T1-weighted coronal section: multiple well defined lesions demonstrating homogeneous and intense enhancement. **b** T2-weighted axial section: it is difficult to distinguish tumor from the surrounding edema

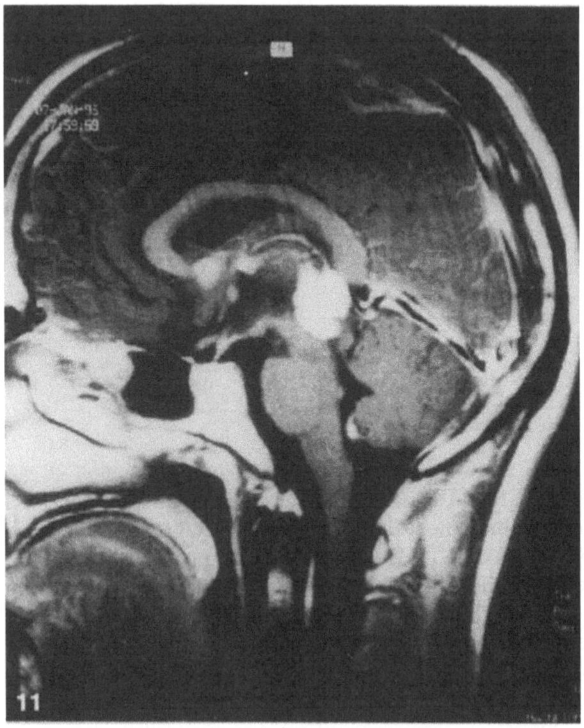

Fig. 3.11. Germinoma on MRI. Post-gadolinium T1-weighted sagittal section exquisitely demonstrates the tumor in the pineal region exhibiting intense homogeneous enhancement. Other small lesions are also shown in the roof of the third ventricle which were not visible on CT

Following the injection of contrast agent, there is almost always homogeneous and well defined enhancement .

Considering the size of these tumors, the indirect signs (mass effect) are generally less marked. The diagnosis of lymphoma is likely if there is marked tumor regression following the treatment with steroids. However, presurgical steroid therapy may complicate the interpretation of the operative biopsy specimens.

MRI

Again the appearances are not characteristic: hypointense on T1, hyperintense on T2, mixing edema and tumor together.

In cases of AIDS, the CT and MR appearances of lymphoma and toxoplasmosis are identical and very often the two conditions coexist. Occasionally their is intracystic hemorrhage in toxoplasmosis.

Pinealoma [1, 27, 35] (fig. 3.11)

Tumors of variable histology are grouped together under the name of pinealoma whose only common characteristic is their development on the pineal region (obstructive hydrocephalus).

CT

In the absence of hydrocephalus, the diagnosis on CT is difficult because the tumor may be very small: excessive calcification in the pineal region (diameter > 1 cm), discrete hypodensity in the pineal region deforming the cisterns, or homogenous enhancement following contrast injection. It is often difficult to confirm the presence of a tumor due to the preexisting pineal calcification, the rich local vascular supply and patient movement.

On CT, the indirect signs are more important: deformity of the posterior aspect of the third ventricle (cupula), deformity of the cisterns, slight dilatation and rounding of the third ventricle indicating early hydrocephalus.

MRI

This is the key examination and also indispensable. In effect, the diagnosis of a tumor in the pineal region is made on the mid-line sagittal T1-weighted image which perfectly demonstrates the anatomy of this region (aqueduct, exit of the aqueduct, posterior part of the third ventricle, etc.). Even small tumors can be demonstrated as is often the case. The diagnosis is confirmed by demonstrating a hyperintense lesion on the axial and coronal T2-weighted images. The indirect signs previously described for CT are equally apparent on MRI.

Extra-axial tumors [3, 12, 22, 26, 34, 37]

These arise from the investing tissues (either from bone and meninges or from the contents of the subarachnoid space, nerve roots, blood vessels, congenital inclusion bodies such as epidermoid or fatty tissue).

Meningioma

CT

In general, the CT diagnosis is easy.

Direct signs:
- well defined iso- or hyperdense mass with a broad dural base. The mass may be calcified (20% of cases),
- marked homogeneous enhancement following contrast injection

Indirect signs:
These are both bony and parenchymal.

The bony signs are most commonly due to an osteoblastic reaction causing hyperostosis in areas in contact with the tumor. Very rarely the meningioma invades the bone: irregular osteolytic appearance rather than hyperostosis.

Bony invasion is more suggestive of malignant meningioma. Even these slow growing benign tumors can be aggressive and frequently recur after surgery.

The parenchymal signs are common to all tumors of a certain size, but in general are characteristic of an extra-axial tumor:
- mass effect: less marked given the size of the tumor.
- edema does not extend into the various digitations of the white matter;
- tumor surrounded by a well defined hypodensity which often represents encysted CSF or «peri-tumoral cyst».

The atypical CT appearances of meningiomas described are:
- hypodense pre- and post-contrast due to myxoid or fatty degeneration;
- totally calcified: psammomatous bodies which do not change density following contrast;
- en plaque which are only detectable on CT by their indirect bony signs: hypertrophy and hyperostosis;
- malignant meningeal tumors are impossible to distinguish from typical meningiomas on CT; hemangiopericytoma, meningeal metastasis, meningeal lymphoma, malignant meningioma.

MRI

MRI is disappointing compared to CT. The tumor is isointense to the adjacent parenchyma both on T1- and T2-weighted imaging. In addition, the calcifications and reactive bone changes are very poorly demonstrated by MR.

However, with the use of gadolinium, MR seems to be superior to CT in the diagnosis of meningiomas en plaque for example, or for assessing tumor extension (cavernous sinus, optic canal, vascular structures, etc.). The excellent contrast as a result of the gadolinium and the multiplanar imaging give a more detailed and precise assessment of tumor extent compared to CT.

Dural metastases

These are enhanced following gadolinium injection in a nodular or infiltrative fashion and are only visible on MRI.

Congenital intracranial tumors

These tumors develop from inclusion bodies of ectoderm, mesoderm or endoderm within the neural tube at the time of its closure, namely during the third to fifth weeks of gestation. The earlier the inclusion, the closer it is to the midline. The later inclusion bodies are situated in the diploe. They are not malignant.

Tumors of the sellar region

Adenomas, craniopharyngiomas and meningiomas do not in general pose any diagnostic problem and their CT and MR appearances will not be described here.

Bony tumors

Epidermoid tumors, hemangiomas, osteomas, chordomas, myeloma, metastases, etc., are all easy to detect and usually can be characterized on the standard radiographs and CT examination.

Tumors of otorhinolaryngological origin

Nasopharyngeal fibromas in children and malignant tumors in adults (carcinoma of the nasopharynx) can infiltrate along the nerve sheaths and extend intracranially. It is necessary to perform coronal CT and particularly MRI in the assessment of these tumors.

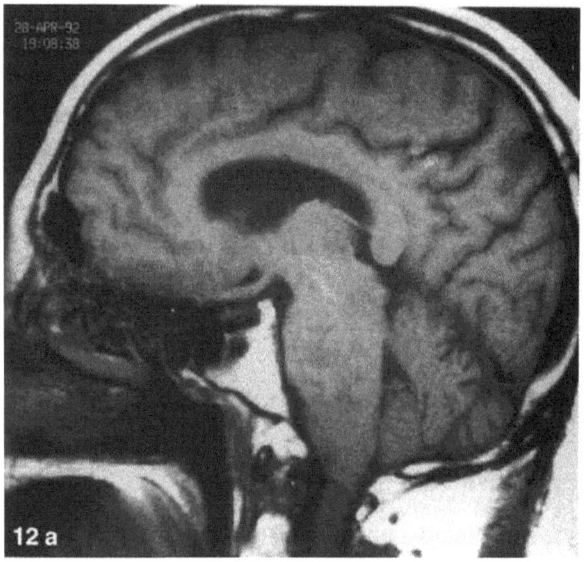

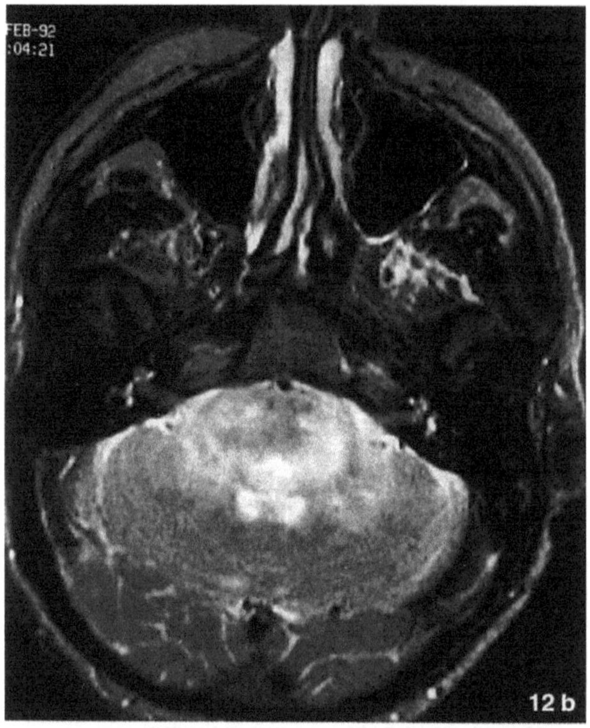

Fig. 3.12. Glioma of the brain stem on MRI. **a** T1-weighted sagittal section: effacement of the normal contours of the brain stem with posterior displacement of the fourth ventricle. **b** Diffuse area of hyperintensity within the brain stem indicating tumor infiltration on T2-weighted imaging

Infratentorial tumors [1, 12, 29, 33, 37]

As with the supratentorial level, these tumors can be divided into intra-axial and extra-axial tumors arising either from a part of the covering layers (bone and meninges) or from elsewhere, the contents of the subarachnoid space (nerve root, blood vessels, congenital inclusion bodies of epidermoid or fatty tissue). The diagnosis of an infratentorial lesion, as with the supratentorial region, is based on the combination of the clinical progression, age of the patient, tumor localization and imaging appearances on CT or MRI.

Infratentorial tumors in children

Axial tumors

The three commonest tumors in children are the brainstem glioma (10% of the all the intracranial tumors of childhood), cerebellar astrocytoma (20%) and primitive neuroectodermal tumor (medulloblastoma 3-20%). Ependymomas are less common (2%). Other various histologies include lymphoma, oligodendroglioma and the ganglioneuroblastoma which are all very rare. Intra-axial metastases in the posterior fossa are also rare in children. The commonest are drop metastases via the subarachnoid space from a primary intra-axial tumor of the brain. Less common are metastases from primary extracranial tumors: hepatoma, osteosarcoma, rhabdomyosarcoma, etc.

Differential diagnosis

The diagnosis of a tumor is usually easy in children but rarely tumors can be confused with:
- vascular malformations which are calcified on CT and enhanced. MRI is also very useful for confirming the diagnosis;
- demyelinating conditions or cerebellar demyelination. These appear hyperintense on T2-weighted imaging and may be enhanced following intravenous contrast on CT in the acute phase. The clinical context is essential for the diagnosis;
- other parasitic or bacterial infections (cysticercosis, tuberculosis) are rarely a consideration in this clinical context.

Brain stem gliomas (fig. 3.12)

These represent 25% of childhood gliomas. The commonest site of origin is the annular protuberance but superior or inferior localizations are not unusual. Hydrocephalus is typically absent or a late sign apart from lesions of the tectum which may appear earlier. These gliomas are generally not calcified but may be partly hemorrhagic.

CT

Brain stem gliomas can be iso-, hypodense or of heterogeneous density on the pre-contrast scan and cause enlargement of the brainstem. Enhancement of these gliomas is present in only 50% of cases. There is no correlation between the degree of malignancy and the CT appearances, particularly the degree of contrast enhancement. A cyst is present in 20% of cases, and an exophytic origin within the basal cisterns and/or around the basilar trunk is seen 30-40% of cases.

In fact, the indirect signs are often the most useful for making the diagnosis because of the frequent artefacts which occur in the posterior fossa. It is difficult to determine whether a change of density within the brainstem is really pathological in the presence of these artefacts. The following indirect signs are suggestive of a brainstem mass: posterior displacement of the fourth ventricle: symmetrical or asymmetrical displacement, deformity of the roof of the fourth ventricle and compression of the prepontine cisterns which are normally very large in children.

MRI

Nowadays it is essential to perform MRI before confirming or suggesting the diagnosis of a brainstem glioma. It is the examination of choice which most often confirms the diagnosis as surgical biopsy is impossible in this situation.

The direct signs are the same as those encountered for all pathologies: hypointense on T1-weighted imaging, hyperintense on T2-weighted imaging, but the sensitivity of MRI is far superior to that of CT and all brainstem lesions can therefore be detected at an early stage.

The indirect signs are much more easily appreciated on MRI than CT. The effacement of the normal contour of the brainstem and posterior displacement of the fourth ventricle are exquisitely demonstrated on the sagittal sections.

The pretreatment assessment of tumor extent can also be well documented on MRI (cranial extent, exophytic nodules in the cisterns, etc.). Finally, MRI is able to confidently exclude the diagnosis of a cavernous haemangioma of the brainstem (central increased signal intensity on T1- and T2-weighted imaging, peripheral ring of hypointensity on T2-weighted imaging due to the presence of hemosiderin).

Cerebellar astrocytomas (fig. 3.13)

These are among the common posterior fossa tumors in children. In the majority of cases, these are benign tumors: benign astrocytomas. They are situated with equal frequency in the cerebellar vermis or hemispheres. Cystic or solid lesions also occur with equal frequency. In the cystic form, the tumor may be represented either by a mural nodule or simply the thin cyst wall.

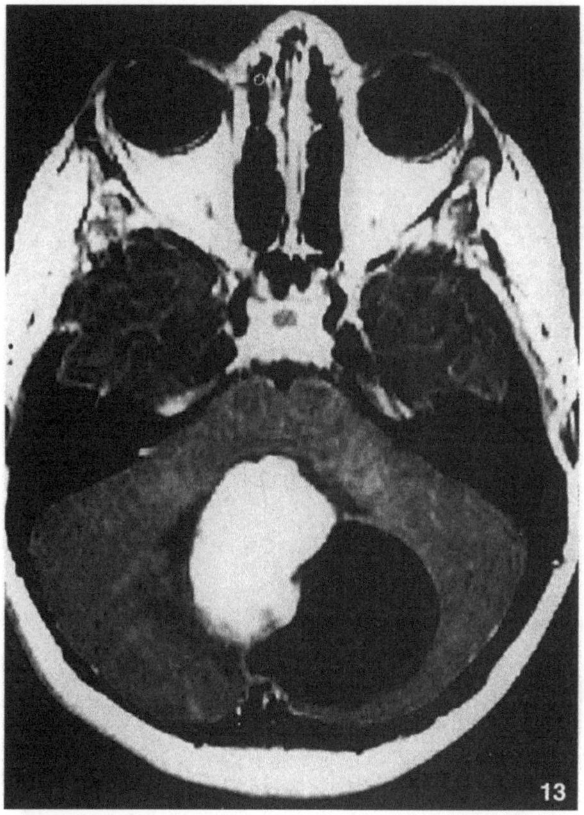
13

Fig. 3.13. Cystic astrocytoma of the cerebellum. MRI, post-gadolinium T1-weighted axial section. Combination of a cystic isointense to CSF mass, and a strongly enhancing mural nodule. Benign astrocytoma confirmed on biopsy

CT

Solid astrocytomas are hypodense on the precontrast CT scan. Cystic astrocytomas are obviously hypodense but have a density which is higher than that of CSF (increased protein content of the cyst fluid). Calcification is relatively rare (10-20%).

Following intravenous contrast, solid astrocytomas become enhanced; the nodule and/or the wall of the cyst also become opacified in cases of cystic astrocytomas. The enhancement pattern is in no way indicative of the histology.

The indirect signs depend on the localization and size of the tumor; effacement of a postero-lateral recess of the fourth ventricle, anterior or lateral displacement of the fourth ventricle, hydrocephalus due to obstruction of the fourth ventricle, herniation of

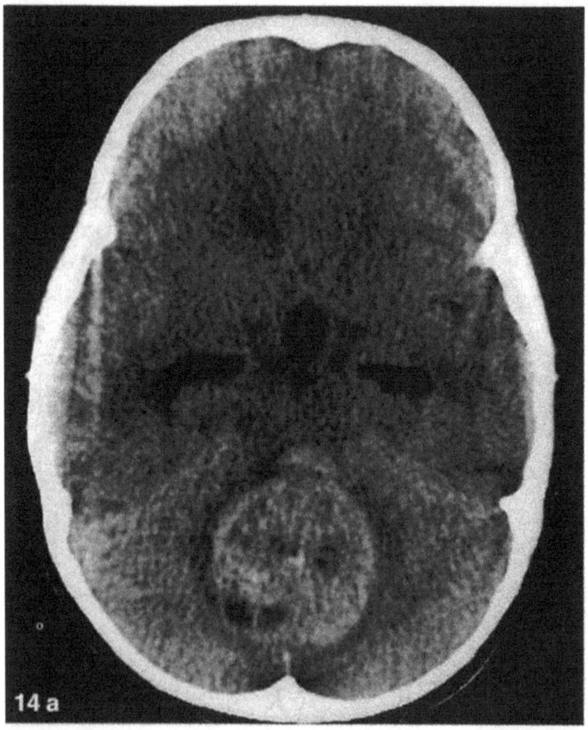

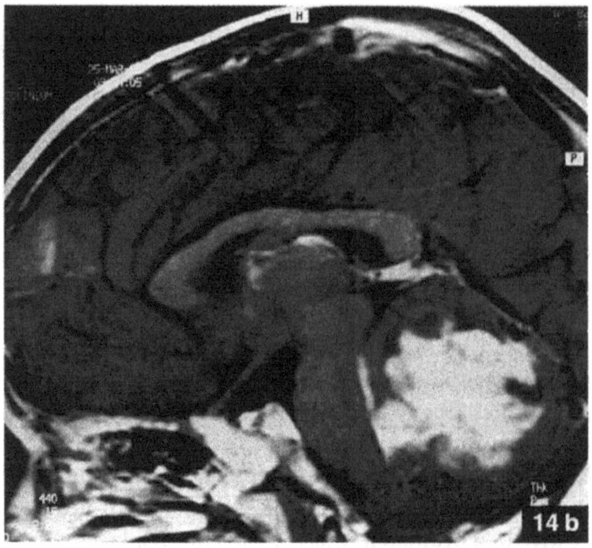

Fig. 3.14 a, b. Medulloblastoma. **a** Pre-contrast CT: intrinsically hypodense area of a well defined tumor in the region of the vermis containing a few small areas of fluid density. **b** MRI, sagittal post-gadolinium T1-weighted image. Mass arising in the cerebellar vermis, compressing the fourth ventricle anteriorly and exhibiting intense enhancement. The poor differentiation posteriorly with the cerebellar vermis is a suggestive but non-specific sign

the cerebellar tonsils or cranio-caudal transtentorial herniation.

MRI

CT examination is very useful both in making the diagnosis and in assessing the extent of the tumor. There are therefore few indications for MRI in the diagnosis of an astrocytoma: hypointense on T1, hyperintense on T2 but this hyperintensity does not change with that of the CSF as the TE is increased either in the case of solid or cystic astrocytomas (high protein content of the fluid).

Medulloblastomas: primitive neuro-ectodermal tumors (fig. 3.14)

CT

The tumor may be intrinsically hyperdense. In certain cases, the tumor contains cystic areas. Calcifications are rare, less frequent than with ependymomas or astrocytomas. Following the injection of contrast agent, medulloblastomas always become enhanced, usually in an homogeneous fashion. The post-contrast scan should include the supratentorial region in a search for secondary deposits.

Indirect signs are usually apparent: collapse of the fourth ventricle, hydrocephalus, ultimate coning.

MRI

MRI signs of medulloblastomas are non-specific. However, MRI appears to be extremely useful in the preoperative assessment of tumor spread:
- within the posterior fossa (sagittal T1-weighted image);
- within the cerebral subarachnoid spaces: effacement of the gyri is well shown on T1-weighted image, or a tumor mass appearing hyperintense on T2-weighted image;
- within the spinal subarachnoid spaces.

This preoperative assessment is of value only following injection of gadolinium.

Therefore, the pretreatment assessment of medulloblastoma nowadays should comprise of: CT examination and/or MRI of the posterior fossa; post-contrast CT or post-gadolinium MRI of the cerebral hemispheres; post-gadolinium MRI of the whole of the spinal cord.

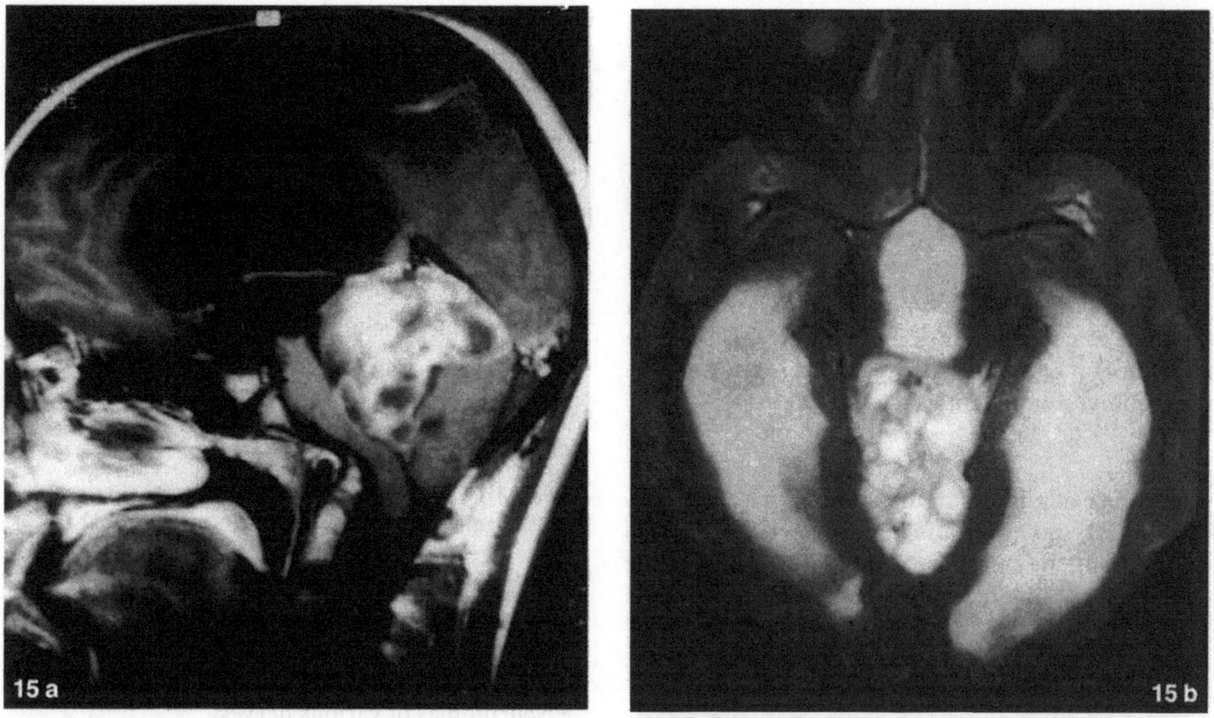

Fig. 3.15 a, b. Ependymoma on MRI. **a** Post-gadolinium T1-weighted section demonstrates a large mass exhibiting heterogeneous enhancement arising primarily in the fourth ventricle and causing significant mass effect on the brain stem. Note the severe hydrocephalus superior to the lesion. **b** T2-weighted section: very heterogeneous appearance of the tumor with punctiform areas of low signal intensity corresponding to the calcification and areas of variable hyperintensity

Ependymoma
(fig. 3.15)

CT

Ependymoma usually appears on CT as an inhomogeneous mass filling the fourth ventricle. In 50% of cases, this mass contains calcifications. Enhancement is invariable following the injection of contrast agent which may or may not be homogeneous.

Indirect signs are apparent: fullness of the posterior fossa, hydrocephalus, eventual coning.

MRI

On the T1-weighted sequence the tumor appears hypointense but also with areas of high signal intensity which correspond to intratumoral hemorrhage. On the T2 sequences the appearances are often heterogeneous: hypointense due to calcifications and blood vessels, moderate hyperintensity due to tumor, more marked hyperintensity due to intertumoral hemorrhage.

In general, the mass remains localized but ependymomas can spread as seedlings to cover the subependymal surface of the ventricular system.

The assessment of tumor spread and post-treatment follow-up should therefore routinely include: a post-contrast CT scan of the posterior fossa and supratentorial level, or an MRI examination with gadolinium.

Papillomas of the choroid plexus

CT

These appear as a hyperdense masses which may contain areas of calcification and fill the fourth ventricle and/or the cerebello-pontine angle. Enhancement in an homogeneous fashion is the rule.

Indirect signs are essentially represented by hydrocephalus which is due to three different but usually associated mechanisms: blockage of the drainage pathways by the mass, over production of CSF, intraventricular and subarachnoid hemorrhage causing compartmentalization of the fluid cavities.

Extra-axial tumors

These are rare and have few specific characteristics compared to those in adults.

Infratentorial tumors in adults

Metastases, acoustic neurinomas and meningiomas are the principle infratentorial tumors encountered in adults.

Intra-axial tumors [1,12,22,36]

Metastases

These are the commonest posterior fossa tumors in the adult. In general, they occur in the cerebellum. The imaging of metastases has already been dealt with in the section on supratentorial lesions.

Gliomas

Occurrence of gliomas in the brains tem is rare (21% of gliomas), and localization in the cerebellum is also uncommon. The cerebellar gliomas are usually cystic and have the same radiological appearances as those in children. They can pose diagnostic problems and be difficult to distinguish from a solitary metastasis or particularly a hemangioblastoma.

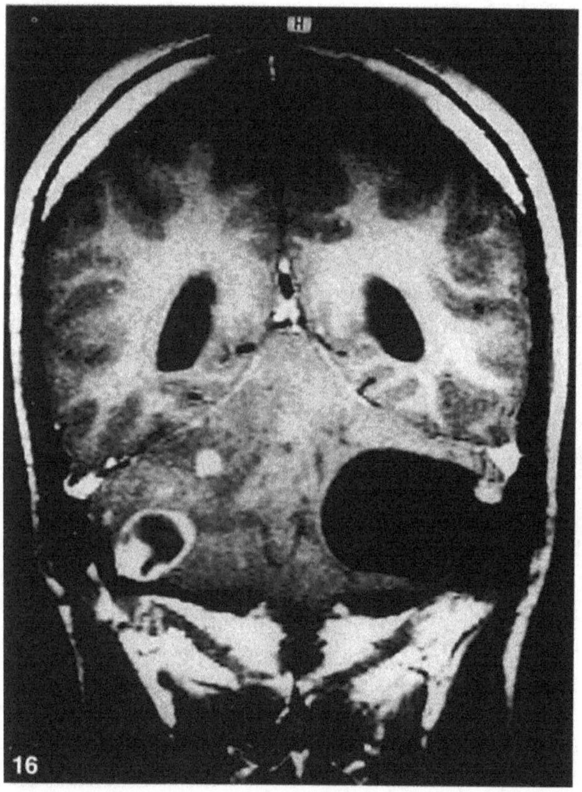

Fig. 3.16. Multiple cerebellar hemangioblastomas occurring in a case of von Hippel-Lindau disease. MRI: post-gadolinium coronal T1-weighted section. The three lesions shown on this section exhibit the three patterns of enhancement seen in hemangioblastomas, namely a cystic lesion with a small mural nodule with completely nodular or limited enhancement of the wall. No perilesional edema

Hemangioblastomas (fig. 3.16)

These are the commonest intra-axial posterior fossa primary tumors in the adult (see chapter 4).

Extra-axial tumors [1,12,13,33]

Tumors of the cerebello-pontine angle are the commonest.

Cerebello-pontine angle tumors: neurinomas, meningiomas, epidermoid tumors.

These extra-axial tumors generally pose no diagnostic problem (see chapter on neurodermatoses).

Other extra-axial posterior fossa tumors

- Meningiomas,
- Tumors of the jugular foramen:
  - Glomus jugulare tumors,
  - Neurinomas of various nerves,
- Clival and retroclival tumors: chordomas and meningiomas.

Pretreatment assessment and management

This assessment determines the choice of treatment: surgery, radiotherapy, chemotherapy or no treatment.

This approach to treatment can only be stopped when the nature of the tumor is known. A certain number of situations are sufficiently diagnostic to allow confirmation of the nature of the lesion based on the clinical and radiological findings.

Multiple lesions in the context of a known cancer are due to metastasis, no further investigation is required.

The tumor is extra-axial; if it is a meningioma then angiography should be performed prior to any treatment; if it is a neurinoma, no further investigation is required.

In the context of an intra-axial tumor, further investigation is necessary. Several illustrative cases are summarized:

- CT examination demonstrates a large glioblastoma of the grey matter and is therefore clearly inoperable. It is unnecessary to complement the CT by an MRI, and angiography is of no value. However, there is some argument as to value of biopsy prior to commencing chemotherapy or radiotherapy;

- CT demonstrates a solitary, well defined lesion which is probably accessible to surgery. In this instance, the performance of MRI is essential. MRI more accurately defines the tumor extent and topography. In certain cases, a diagnostic error may be rectified by MRI (cavernous hemangioma, detection of multiple lesions, meningeal carcinomatosis, etc.);
- in children, the MRI examination is invaluable for the pretreatment assessment at the following situation: posterior fossa tumor, tumor of the pineal region, craniopharyngioma, hypothalamic tumor, etc.

Again, angiographic examination is of no diagnostic value and no longer indicated even if surgical intervention is contemplated.

However, let us not forget that, although angiography has lost its role as a diagnostic examination, it still has a specific indication in some elderly patients in whom neither CT nor MRI have excluded the possibility of a glioblastoma and the localization of the lesion is a contraindication to surgery and renders the biopsy hazardous. In these cases, before proposing palliative radiotherapy treatment, angiography may help in reaching a decision by demonstrating arteriovenous shunts and/or a pathological hypervascularization indicating malignancy.

The value of CT and MRI must be emphasized in the pretreatment and assessment of cerebral tumors prior to radiotherapy. Accurate localization of the tumor from the CT or MRI findings is now possible thanks to computer programs which can perform 3D reconstructions of the tumor and precisely localize it relative to the bony structures. Very accurate dosimetry can be calculated, focusing onto a target and thus protecting the neighboring healthy structures. Treatment levels to the tumor bed up to 70 grays are possible.

Follow-up and post-treatment appearances of intra-axial tumors

[1, 8, 12, 28, 32]

The follow-up of cerebral tumors depends on the comparison of the clinical and radiological findings. This is vital for the image interpretation, particularly in patients following treatment. In effect:

- neurological deterioration is not synonymous with neoplastic progression;
- certain focal radiological changes, particularly iatrogenic, may simulate tumor growth;
- conversely, CT sometimes underestimates the volume or the spread of the tumor.

- In about 70% of cases, neurological deterioration corresponds to an increase in the tumor volume which is visible on CT. Even if the lesions are in clinically sensitive zones, the neurological deficit can precede the deterioration in the radiological signs by up to several weeks. Tumor progression is much more commonly focal than multifocal (5%). It may be complicated by a cyst under pressure which is amenable to puncture, or intra- or peritumoral hemorrhage responsible for the sudden onset of a neurological deficit.

However as already indicated, neurological deterioration is not synonymous with tumor progression. A focal or diffuse neurological deterioration occurring several weeks or months or even later after radiotherapy is most likely to be due to an early or late encephalopathy [15]. This is characterized by involvement of the white matter, better shown on MRI than CT as areas of high signal intensity on T2-weighted imaging, usually involving the area receiving the largest radiation dose. The clinical symptoms are usually reversible in one or two months. In the weeks or months following intra-arterial chemotherapy, a focal neurological deficit may be noted, corresponding to the territory supplied by the injected artery. CT demonstrates a hypodense zone, sometimes with an associated mass effect. MRI (fig. 3.17), which is more sensitive than CT, demonstrates areas of high signal intensity on T2-weighted imaging corresponding to areas of edema, demyelination and/or necrosis of the white matter.

Delayed intellectual impairment is observed in about 10% of cases of metastases or supratentorial gliomas treated by radiotherapy and possibly chemotherapy. MRI will usually show cortical atrophy which is rarely isolated but often associated with high signal intensity on T2-weighted imaging within the white matter, and ventricular dilatation. At the same time, the possibility of recurrent disease is excluded [16].

- Some focal radiological changes can simulate a progressive tumor. During the post-operative period, the mechanical effect of excising the tumor causes a reversible breakdown of the blood brain barrier (BBB) with the appearance of enhancement of the limits of the surgical cavity. This enhancement appears between the fifth and maximum fifteenth day, and spontaneously regresses within several months [6]. Failure to appreciate this phenomenon can lead to an underestimation of the true extent of the surgical cavity or early recurrence. In order to avoid this error, Cairncross et al [6] advise the performance of a post-operative baseline CT within 48 hours of the surgical intervention. Similarly, the effect of radiation on the BBB [15] can induce or increase enhancement in a region of the

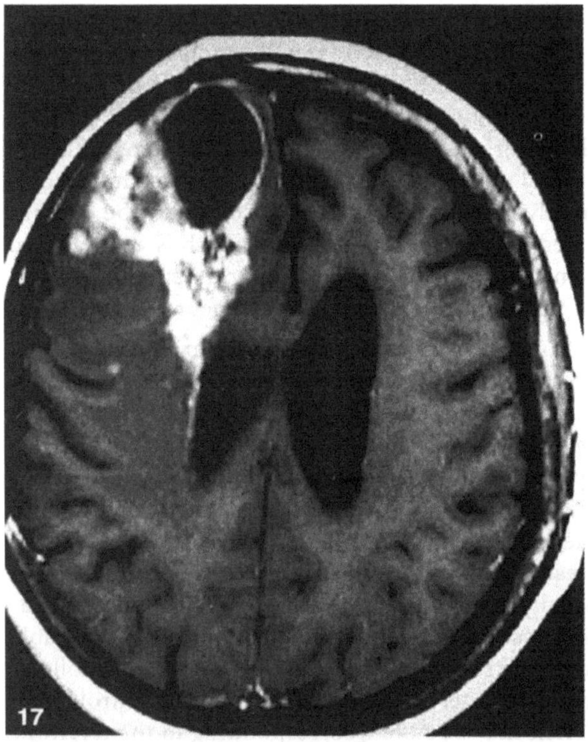

Fig. 3.17. Biopsy proven radionecrosis. This patient had undergone operation and radiotherapy for a grade II astrocytic glioma of the right frontal lobe. It is extremely difficult to distinguish between radionecrosis and recurrent tumor on this post-gadolinium T1-weighted section

tumor bed which simulates recurrence or neoplastic progression. However, in these both situations, the CT appearances do not show any evidence of mass effect and remain clinically silent.

When radiotherapy is given in conventional fractionated doses, the risk of radionecrosis is less than 5% , although this is increased by certain risk factors of cardiovascular disease, such as hypertension or diabetes. The great majority of radionecrosis occur in areas which have received the highest radiation dose, i.e. the tumor bed, and become apparent in the first two years following radiotherapy [17]. Neither the location nor the intrinsic appearances of the radionecrosis on CT or MRI allow differentiation from recurrent tumor. The diagnosis depends on biopsy or better still on the neuropathological examination of the operative specimen.

The pathological significance of residual lesions sometimes seen anteriorly in the region of the tumor bed after radiotherapy and chemotherapy remains a difficult problem to resolve. These lesions usually appear in the form of calcification surrounded by an area of discrete enhancement or enhancement in a heterogeneous fashion without mass effect. They can remain unchanged for years without any clinical symptoms. The rare cases with pathological correlation suggest that they correspond to glial scar tissue which contains of a certain amount of vascularization.

- CT may underestimate the volume or spread of a tumor. Steroids may decrease the degree of enhancement or the diameter of the lesion by a simple effect on the BBB without any anticancer effect. In malignant gliomas, Cairncross et all [7] have reported reductions in the diameter of contrast enhancement by between 30 to 50%. This effect reaches its maximum between the 10th and 15th days. In order to avoid attributing these changes to the action of the antitumor treatment, it is advisable to perform a pretherapeutic baseline CT scan 15 days after the commencement of corticosteroids.

In cases of large hemispheric tumors, CT appearances do not always explain the deterioration in the neurological deficit. In fact, there is a risk that CT will underestimate neoplastic infiltration of the diencephalon or corpus callosum, especially if the lesion is not enhanced. MRI, since it is much more reliable in the detection of the morphological changes in large structures or in the midline, is therefore indicated.

Disseminated neoplastic involvement of the meninges is associated with cerebral metastasis and complicates the evolution of a glioma in about 5 to 10% of cases [14, 18]. This may result in deterioration in the neurological state without any morphological change in the tumor, or even occur after tumor regression in a patient apparently in remission. In cases of glioma, the commonest indirect radiological sign of leptomeningeal involvement is ventricular dilatation which occurs in approximately 50% of patients. Gadolinium enhanced MRI of the brain and spine demonstrates leptomeningeal spread of the tumor over the convexity, at the skull base or in the perimedullary spaces as areas of linear or multinodular enhancement.

- The neuroradiological findings are also essential in order to evaluate the response to treatment. The radiological examinations performed at regular intervals must fulfill certain conditions mentionned above, and the necessity of using the same injection protocol and scan plane for each examination.

Conclusion

Medical imaging and notably CT are indispensable in the diagnosis and treatment planning of intracranial

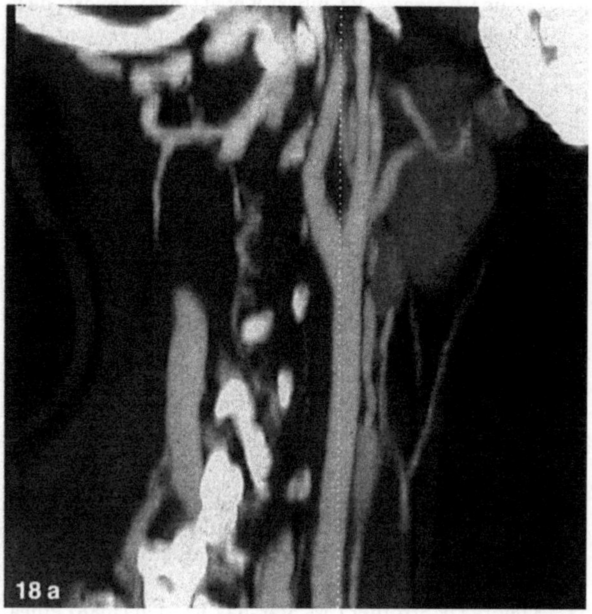

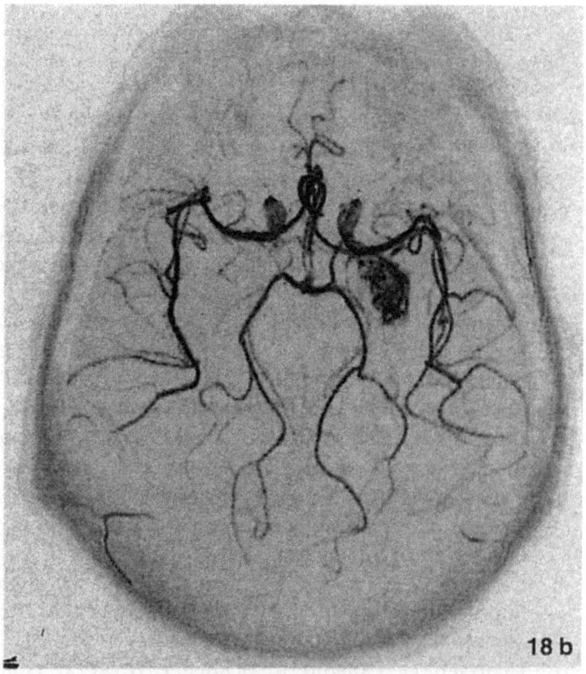

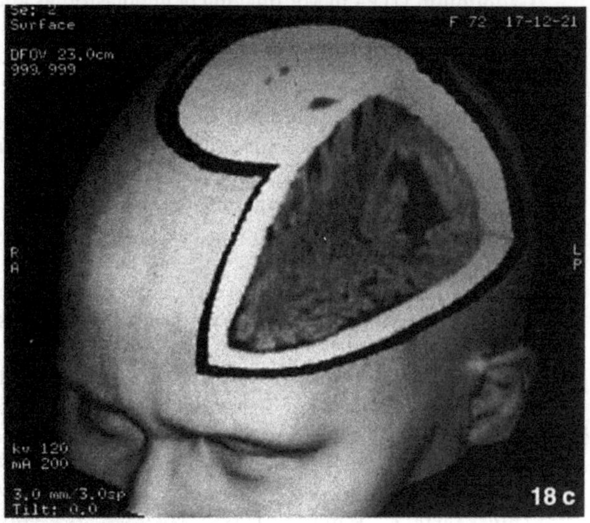

Fig. 3.18 a-c. New imaging techniques in CT and MRI. **a** 3D volumetric helical CT of the normal carotid vessels shown in a sagittal reconstruction. **b** MR angiogram (reverse contrast) without any injection demonstrating a hypervascular left temporal metastasis (image courtesy of D. Buthiau, Centre RMX). **c** 3D volumetric reconstruction of the CT in cerebral lymphoma (pre-radiotherapy): the value of a direct link with the radiotherapy console is still under study (image courtesy of General Electric)

tumors. There are multiple indications for CT which should be performed in the presence of any suspicious neurological signs. A normal CT scan is highly cost efficient and remains the cheapest option for society. Due to limited access and availability, the indications for MRI are still limited. In the future, in view of its diagnostic value, MRI may well replace CT for diagnosis and treatment follow-up of intracranial tumors. The new imaging techniques (fig. 3.18) will bring new attributes in the evaluation of cerebral tumors.

References

1. Atlas SW (1991) Magnetic Resonance Imaging of the brain and spine. Raven Press, New York
2. Brant-Zawadski M, Normand D (1987) MRI of the central nervous system. Raven Press, New York
3. Byder G, Kingsley P, Brown J, Niendorf H, Young IR (1985) MR imaging of meningiomas including studies with and without Gadolinium DTPA. J Comput Assist Tomogr 9: 690-697

4. Caillé JM, Guibert F (1981) Les gliomes astrocytaires malins hémisphériques de l'adulte: limites du scanner. Neurochir 27: 261-267
5. Caillé JM, Lemanceau B, Bonnemain B (1983) Gadolinium as a contrast agent of NMR. AJNR 4: 1041-1042
6. Cairncross JG, Pexman JMW, Radthbone MP, Del Maestro RF (1985) Post-operative contrast enhancement in patients with brain tumors. Ann Neurol 17: 570-572
7. Cairncross JG, Mc Donald DR, Pexman WJH, Ives JF (1988) Steroid-induced CT changes in patients with recurrent malignant glioma. Neurology 38: 724-726
8. Castel JG, Kien P, Caillé JM (1989) Imagerie des tumeurs cérébrales irradiées. Intérêt de l'imagerie par résonance magnétique. J Neuroradiol 16: 81-132
9. Cellerier P, Chiras J, Gray F, Metzger J, Bories J (1984) Computed tomography in primary Iymphoma of the brain. Neuroradiology 26: 485-492
10. Centeno RS, Lee AA, Winter J, Barba D (1986) Supratentorial ependymomas: neuroimaging and clinicopathological correlation. J Neurosurg 64: 209-215
11. Claussen C, Lanadio K, Schorner W, et al (1985) Gadolinium DTPA in MR imaging of glioblastomas and intracranial metastases. AJNR 6: 669-674
12. Cohadon F (1989) Tumeurs du système nerveux et de ses enveloppes. Flammarion Médecine-Sciences, Paris
13. Curati WL, Graif M, Kingsley DPE, Niendorf HP, Young IR (1986) Acoustic neurinomas: Gd-DTPA enhancement in MR imaging. Radiology 158: 447-451
14. Davila G, Duyckacrts C, Lazareth JP, Poisson M, Delattre JY (1993) Diffuse primary loptomeningeal gliomatosis. J Neurooncol 15: 45-49
15. Delattre JY, Poisson M (19907 Etude expérimentale des effets de la radiothérapie cérébrale. Bull Cancer 77: 715-724
16. Delattre JY, Poisson M (1991) Syndromes démentiels post-radiques et post-radio-chimiothérapie. In: Maladie d'Alzheimer et autres démences. Flammarion Médecine-Sciences, Paris, pp 357-363
17. Delattre JY, Poisson M, Pertuiset BF, Touati M, Duyckaerts C, Hauw JJ (1986) Nécrose des voies optiques, de l'hypothalamus et du tronc cérébral après irradition d'un adénome hypophysaire. Rev Neurol (Paris) 142: 232-237
18. Delattre JY, Walker RW, Rosenblum MK (1989) Leptomeningeal gliomatosis with spinal cord or cauda equina compression: a complication of supratentorial gliomas in adults. Acta Neurol Scand 79: 133-13919. Dubbelaere P, Clarisse J (1982) Tumeurs cranio- encéphaliques. Scanographie. Encycl Med Chir Paris, 31 660 F20, 5
20. Eresué J, Casenave P, Guibert F, et al (1983) Apports de la radiologie dans les tumeurs du IIIème ventricule. J Neuroradiol 10: 345-354
21. Ferrey G, Jedynak CP (1981) Troubles psychiques au cours des tumeurs cérébrales. Encycl Med Chir Paris Psychiatrie 37510 A10, 10
22. Gardeur D, Metzger J (1978) Tomodensitométrie en pathologie tumorale intracrâniehne. Doin, Paris
23. Gentry LR, Jacoby CG, Turski PA, et al (1987) Cerebellopontine angle-petromastoid mass lesions: comparative study of diagnosis with MR imaging and CT. Radiology 162: 513-520
24. Graif M, Bydder GM, Steiner RE, et al (1986) Contrast-enhanced MR imaging of malignant brain tumors. AJNR 6: 855-862
25. Holland BA, Brandt-Zawadski M, Normand D (1985) Magnetic resonance imaging of primary intracranial tumors: a review. Int J Radiat Oncol Biol Phys 121: 315-321
26. Karnaze MG, Sartor K, Winthrop JD, Godo MH, Hodges JF (1986) Suprasellar lesions: evaluation with MRI. Radiology 161: 77-82
27. Kilgore DP, Strother CM, Starshak RJ, et al (1986) Pineal germinoma: MR imaging. Radiology 158: 435-438
28. Kingsley DPR, Kendall BE (1981) CT of the adverse effects of therapeutic radiation of the central nervous system. AJNR 2: 453-460
29. Lee BCP, Kneeland JB, Alter RW, et al (1985) MR imaging of brain stem tumors. AJNR 6: 159-163
30. McMurdo SK, Moore 5G, Brant-Zawadsi M, et al (1987) MR imaging of intra-cranial tuberous sclerosis. AJNR 8: 72-82
31. Morrison G, Sobel DF, Kelley WM, et al (1984) Intraventricular mass lesions. Radiology 153: 435-442
32. Ouchi T, Steiner RE, Mc Kenzie CG (1984) MR imaging of central nervous system diseases before and after therapy. Radiat Med 2: 37-43
33. Packer RJ, Zimmerman RA, Bilaniuk LT, et al (1985) Magnetic resonance imaging of lesions of the posterior fossa and upper cervical cord in childhood. Pediatrics 76: 84-90
34. Spagnoli MV, Goldgerg HI, Grossman RI, et al (1986) Intracranial meningiomas: high field MR imaging. Radiology 16: 369-376
35. Vorkapic P, Pendl G (1985) Neuroimaging of mass lesions of the pineal region in infancy and childhood. Acta Neurochir 35 suppl: 65-69
36. Zimmerman RA (1987) Infratentorial neoplasms. Diagnostic Radiology, Neuroradiology, November 29 - December4, 1987
37. Zimmerman RA, Fleming CA, Saint-Louis LA, Lee BCP, Manning JJ, Deck MDF (1985) MRI of meningiomas. AJNR 6: 149-157

CHAPTER 4

Tumors associated with the neurodermatoses

Clinicians
R. Grob, F. Bolgert, J.-V. Chantelard, L. Zelek, J. de Recondo

Radiologist
D. Buthiau

The neurodermatoses or neuroectodermal dysplasias are usually genetically determined familial conditions inherited in an autosomal dominant fashion.

The tumors associated with the neurodermatoses are characterized by their polymorphism and are often the most important feature of the disease requiring complete assessment and follow-up of the patient. This predisposition to tumor development is one of the characteristics of these conditions. The tumors may be congenital, commonly associated with other malformations, and represent one of the essential elements for the diagnosis. In fact, this association as well as the small proliferative tendency differentiates these congenital tumors from the usually encountered neoplasms. The organs most commonly effected are the skin, central and peripheral nervous systems, the viscera and bone. MRI and CT have a fundamental role in the diagnosis and assessment of CNS involvement, and act as an aid in the diagnosis of the initial lesions or «formes frustes» thus guiding the clinical examination and genetic diagnosis.

Neurofibromatosis (table 4.1)

In the type 1 form (NF1) called von Recklinghausen's disease, the gene is situated on chromosome 17 and causes a peripheral neurofibromatosis. Often familial, it is characterized by the appearance of mainly cutaneous tumor malformations ("café au lait" patches), neurofibromas, gliomas and hamartomas.

Table 4.1. Distinction between NF1 and NF2

Distinctive features	NF1	NF2
Localization on gene	chromosome 17	chromosome 22
Frequency	1 per 2,500-4,000	1 per 50,000
Cutaneous marks	multiple and common	rare
Lesions affecting the CNS	- gliomas of the optic pathways - astrocytomas - hamartomas	- neurinomas of VIII or other paired cranial nerves - meningiomas

Type 2 neurofibromatosis (NF2) is transmitted on the chromosome 22 and corresponds to the classical «central form» [6, 15, 16]. It is at least 10 times rarer than NF1 and is characterized by bilateral acoustic neurinomas, which may or may not be associated with other spinal or intracranial schwannomas, hamartomas or meningiomas (table 4.1).

Neurofibromas

These multiple tumors affecting the peripheral nervous system characterize NF1. They may arise from any of the constitutive elements of the nerve, but hyperplasia of the nerve sheath (Schwann cells and fibroblasts) is characteristic. The tumors may cause problems in the CNS either intracranially or within the spine by compressing the cranial nerve roots or spinal nerves.

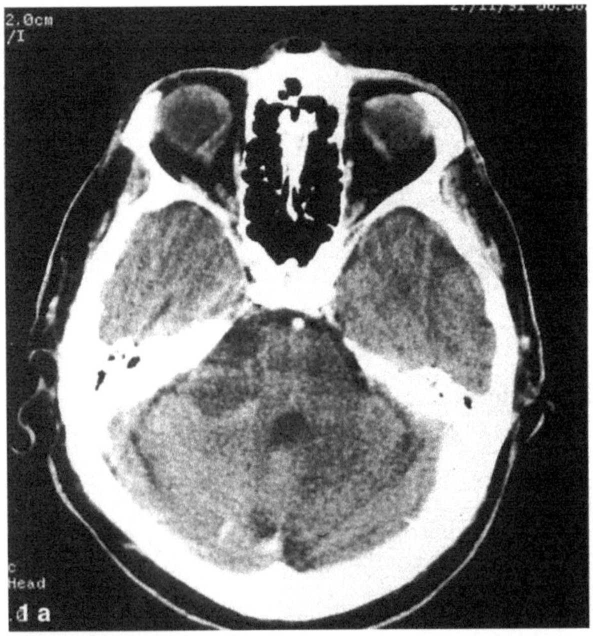

Fig. 4.1 a-c. Acoustic neurinoma on CT and MRI. **a** Post-contrast CT: this demonstrates a hypodensity in the right cerebello-pontine angle causing extrinsic compression of the fourth ventricle. The lesion is hypodense (presumably cystic) with relatively regular contours and exhibits both thin peripheral and internal enhancement due to a fine septum; **b** axial T1-weighted MRI: the lesion is well defined and hypointense; **c** post-gadolinium T1-weighted coronal MRI in same patient demonstrating thin peripheral enhancement *(arrows)* and a band of enhancement within the lesion. The appearances are those of a predominantly cystic and essentially extracanalicular neurinoma with minimal intracanalicular extension

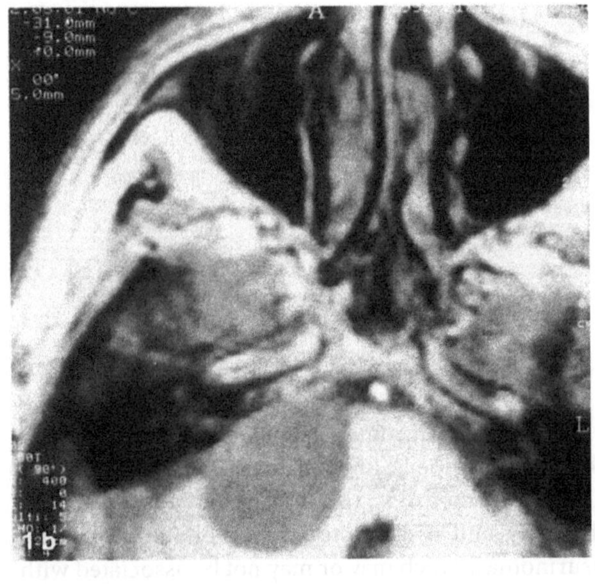

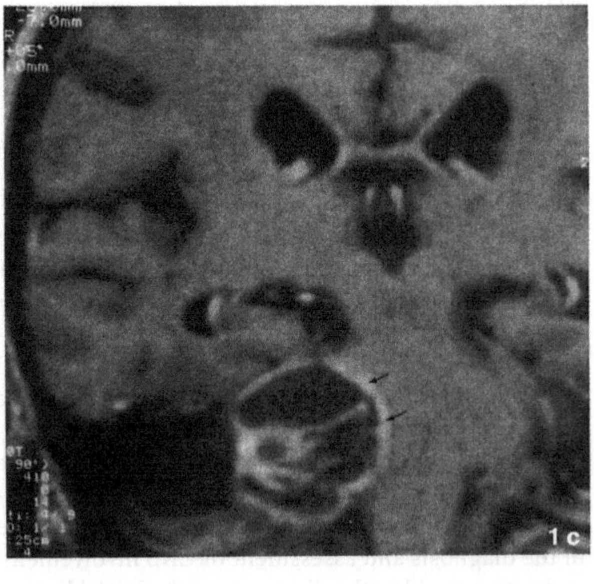

Neurinomas

(fig. 4.1) (see chapter 7)

Schwannomas or neurinomas are due to proliferation of the Schwann cells. They most commonly involve the nerve VIII, but the nerves III to XII, notably V, IX, X, XI and oculomotor nerves are equally affected.

Dermatological, ophthalmological and audiometric examinations precede the radiological investigation. MRI has a particularly important role in the demonstration of the intracranial and spinal neurinomas.

In cases of spinal involvement, the multiplanar capability of contrast enhanced MRI is able to diagnose the neurofibromas and accurately demonstrate the extent of the multilevel involvement. It is currently the most accurate imaging modality for this pathology.

Glial tumors

These may be astrocytomas, polymorphic glioblastomas or ependymomas, and may be localized or diffuse and occur anywhere in the CNS. They are characterized by their multiplicity and association with other CNS tumors. There is a predilection for certain sites.

Hemispheric gliomas

The central grey matter and cerebellar hemispheres are common sites for astrocytomas and glioblastomas.

CT appearances are identical to those seen in any glioma, and there are no specific features.

MRI gives a much better evaluation of these lesions [4] with improved differentiation of edema from the tumor itself, better assessment of the composition (cystic, haemorrhagic) and tumor extent. In general, the lesions appear hypo- or isointense on T1-weighted imaging and hyperintense on T2-weighted imaging. Enhancement following gadolinium is more marked in the poorly differentiated high grade lesions and indicates breakdown of the blood brain barrier.

Gliomas of the optic pathways

(see fig. 5.8, chapter 5)

Particularly common in children, these are either pre-chiasmatic (predominantly orbital), or chiasmatic, developing either posteriorly near the third ventricle or anteriorly towards the orbit (see chapter 5).

Meningo-encephalic gliosis

This central and meningeal gliomatosis is rare and is suggested on CT by bilateral hypodense areas associated with cerebral edema. Meningeal involvement is difficult to detect.

Gliomas of the spinal cord

Ependymomas are the commonest (fig. 4.2), astrocytomas rarer. Ependymomas are often multiple, more than 50% occurring at the level of the conus and are frequently associated with multiple meningiomas and bilateral acoustic neuromas in cases of NF2.

CT is non-contributory in making the diagnosis. On the other hand, MRI is the investigation of choice because it can make the diagnosis and assess the extent of the lesion preoperatively. These tumors always manifest as enlargement of the spinal cord appearing hypointense on T1-weighted imaging, enhancement with gadolinium (o. 4.2), and hyperin-

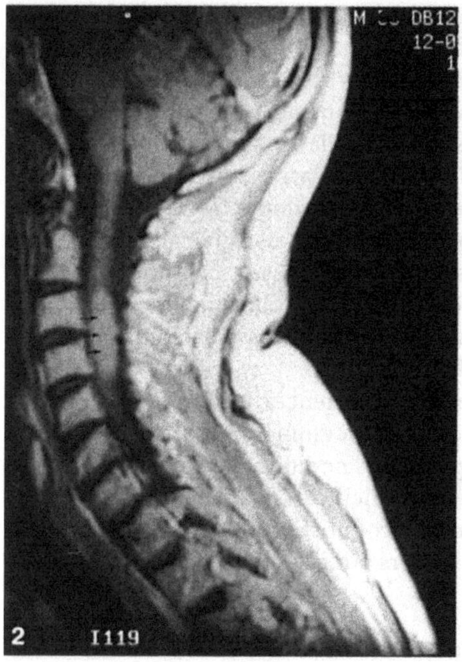

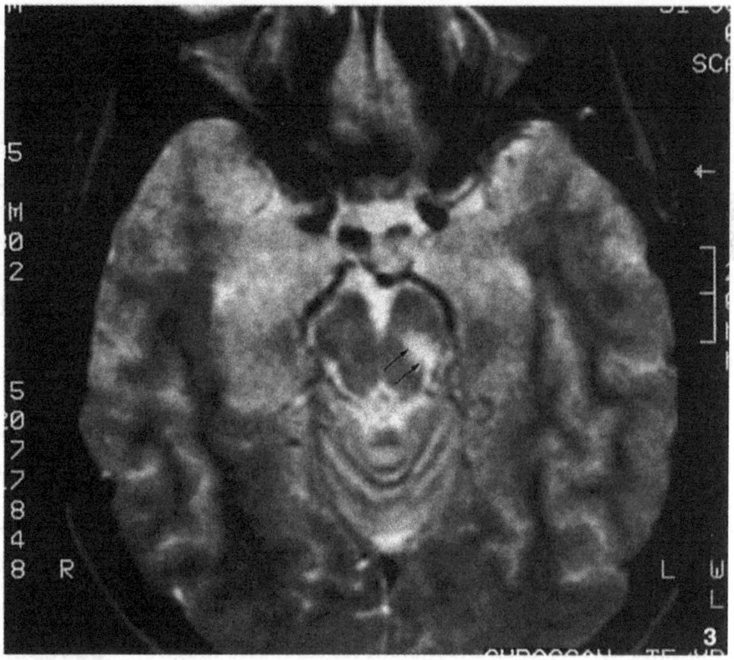

Fig. 4.2. Ependymoma of the cervical cord on post-gadolinium sagittal T1-weighted MRI: expansion of the cord by enhancing tissue without any cystic change at the pole of the lesion

Fig. 4.3. Hamartoma of the brain stem on axial T2-weighted MRI: significant non-specific areas of hyperintensity in the left cerebellar peduncle *(arrows)*

tense on T2-weighted imaging; paradoxical areas of low signal intensity are sometimes seen on T2 WI due to a chronic hemosiderin deposition. The tumor is associated with cystic change at the two poles of the lesion appearing isointense to CSF. These tumoral cysts may be hemorrhagic which would appear hyperintense on T1- and T2-weighted imaging. There is often a chronic hematomyelia adjacent to the upper and lower limits of the tumor appearing as a narrow hypointense band on T1- and T2-weighted imaging.

Hamartomas

These mass lesions are malformations which have a «blastomatous potential». They may be detected incidentally, the zones of gliosis being difficult to demonstrate on CT. MRI may show hyperintense areas on T2-weighted imaging within the central grey matter nuclei, brain stem (fig. 4.3), cerebellar peduncles and sometimes the white matter [1, 3, 4].

Meningiomas

These lesions are benign, and meningiomatosis is rare but may occur. There is often marked calcification.

Other lesions

Unusual cerebral neurinomas are described in the literature (P. Chaine) [6]. Subependymal gliofibrillar nodules have been reported, infiltrating the ventricular walls and occasionally causing aqueduct stenosis. These lesions are sometimes associated with a diffuse glial proliferation. They are difficult to differentiate from pilocytic astrocytomas.

Tuberous sclerosis of Bourneville

The abnormal gene for this entity is localized on the chromosome 9. The condition is characterized by three fundamental clinical signs - epilepsy, mental retardation and facial adenoma sebaceum. It is very uncommon, occurring in approximately 1:100,000. Familial history is an inconstant feature. The diagnosis is essentially clinical, sometimes aided by imaging in children.

Intracerebral tumors are very suggestive when associated with specific lesions, notably subependymal nodules (fig. 4.4) and cortical tubers.

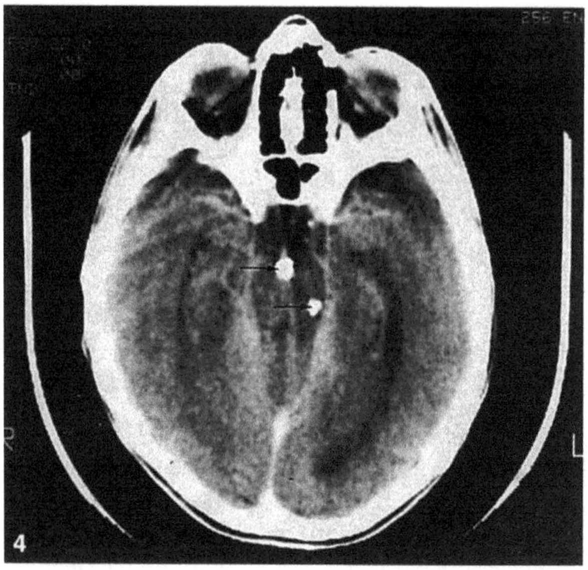

Fig. 4.4. Tuber nodules *(arrows)* in a case of tuberous sclerosis of Bourneville on post-contrast CT

Intracerebral tumors

Astrocytomas are the commonest and almost certainly correspond to a malignant transformation of the subependymal nodules (fig. 4.5). They can be differentiated from them by their size and associated signs of intracranial hypertension due mainly to the preferential localization close to the foramina of Monro causing secondary hydrocephalus. These tumors tend to have a relatively benign progression but may be large and extend into the ventricles.

On CT, these lesions are usually calcified, always with an associated soft tissue component which strongly become enhanced following the injection of contrast agent. There may be associated intraventricular hemorrhage.

On T2-weighted sequences, MRI can differentiate the hyperintense astrocytoma from the hypo- or isointense subependymal nodules, allowing early diagnosis. Small areas of calcification are better seen on CT. MRI may have a prognostic value in demonstrating not only the tumors but also the areas of heterotopia.

Subependymal nodules

The demonstration of subependymal nodules, frequently multiple and bilateral, located along the ventricular wall or aqueduct of Sylvius, as well as cortical tubers will assist in the diagnosis. CT is more sensitive

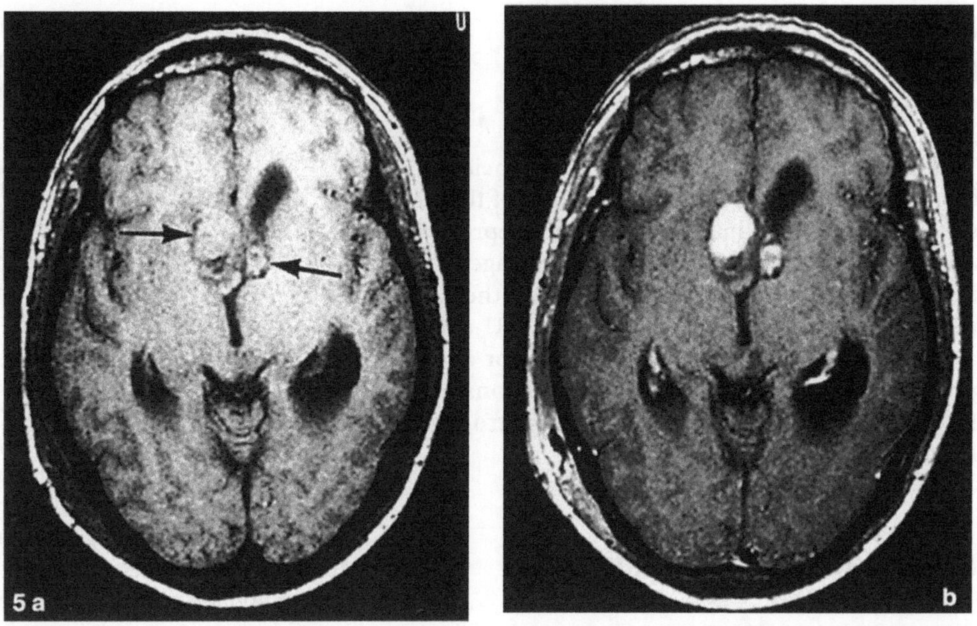

Fig. 4.5 a-b. Tuberous sclerosis of Bourneville on MRI: subependymal astrocytomas showing as nodular lesions close to the lateral ventricles with nodular intraventricular projections (**a**, *arrows);* these lesions are responsible for causing obstruction of the left foramen of Monro. On the T1-weighted sequence (**a**) the lesions are isointense and enhanced following gadolinium injection (**b**) (images courtesy of Prof. D Balériaux, Brussels)

in the detection of calcified nodules and MRI for the demonstration of cortical tubers.

Both examinations will demonstrate the associated visceral tumors, particularly renal and more rarely cardiac or pulmonary tumor.

Pigmented neurodermatoses

Neurocutaneous melanosis

This childhood condition is an association of cutaneous and leptomeningeal infiltration with or without meningeal hemorrhage. This infiltration essentially occurs at the skull base, cranial nerves and 4th ventricle, and is often associated with hydrocephalus (fig. 4.6). The experience to date with CT and MRI in this condition is limited. Melanoblastic tumors resulting from a neoplastic transformation of the meningeal infiltration, may result in a diffuse infiltration or focal lesion similar to a melanoma. Primary or secondary melanomas may be differentiated by the presence of meningeal infiltration and the benign character of the cutaneous lesion (malignant cutaneous transformation is nonetheless possible in 10% of cases).

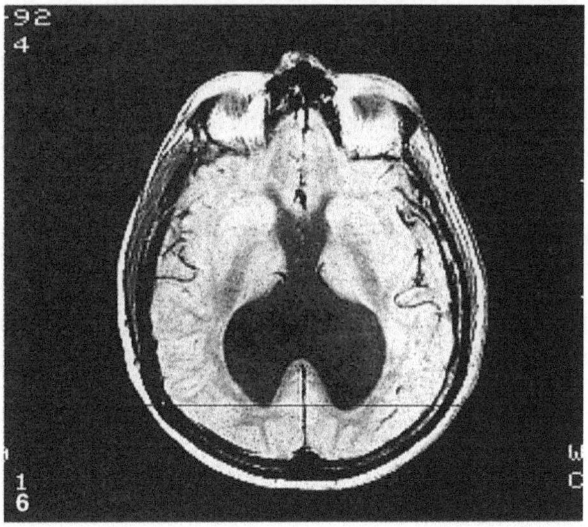

Fig. 4.6. Proton density weighted axial MRI. Hydrocephalus due to infiltration of the base of the fourth ventricle in a case of neurocutaneous melanosis

Among the other pigmented neurodermatoses, encephalo-trigeminal melanosis (Ota's syndrome) and the possibility of intracranial melanomas should be mentioned.

Basal cell nevomatoses (Gorlin's syndrome)

This syndrome is characterized by the association of basal cell epithelioma with abnormalities of the CNS, skull and face. The malformations are represented above all by congenital hydrocephalus and agenesis of the corpus callosum. Medulloblastoma is the dominant tumor in this condition. CT and MRI appearances are dependent on the type of tumor and the presence elsewhere of lamellar calcifications of the falx, dura mater, tentorium cerebelli and petro-clinoid ligaments.

Angiomatous neurodermatoses

Characterized by the presence of capillary hemangiomas, these neurodermatoses are not true tumors of the CNS. Nonetheless, an associated tumor is seen in the Louis-Bar syndrome (non-neurological lymphoreticular neoplasia, atypical cerebellar medulloblastoma and gliomas), the «Bean Blue Rubber Bled Nevi Syndrome» (cerebellar medulloblastoma), and the Maffuci and Kast syndrome (chondro-fibro-angiosarcoma which may affect any organ). It should be remembered that the Sturge-Weber angiomatous syndrome is not associated with any tumor.

von Hippel-Lindau syndrome (VHL)

This condition, often hereditary, is characterized by hemangioblastomas of the cerebellum, retina, other intracranial sites and spinal cord, and by visceral (renal and pancreatic lesions). The gene responsible is situated on chromosome 3.

Intracranial hemangioblastomas

(see fig. 3.16, chapter 3)

Although cerebellar involvement is the most frequent, the retinal lesions often present earlier and may be bilateral and multiple.

In the presence of a solitary lesion (usually cerebellar), it is imperative to perform a systematic and, if necessary, repeated search for lesions at other sites by non-invasive complimentary investigations. Cerebral and whole body CT and MRI of the spinal cord are the examinations of choice. In hemangioblastomas of the posterior fossa, CT clearly demonstrates the low density of the cystic component and contrast enhancement of the tumor component. Nonetheless, CT may miss small lesions or punctiform mural lesions which are well shown by angiography [17, 19].

A normal CT does not rule out the diagnosis but is always contributive as soon as clinical symptoms are present.

MRI demonstrates more clearly both the cystic and soft tissue components, and the vascular nidus appearing as low or intermediate signal on T1-weighted imaging and high signal on T2-weighted imaging, with enhancement following gadolinium. The cyst contents may be slightly hyperintense on T1- and T2-weighted imaging. The demonstration of dilated vessels close to the tumor differentiates hemangioblastoma from other neoplastic cysts. These vessels appear as serpiginous hypointensities on T1- and T2-weighted imaging and hyperintense on the fast imaging techniques.

Supratentorial hemangioblastomas are rare, and few are cystic. Involvement of the intraorbital portion of the optic nerve is itself very rare and not documented.

Hemangioblastomas of the spinal cord

(see fig. 7.9, chapter 7)

Usually intradural, intra- or extramedullary, or much more rarely extradural, these tumors as a rule develop on the posterior aspect of the cervico-thoracic cord. The presence of a frequently associated syringomyelia may complicate the interpretation of the cystic lesions (cf chapter 7).

The value of CT must be remembered in the detection of visceral lesions, renal or pancreatic tumors (clear cell renal carcinomas, metastasis in more the 50% of cases). These tumors may occur exceptionally at other sites such as adrenals, liver, spleen, lungs or gastrointestinal tract.

Conclusion

CT and MRI have a particularly important role in pathological tumors occurring in the neurodermatoses:

- in the neurofibromatoses, these two modalities are most reliable for the evaluation and follow-up of patients with this disease. Calcification is better

shown on CT, but MRI is superior for tumor assessment;
- in tuberous sclerosis of Bourneville, CT is very sensitive for the detection of calcified nodules, and MRI for the demonstration of cortical tubers. Both examinations are useful for the detection of intracerebral tumors although MRI is superior to CT in differentiating tumors from simple subependymal nodules;
- in cases of von Hippel-Lindau disease, a complete and early radiological study is justified by the severity of the CNS involvement and improvements in the surgical results. These investigations, particularly MRI following gadolinium injection, can guide the surgical management of all the lesions, mainly by differentiating the cysts from the tumor nodule, and avoiding recurrences. Preoperative angiography is still indispensable.

References

1. Aoki S, Barkovich J, Nishimura K, et al (1989) Neurofibromatosis type I and 2. Cranial MR findings. Radiology 172: 527-534
2. Bertrand JL, Salaniand P, Arnault G, et al (1988) Imagerie médicale et principales phacomatoses. Feuillets de Radiologie 3: 239-246
3. Bognanno JR, Edwards MK, Lee TA, et al (1990) Cranial MR Imaging in Neurofibromatosis. AJNR 9: 461-468
4. Braffman BH, Bilaniuk LT, Zimmerman RA (1988) The central nervous system manifestations of the phakomatoses on MR. Radiol Clin North Am 4: 773-800
5. Brant-Zawadzki M, Norman D (1987) Common congenital malformations of the brain. Magnetic resonance imaging of the central nervous system. Raven Press, New York, pp 131-150
6. Chaine P, Brachet P, Haguenau M, Ziller C (1989) Tumeurs du système nerveux des phacomatoses. Encycl Med Chir (Paris), Neurologie, 17260 D10: 7-23
7. Enomoto H, Shibata T, Ito A, et al (1984) Multiple hemangioblastomas accompanied by syringomyclia in the cerebellum and the spinal cord. Surg Neurol 22: 197-203
8. Fryer AE, Connor JM, Povey S, et al (1987) Evidence that the gene for tuberous sclerosis is on chromosome 9. Lancet 2: 659-661
9. Gardeur D (1983) Pathologies malformatives et néonatales. Livre VI. Tomodensitométrie intracrânienne. Ellipse, Paris
10. Grégoire N, Momose T, Rumeau C, et al (1990) Apport du gadolinium-DTPA à l'étude des tumeurs intracrâniennes de l'adulte. Rev Neurol (Paris) 46: 133-143
11. Halimi Ph, Marcus C. Doyon D, et al (1987) L'imagerie par résonance magnétique de la moelle. Radiologie J Cepur7: 271-280.
12. Idir ABC, De Recondo J, Husson B, Doyon D (1990) Les phacomatoses. In: D Buthiau (ed) TDM et IRM Cliniques. Frison-Roche, Paris, pp 257-266
13. Kingsley DPE, Kendall BE, Fitz CR (1986) Tuberous sclerosis: a clinico-radiological evaluation of 110 cases with particular reference to atypical presentation. Neuroradiology 28: 38-46
14. Mayfrank L, Mohadjer, M. Wullich B (1990) Intracranial calcified deposits in neurofibronsatosis type 2: a CT study of 11 cases. Neuroradiology 32: 33-37
15. National Institutes of Health Consensus Development (1988) Neurofibromatosis. Arch Neurol 45: 575-578
16. de Recondo J (1989) Phacomatoses. In: F Cohadon (ed) Tumeurs du système nerveux et de ses enveloppes. Flammarion Médecine-Sciences, Paris
17. Sarwar M (1985) Neurocutaneous syndromes (phakomatoses) Computed Tomography of congenital brain malformations. Nijhoff Publishing, pp 127-143
18. Sato Y, Waziri M. Smith W, et al (1988) Hippel-Lindau disease: MR Imaging. Radio]ogy 166: 1-6
19. Seeper JF, Burke DP, Knake JE, et al (1981) Computed tomography and angiographic eva]uation of hemangioblastomas. Radiology 138: 65-73
20. Seizinger BR, Rouleau GA, Ozelius LJ, et al (1988) von Hippel-Lindau disease maps to the region of chromosome 3 associated with renal celı carcinoma. Nature 332: 268-269
21. Waga S, Yamamoto Y, Kojima P, et al (1977) Massive hemorrhage in tumor of tuberous sclerosis. Surg Neurol 8: 99-101
22. Welch K, Naheedy MH, Abroms IF, et al (1980) CT of Sturge-Weber syndrome in infants. J Comput Assist Tomogr 4: 33-36

CHAPTER 5

Tumors of the optic nerve, eye and orbit

Clinician
Ch. Billote

Radiologists
P. Courtheoux, L. Boiteau

Due to its anatomical and histological composition, the orbit is an area where many tissues of different nature and origin are juxtaposed (bone, ocular globe, muscles, nerves, meninges, fat, vessels, lacrymal gland...). This diversity of tissue types is the reason for the multiplicity of disease processes encountered.

Tumors of the orbit are fairly uncommon although the exact incidence is difficult to define. In fact, the incidence varies in the published series depending on the origin of each team. Malignant tumors are consistently less common than benign processes.

The radiological investigation of orbital tumors depends primarily on CT and MRI. CT remains essential due to its ability to perform thin sections allowing simultaneous visualization of the orbital bones, orbital contents, adjacent sinuses and intracranial cavity in order to define accurately the site and extent of the tumor.

MRI can provide supplementary information but is sensitive to movement and especially chemical shift artefacts which are related to the numerous tissue interfaces encountered in this region.

Clinical signs

Exophthalmos is the most constant sign and its direction is dependent on the exact intraorbital location of the tumor, namely in an axial direction if the tumor is retro-ocular, and lateral or vertical for tumors elsewhere. The exophthalmos may be associated with keratitis due to corneal exposure.

Oculomotor problems are also very common either due to mass effect or by compression of one of the oculomotor nerves.

Signs of inflammation such as palpebral edema or a chemosis may be present from the outset or occur during the course of the disease.

A reduction in visual acuity occurs much earlier if the tumor involves the optic nerve. There is often an associated visual field loss.

Fundoscopy may reveal puckering of the choroid due to mass effect, involvement of the optic nerve, edema, atrophy, and congestion of the retinal veins.

Pain is an inconstant feature.

Techniques of investigation

CT

The reference plane utilized is the neuro-ocular plane (PNO) which is parallel to the line between the outer canthus and tragus. This is the only plane which biometrically aligns the lens, the optic nerve head and the optic canal. The slice thickness can vary between 1 and 5 mm, and sections should be contiguous to allow 3-dimensional reconstructions. The examination is performed both before and after the administration of iodinated contrast. Complimentary sections may be necessary to demonstrate the adjacent structures such as the sinuses and skull base.

Examinations in the axial and even the coronal planes can also be added to this standard technique in the investigation of a deficit.

MRI

The initial MRI examination should be performed using the standard head coil and secondarily with a specific orbital surface coil in order to define more accurately the relationship of the tumor to the adjacent structures. Prior to the examination, it is beneficial to exclude all contraindications to MRI and request the patient to avoid using any make-up which may contain paramagnetic materials.

The initial acquisition is also performed in the axial neuro-ocular plane. This can be complemented by orthogonal coronal or sagittal sections. Spin echo sequences are the most commonly utilized because the gradient echo sequences are particularly sensitive to movement artefacts.

Usually pre- and post-gadolinium T1-weighted sequences are performed, supplemented by a delayed late echo T2-weighted sequence to demonstrate retinal detachment.

In pediatric practice, sedation or general anesthesia may be necessary.

Classification of orbital tumors

Orbital tumors can arise from a variety of structures. The commonest is an extraocular intraorbital lesion; other possibilities include tumors of extraorbital origin with secondary intraorbital extension (ENT or intracranial or palpebral tumors) or lesions of the globe involving the orbit.

Orbital tumors can be divided into primary or secondary lesions which in turn may be metastatic or due to invasion from a neighboring primary tumor.

The tumors afflicting children and adults are often of different etiologies and will be dealt with separately.

Orbital tumors in children

Rhabdomyosarcoma (fig. 5.1 a-f)

This is the commonest malignant orbital tumor in a child under 10 years of age, characterized by a non-axial exophthalmos, very rapid evolution and inflammation with preservation of visual acuity until a late stage. Pulmonary and bone marrow metastases are encountered primarily in the alveolar forms.

It is a malignant connective tissue tumor. Histological diagnosis depends on biopsy which most frequently reveals an embryonic-type tumor. The prognosis depends on the earliness of the diagnosis, histological degree of differentiation and presence of metastases.

Treatment is usually a combination of radiotherapy and chemotherapy.

CT demonstrates a mass within the preseptal space which is iso- or hypodense to the muscles and strongly enhances following injection of iodinated contrast. This well or poorly defined lesion most often arises from the superior or lateral rectus muscles. The bony windows are used to look for bone erosion or lytic change. The degree of unilateral exophthalmos can be appreciated relative to the bicanthal line.

Direct or 3-D reconstruction coronal sections are used to evaluate the presence of extension into the nasal fossa, pterygo-maxillary fossae, the sinuses and skull base.

MRI demonstrates an homogeneous tumor on the T1-weighted sequences whereas the tumor appears heterogeneous on T2-weighted images. Rhabdomyosarcomas exhibit intense enhancement with gadolinium. MRI provides a very accurate analysis of the spread of the tumor to the soft tissues and intracranial cavity. The rare leptomeningeal tumor dissemination may also be shown.

MRI is more useful than CT for the post-treatment follow-up in the detection of tumor recurrence and radiation changes.

Optic nerve glioma (fig. 5.2 a-d)

This is primarily a childhood tumor which rarely effects adults. There is no sex preponderance. It is characterized clinically by a slowly developing axial exophthalmos without any associated signs of inflammation. A reduction in visual acuity is an inconstant feature, sometimes only manifested by an absence of the photomotor reflex in the very young infant. Strabismus is often an associated feature due to the amblyopia or the tumor mass.

The optic nerve glioma occurs in children aged between 5 and 10 years in 75% of cases. It is a slowly growing benign tumor arising from the axonal supporting tissues of the optic nerve. The astrocytoma is the commonest, and the rarer oligodendrocytoma is a higher grade tumor which breaks through the meningeal sheath around the optic nerve. It is associated with von Recklinghausen's disease in a quarter of cases necessitating a search for involvement of the optic chiasma and the contralateral optic nerve.

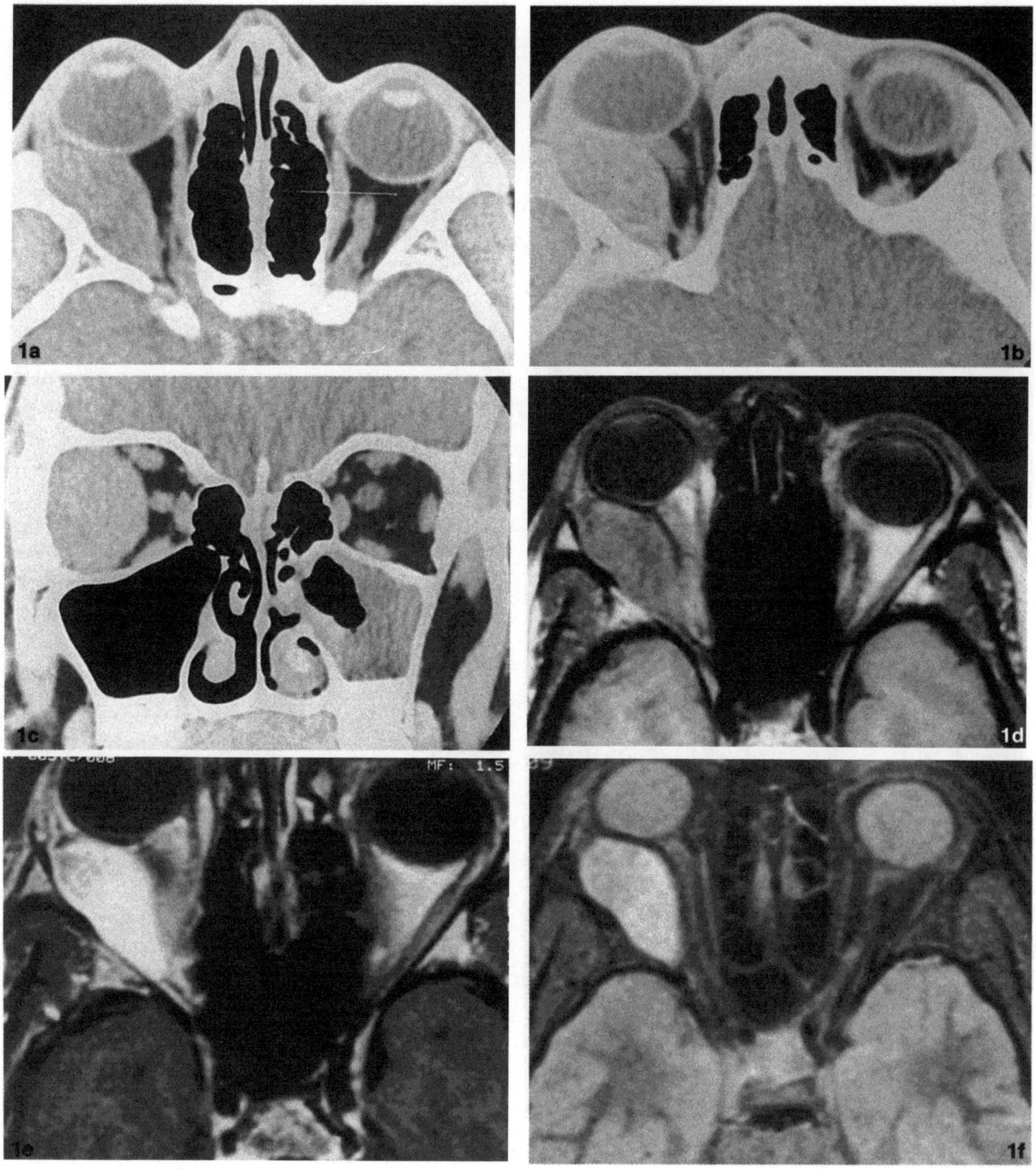

Fig. 5.1. 14 year old child with rhabdomyosarcoma of the lateral rectus. CT: **a** axial section: oval shaped, laterally placed, retrobulbar, isodense, homogeneous lesion. The lateral rectus itself cannot be identified. Note the scalloping of the sphenoidal wall; **b** axial section: the lesion enhances homogeneously after contrast injection; **c** post-contrast coronal section: note the medial displacement of the optic nerve. MRI: **d** axial T1 section pre-gadolinium: the lesion appears isointense; **e** axial T1 section post-gadolinium: heterogeneous enhancement of the tumor, particularly in its anterior pole; **f** axial T2 section: the lesion appears markedly hyperintense, especially posteriorly

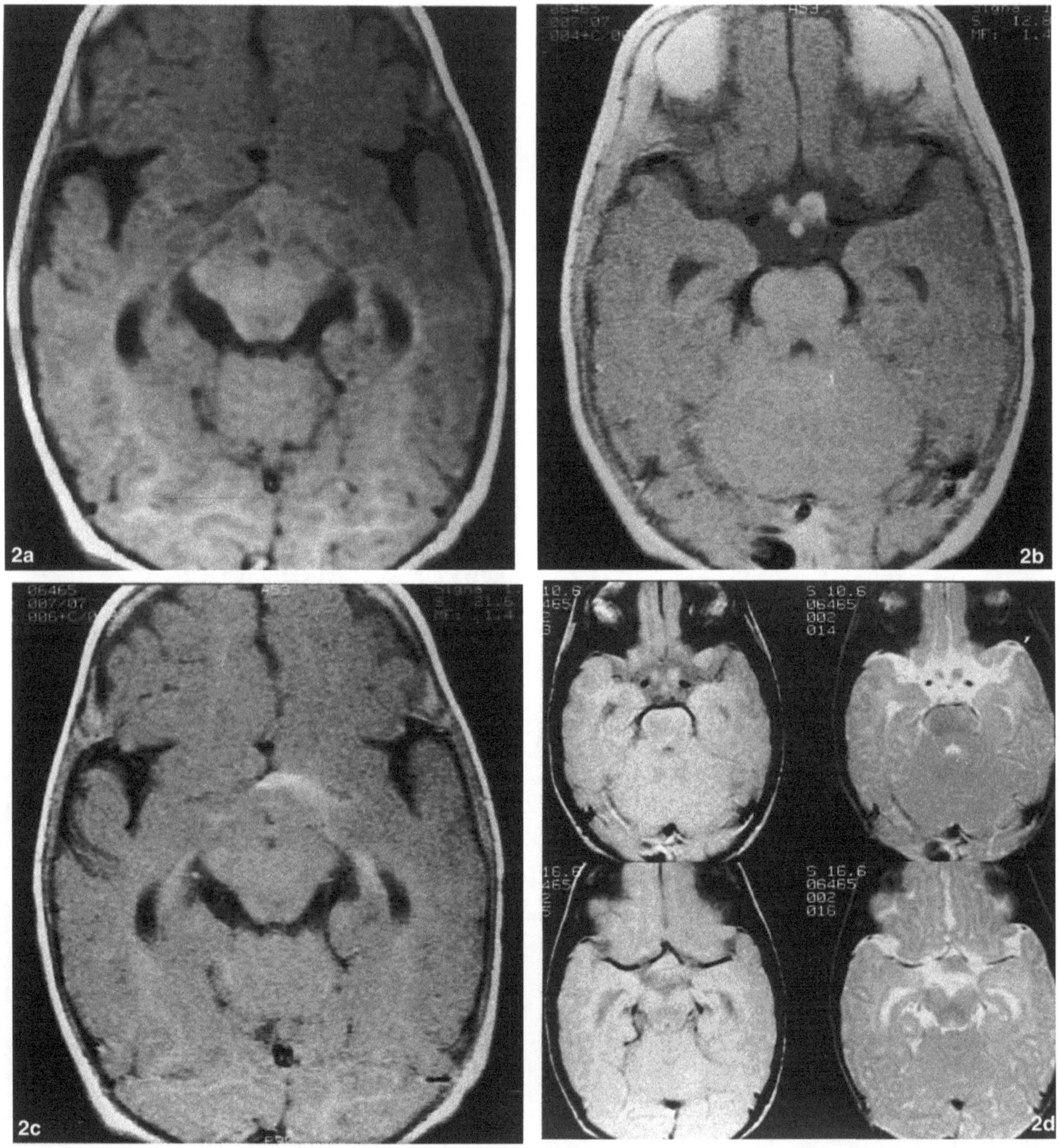

Fig. 5.2. 9 year old child with a glioma of the optic tract. MRI **a** axial T1 section pre-gadolinium: enlargement of the optic chiasma, mainly on the left; **b** axial T1 section post-gadolinium: enhancement with infiltration of the left optic tract, the anterior part of the globus pallidus and left uncus; **c** axial T2 section: enlargement of the optic chiasma is all that is visible

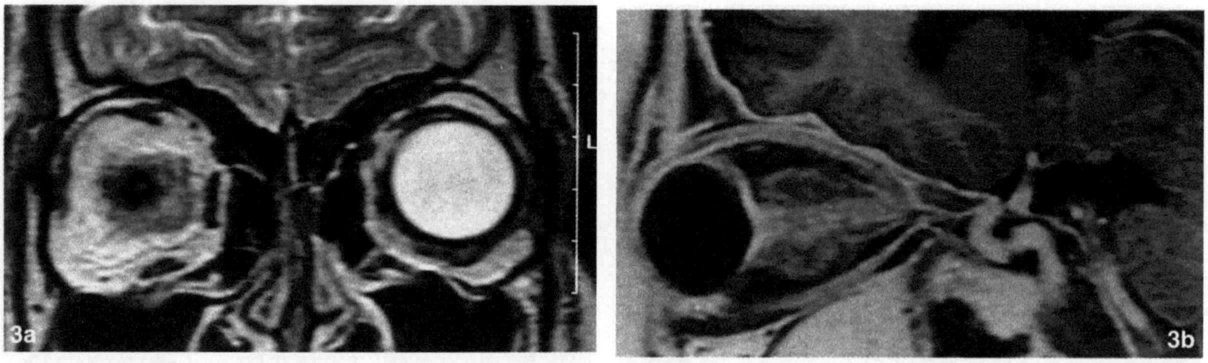

Fig. 5.3. Young 17 year old man with exophthalmos due to a meningioma of the optic nerve. MRI: coronal and axial T2-weighted images: the lesion is isointense and encases the optic nerve. It extends from the posterior aspect of the globe to the optic canal. Note the enlargement of the orbit

Two histopathological types have been described: the low grade, pilocytic, slow growing, type I astrocytoma, and the type II astrocytoma occurring in cases of von Recklinghausen's disease.

CT

On the pre-contrast CT scan, there is truncal or fusiform enlargement of the optic nerve which isodense to the contralateral optic nerve. Moderate enhancement is seen following contrast injection.

MRI

MRI is the essential examination for the investigation of an optic nerve tumor. The lesion appears isointense on the T1-weighted and hyperintense on T2-weighted sequences. A variable degree of enhancement occurs after gadolinium administration. MRI is of particular value in the assessment of posterior extension towards the chiasma and the retrochiasmatic optic pathways, which determines the therapeutic options.

It remains the examination of choice for the post-treatment follow-up of optic nerve gliomas. Dilatation of the fluid filled subarachnoid spaces around the optic nerve is frequently encountered giving a "railway track" appearance.

Teratoma

Occurring at any time from birth, this tumor results in a rapidly evolving exophthalmos associated with orbital enlargement.

Histologically it is composed of tissue elements of ectopic origin. Its malignant potential is much greater if the component tissues are immature.

Meningioma (fig. 5.3 a-b)

Rare in children, commoner in adults, this tumor results in a progressive diminution in visual acuity, optic atrophy and non-inflammatory axial exophthalmos.

Dermoid cyst (fig. 5.4 a-e)

This is an extremely common tumor of embryonic origin which mainly affects children and young subjects. It is a rare cause of exophthalmos. The commonest localization is the anterior orbital margin. It may sometimes extend posteriorly or arise within the orbit.

The lesion comprises a cystic mass of epidermal origin with the structures indicative of epithelial elements including hair, teeth as well as microcalcifications. There may be associated bone lesions, either a reactive sclerosis or more rarely, bone lysis.

CT demonstrates a cystic mass of fatty density, most frequently in an extraorbital location at the outer angle.

On MRI, the tumor appears hyperintense on the T1- and hypointense on the T2-weighted images. The microcalcifications are better assessed by CT.

Meningoencephalocele

Meningoencephalocele is a congenital anomaly resulting in ptosis of intracerebral structures into the orbit by herniation through a bony defect. It causes a non-axial exophthalmos. This is a palpable cystic tumor at the inner angle which reducibly increases in size on crying.

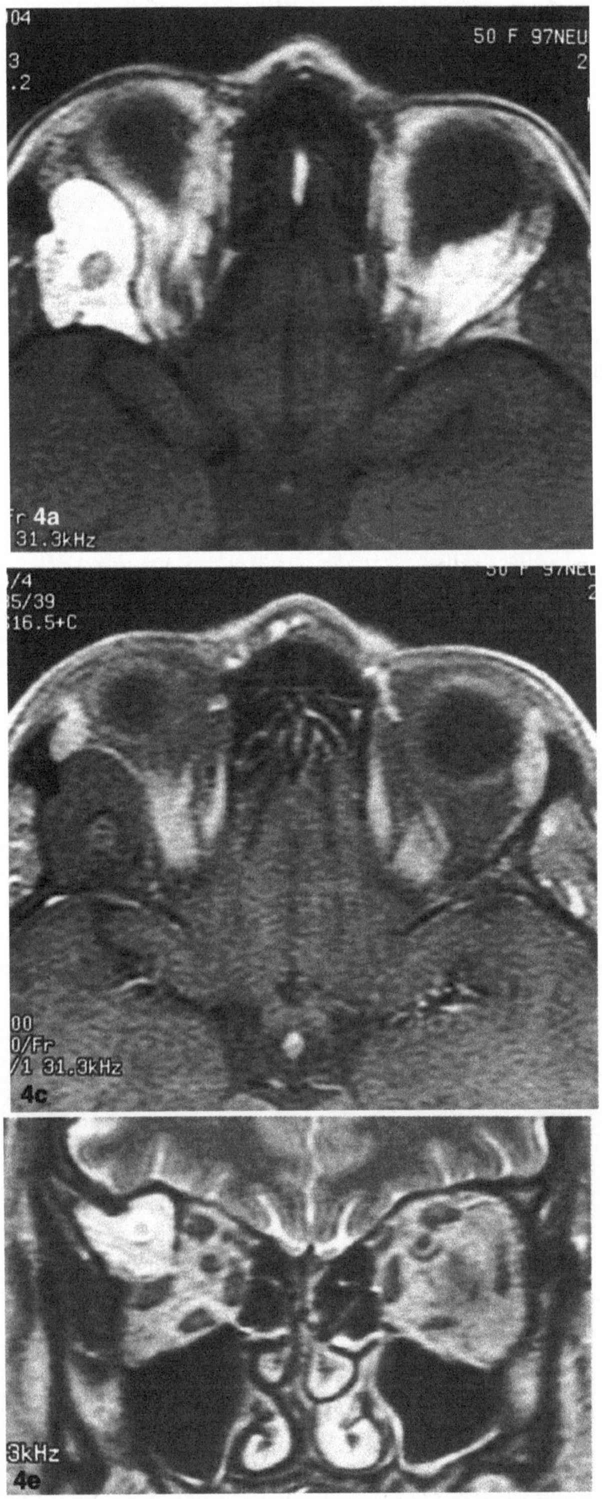

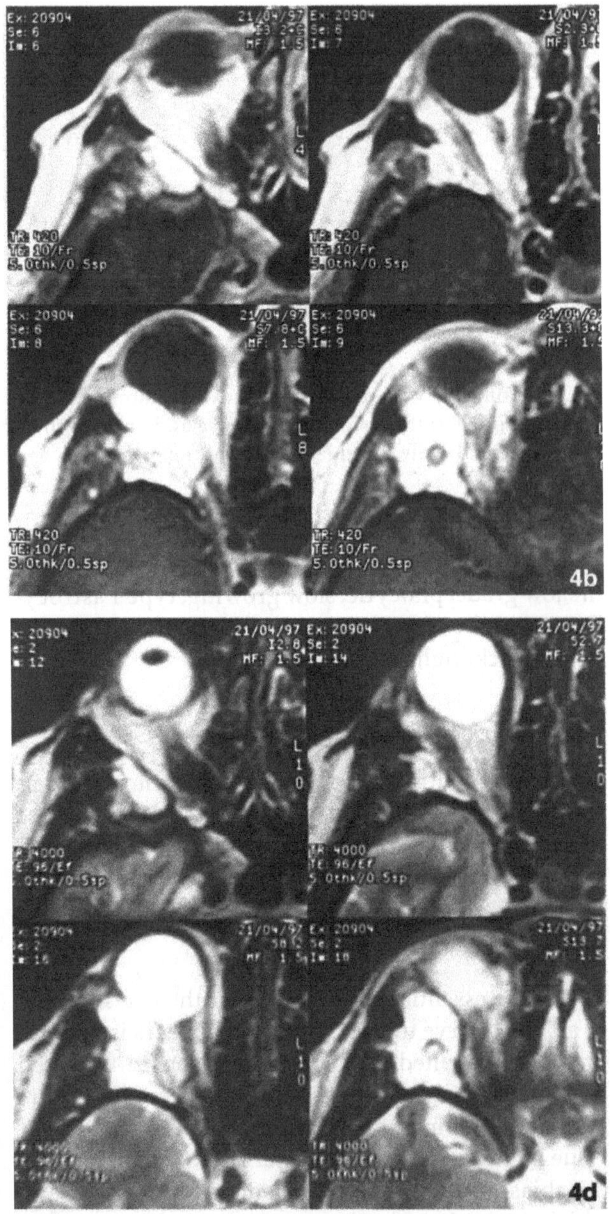

Fig. 5.4. 50 year old patient with a dermoid cyst. MRI: **a** axial T1 section: intra- and extraconal mass laterally eroding the sphenoid. The cyst appears hyperintense (fat) with an area of central low signal intensity corresponding to an epithelial structure; **b** axial T1 section post-gadolinium: weak peripheral enhancement; **c** axial fat sat T1 section: this sequence confirms the fatty origin of the lesion with nulling of the normally high fat signal; **d, e** coronal and axial T2 sections: the coronal images show the medial displacement of the intraconal structures

Surgical treatment consists of resection of the hernia and closure of the bony defect.

On CT and MRI, a meningoencephalocele has all the characteristics of normal cerebral tissue.

Retinoblastoma

This is a malignant intraocular tumor of children between the ages of 6 months and 3 years. It presents with a rapid reduction in visual acuity, often with an associated strabismus and leucoria. Although usually unilateral, it may be bilateral at presentation, either in the familial forms or in cases effecting very young children. It is a genetic disorder linked to an anomaly on chromosome 13.

The diagnosis depends on examination of the eye of the infant under general anesthesia.

MRI should form a part of the routine investigation to determine whether the lesion is unilateral or bilateral. This also may need to be performed under anesthesia.

On T1-weighted images, a retinoblastoma generally appears as an homogeneous mass, more rarely heterogeneous with discrete areas of hyperintensity. On T2-weighted sequences, the tumor is hypointense and of variable heterogeneity depending on the amount of intratumoral calcification.

There is often an associated retinal detachment, better appreciated on the gradient echo sequences.

MRI, in association with fundoscopy, is the examination of choice for post-treatment follow-up.

CT demonstrates hyperdense areas on the retina which enhance following contrast. CT clearly identifies the frequently occurring intratumoral zones of calcification.

The principle differential diagnosis of retinoblastoma in a child is Coat's disease. This is a condition effecting the retina which is a combination of retinal vascular dysplasias, telangiectasia and large exudates.

The diagnosis is easily made on MRI with the hyperintensity relative to the vitreous on the T1-weighted sections and the hyperintensity particularly on the late echo T2-weighted images.

Rare orbital tumors of childhood

- Capillary hemangioma arising posteriorly,
- orbital histiocytosis,
- orbital mucocele arising from the sinuses,
- spontaneous hematoma,
- orbital metastases (abdominal neuroblastoma, osteosarcoma, hematological disorders).

Orbital tumors of adults

Vascular tumors

Cavernous hemangioma (fig. 5.5 a-e)

Cavernous hemangioma is a common slowly growing benign orbital tumor which may be the cause of axial or non-axial exophthalmos, depending on whether it situated intra- or extraconally. This well defined encapsulated lesion does not have a tendency to regress spontaneously, unlike the capillary hemangioma of childhood. It is made up of large vascular spaces lined by endothelial cells forming intratumoral septa. The tumor is characterized by extremely slow flowing blood, explaining its occult nature on angiography.

On CT, the cavernous hemangioma appears hyperdense and enhances strongly after contrast.

On T1-weighted MRI images, the lesion is characteristically hypointense relative to the intraconal muscles and markedly hyperintense on the T2-weighted images. In addition, there is significant enhancement on T1 after gadolinium injection. MRI can demonstrate the intratumoral hemorrhagic changes as well as phleboliths.

The other vascular tumors are rarer: hemangiopericytoma, hemangioendothelioma, vascular leiomyoma.

Orbital varices

Orbital varices are formed by venous dilatation causing increased exophthalmos on internal jugular vein compression, Valsalva maneuver, physical exertion and inclination of the head.

Often no treatment is required due to the minimal symptomatology caused.

The different maneuvers required to make the diagnosis explain the diagnostic difficulties encountered during assessment by CT and MRI.

The MRI examination may be normal, or only a paroxysmal enophthalmos is seen. In the more advanced cases, a mass is seen isointense relative to muscle on the T1-weighted sections and hyperintense on T2. The phleboliths are better appreciated on CT. Conversely, thrombosed areas are better shown by MRI.

CT sections can be performed with the patient prone which significantly increase the size of the lesion, thus increasing the sensitivity of the technique.

If surgical intervention is being contemplated, orbital venography should be performed in order to obtain a map of the whole of the venous drainage of the orbit.

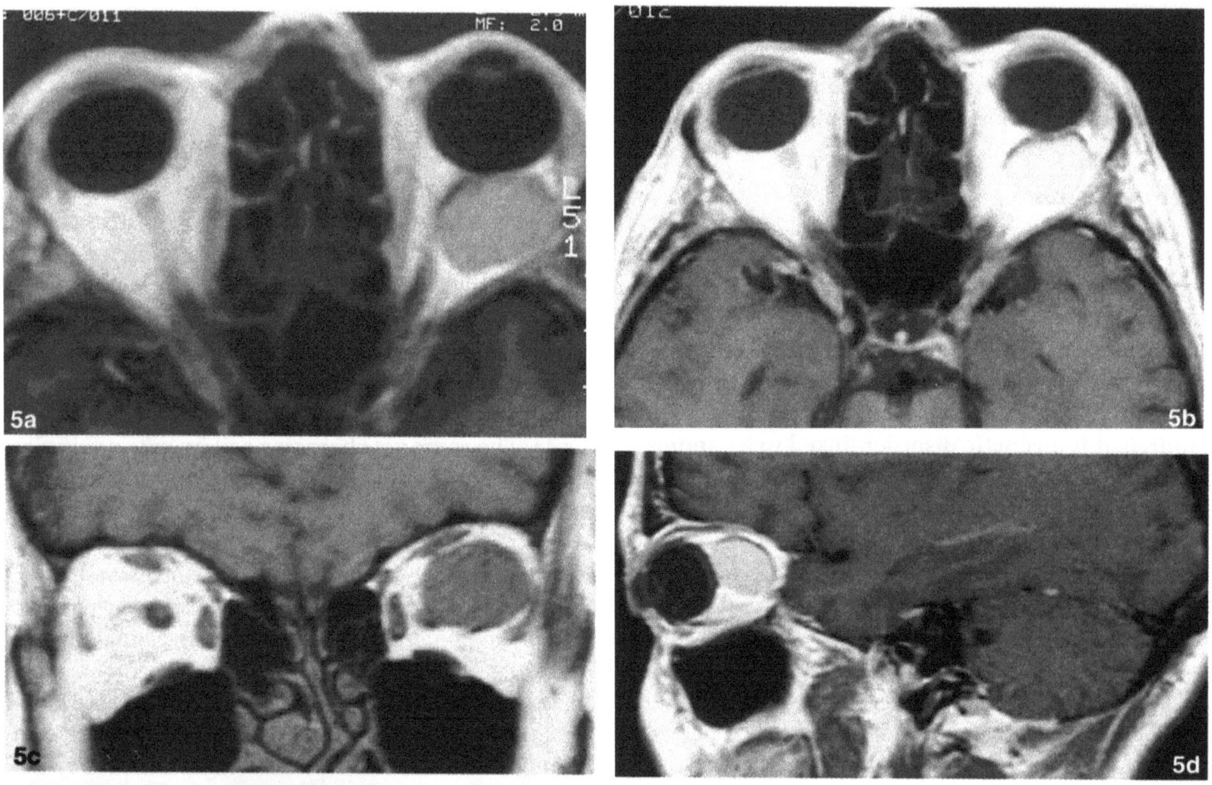

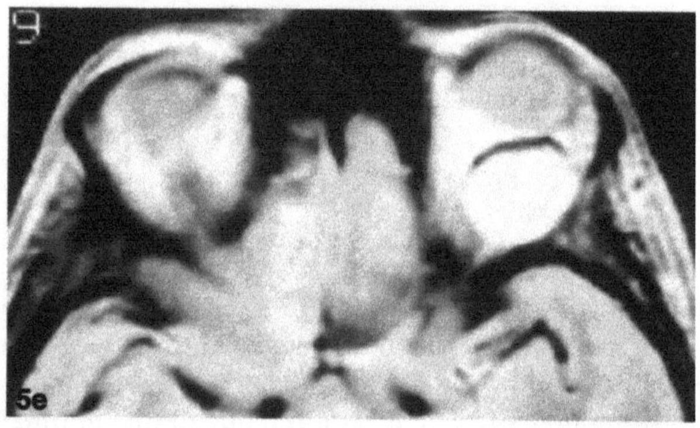

Fig. 5.5. 45 year old patient with a cavernous hemangioma. MRI: **a** axial T1 section: oval, intraconal lesion situated laterally appearing isointense and homogeneous and separate to the oculomotor muscles and optic nerve; **b-d** axial, coronal and sagittal T1 images post-gadolinium: the cavernous hemangioma enhances strongly in a homogeneous fashion. The intraconal fat appears normal; **e** axial T2 section: the cavernous haemangioma appears isointense. Note the significant chemical shift at the periphery of the tumor

Orbital arterio-venous fistulae

These congenital or post-traumatic fistulae may be the cause of a pulsatile exophthalmos with a vascular discernible hum on auscultation, and dilatation of the episcleral vessels into a medusa head formation.

Traumatic carotido-cavernous fistulae

These fistulae are due to a connection between the intracavernous internal carotid artery and the cavernous sinus. They are of traumatic origin and result in marked pulsatile exophthalmos with conjunctival hyperemia and chemosis. Urgent treatment is necessary in order to avoid loss of the eye. Treatment is usually by endovascular occlusion of the drainage veins or, more rarely, by occlusion of the internal carotid artery opposite the hole in the vessel.

Both CT and MRI demonstrate a significant dilatation of the superior ophthalmic vein, crossing the path of the optic nerve. The definitive diagnosis can only be made angiographically.

Congenital carotido-cavernous fistulae

These are due to the opening of meningeal arterio-venous shunts between branches of internal and external carotid arteries and the cavernous sinus. They present clinically with a slightly pulsatile exophthalmos and conjunctival hyperemia resulting in a "red eye". Frequently there is an associated reduction in visual acuity.

Treatment is essentially by embolization of the arterial meningeal branches or endovascular occlusion of the drainage veins.

MRI and CT show a moderate dilatation of the superior ophthalmic vein which appears dilated and hypointense on MRI due to the rapid blood flow within the vessel. This dilatation may be absent when the venous return is predominantly into the inferior petrosal sinus.

Rare vascular tumors

- Paragangliomas (fig. 5.6 a-f),
- hemangiopericytomas,
- malignant hemangiothelioma,
- aneurysm of the ophthalmic or lachrymal artery.

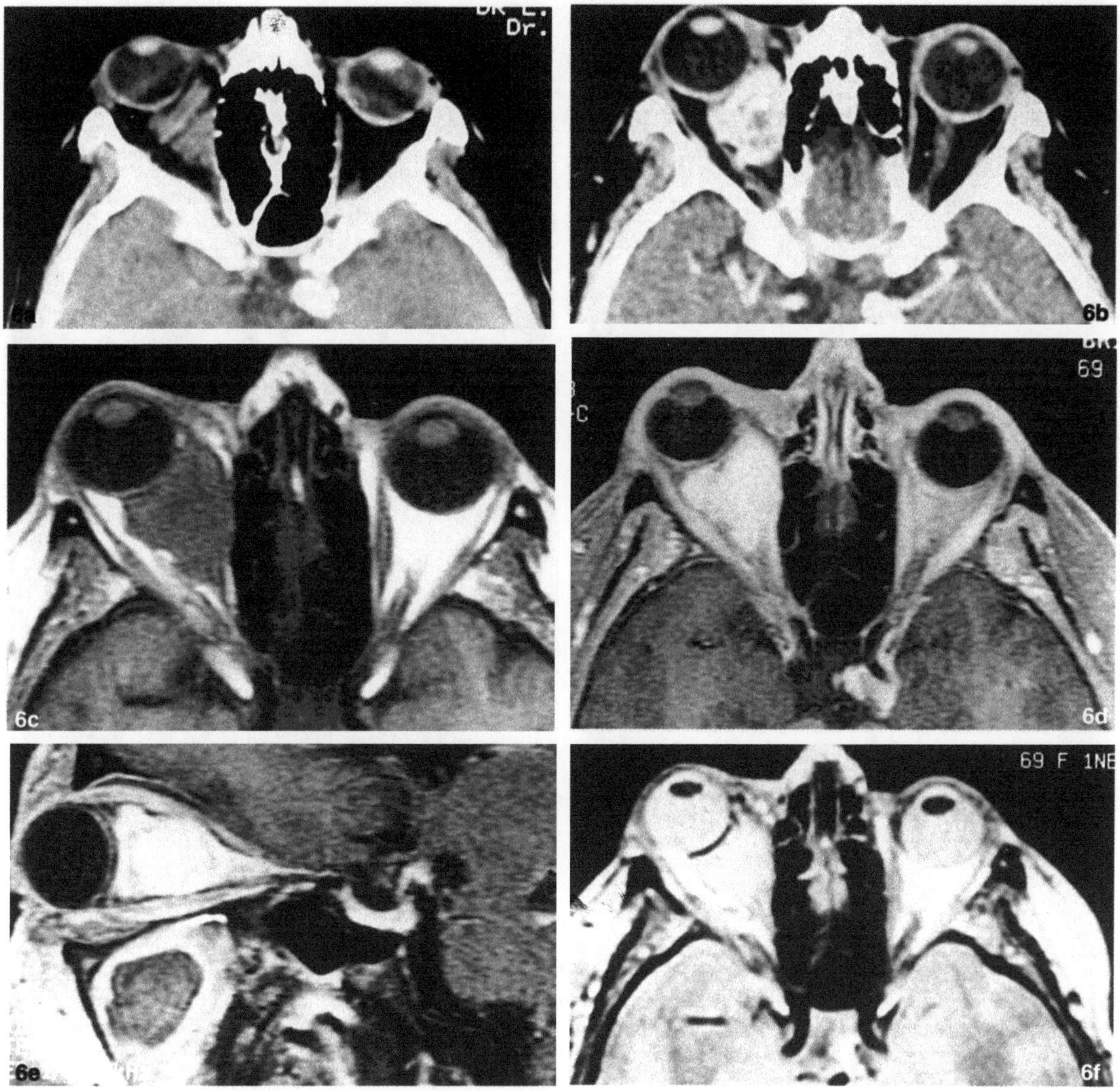

Fig. 5.6. 69 year old patient with an orbital paraganglioma. CT: **a** pre-contrast axial section; the paraganglioma is seen as an isodense mass with irregular margins situated medially; **b** post-contrast axial section: heterogeneous enhancement is noted, mainly in the periphery of the lesion. MRI: **c** axial T1 section: the paraganglioma appears homogeneously iso- or hypointense; **d** axial T1 section post-gadolinium: there is intense, heterogeneous enhancement; **e** sagittal T1 section post-gadolinium (STIR sequence): this sequence demonstrates the extent of the lesion from the superior pole of the eye to the sphenoidal fissure. Note the elevation of the superior rectus muscle; **f** axial T2 section: the lesion is slightly hyperintense

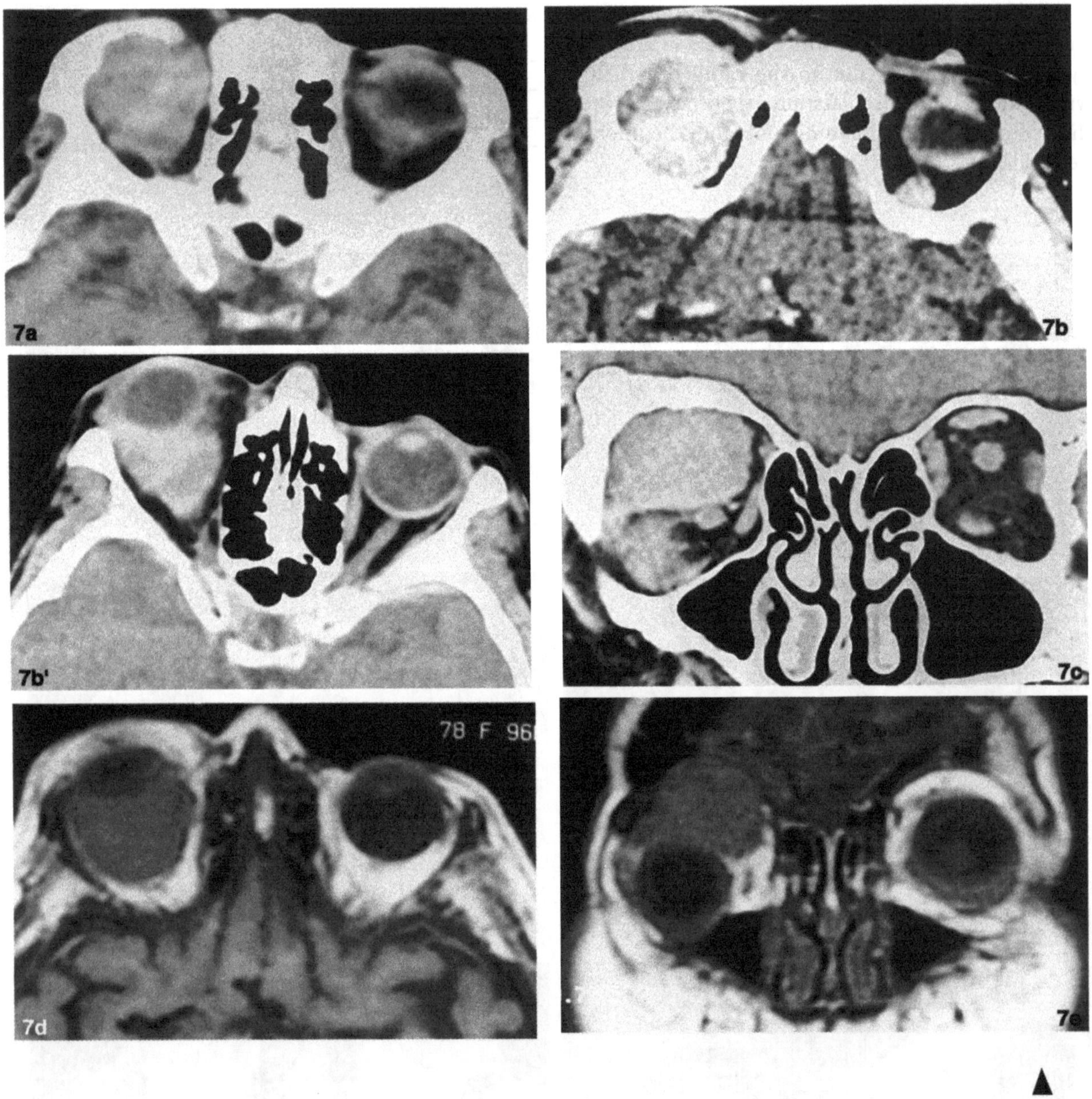

Fig. 5.7. 78 year old patient operated on 15 years previously for a prefrontal meningioma presenting now with exophthalmos due to orbital meningioma. CT: **a** axial section: slightly hyperdense mass lesion in the superior aspect of the orbit causing a moderate exophthalmos; **b, b'** post-contrast axial section: intense and homogeneous enhancement; **c** post-contrast coronal section: the meningioma is pushing down the exophthalmic eyeball and optic nerve. Note the significant bony thickening of the superior orbital margin. MRI: **d, e** axial and coronal T1 sections: the meningioma appears homogeneously isointense; **f-h** axial, coronal and sagittal T1 sections: homogeneous enhancement pattern post-gadolinium with a central low signal intensity indicating necrosis; **i** axial T2 section: the meningioma is slightly hyperintense

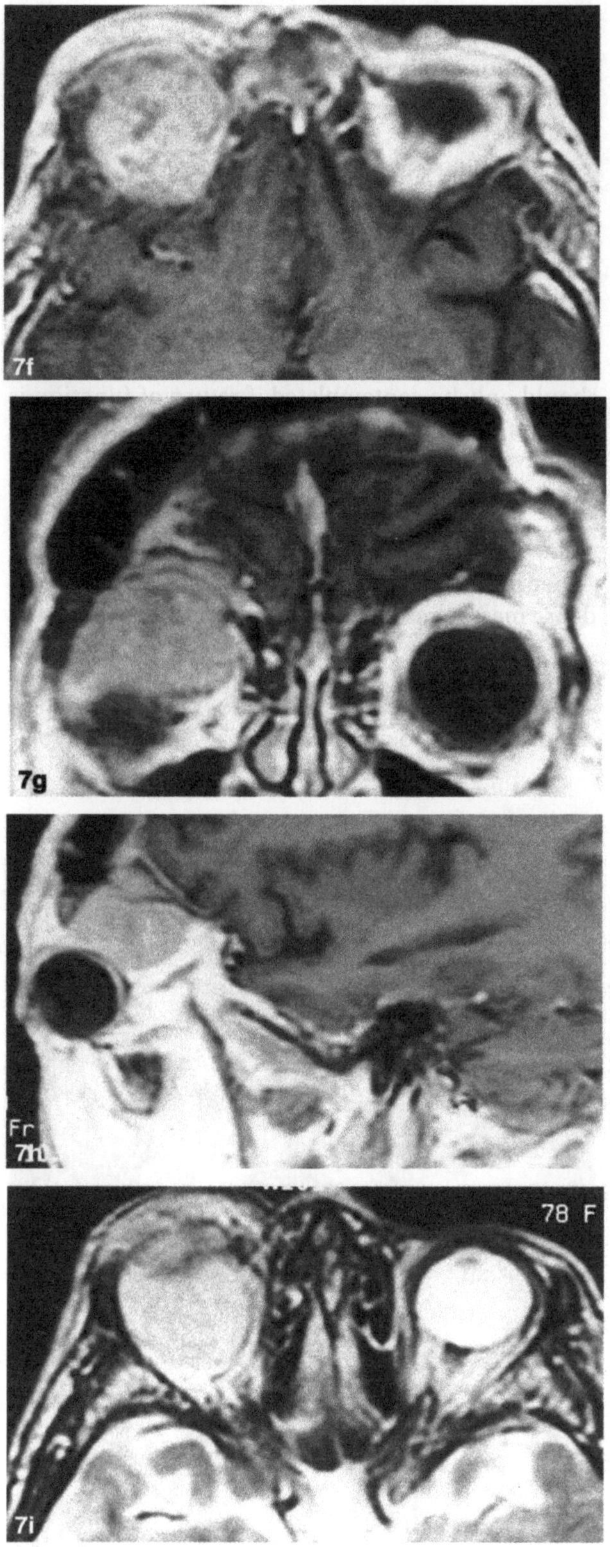

Meningeal or nerve tumors

Meningioma

Meningioma of the optic nerve sheath (fig. 5.7 a-i)

Meningioma is a tumor which has a female preponderance and occurs mainly in the fourth and fifth decades. It may either arise as a primary lesion of the optic nerve sheath or, more commonly, as an extension of a skull base meningioma (most often sphenoidal). The tumor is slowly evolving and may occur bilaterally. Exophthalmos occurs usually after the reduction in visual acuity.

The optic nerve meningioma is a benign, slowly growing, intraconal tumor arising from the meninges which spares the optic nerve, unlike a glioma, but causes a progressive optic atrophy. The treatment is surgical but complete excision is rarely possible and recurrences are frequent.

CT

A meningioma appears slightly hyperdense before contrast injection, with tubular extension in relationship to the optic nerve. There is significant enhancement of the nerve sheath following iodinated contrast. Calcifications are common, sometimes of a large pseudotumoral nature becoming psammomatous.

Bone windows are required to look for spread into the optic canal seen as enlargement or expansion of this structure.

MRI

On the T1-weighted images, the lesion appears hypo- or isointense relative to muscle and surrounds the optic nerve fibers. There is marked enhancement following gadolinium injection resulting in a "railway track" appearance due to the high signal intensity of the meningioma and the central low signal intensity of the optic nerve. On the T2-weighted images, the signal intensity depends on the histological type and may be either hypo- or hyperintense. Sagittal oblique sections are useful to look for spread into the optic canal towards the chiasma. Intra- or peritumoral calcifications are more difficult to appreciate on MRI compared to CT.

In children, a complete cervico-cranial examination should be performed to detect other lesions in cases of von Recklinghausen's disease.

Meningioma of the spheno-orbital ridge

These slowly growing tumors may cause exophthalmos which progress on to a true exorbitism. The role of CT and MRI is to make the diagnosis and define any spread particularly into the optic canal and sphenoidal fissure.

CT

The tumor appears hyperdense and exhibits strong homogeneous enhancement following injection of contrast agent. This lesion astride the spheno-orbital ridge displaces equally the intraorbital and intracranial structures of the anterior temporal fossa.

MRI

A meningioma may be iso- or hypointense on the T1- and T2-weighted sections and enhances strongly after gadolinium injection. There is often associated significant enhancement of the thickened adjacent meninges.

These spheno-orbital meningiomas can appear similar to fibrous dysplasia and en plaque meningiomas which cause significant thickening of the spheno-orbital ridge. This thickening, best appreciated on CT, appears on MRI as heterogeneous areas of hypo- and hyperintensity on the T1- and T2-weighted sections with heterogeneous enhancement following gadolinium injection.

Neurofibroma

This tumor is usually associated with von Recklinghausen's disease. It is a benign condition effecting the peripheral nerves.

In the solitary form, it constitutes a slowly growing, single entity, soft tissue tumor occurring as a single entity. The plexiform neuroma, characteristic of von Recklinghausen's disease, is diffuse and invades the orbit.

Surgical excision is possible in the well-defined solitary forms. However, this may be incomplete and should only be contemplated if return of function is important. These neurofibromata are often associated with dysplasias of the sphenoidal fissure, opto-chiasmatic gliomas or intracerebral astrocytic lesions.

CT

A neurofibroma appears as an intrinsically hyperdense mass which exhibits moderate enhancement.

MRI

The lesion is characteristically iso- or slightly hyperintense relative to muscle on the T1- and more hyper-

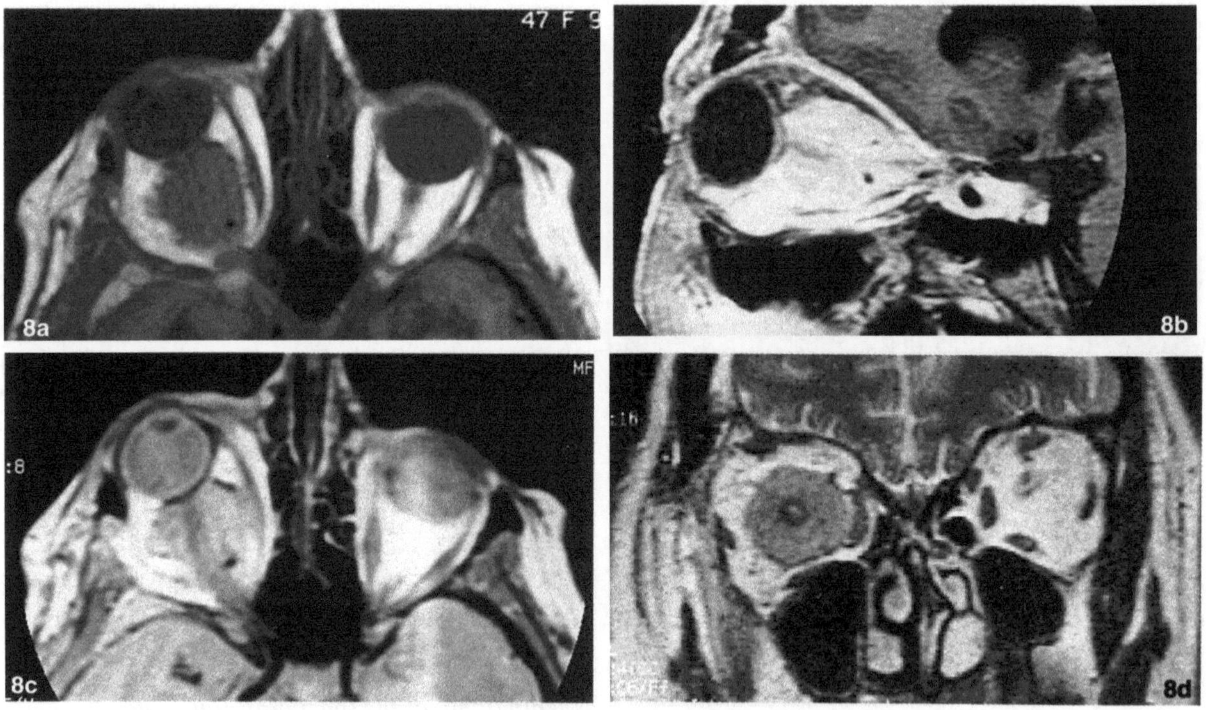

Fig. 5.8. 47 year old patient with a solitary neurofibroma. MRI: **a** axial T1 section: the oval, retro-ocular lesion appears isointense and surrounds the optic nerve; **b** sagittal T1 section post-gadolinium: homogeneous enhancement; **c-d** axial and coronal T2 sections: the two images demonstrate well the involvement of the optic nerve by the schwannoma

intense but less homogeneous on the T2-weighted images. Moderate enhancement is seen following gadolinium injection.

MRI will demonstrate any spread into the pterygomaxillary fossa or intracranial extension.

Optic nerve glioma

This has already been discussed in children and is rare in adults in whom it is particularly malignant (glioblastoma).

Other rare nerve tumors

- Benign or malignant schwannoma (fig. 5.8 a-d),
- ganglioneuroma,
- alveolar sarcoma.

Tumors of hematological origin

Non-Hodgkin's lymphoma (NHL) (fig. 5.9 a-d)

This is a fairly common condition affecting adults after the age of 50, causing a slowly progressive, uni- or bilateral, painless exophthalmos.

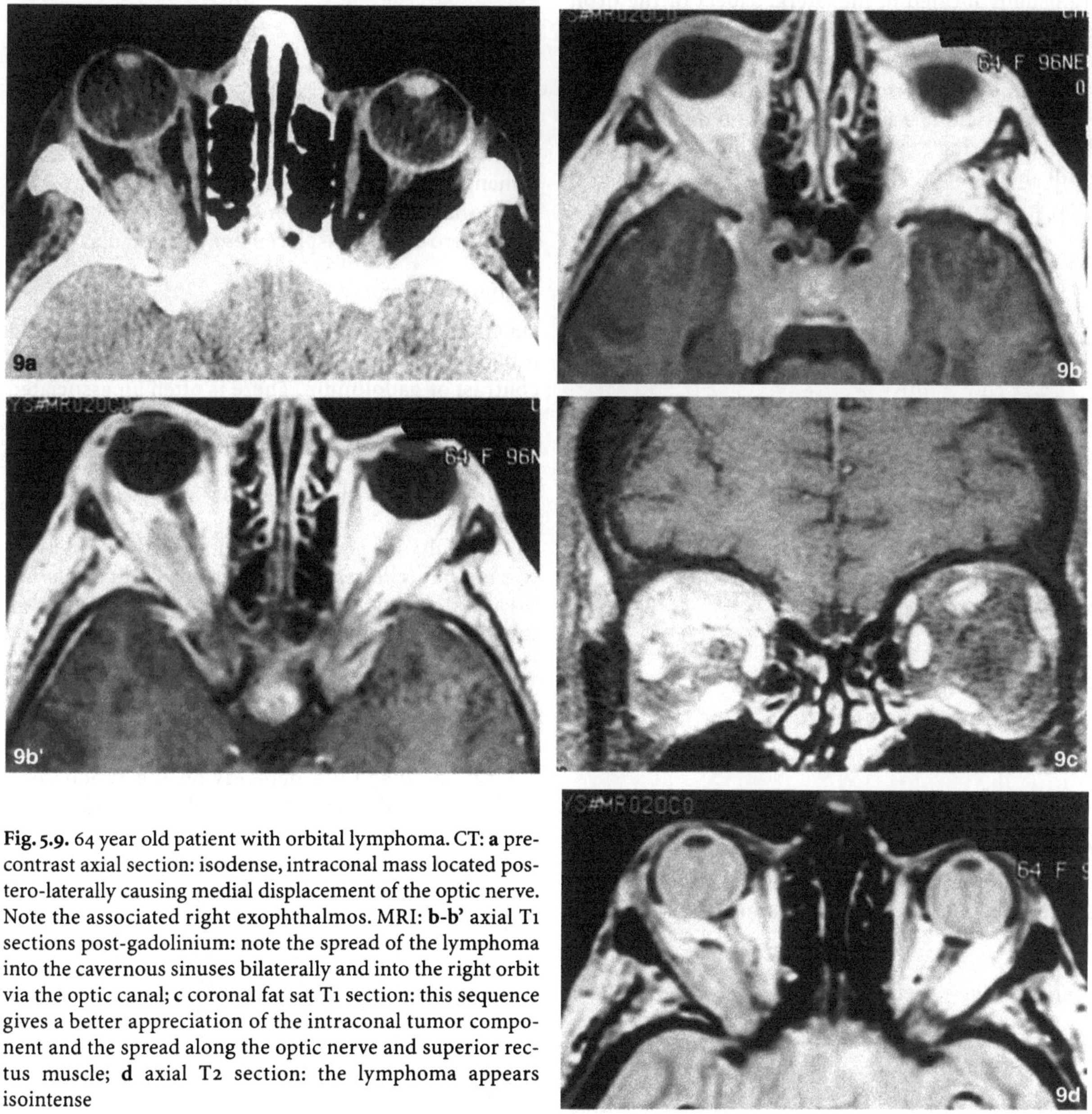

Fig. 5.9. 64 year old patient with orbital lymphoma. CT: **a** precontrast axial section: isodense, intraconal mass located postero-laterally causing medial displacement of the optic nerve. Note the associated right exophthalmos. MRI: **b-b'** axial T1 sections post-gadolinium: note the spread of the lymphoma into the cavernous sinuses bilaterally and into the right orbit via the optic canal; **c** coronal fat sat T1 section: this sequence gives a better appreciation of the intraconal tumor component and the spread along the optic nerve and superior rectus muscle; **d** axial T2 section: the lymphoma appears isointense

There is a diffuse invasion of the intraorbital soft tissues.

The main diagnostic problem is the differentiation from an inflammatory pseudotumor. The histological classification, obtained by biopsy, depends on the malignant potential and guides the chemotherapy and/or radiotherapy. Two types are distinguishable radiologically: the well-defined pseudotumoral form and the infiltrative form involving the whole of the retrobulbar space and infiltrating the optic nerve and conal muscles.

CT

The well-defined forms appear slightly hyperdense, are usually located in the lateral aspect of the orbit and enhance strongly and in a homogeneous fashion after injection of contrast agent.

The infiltrative forms involve the optic nerve, muscles and fat. Bone lysis is best seen on the bone windows, occurring especially in the lymphomas of high grade malignancy.

MRI

Lymphoma usually appears isointense relative to muscle on the T1-weighted image and hypointense on the T2-weighted sections. Homogeneous enhancement is seen following gadolinium injection.

Sagittal oblique sections will demonstrate extraorbital spread.

Myeloma

This usually occurs in association with Kaller's disease with diffuse bone involvement and biological stigmata.

Rare hematological disorders

- Hodgkin's lymphoma,
- isolated plasmocytoma,
- leukemic orbital infiltration.

Tumors of the lacrymal gland

Located in the supero-lateral angle of the orbit, these tumors are responsible for an exophthalmos characterized by infero-nasal displacement of the ocular globe.

Epithelial lacrymal tumors

These are the commonest (fig. 10a-d):
- either mixed, benign, encapsulated, well-defined, slowly growing, without associated bone lysis,
- or malignant tumor ,cylindroma, adenocarcinoma, more rapidly progressive, with capsular breech and signs of peritumoral bone invasion.

Other conditions include a lacrymal gland cyst, lymphoid hyperplasia (Mikulicz syndrome), and lymphoma. Dacro-adenitis, a pseudo-inflammatory syndrome or Besnier-Boeck-Schaumann's syndrome should be excluded before proposing a benign tumor of the lacrymal gland.

CT

The mixed tumors appear as uni- or multinodular, extraconal lesions, isodense to muscle, which may cause a curvilinear erosion of the bony wall. There is moderate, sometimes heterogeneous enhancement after contrast injection.

MRI

On the T1-weighted images, the tumor is iso- or hyperintense relative to muscle and heterogeneously hyperintense on the T2-weighted images. Marked enhancement is noted following gadolinium injection.

Coronal sections demonstrate the exophthalmos with infero-medial displacement of the ocular globe.

Malignant tumors

On CT and MRI, there is a diffuse extra- or intraconal infiltration with enhancement following iodinated contrast or gadolinium. There is often an associated orbital inflammation.

Ocular tumor with orbital spread

In the adult, this is essentially due to advanced uveal melanoma (ciliary body, choroid) which, having breached through the wall of the sclera, has invaded the orbital tissues causing exophthalmos. Tumor recurrence may be seen following enucleation.

Orbital melanoma is a therapeutic emergency because of the risk of metastases. Clinically melanoma manifests as a rapid deterioration in visual acuity. The diagnosis depends on the fundoscopy findings and ultrasound, particularly for the small tumors.

Color Doppler ultrasound is able to confirm the hypervascular nature of the melanoma. The combination of all these examinations can exclude a benign tumor, notably the benign melanocyte type of tumor, choroidal hemangioma or astrocytic hamartoma. More rarely, sarcoid and other granulomatous conditions need consideration.

CT and MRI are useful mainly in the search for metastases.

CT

Melanoma is characterized by a well-defined, intravitreous hyperdensity which exhibits intense, homogeneous enhancement following contrast injection. There is often an associated retinal detachment.

MRI

On the T1-weighted images, melanoma appears hyperintense relative to the vitreous and hypointense on the T2-weighted sections. Moderate enhancement is seen after gadolinium administration. The MRI examination should include a study of the whole brain to look for metastases.

CT and MRI are of little value in the local follow-up of melanomas. This rests principally on the fundoscopy findings.

Rare primary orbital tumors

Tumors of bone origin

- Osteoma, osteosarcoma, eosinophilic granuloma (histiocytosis X),
- vascular bony anomaly,
- giant-cell tumor (osteoblastoma),
- fibrous dysplasia, Paget's disease.

Tumors of cartilaginous origin

- Chondroma,
- chondrosarcoma.

Connective tissue tumors

- Fibroma,
- fibrosarcoma,
- rhabdomyoma,

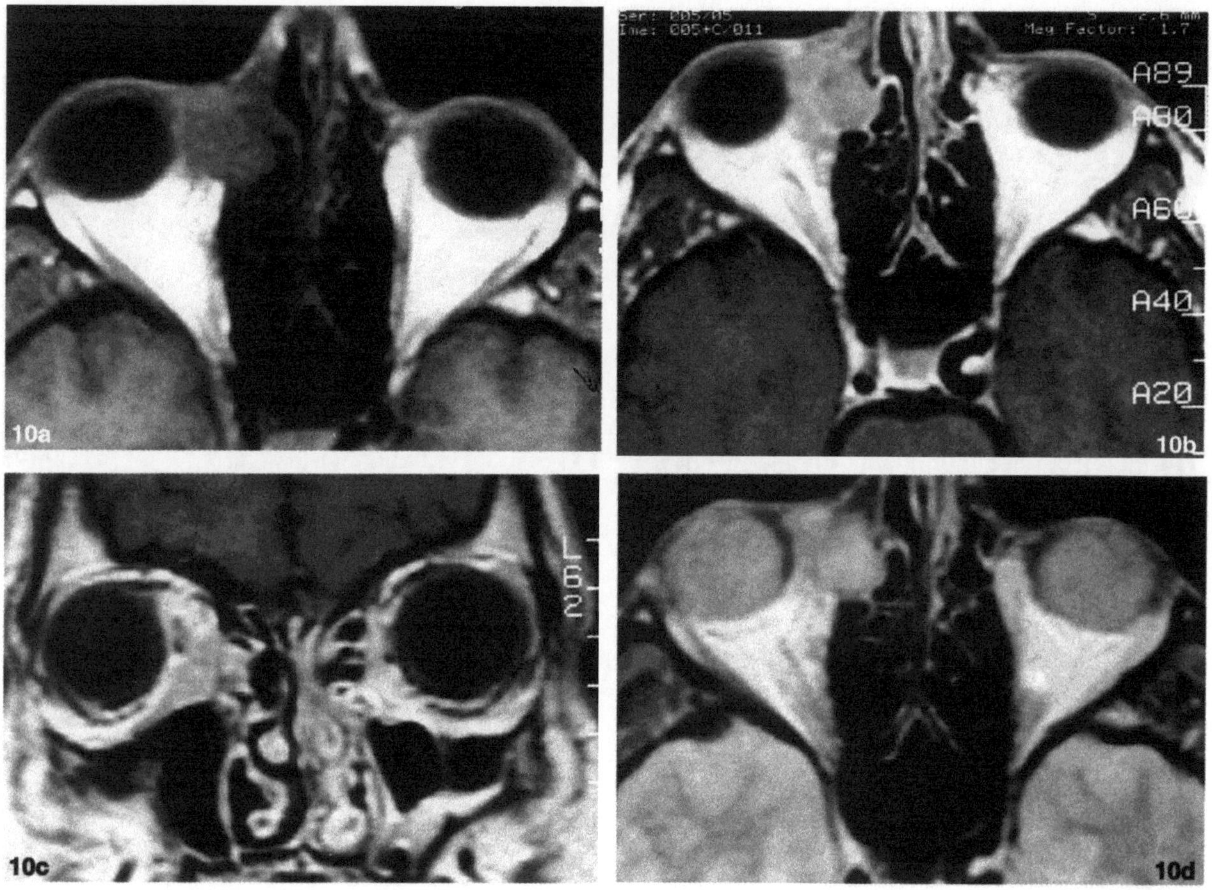

Fig. 5.10. 32 year old patient with lymphoma of the right lacrymal gland. MRI: **a** axial T1 section: the lesion appears slightly hypointense and involves the lacrymal gland and naso-lacrymal duct. It is invading the intraorbital fat and adjacent ethmoid sinuses; **b, c** axial and coronal T1 sections post-gadolinium: clear and homogeneous enhancement is seen; **d** axial T2 section: the lymphoma appears isointense

- leiomyoma, leiomyosarcoma,
- lipoma, liposarcoma,
- primary melanoma,
- tumor of parasitic origin.

Epidermoid cyst

See fig. 5.11 a-d

Secondary orbital tumors by direct spread.

These are common tumors.

- Palpebral or conjunctival tumors. All neoplastic lesions of the eyelids may secondarily invade the orbit (spinocellular epithelioma, melanoma).
- The same is true of ENT tumors:
  • benign: mucocele of the sinus, osteoma,
  • malignant: sinus, ethmoid, cavum.
- Intracranial meningiomas

Meningiomas of the medial and inferior temporal region may invade the orbit. This invasion may only cause subtle changes and is difficult to appreciate. It is imperative to look for bone invasion on the bone windows and use fine sections for orbital invasion.

Secondary metastatic orbital tumors (fig. 12 a-g)

An orbital metastasis can sometimes be the first manifestation of an previously unknown cancer, triggering the search for a primary lesion.

The lesion may be solitary or multiple, uni- or bilateral, and usually rapidly progressive. There are often the accompanying radiological signs of bone destruction. Certain metastases provoke an enophthalmos rather than the expected exophthalmos.

The commonest primary tumors are breast, bronchus, prostate and gastrointestinal tract. Metastatic

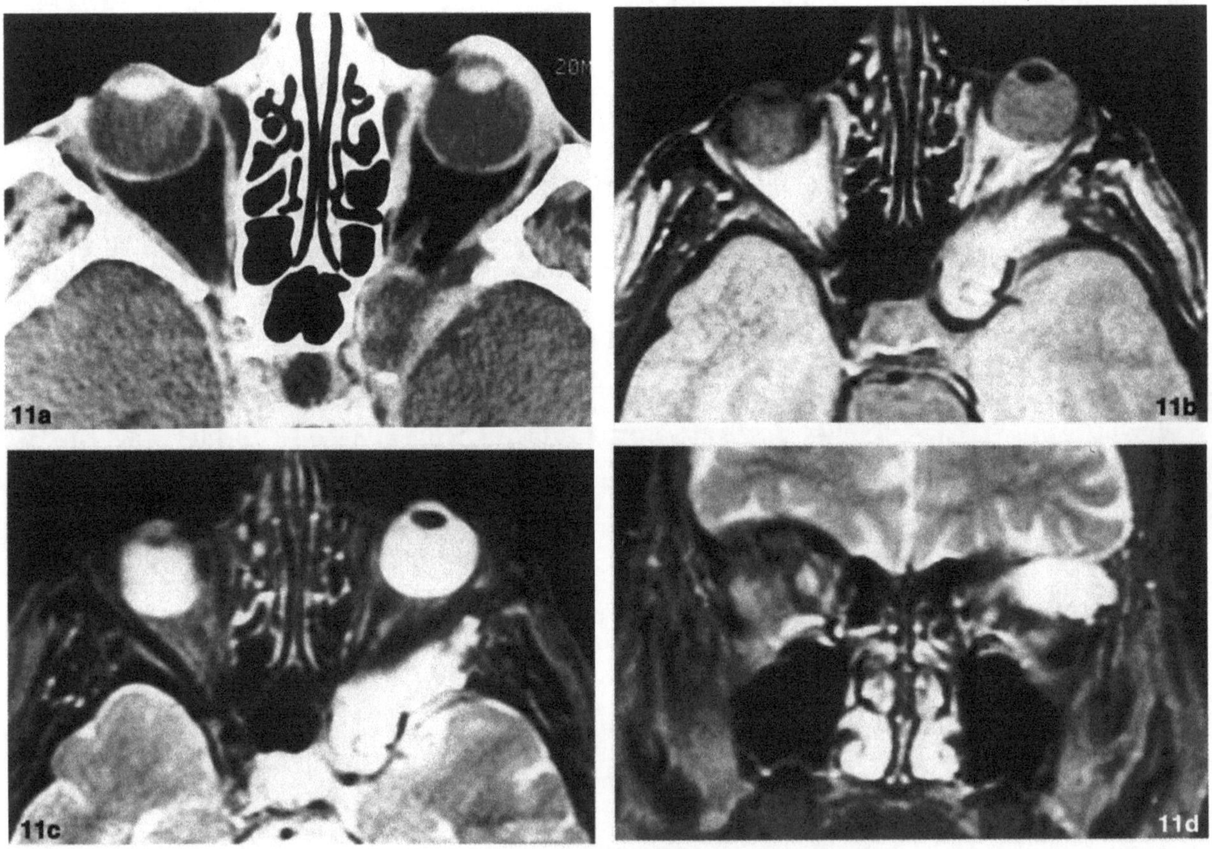

Fig. 5.11. 59 year old patient with an epidermoid cyst. CT: **a** post-contrast axial section: hypodense lesion showing peripheral enhancement, destroying the posterior aspect of the orbital wall and invading the posterior intraconal fat. MRI: **b, c** axial dual echo T2 sections: the cyst is heterogeneously hyperintense. The extension towards the cavernous sinus is well appreciated. **d** Coronal T2 section: this section demonstrates the inferior displacement of all the intraconal structures

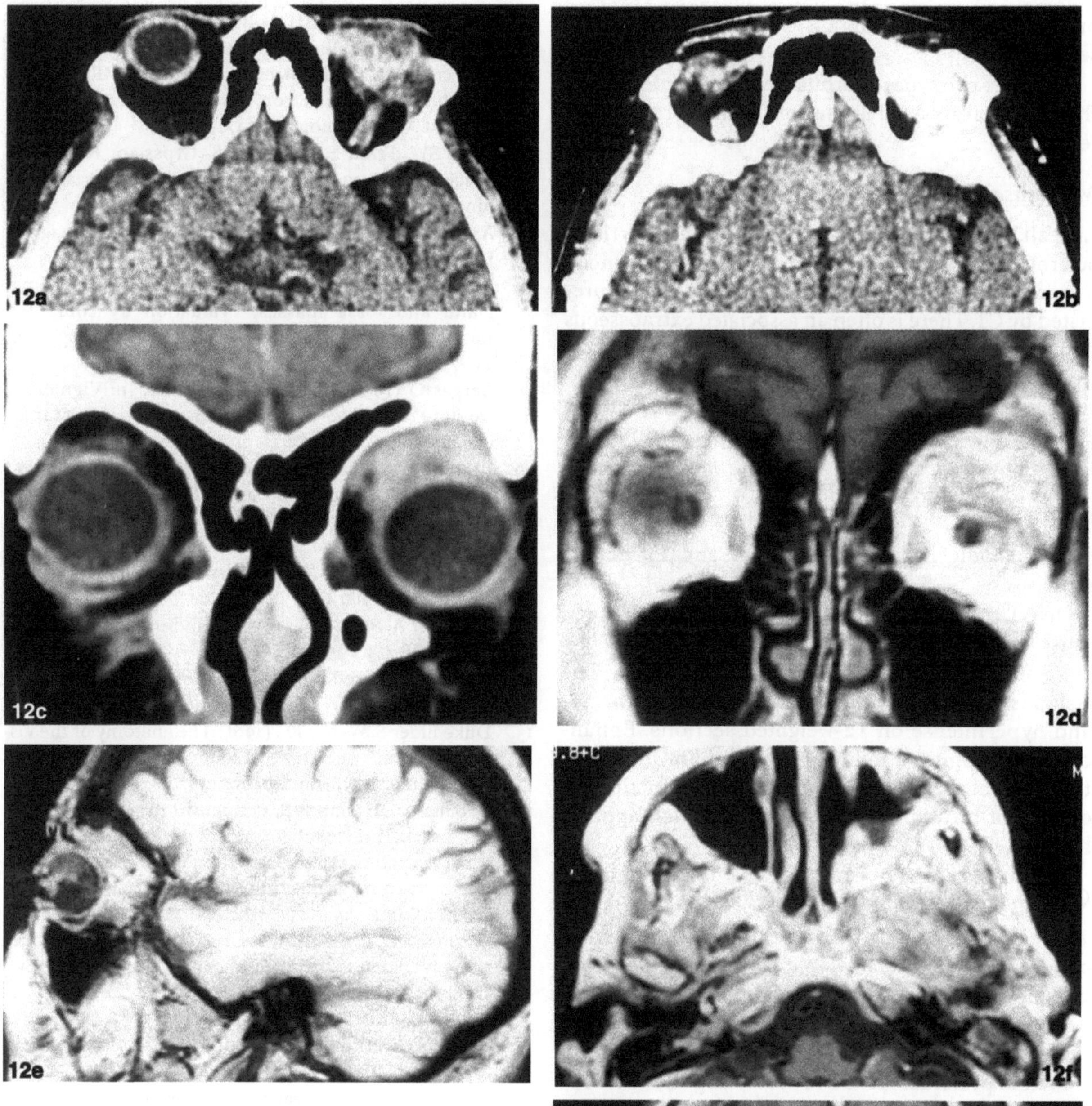

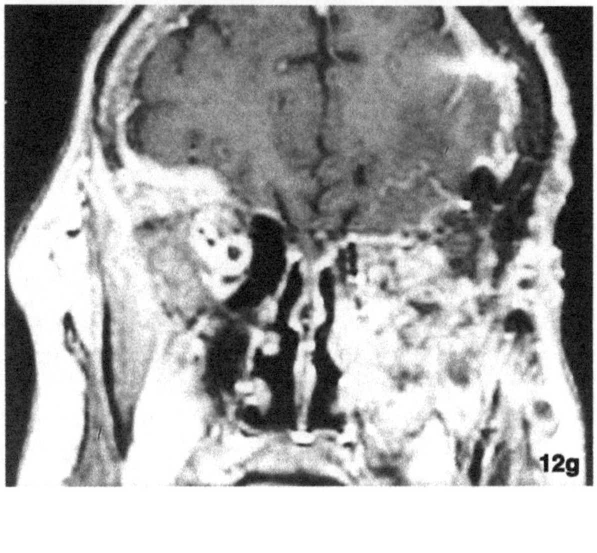

Fig. 5.12. 56 year old patient with an intraorbital metastasis from an adenocarcinoma. CT: **a, b** pre- and post-contrast sections: soft tissue lesion in the left supraocular region, encasing the superior and lateral rectus muscles. Homogeneous enhancement pattern; **c** direct coronal post-contrast section: this section demonstrates the inability to individually identify the superior rectus muscle; **d, e** coronal and sagittal T1 sections post-gadolinium: there is a better definition of the posterior extent of the lesion and invasion of the superior and lateral rectus muscles on the images. MRI: **f-g** two years after excision of the orbital metastasis showing very advanced invasion of the operative site, the pterygo-maxillary fossa, the meninges and the subdural spaces

orbital sympathoblastoma is an extremely unusual, separate entity.

There are two types of orbital secondaries: lesions of the bony margins and lesions of the intraorbital contents.

Metastases of the bony margins

Like all bone metastases, they may present as lytic or sclerotic areas depending on the primary cancer. These lesions of the orbital margins are best appreciated by CT. There is often an associated extraosseous soft tissue extension, better seen on MRI and appearing usually iso- or hypointense on T1- and hyperintense on T2-weighted images. Heterogeneous enhancement is most often seen after gadolinium injection.

Metastases to the intraorbital structures

These usually involve the muscles and intraconal structures.

On CT, they appear as a soft tissue mass, isodense to muscle, and enhancing after contrast injection.

No specific MRI features have been reported. The lesion is usually iso- or hypointense to muscle on T1- and hyperintense on T2-weighted sections. Enhancement is common following gadolinium injection. Intraorbital metastases are characterized by the frequency of intratumoral hemorrhage which appears hyperintense on T1.

Orbital metastases from sympathoblastoma

These arise from retroperitoneal neuroblastoma in children and are characterized by an important clinical syndrome comprising of exophthalmos and periorbital ecchymoses. Orbital metastases from neuroblastoma tend to occur frequently.

MRI is preferable to CT for assessing the extent of the lesion which appears hypointense on T1- , hyperintense on T2-weighted images, and enhances post-gadolinium injection.

References

1. Abramson DH, Ellsworth R, Kitchin S (1984) Second non ocular tumors in retinoblastoma survivors. Ophthalmology 91: 1351-1355
2. Atlas SW, Bilaniuk LT, Zimmermann RA (1988) MR imaging of the orbit. In: Stark D, Bradley WG (eds) Magnetic Resonance Imaging. Mosby, St-Louis
3. Atlas S, Bilaniuk LT, Zimmerman RA et al (1988) Orbit: initial experience with surface coil spin-echo MR Imaging at 1.5 T. Radiology 164: 501-509
4. Atlas SW, Braffman BH, LoBrutto R, Elder D, Herlyn D (1990) Human malignant melanomas with varying melanin content in nude mice: correlations of MR with histopathology and electron paramagnetic resonance. J Comput Assist Tomogr 14: 547-554
5. Atlas SW, Fram EK, Mark AS. Grpss,am RO (1988) Vascular intracranial lesions: applications of fast scanning. Radiology 169: 455-461
6. Axel L (1984) Surface coil magnetic resonance imaging. J Comput Assist Tomogr 8: 381-384
7. Balchunas WR, Quencer RM, Byrne SF (1983) Lacrimal gland and fossa masses: evaluation by computed tomography and A-mode echography. Radiology 149: 751-758
8. Berges O (1988) Pathologie orbitaire. In: Vignaud J, Boulin A (eds) Tomodensitométrie cranio-encéphalique. Vigot, Paris, pp 503-550
9. Bradley WG (1987) MR appearance of flowing blood and CSF. In: Brant-Zawadzki M, Norman D (eds) Magnetic Resonance Imaging in the Central Nervous System. Raven Press, New York, pp 93-96
10. Brateman L (1986) Chemical shift imaging: a review. AFT 146: 971-980
11. Danziger A, Price HI (1979) CT findings in retino-blastoma. AFR 133: 695-697
12. Dufier JL, Pierre Kahn A (1986) Les tumeurs orbitaires de l'enfant. Archives Françaises de Pédiatrie 43: 133-139
13. Duke Elder S, Wybar KC (1961) The anatomy of the visual system. In: Duke Elder S (ed) System of Ophthalmology. Kimpton, London
14. Enochs WS, Hyslop WB, Bennett JF, Brown RD, Koenig SH, Swartz HM (1989) Sources of the increased longitudinal relaxation rates observed in melanotic melanoma and in vitro study of synthetic melanins. Invest Radiol 24: 794-804
15. Enzmann D, Donaldson S, Kriss JP (1979) Appearance of Graves' disease on orbital computed tomography. J Comput Assist Tomogr 3: 815-819
16. Fries PD, Char DH, Norman D (1987) MR imaging of orbital cavernous hemangioma. J Comput Assist Tomogr 11: 418-421
17. Gardner TW, Zaparackas ZG, Naidich TP (1984) Congenital optic nerve colobomas: CT demonstration. J Comput Assist Tomogr 8: 95-102
18. Holland, BA, Kucharcyzk W, Brant-Zawadzki M, Norman D, Haas DK, Harper PS (1985) MR imaging of calcified intracranial lesions. Radiology 157: 353-356
19. Hoyt WF, Imes RK (1990) Optic gliomas of neurofibromatosis: contemporary perspectives. In: Ishibashi Y, Hoti Y (eds) Tuberous sclerosis and neurofibromatosis: epidemiology, biology and management. Elsevier Science Publisher
20. Johnson G, Mill DH, Mac Manus D, et al (1987) Stir sequences in NMR imaging of the optic nerve. Neuroradiology 29: 238-245
21. Knowles DMI, Jakobiec FA (1980) Orbital lymphoid neoplasms: a clinicopathologic study of 60 cases. Cancer 46: 579-589

22. Koenig SH, Brown RD (1988) The raw and the cooked, or the importance of the motion of water for MRI revisited. Invest Radiol 23: 495-497
23. Linder B, Campos M, Schafer M (1987) CT and MRI of orbital abnormalities in neurofibromatosis and selected craniofacial anomalies. Radiol Clin North Am 25: 787-802
24. Lloyd GAS (1975) Radiology of the orbit. Saunders, London
25. Mafee MF, Peyman GA, McKusick MA (1985) Malignant uveal melanoma and similar lesions studied by computed tomography. Radiology 156: 403-408
26. Nugent RA, Lapointe JS, Rootman J, Robertson WD, Graeb DA (1987) Orbital dermoids features on CT. Radiology 165:475-478
27. Peyster RG, Augsburger JJ, Shields JA, Hershey BL, Eagle R Jr, Haskin ME (1988) Intraocular tumors: evaluation with MR imaging. Radiology 168: 773-779
28. Peyster RG, Shapiro MD, Haik BG (1987) Orbital metastasis: role of magnetic resonance imaging and computer tomography. Radiol Clin North Am 25: 647-662
29. Rootman J, Damji KF, Dimmick JE (1989) Malignant rhabdoid tumor of the orbit. Ophthalmology 96: 1650-1654
30. Sandberg-Wolheim M, Bynke H, Cronqvist S, Holtas S, Platz P, Ryder LP (1990) A long-term prospective study of optic neuritis: evaluation of risk factors. Ann Neurol 27: 386-393
31. Shields JA, Shields CL, Lieb WE, Eagle RC (1990) Multiple orbital neurofibromas unassociated with von Recklinghausen's disease. Arch Ophthalmol 108: 80-83
32. Sobel DF, Mills C, Char D, et al (1984) NMR of the normal and pathologic eye and orbit. Am J Neuroradiol 5: 345-350
33. Sobel DF, Kelly W, Kjos BO, et al (1985) MR imaging of orbital and ocular disease. Am J Neuroradiol 6: 259-264
34. Stem J, Jakobiec FA, Housepien EM (1980) The architecture of optic nerve gliomas with and without neurobibromatosis. Arch Ophthalmol 98: 505-511
35. Sullivan JA, Harms SE (1986) Surgace-coil MR imaging of orbital neoplasms. Am J Neuroradiol 7: 29-34
36. Pasztor E, Remenar L (1978) Optic nerve gliomas. 1 - Clinical diagnosis and pathology. Acta Neurochir 41: 191-203
37. Pigeau I, Guinet C, Meary, et al (1990) IRM du globe et de l'orbite: comparaison des séquences en échos de gradient et échos dde spin. apport du gadolinium. Rev Imagerie Médicale 2: 299-307
38. Sobel DF, Salvolini U, Newton TH (1988) Ocular and orbital pathology in computed tomography of the head and neck. In: Newton TH, et al (eds) Modern neuroradiology. Clavadel Book. Raven Press, New York, pp 91-694
39. Ulshafer RJ, Allen CB, Rubin ML (1990) Distributions of elements in the human retinal pigment epithelium. Arch Ophthalmol 108: 113-117
40. Vade A, Armstrong D (1987) Orbital rhabdomyosarcoma in childhood in imaging in ophthalmology. Radiol Clin North Am: 701-714
41. Wolter JR, Knoblich RR (1965) Pathway of centrifugal fibres in human optic nerve, chiasm and tract. Br J Ophthalmol 49: 246-250
42. Zimmermann RA, Bilaniuk LT, Metzger RA, et al (1983) Computed tomography of orbital facial neurofibromatosis. Radiology 146: 115-116

CHAPTER 6

Malignant sellar, parasellar and skull base tumors

Clinicians
R. Grob, J.-V. Chantelard, E.-Ch. Antoine, J. de Recondo, B. Charbonnel, D. Khayat

Radiologists
B. Dupas, J.-M. Mussini, M. Gayet-Delacroix, D. Buthiau

Accurate imaging by CT and particularly MRI is indicated in cases where the endocrinological and /or secondary neurological signs point to a tumor involving the sellar, parasellar regions or the skull base.

Endocrine signs

Hypersecretion of the anterior pituitary hormones causes the clinical features which necessitate imaging of the hypothalamo-pituitary region to determine the etiology. Hyperprolactinemia is the commonest, but acromegaly due to growth hormone hypersecretion, Cushing's disease and exceptionally gonadotrophin and thyrotrophin secreting adenomas are also encountered. Insufficiency of the anterior and posterior pituitary is frequently associated with tumors and is an indication for imaging. Diabetes insipidus and polydipsia are often associated with a hypothalamic lesion which first excludes simple causes such as diabetes mellitus or hypercalcemia.

Neurological signs

Involvement of cranial nerves

Cranial nerve involvement may be isolated or include several contiguous or even topographically remote nerves. In the latter case, it is useful to describe the associated syndromes according to the localization (table. 6.1): syndrome of the sphenoidal fissure, jugular foramen, petrous apex... These syndromes comprising of various cranial nerve deficits should always immediately raise the suspicion of an underlying tumor. Clinical examination at this stage is a useful guide to the radiological investigations.

Similarly, syndromes of the anterior, midportion or posterior wall of the cavernous sinuses are defined by the associated cranial nerve deficits and have the same valuable feature of localizing signs. These are very similar or even identical to the so-called parasellar syndromes. They are likely to be due to arterial or venous abnormalities, either acute or chronic, or local inflammatory lesions as tumors.

Isolated cranial nerve involvement is much less specific both for localization and etiology. For instance, oculomotor nerve paresis, pure hemifacial spasm,

Table 6.1. The principal clinical syndromes of multiple cranial nerve involvement

Semiology	Name of syndrome
II, III, IV, V, VI	Syndrome of the orbital apex
III, IV, V, VI	Syndrome of the sphenoidal fissure
III, IV, VI, ± 2 or 3	Syndrome of the cavernous sinus
V, VI	Syndrome of the petrous apex, called Gradenigo's syndrome
V, sympathetic	Syndrome of the paratrigeminal space, called Raeder's syndrome
VII, VIII, ± other nerves	Syndrome of the cerebello-pontine angle
IX, X, XI	Syndrome of the jugular foramen
IX, X, XI, XII	Syndrome of the anterior condyle
I ± II ± III ± IV...XII	Garcin's syndrome

regardless of the speed of onset, can be due to a multitude of etiologies. Neoplastic disease is not always the commonest. The most extreme example is palsy of the VIth cranial nerve which is the least specific of all the lesions in the CNS (the "Cinderella of Neurology" according to J. Lapresle). This explains the necessity and value of imaging over a large area if there are no preexisting localizing clinical signs.

Painful syndromes indicating a tumor of the skull base or parasellar region result from the sensory or very rich sympathetic innervation of certain areas of the meninges and should be considered separately. Such is the case for retro-orbital and parasellar lesions simulating painful ophthalmoplegia (Tolosa-Hunt) or ophthalmoplegic migraine; this also applies to certain lesions of the petrous bone invading the tentorium cerebelli and readily causing headaches suggestive of migraine or facial pain of vascular origin.

The sequelae of parenchymal involvement

These have become rare as presenting features and are avoided by the early use of modern imaging techniques in the majority of cases. Nevertheless, focal signs may occur during the clinical progression of such a tumor: epileptic fit, usually focal and especially "temporal", uncinate or hallucinatory, pyramidal motor deficit, signs of compression or distortion of the metencephalon or mesencephalon... the mechanisms are variable. A meningioma of the lesser wing of the sphenoid elevates the temporal cortex, whereas the same tumor in a more medial location, e.g. parasellar, may encase the internal carotid artery causing thrombosis and subsequent infarction.

CSF flow disturbances

Intracranial hypertension is rare in these tumors. Headaches are most commonly due to bone pain or related to invasion of sensory nerves such as the trigeminal nerve. Tumor expansion is rarely sufficient to cause pure intracranial hypertension. True hydrocephalus remains the exception:

- tumor of the skull base associated with an inflammatory reaction or tumor invasion of the arachnoid space which produces a communicating hydrocephalus;
- large lesion of the clivus and foramen magnum, complete obstruction to the circulation of CSF.

In these rare situations, the signs of intracranial hypertension may dominate the clinical picture at presentation.

Diagnosis of an anterior pituitary tumor

Pituitary adenomas

These represent 10% of intracranial tumors. They either present with hormonal hypersecretion (most common in young patients) or are non-functioning and are clinically silent until the onset of a complication (patients more than 50 years old) due to compression of the chiasm, hypopituitarism or hemorrhagic complications and/or acute necrosis [17, 27]. Rarely, adenomas arise in the context of a familial multiple endocrine neoplasia syndrome (MENS). The radiological classification is based on size criteria: a microadenoma is less than 10 mm and a macroadenoma greater than 10 mm. It is sometimes difficult to identify a microadenoma within a healthy pituitary and conversely to differentiate the normal pituitary parenchyme compressed by a macroadenoma.

Diagnosis of microadenomas (figs 6.1 & 6.2)

These benign lesions will not be described here.

Diagnosis of macroadenomas

Imaging is able to assess the extent of an intra- and/or suprasellar tumor of greater than 10 mm in diameter, but the differentiation between an expanding and invasive macroadenoma may sometimes be difficult. Pretherapeutic investigation is essential, examination in three planes is possible with MRI, the post-gadolinium T1-weighted sequence is indispensable to appreciate the limits and extent of the tumor and particularly its relationship to the cavernous sinus.

CT is still useful for the diagnosis of calcifications. MRI would appear from now on to be superior to CT in the diagnosis, preoperative assessment and follow-up, either during medical treatment or post-operatively.

Findings

CT

Calcifications are visible in the sellar region on the pre-contrast examination; the enhancement following contrast injection is heterogeneous and depends on the consistency of the tumor, i.e. solid, partially necrotic or hemorrhagic. Following the injection, the contours of the tumor are generally best defined relative to the adjacent structures; but the extension of the

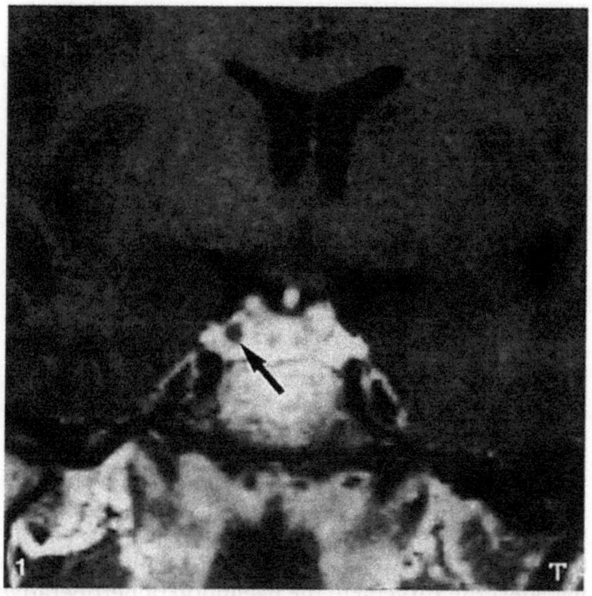

Fig. 6.1. Hyperprolactinemia (120 ng/ml) in a 25 year old female. Ectopic intracavernous microadenoma on the right appearing hypointense on post-gadolinium MRI, measuring 4 mm in diameter *(arrow)*

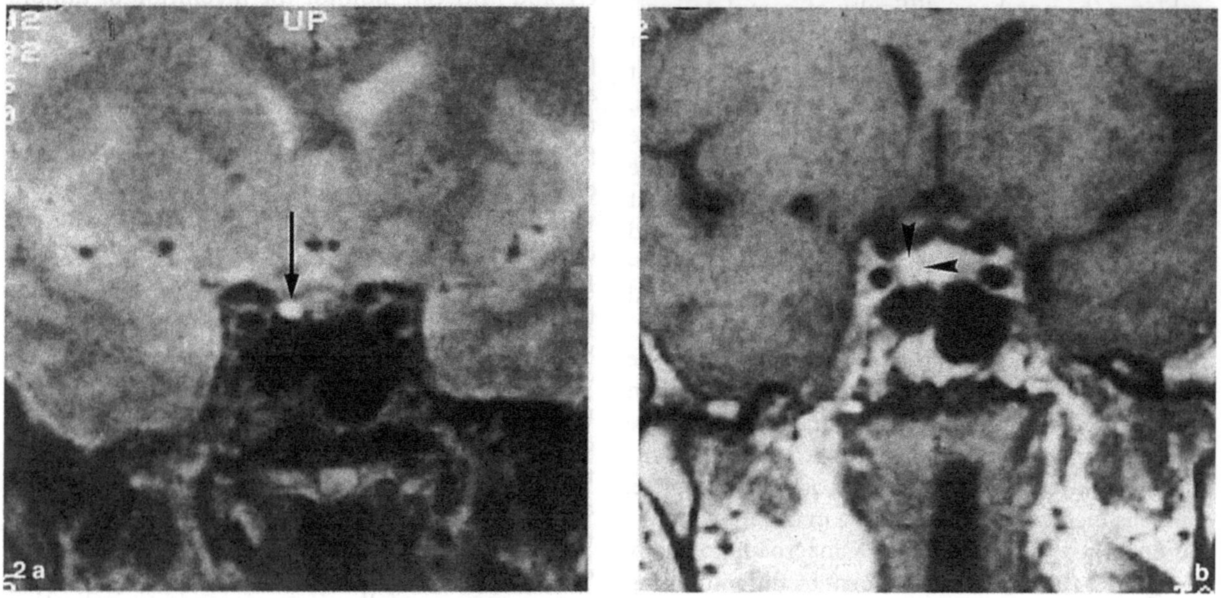

Fig. 6.2 a, b. Cushing's disease in a 31 year old male. MRI of a 5 mm microadenoma in the right lobe of the pituitary appearing hyperintense on T2-weighted imaging (**a**, *arrow*), and hyperintense on T1-weighted imaging following gadolinium injection (**b**, *arrow*)

tumor into the suprasellar cisterns, cavernous sinuses or skull base is more accurately assessed by MRI.

MRI

The signal intensity (table 6.2) of the tumor is often mixed due to the heterogeneous composition of the tumor which comprises of areas of cystic degeneration or necrosis. There may be associated hemorrhagic complications which sometimes cause a sudden onset of clinical symptoms ("pituitary apoplexy"). However, the majority of macroadenomas are isointense to brain tissue on T1- and T2-weighted imaging. Hence the gadolinium enhances the borders of the lesion. There is no correlation between the signal intensity and hormonal activity of the pituitary macroadenoma. When the tumor is enlarged, it is impossible to identify the normal residual pituitary tissue in the pituitary fossa.

Limits and extent of the tumor

The contours of the tumor are defined in relation to the suprasellar cisterns, and its limits relative to the brain parenchyme, optic chiasma and carotid vessels.

Table 6.2. Significance of signal intensities on MRI

T1-weighted sequence		T2-weighted sequence	
Hyperintense	Hypointense	Hyperintense	Hypointense
Methemoglobin (chronic and subacute hemorrhage)	Hemosiderin Calcifications	Methemoglobin (chronic and subacute hemorrhage)	Hemosiderin Calcifications
Fat	CSF	CSF	Fat
Mucopolysaccharides and certain proteins	Cyst contents (depending on chemical composition)	Cyst contents (depending on chemical composition)	Melanin
Melanin	Necrotic contents	Necrotic contents	Solid tumor
Solid tumor	Solid tumor	Solid tumor	

An hour glass deformity may be present due to constriction of the tumor by the diaphragma sella. This will alert the surgeon to the likelihood of peroperative problems (hemorrhage, difficulty of complete excision, CSF leak). The optic chiasma in better seen on MRI than CT may be deformed and displaced without necessarily any resultant visual field disturbances. Non-visualization or encasement of the chiasma are features suspicious of a tumor not arising from the pituitary. MRI accurately defines the superior extent of the tumor by its relationship to the floor and recesses of the 3rd ventricle and by assessment of displacement or encasement of the anterior cerebral arteries.

Invasive macroadenomas (fig. 6.3) may invade the dura mater of the sellar floor, diaphragma sella (when the superior borders are irregular) or laterally into the cavernous sinuses. Encasement of the intracavernous portion of the carotid artery, either partial or complete, confirms the invasive nature of the macroadenoma.

Preoperative assessment of a macroadenoma by MRI guides the choice of treatment by differentiating invasive from non-invasive adenomas, and the macroadenoma is usually inaccessible via the transphenoidal approach. However, some lesions are surgically inaccessible via the skull base (subfrontal extension above the jugum, temporal extension, retroclival extension, narrow collar at the level of the diaphragmatic orifice),and necessitate a transcranial approach as either the initial or secondary procedure.

MRI is therefore the examination of choice in the preoperative assessment of macroadenomas. It can precisely determine whether the adenoma is well defined or invasive, thus guiding the surgical approach. The information obtained from the MRI usually removes the need for preoperative arteriography.

Follow-up of macroadenomas on medical treatment, post-surgery or radiotherapy

CT and MRI can monitor the involution of tumors under medical treatment, bromocriptine for macroprolactinomas or somatostatin for GH secreting adenomas. The effect of bromocriptine in reducing the size of the tumor may be significant even after the first week of treatment [18] but can persist over several years. Similarly, signal changes may be seen within the tumor corresponding to subacute or chronic hemorrhage associated with necrosis. Invagination of the chiasma with intrasellar herniation of the suprasellar cisterns is common but does not result in any visual disturbance. Periodic follow-up by MRI during medical treatment of prolactinomas is essential for detection of possible re-expansion of the tumor which may occur without elevation of the prolactin level. It is advisable to scan the patient at 6 months following surgery [32] due to the difficulties of image interpretation in the immediate post-operative period. The diagnosis by MRI of residual or recurrent tumor following surgery is an indication for radiotherapy, particularly in the case of residual intracavernous tumor. Intra- and parasellar calcifications following surgery and/or radiotherapy are visualized only on CT.

Other lesions

Metastases

Hypophyseal metastases are rarely symptomatic. Symptoms arise from anterior pituitary dysfunction (usually hypopituitarism) or diabetes insipidus due to infiltration of the infundibulum [30]. They may be invasive and cause an oculomotor disturbance by

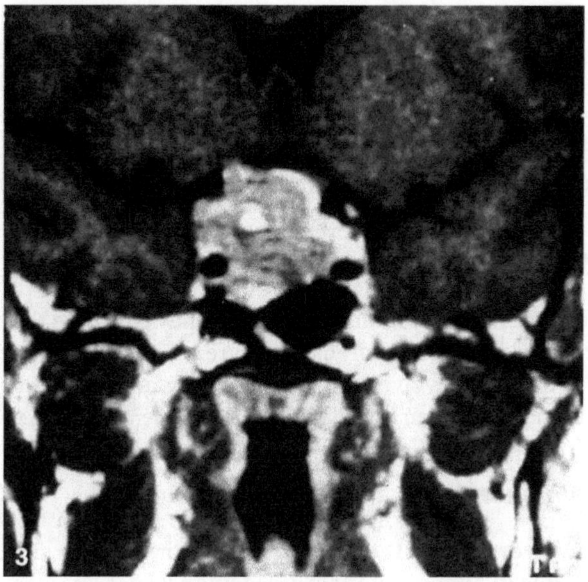

Fig. 6.3. Marked reduction in visual acuity for 6 months in 33 year old male. Suspicion of a retrobulbar neuritis on the right. Visual field defect and reduced libido. MRI, coronal T1-weighted sequence following the gadolinium injection: intra- and suprasellar tumor displacing the optic chiasma, eroding the walls of the sella turcica, appearing hyperintense in its upper border. The lesion measures 25 mm in height; the tumor is invading the right cavernous sinus with hemicircumferential encasement of the intracavernous portion of the carotid artery. Hormonal assay performed after imaging revealed a hyperprolactinemia of 200 ng/ml. This was a macroprolactinaemia which was treated medically with high dose bromocriptine

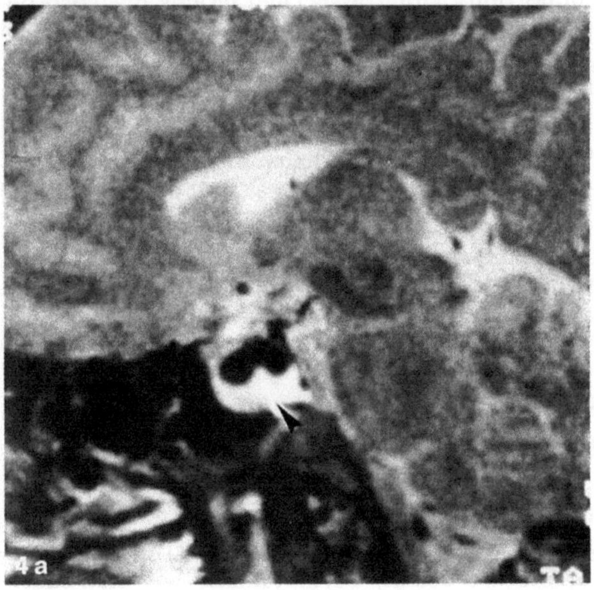

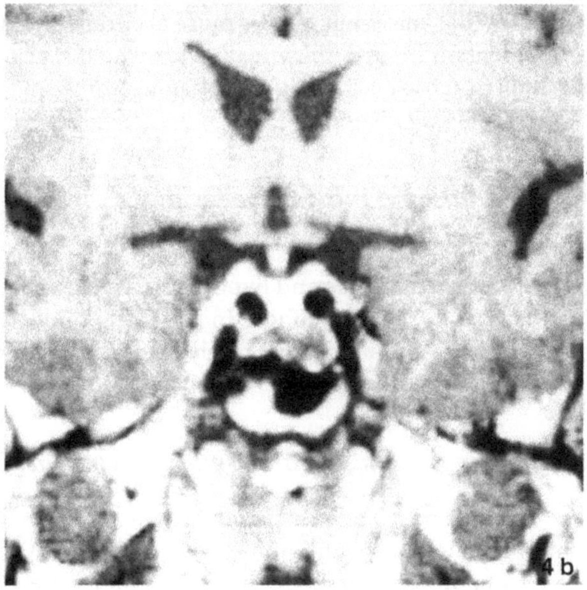

Fig. 6.4 a, b. 35 year old female presenting with type 1 mdultiple endocrine neoplasia and hyperprolactinemia. Previous parathyroidectomy, right adrenalectomy and resection of the pancreatic tale with splenectomy for Zollinger-Ellison syndrome. **a** MRI sagittal T2-weighted sequence. Hyperintense infrasellar macroadenoma (15 mm) (arrowhead). **b** Coronal T1-weighted sequence following the gadolinium injection: the infrasellar adenoma appears hypointense, and is eroding the sellar floor and comes into contact with the carotid artery

involvement of the cavernous sinus (compression of the III, IV, and VI cranial nerves). The commonest primary tumors to cause hypophyseal and hypothalamic metastasis are carcinoma of the breast and bronchus [20].

CT and MRI demonstrate intra- and/or suprasellar tumor masses. On MRI, the lesion is usually isointense on T1-weighted imaging and moderately hyperintense on T2-weighted imaging. Following the injection of gadolinium the enhancement is homogeneous or "ring like". The suprasellar lesions often have an hour glass appearance due to narrowing at the diaphragma sella and may invade the floor of the 3rd ventricle. The rapidly invasive nature of metastasis is also apparent by involvement of the skull base with extension to the clivus and petrous apex with irregular borders due to the rapid growth. Metastasis from melanoma may appear hyperintense on a T1-weighted sequence [7] due to the paramagnetic effect of melanin and must be differentiate from a hemorrhagic lesion (adenoma), or lipid contents, cholesterol (epidermoid cyst) or mucopolysacharrides (cyst of Rathke's pouch).

Multiple endocrine neoplasia

This multi-organ familial condition may effect the thyroid, parathyroids, adrenals, pancreas, liver and lungs.

Pituitary involvement appeared as an intrasellar tumor mass, often causing hyperprolactinemia (fig. 6.4).

Lymphoma

Involvement of the anterior pituitary is rare and results in hypopituitarism. CT demonstrates an intra- or suprasellar mass, but MRI is more accurate in the assessment of this area showing a lesion which is usually hyperintense on T2-weighted imaging, sometimes with direct bony invasion.

Granulomas and infiltrative lesions

Non-infectious granulomas can involve simultaneously the hypothalamus and hypophysis. In children, histiocytosis is the commonest. In adults, sarcoidosis and Wegener's granulomatosis rarely involve the anterior pituitary.

Pseudotumors and hypophyseal hyperplasia

The diagnosis is made in patients with functional hyperprolactinemia with symmetrical enlargement of the pituitary, a convex superior border and homogeneous enhancement following gadolinium injection on MRI. The prolactin levels are moderately elevated and increased further following the TRH stimulation test as the pituitary is still responsive. Hypothyroidism can also result from pseudotumoral hypophyseal hyperplasia which regresses following treatment with thyroid hormones [14].

Diagnosis of a tumor of the pituitary stalk and/or posterior pituitary

Growth problems (growth retardation, congenital hypopituitarism) and diabetes insipidus are the principle indications for investigation of the pituitary stalk and posterior pituitary. Numerous authors have emphasized the need for repeated MRI examination in cases of diabetes insipidus with or without associated involvement of the anterior pituitary. Diabetes insipidus may be primary (idiopathic, sporadic or familial) or acquired, secondary to a hypothalamo-hypophyseal tumor, trauma with transection of the pituitary stalk, an inflammatory lesion or autoimmune neuro-hypophysitis.

Tumors of the hypothalamo-hypophyseal axis

Absence of the hyperintensity of the posterior pituitary on a T1-weighted sequence is a constant feature and usually associated with thickening of the infundibulum and pituitary stalk (greater than 3 mm in its midportion). Other associated lesions may also be demonstrated: invasion of the floor of the third ventricle and/or hypothalamus, pineal tumor.

The etiology of a hypothalamo-hypophyseal tumor [35, 36] includes germinomas, teratomas, craniopharyngiomas, hypothalamic gliomas, metastasis and histiocytosis X. Histiocytosis X in children appears as symmetrical thickening of the pituitary stalk with loss of the high signal intensity of the posterior pituitary. The differential diagnosis consists of tuberculosis and sarcoidosis of the pituitary stalk.

Primary tumors of the neurohypophysis and infundibulum

These are extremely rare. Two types are recognized: glioma (or pituicytoma) and choristoma. These tumors are usually asymptomatic but may cause symptoms if sufficiently large: headaches, visual disturbances, reduced libido, infertility. Authors have described a mass appearing isointense on T1- and T2-weighted imaging [8] in the rare published cases.

Diagnosis of a juxtasellar tumor: supra-, latero-, infra- and/or retrosellar

Lesions of the cavernous sinuses

Lesions involving the cavernous sinuses are classified as inflammatory (thrombo-phlebitis of the cavernous sinuses), vascular (carotid-cavernous fistula, carotid artery aneurysm), neoplastic (neurinoma, meningioma, metastasis), and secondary tumor extension into the cavernous sinus (pituitary adenoma). Some lesions of the cavernous sinuses can, in the future, be approached using the latest neurosurgical techniques and hence the primary interest in tumor evaluation by MRI which is superior to CT. Whatever the cause, involvement of the cavernous sinus appears as an expansive enlargement of the cavernous sinus: convexity of the lateral wall of the cavernous sinus, bony erosion of the sphenoid sinus. These two signs are well seen on CT and MRI, but the bony signs are better shown on CT. If the lesion is unilateral, asymmetry of the cavernous sinuses is apparent. Gadolinium injection is indispensable in order to improve the definition of the borders of the tumor and meningeal involvement.

CT

Coronal sections (3 mm) with a high dose of intravenous contrast are essential for demonstrating the hypodense intracavernous cranial nerves and Meckel's cave. Involvement of the cavernous sinuses on CT (fig. 6.5) appears as effacement of the normal hypodensity of Meckel's cave associated with filling defects within the cavernous sinus.

MRI

This is complementary to CT; injection of gadolinium gives better definition of the tumor boundaries. However, small isointense meningiomas may be missed, and CT is more sensitive due to the presence of calcification and/or hyperostosis.

The Tolosa-Hunt syndrome presents clinically as a painful ophthalmoplegia caused by inflammation of the cavernous sinus and is one of the differential diagnoses of cavernous sinus tumors. It is an inflammatory lesion and resolves on steroid treatment appearing on MRI as a mass of the cavernous sinus. On the T1 sequence it is hypointense to fat and isointense to muscle; the signal of this pseudotumor (similar to orbital pseudotumors) is isointense to fat on T2-weighted imaging [41].

Parasellar tumors

Craniopharyngiomas

The commonest cause of acquired hypopituitarism; these are benign embryological tumors characterized

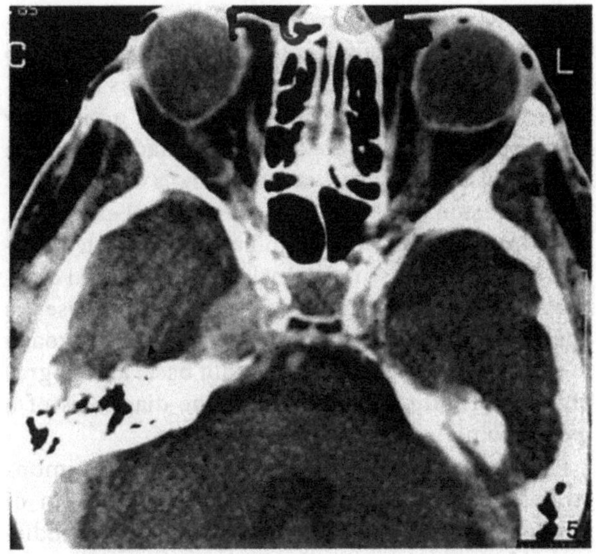

Fig. 6.5. Paresis of the right 5th and 6th nerves of sudden onset in an 82 year old female. Contrast enhanced shows an axial CT metastasis in the right cavernous sinus on both sides of the petro-clinoid ligament. The lateral border of the right cavernous sinus is convex

histologically by three components (cystic, soft tissue and calcium, the latter better seen on CT), the majority being predominantly cystic.

Craniopharyngiomas [1, 2] are either both intra- and suprasellar (70%), or suprasellar (20%) or purely intrasellar (10%). They may be detected incidentally or present with pituitary insufficiency, delayed puberty, diabetes insipidus, signs of chiasmatic compression or intracranial hypertension.

Meningiomas of the sellar region

The diagnostic accuracy of contrast enhanced CT for a meningioma approaches 90%, but MRI gives a better assessment of the extent of the tumor preoperatively relative to the adjacent structures [13].

Unlike meningiomas in adults, the meningiomas in children principally occur in boys, with a rapid growth rate and a tendency to sarcomatous degeneration [6]. Meningiomas represent 15 to 20% of all intracranial tumors and 5% occur in suprasellar region and may have an intrasellar extension [23].

On pre-contrast CT, the typical signs are those of an intrinsically hyperdense tumor which may contain calcification and be associated with hyperostosis. Following injection, the tumor becomes enhanced intensely and blended with the adjacent dura mater.

On MRI, it is isointense with the adjacent parenchyme on T1 WI. Gadolinium injection is essential to demonstrate the very definite homogeneous hyperintensity of the tumor, greater than that of a pituitary macroadenoma. The thickening of the adjacent dura mater is also well shown, as well as signs of cavernous sinus invasion. MRI evaluates locoregional extension. The rare intrasellar meningiomas can simulate pituitary adenomas. It is vital to make the differential diagnosis between meningioma and adenoma because the operative approach is different: the surgical approach to meningiomas is not via the skull base; arteriography is still indicated to confirm the diagnosis of a meningioma.

Finally, in the case of a meningioma, CT demonstrates the hyperostosis, MRI assesses invasion of adjacent structures and arteriography remains indispensable in the preoperative assessment. Post-operative follow-up of meningiomas is essential using MRI with or without gadolinium injection in order to detect residual or recurrent tumor [39] which may indicate a very aggressive lesion.

Meningoangiomatosis

This is a rare benign hamartoma of the leptomeninges. Some authors consider it to be an unrefined form of neurofibromatosis. On CT, the lesion contains psammomatous calcifications, and on MRI there is a peripheral hyperintensity of the mass associated with edema of the white matter on the T2-weighted sequence.

Gliomas of the sellar region

MRI is the investigation of choice for the assessment of these lesions. Opto-chiasmatic glioma is a tumor of children which is associated in a third of cases with von Recklinghausen's disease. The chiasma is enlarged (fig. 6.6), usually isointense on T1- weighted imaging, hyper- or isointense on T2-weighted imaging. These signal changes are not characteristic, but MRI allows an assessment of the tumor in three dimensions relative to the other parasellar structures.

Hypothalamic glioma is a tumor of adults and occurs in the wall of the 3rd ventricle; MRI is the investigation of choice to demonstrate the position and extent of this infiltrative and poorly defined lesion.

Hypothalamic hamartomas, lipomas of the tuber cinereum, epidermoid cysts

These form a part of the differential diagnosis.

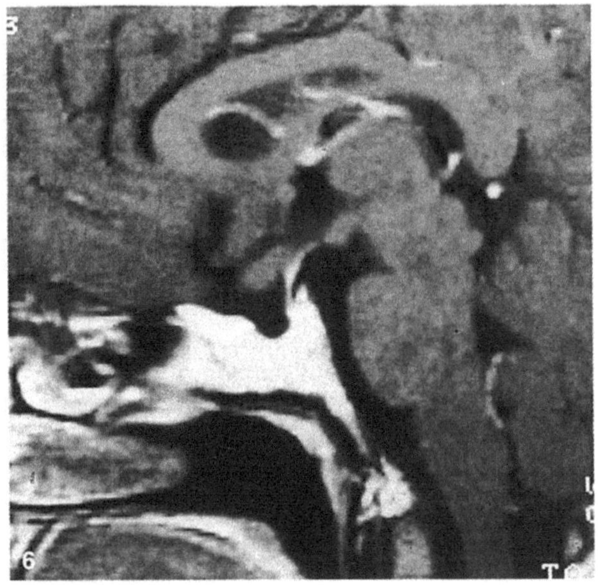

Fig. 6.6. Pituitary insufficiency in an 18 year old female. MRI: T1-weighted sequence following the gadolinium injection. Thickening of the optic chiasma due to a glioma. The pituitary stalk is normal. Non-visualization of the anterior pituitary explaining the pituitary insufficiency

Other parasellar tumors

Juxtasellar neurinomas (tumors of the cranial nerves within the cavernous sinuses), metastasis and malignant lymphomas may invade the suprasellar cisterns [29].

Cystic lesions

Whether a cyst of Rathke's pouch, an arachnoid cyst or colloid cyst, these lesions are all benign and should be included in the differential diagnosis.

Mucocele of the sphenoid sinus

A sphenoidal mucocele occurs as a result of accumulation of mucus secretions in the sinus which may be due to a benign or malignant cause. The signal characteristics are very variable depending on the age of the lesion, its degree of hydration and chemical composition. The signal is hypointense on T1-weighted imaging and hyperintense on T2-weighted imaging if the content is predominantly water, hyperintense on T1-weighted imaging if the contents are proteinaceous. There is always regular expansion of the bony walls occasionally with postero-superior displacement of the pituitary.

Diagnosis of a skull base tumor

Assessment of extent

CT and MRI are complementary in the initial diagnosis and give a precise assessment of size, localization and extent of the tumor mass.

MRI has a role in planning the surgical approach for complete resection of large tumors. It is also essential in the follow-up after surgical excision and/or radiotherapy.

CT can demonstrate extension into the adjacent bony structures, namely the sphenoid, ethmoid and petrous bones. The anatomical relationships with vessels and nerves are defined on MRI. MRI is superior to arteriography for assessing vascular invasion. It is impossible to give a definitive diagnosis as to the exact nature of the tumor based solely on the CT and MRI appearances: the role of imaging is to accurately define the locoregional extent by showing extension into the cavernous sinus, the sella turcica, sphenoid sinus and parapharyngeal space. This assessment is important since radical resection of certain tumors may in future be possible with the advent of new surgical techniques. A large number of primary or secondary tumors can affect the skull base.

Assessment of etiology

Chordomas

Slowly growing embryonic tumors derived from the notochord, chordomas are rare tumors representing less than 1% of all intracranial tumors and only 3 to 4% of primary bone tumors [10]. They are locally invasive, rarely metastasize and primarily affect the clivus. They are radio-resistant, and preoperative evaluation by imaging is therefore important in order to assess the extent of the tumor.

CT and MRI are equally sensitive in tumor detection, but MRI is superior for the evaluation of the extension of the lesion, particularly the encasement of vascular structures and the degree of intracranial spread.

CT demonstrates intratumoral calcification and the degree of bony destruction. On MRI, chordomas are isointense on T1-weighted imaging and hyperintense on T2-weighted imaging, the hypointense zones corresponding to calcification. Cystic or hemorrhagic areas have been described within the tumor, responsible for increased hyperintensity on T2-weighted imaging. No significant difference in the signal characteristics on MRI has been demonstrated between the typical chordomas and chondroid chordomas.

The two types of tumors are enhanced in a heterogeneous fashion following the injection of gadolinium. Displacement and/or encasement of vessels is common, and extension into adjacent structures is often towards the cavernous sinus, sella turcica, petrous bone, nasopharynx and hypoglossal canal [22].

Cartilaginous tumors

Chondromas

Rare, benign cartilaginous tumors representing less than 1% of all intracranial tumors [33]. The tumor may be solitary or multiple and associated with multiple enchondromatosis of Ollier and Maffucci's syndrome. On pre-contrast CT, chondromas are hypo- or hyperdense and exhibit moderate, late enhancement following the contrast injection. Intratumoral calcifications may result in the mass appearing hyperdense on the pre-contrast scan and are present in more than 60% of chondromas. The preoperative differential diagnosis between intracranial chondroma and meningioma is difficult, and the latter tumors is enhanced earlier following contrast injection.

Chondrosarcomas

Chondrosarcomas are slowly growing cartilaginous tumors which constitute approximately 6% of all lesions of the skull base. They may be primary or secondary to a preexisting bony lesion (fibrous dysplasia, Pagets's disease, osteochondroma). They are locally invasive and have a predilection for the parasellar region, cerebello-pontine angle, sphenoid and ethmoid bones. The histological distinction between chondrosarcoma, benign chondroma and chondroid chordoma is sometimes difficult.

CT is useful in the evaluation of intratumoral calcification and bony erosion. Following the intravenous contrast injection, the soft tissue component of the tumor becomes enhanced. On MRI, the tumor is hypointense on T1-weighted imaging hyperintense on T2-weighted imaging, heterogeneous areas correspond to calcifications and enhancement following the

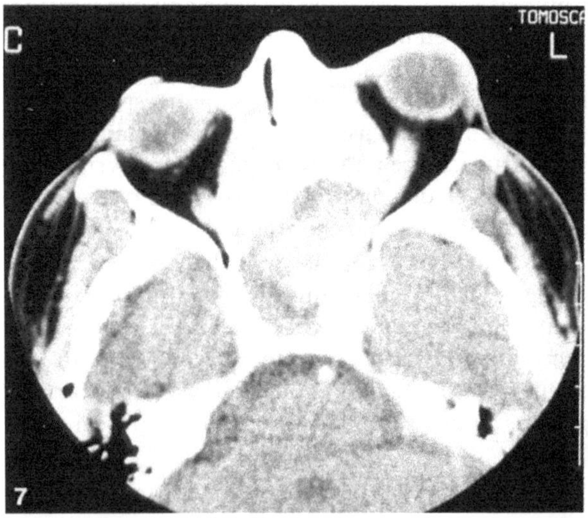

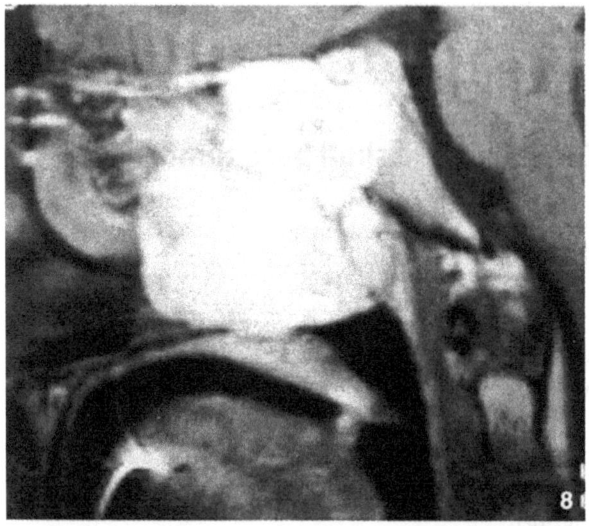

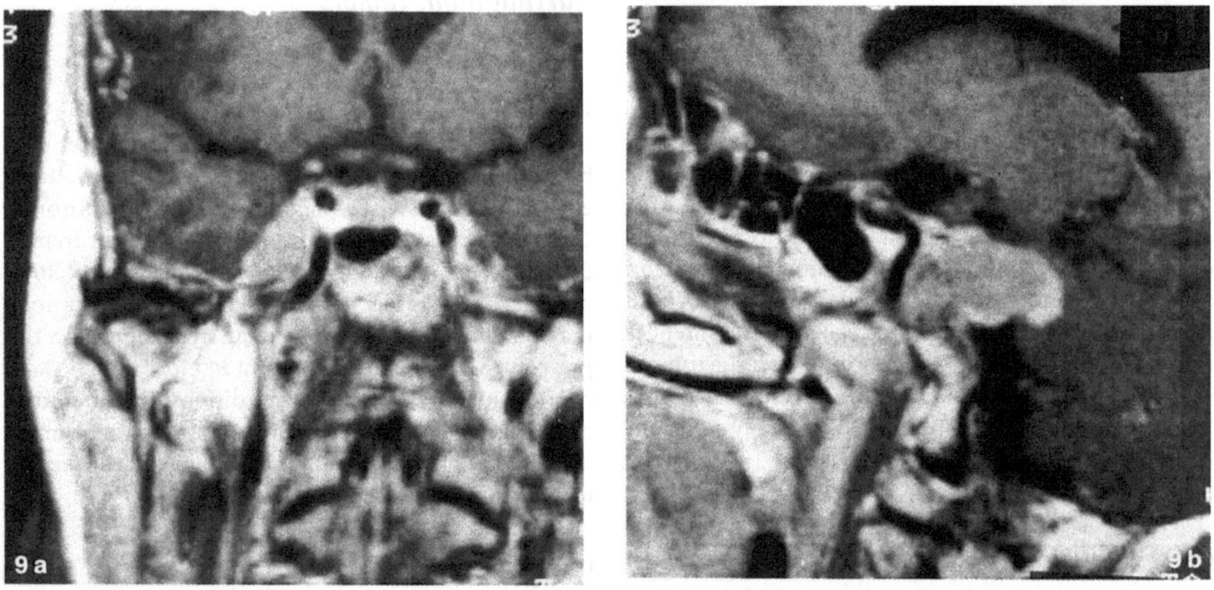

Fig. 6.7. Metastasis of the ethmoid and anterior cranial fossa from a melanoma with invasion of the sphenoid. Axial contrast enhanced CT: invasive tumor causing osteolysis

Fig. 6.8. Nasopharyngeal tumor in a 16 year old boy. MRI, sagittal T1-weighted image following the gadolinium injection: marked hyperintensity with numerous vascular structures; invasion of the cavum and sphenoid sinus

Fig. 6.9 a, b. Follow-up of a 60 year old female with myeloma. Hypoesthesia of the cheek complicated 8 days later by diplopia due to a right VIth nerve paresis. MRI, coronal and sagittal and T1-weighted sequences following gadolinium injection: hyperintense tumor invading the right cavernous sinus, effacement of the Gasserian ganglion (**a**) and expansion into the cerebello-pontine angle (**b**)

injection of gadolinium is heterogeneous for the same reason. MRI is better than CT for the evaluation of these tumors because chondrosarcomas, being locally invasive, often extended into the cavernous sinus, the sella turcica, the sphenoid sinus and the parapharyngeal space. Total or subtotal surgical resection is the best treatment, and this has been facilitated by the development of new surgical approaches to the skull base. Supplementary radiotherapy to residual lesions is indicated following surgery. [21].

Invasive pituitary adenomas

These may be extended laterally into the cavernous sinuses or inferiorly into the sphenoid sinus and skull base. This can present diagnostic difficulties and result in confusion with other skull base lesions when there is only infrasellar extension, although there is usually an intra- and suprasellar component to the tumor. In the case of infrasellar extension, CT demonstrates enhancement of the soft tissue components following the contrast injection and bony destruction. On MRI, the coronal and sagittal sections give a better assessment of tumor extension than on CT.

Meningiomas

These represent approximately 15% of primary intracranial tumors, and 33% occur in the skull base [10]. CT demonstrates the hyperostosis, and MRI assesses tumor extent. On T1-weighted imaging, meningiomas are generally isointense or slightly hypointense relative to the grey matter, and on T2-weighted imaging, 10% of lesions are hypointense, 50% are isointense and 40% hyperintense relative to the cerebral parenchyme. The tumors exhibit homogeneous and intense enhancement following intravenous injection of gadolinium.

Metastases

These are commoner skull base lesions than the primary bone tumors. The commonest primary tumors which metastasize to the skull base arise from the prostate, lung, breast and kidney. CT demonstrates areas of bone destruction (fig. 6.7) from metastases of prostatic cancer which are osteoblastic. On MRI, these lesions are hypointense on T1-weighted imaging and the normal hyperintense fatty marrow is effaced. They are hyperdense on T1-weighted imaging when compared to normal marrow. Usually there are other bony metastases demonstrated by scintigraphy.

Nasopharyngeal tumors

On CT, these carcinomas are enhanced and appear hyperdense following the intravenous contrast injection. Invasion of the skull base with associated bone destruction is clearly demonstrated. MRI assess the locoregional extension of the disease (fig. 6.8), particularly the involvement of adjacent blood vessels and nerves.

Metastases, lymphoma [11] and primary bone tumors can also cause bone destruction at the skull base and extend into the soft tissues of the nasopharynx which sometimes cause difficulties in the differential diagnosis.

Benign sino-nasal tumors

These may extend into the sphenoid sinus [31] or cause destructive bone changes suggestive of a carcinoma as is the case for extensive nasal polyposis or inverted papillomas. In the presence of bony erosion of the skull base, CT is unable to differentiate a benign from a malignant lesion.

Other tumors

Plasmocytomas (fig. 6.9), giant cell tumors, osteosarcomas, histiocytosis X and fibrosarcomas are rare tumors of the skull base. CT and MRI can assess tumor extension but there are no specific signs which will diagnose the histological type of tumor. These two modalities are complementary in the initial assessment and follow-up of the progression of these neoplastic skull base lesions on treatment.

Fibrous dysplasia

On CT, the affected bone is hyperdense or lytic. On MRI, the signal is hypointense or of intermediate signal intensity on T1- and T2-weighted imaging, but there may be small hyperintense areas on both sequences. The lesion enhances following the injection of gadolinium [5].

References

1. Akimura T, Kameda H, Abiko S, Aoki H, Kido T (1989) Infrasellar Craniopharyngioma. Neuroradiology 31: 180-183
2. Benitez WI, Sartor KJ, Angtuaco EJC (1988) Craniopharyngioma Presenting as a Nasopharyngeal Mass: CT and MR Findings. J Comput Assist Tomogr 12: 1068-1072
3. Boyko OB, Curnes JT, Oakes WJ, Burger PC (1991) Hamartomas of the Tuber Cinereum: CT, MR and Pathologic Findings. AJNR 12: 309-314
4. Carsin M, Carsin-Nicol B, Rolland Y, Vernouillet S, Gandon Y, Brassier G (1990) Apport de l'IRM au Diagnostic des Adénomes Hypophysaires Corticotropes. J Neuroradiol 17: 255-275
5. Casselman JW, De Jonge I, Neyt L, De Clercq C, D'Hont C (1993) MRI in Craniofacial Fibrous Dysplasia. Neuroradiology 35: 234-237
6. Castillo M, Davis PC, Ross WK, Hoffman JC (1989) Meningioma of the Chiasma and Optic Nerves: CT and MR Findings. J Comput Assist Tomogr 13: 679-681

7. Chappell PM, Kelly WN, Ercius M (1990) Primary Sellar Melanoma Simulating Hemorragic Pituitary Adenoma: MR and pathologic findings. AJNR 11: 1054-1056
8. Cone L, Srinivasan M, Romanul FCA (1990) Granular Cell Tumor (Choristoma) of the Neurohypophysis: Two Cases and a Review of the Literature. AJNR 11: 403-406
9. Dupas B, Gayet-Delacroix M, Charbonnel B, Buthiau D, Derome PJ, Grob R (1991) Pathologie sellaire et parasellaire. In: D Buthiau (ed) TDM et IRM Cliniques. Frison-Roche, Paris
10. Ginsberg LE (1992) Neoplasic Diseases Affecting the Central Skull Base, CT and MR Imaging. AJR 159: 581-589
11. Han MH, Chang KH, Kim IO, Kim DK, Han MC ( ] 993) Non-Hodgkin Lymphoma of the Central skull base: MR Manifestations. J Comput Assist Tomogr, 117: 567- 571
12. Henkelman RM, Watts JF, Kucharczyk W (]99]) High Signal Intensity in MR Images of Calcified Brain Tissue. Radiology, 179: 199-206
13. Hirsch WL, Sekhar LN, Lanzino G, Pomonis S, Sen CN (1993) Meningiomas involving the Cavernous Sinus: Value of Imaging for Prediction Surgical Complications. AJR 160: 1083-1088
14. Hutchins WW, Crues JV, Miya P, Pojunas KW (1990) MR Demonstration of Pituitary Hyperplasia and Regression after Therapy for Hypothyroidism. AJNR 11: 410
15. Korogi Y, Takahashi M, Sakamoto Y, Shinzato J (1991) Cavernous Sinus: Correlation between Anatomic and Dynamic Gadolinium-enhanced MR Imaging Findings. Radiology, 180: 235-237
16. Kulkarni M, Lee KF, McArdle CB, Yearkley JM, Haar FL (1989) 1,5 T MR Imaging of Pituitary Microadenomas: Technical Considerations and CT Correlation. AJNR 9: 511
17. Kyle CA, Laster RA, Burton EM, Sanford RA (1990) Subacute Pituitary: MR and CT appearance. J Comput Assist Tomogr 14: 40-44
18. Lundin P, Bergstrom MK, Nyman R, Lundberg PO, Muhr C (1992) Macroprolactinomas: serial MR Imaging in long-term Bromocriptine therapy. AJNR 13: 1279-1291
19. Maeder PP, Holtas SL, Basibuyuk LN, Salford LG, Tapper UAS, Brun A (1990) Colloid Cysts of the Third Ventricule: Correlation of MR and CT Findings with Histology and Chemical Analysis. AJNR 11: 575-581
20. Mayr NA, Yuh WTC, Muhonen MG, et al (]993) Pituitary Metastases: MR Findings. J Comput Assist Tomogr 17: 432-437
21. Meyers SP, Hirsch WL, Curtin HD, Barnes L, Sekhar LN, Sen C (1992) Chondrosarcomas of the skull base: MR Imaging Features. Radiology 184: 103-108
22. Meyers SP, Hirsch WL, Curtin HD, et al (1992) Chordomas of the Skull Base: MR Features. AJNR 13: 1627-1636
23. Michael AS and Paige ML (1988) MR Imaging of Intrasellar Meningiomas Simulating Pituitary Adenomas. J Comput Assist Tomogr 12: 944-946
24. Miki Y, Matsuo M, Nishizawa S, et al (]990) Pituitary Adenomas and Normal Pituitary Tissue: enhancement Patterns on Gadopentetate-enhanced MR Imaging. Radiology 177: 35-38
25. Mize W, Ball WS, Towhin RB, Han BK (1989) Atypical CT and MR Appearance of a Rathke's Cleft Cyst. AJNR 10: 83-84
26. Nemoto Y, Inoue Y, Fukuda T, et al (1988) MR Appearance of Rathke's Cleft Cysts. Neuroradiology 30: 155-159
27. Ostrov SG, Quencer RM, Hoffman JC, Davis PC, Hasso AN, David NJ (1989) Hemorrhage within Pituitary Adenomas: How often Associated with Pituitary Apoplexy Syndrome ? AJR 153: 153-160
28. Sakamoto Y, Takahaschi M, Korogi Y, Bussaka H, Ushio Y (1991) Normal and Abnormal Pituitary Glands: Gadopentetate Dimeglumine-enhanced MR Imaging. Radiology. 178: 441-445
29. Sartor K, Karnaze MG, Winthrop JD, Gado M, Hodges FJ (1987) MR Imaging in infra, para and retrosellar mass lesions. Neuroradiology 29: 19-29
30. Schubiger O, Haller D (1992) Metastases to the Pituitary Hypothalamic Axis, an MR study of 7 symptomatic patients. Neuroradiology 34: 131-134
31. Som PM, Lawson W, Lidov MW (1991) Simulated Aggressive Skull Base erosion in Reponse to Benign Sinonasal Disease. Radiology 180: 755-759
32. Steiner E, Knosp E, Herold C, et al (1992) Pituitary Adenomas: Findings of post operative MR Imaging. Radiology 185: 521-527
33. Tanohata K, Macharat, Aida N, et al (1987) Computed Tomography of Intracranial Chondroma with emphasis on delayed Contrast enhancement. J Comput Assist Tomogr 11: 820-823
34. Tien RD (1992) Sequence of enhancement of Various portions of the Pituitary Gland on Gadolinium-enhanced MR Images: Correlation with Regional Blood Supply. AJR 158: 651-654
35. Tien RD, Kucharczyk J, Kucharczyk W (1991) MR Imaging of the Brain in Patients with Diabetes Insipidus. AJNR 12: 533-542
36. Tien RD, Newton TH, Mc Demmott MW, Dillon WP, Kucharczyk J (1990) Thickened Pituitary Stalk on MR Images in Patients with Diabetes Insipidus and Langerhans Cell Histiocytosis. AJNR 11: 703-708.
37. Truwitt CL, Barkovich AJ (1990) Pathogenesis of Intracranial Lipoma: an MR Study in 42 patients. AJNR 11: 665-674
38. Vion-Dury J, Vincentelli F, Jiddane M, et al (1987) MR Imaging of epidemmoid Cysts. Neuroradiology 29: 333-338
39. Weingarten K, Ernst RJ, Jahre C, Zimmerman R (1992) Detection of Residual or Recurrent Meningioma after Surgery: Value of enhanced vs unenhanced MR Imaging. AJNR 158: 645-650
40. Youssem DM, Arrington JA, Zinreich SJ, Kumar AJ, Bryon RN (1989) Pituitary Adenomas: Possible Role of Bromocriptine in intratumoral Hemorrhage. Radiology 170: 239-243
41. Youssem DM, Atlas SW, Grossman RI, Sergott RC, Savino PJ, Bos]ey TM (1989) MR Imaging of Tolosa-Hunt Syndrome. AJNR 10: 1181-1184

CHAPTER 7

Malignant tumors of the spine and spinal cord

Clinicians
G. Missenard, P. Lapresle, R. Grob, E.-Ch. Antoine, D. Grosskopf, F. Guinet, C. Borel, P. Brunet

Radiologists
M. Sahel, D. Dormont, B. Marro, S. Gerber, A. Biondi, C. Marsault

The investigation of spinal pathology has changed dramatically with the widespread use of magnetic resonance imaging (MRI). For intraspinal tumors, MRI (with and without the injection of a paramagnetic contrast agent), has become the examination of choice, particularly for suspected spinal cord compression. In fact, conventional myelography (which may or may not be complemented by CT myelography) is an invasive technique which may cause a deterioration in the neurological signs in a high percentage of cases. The indications for myelography should therefore be limited to cases in which the performance of MRI is not possible. The role of computed tomography (CT) for intraspinal pathology remains limited.

CT is useful in the assessment of bone trauma (apart from the problems caused by the effect of these lesions on the neural axis). However, there has been a renewed interest in this technique due to the development of 3D CT imaging techniques. MRI (with and without the injection of a paramagnetic contrast agent) is of great value in the investigation of primary and secondary tumors of the vertebrae, giving direct visualization of the spine in three planes with excellent contrast between healthy tissue and tumor.

By far the commonest spinal tumors are metastases which are also most often responsible for the neurological complications. The diagnosis can only be confirmed by histology.

Spinal tumors

Benign vertebral tumors (figs 7.1 & 7.2)

The commonest benign tumors of the spine are vertebral hemangioma, aneurysmal bone cyst and giant cell tumors (the latter lesions are relatively benign due to their tendency to recur locally). The differential diagnosis of these lesions is a malignant tumor.

Primary malignant tumors

Osteosarcoma

This is a malignant tumor occurring between 10 and 20 years of age. Of all the bone tumors, osteosarcoma is one of the commonest, and the spine is an uncommon site [8]. CT demonstrates a solid soft tissue mass, and usually osteolytic, more rarely osteosclerotic or mixed bone lesion. There is associated infiltration of the prevertebral soft tissues anteriorly and the epidural space posteriorly. MRI clearly demonstrates the neoplasm (hypointense on T1-weighted imaging and hyperintense on T2-weighted imaging) and its relationship to adjacent structures (soft tissues and spinal cord) (fig. 7.3). Effacement of the fat planes is a good sign of invasion of the soft tissues. The lesion becomes enhanced strongly following contrast injection indicating its highly vascular nature.

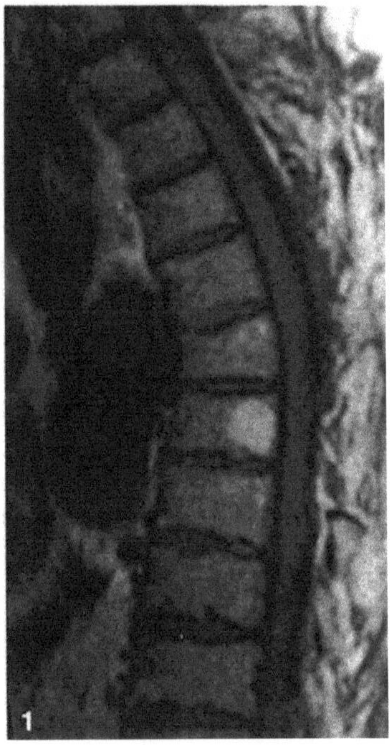

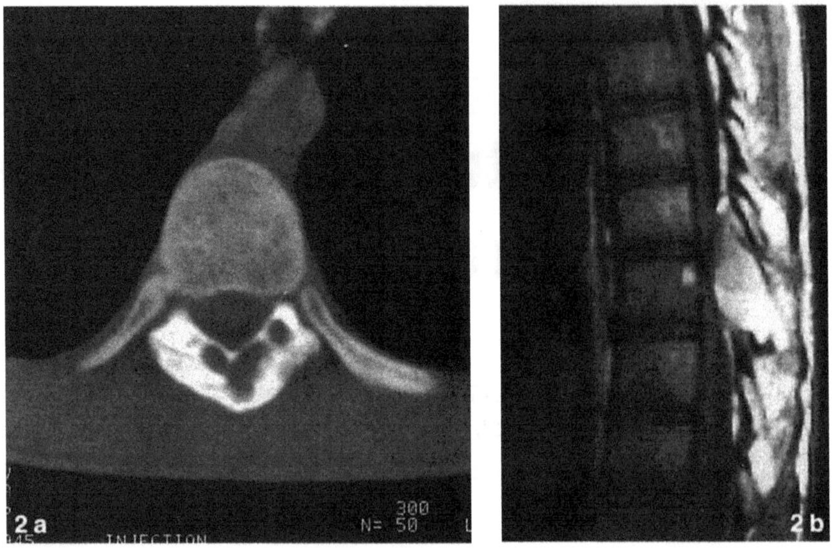

Fig. 7.1. MRI of a vertebral hemangioma discovered as an incidental finding in a 64 year old patient. Sagittal T1-weighted image without gadolinium. There is a rounded area of intrinsically high signal intensity in the posterior aspect of the body of T8. Note the appearance of the vertebral body immediately above (T7) as a result of osteoporotic collapse

Fig. 7.2 a, b. Aneurysmal bone cyst in a 16 year old patient. a CT demonstrating a lytic lesion in the posterior neural arch of the T9 vertebra. b MRI in the same patient, sagittal T1-weighted image. The lesion expands in the posterior neural arch and has a heterogeneous signal intensity with areas of hyperintensity indicating the presence of blood breakdown products

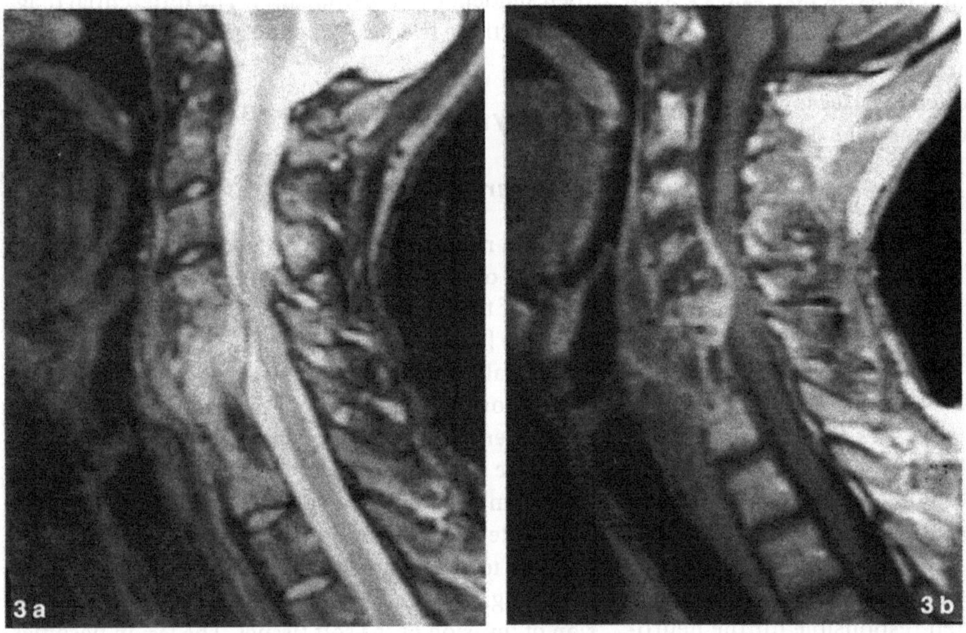

Fig. 7.3 a, b. MRI in a 26 year old patient presenting with recurrent osteosarcoma of the cervical spine. a Sagittal T1-weighted section. Lesion involving the C4, C5 and C6 vertebrae appearing heterogeneously hyperintense and causing early spinal cord compression. b Sagittal post-gadolinium T1-weighted section. Heterogeneous tumor enhancement with significant prevertebral extension

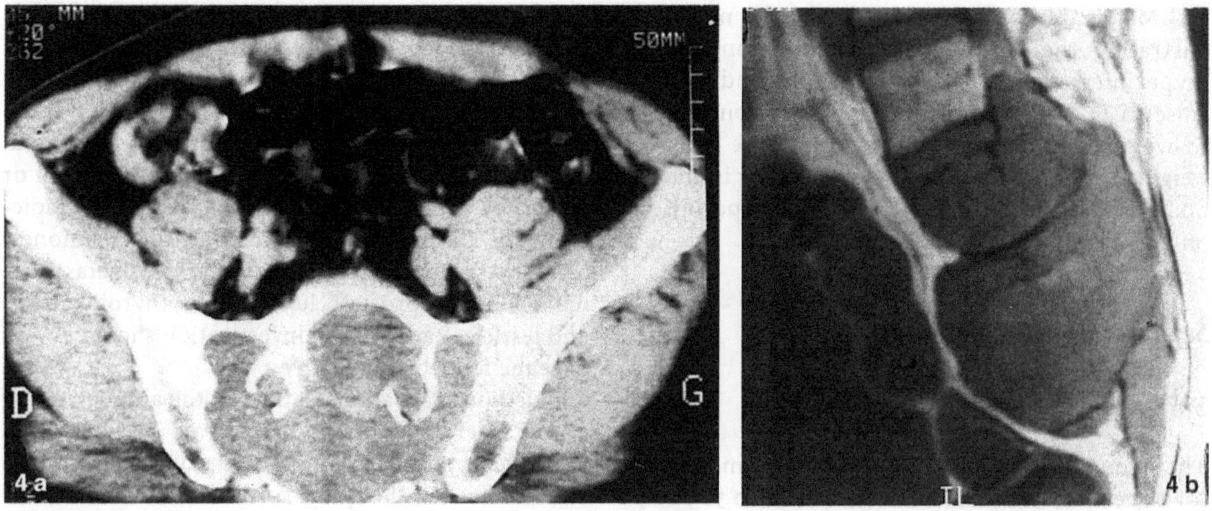

Fig. 7.4 a, b. Chordoma in a 31 year old man. **a** CT demonstrates a large osteolytic lesion invading the sacrum. **b** MRI in the same patient, sagittal T1-weighted image clearly defining the extent of the lesion which is invading the whole of the sacrum with a significant anterior extension

Chondrosarcoma

This is a tumor which occurs in older adults (30 to 60 years) with a cartilaginous proliferation [8]. The CT appearance is one of irregular vertebral osteolysis of variable extent containing diffuse calcifications [10]. MRI is less sensitive in the detection of calcification but clearly demonstrates the tumor and its extension.

Ewing's sarcoma

This malignant tumor of young adults (less than 30 years) commonly occurs in the long bones and flat bones (the pelvis and scapula) but much more rarely in the spine. On CT, there is an irregular osteolysis (without reactive osteosclerosis) with a significant soft tissue component. Intense enhancement is noted following contrast injection. The MRI appearances are identical to those of osteosarcoma.

Clear cell sarcomas, fibrosarcomas

These soft tissue tumors very rarely occur in the spine.

Tumors of embryonic origin

Neuroblastomas

These are common tumors of infancy which arise in the paraspinal sympathetic chains and adrenal medulla. The tumor is often associated with metastases to the lymph nodes, bones and particularly the spine. Spinal involvement occurs initially by direct spread into the epidural spaces causing spinal cord compression. CT demonstrates a solid paraspinal soft tissue mass containing areas of calcification. MRI more clearly demonstrates the extension of the tumor, particularly if there is intraspinal involvement in the form of an "hour glass" lesion.

Chordomas

Spinal chordomas arise from remnants of the notochord. These tumors occur in the sacrum (50%), clivus (35%) or a vertebra (15%). Chordomas progress very slowly, but only very rarely they are totally curable (fig. 7.4) due to the extension into the spinal canal.

CT demonstrates a vertebral and paravertebral solid tumor mass, markedly osteolytic and sometimes containing irregular calcifications. The lesion becomes enhanced following contrast injection which improves definition of its extension. MRI is less sensitive in its detection of calcifications but allows direct visualization of the tumor expansion and particularly its relationship with the spinal cord. Chordomas appear isointense or hypointense on T1-weighted imaging and hyperintense on T2-weighted imaging [28].

Sacrococcygeal teratoma

This is a tumor of the neonate arising in the sacral region, which is of a solid or partially cystic nature

[25]. MRI is able to characterize the neoplasm by demonstrating the various different components: fat (hyperintense on T1-weighted imaging and hypointense on T2-weighted imaging), cystic (hypointense on T1-weighted imaging and hyperintense on T2-weighted imaging) and soft tissue (hypo- or isointense on T1-weighted imaging and relatively hyperintense on T2-weighted imaging).

Secondary vertebral tumors

Spinal metastases

The spine, after the skull, is the second commonest site for bone metastasis in adults aged between 50 and 70 years [8]. The dissemination of tumor to the spine is by hematogenous spread and is explained by the markedly rich blood supply of the vertebrae. However, metastatic disease in fact is still poorly understood; it is probable that the diffusion occurs via the venous system and by retrograde flow due to the pressure changes within the vertebral veins during respiration. The vertebral body is often the bony element involved at an early stage; extension by direct spread into the epidural spaces and towards the posterior neural arch occurs later [11]. Pain (dorsalgia in 70% of cases) is the commonest presenting clinical feature of a spinal metastasis [29] and may be an isolated symptom or associated with neurological symptoms, notably radiculopathy. The osteophylic cancers are the commonest primary tumors responsible for spinal metastases, namely breast, prostate, lung, kidney, thyroid, uterus and testicle. Radiological investigation should always have the following objectives:

- to demonstrate abnormalities in the architecture of one or several pathological vertebrae;
- to detect possible associated epidural infiltration and its effect on the spinal cord;
- to define accurately the spread of tumor into the paraspinal soft tissues.

In the presence of a known primary tumor and multiple associated spinal lesions, the diagnosis of metastasis is usually easy. However, in the case of a solitary vertebral lesion and no known primary cancer, it is more difficult to confirm the diagnosis. In this

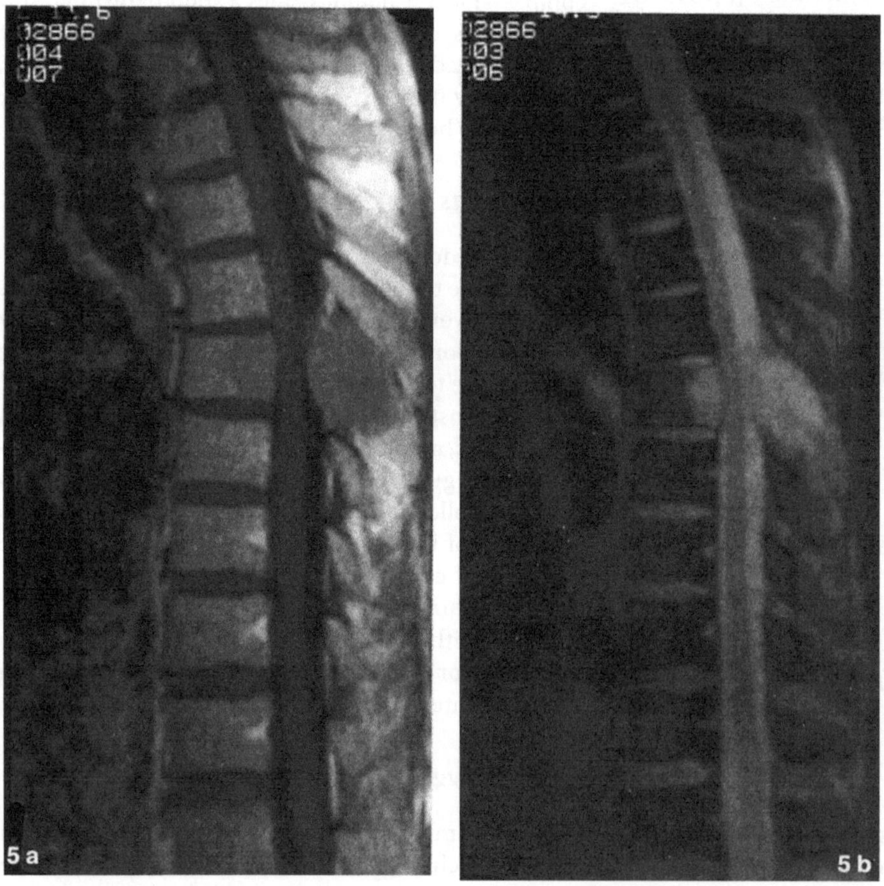

Fig. 7.5 a, b. Vertebral metastasis from a primary lung cancer in a 46 year old male. **a** Sagittal T1-weighted image demonstrating a hypointense lesion in the posterior aspect of the vertebral body and posterior neural arch of T7; **b** sagittal T2-weighted image, the metastasis appears hyperintense

instance, it is sometimes necessary to resort to vertebral biopsy in order to obtain histological proof of the metastatic nature of the lesion.

CT provides an excellent assessment of secondary tumors of the spine [10]. The metastatic bone destruction and extraspinal extension are particularly well shown on CT. Localized osteolysis of a vertebral body without any reactive osteosclerosis is the commonest finding. Sclerotic metastases are rare and usually arise from primary prostatic or breast carcinomas [2, 29]. These tumors often become enhanced intensely following contrast, thus giving improved tumor delineation and better appreciation of the spread into the paravertebral soft tissues.

MRI is a highly sensitive technique for the diagnosis of vertebral metastases (fig. 7.5) [12, 16, 27]. Replacement of the vertebral marrow fat [16], which normally appears hyperintense on T1-weighted imaging, by neoplastic tissue results in a hypointensity on T1-weighted imaging and hyperintensity on T2-weighted imaging [27]. However, the diagnosis of metastasis may be difficult in an elderly patient due to the normally heterogeneous signal intensity of the vertebrae on T1-weighted imaging. The tumor is enhanced in a homogeneous fashion following the injection of gadolinium which may result in the signal intensity of the pathological vertebra becoming isointense to the normal adjacent vertebrae. Post-contrast sequences equally mask a vertebral metastasis within a previously irradiated spine which causes hyperintense vertebral bodies [11]. It is, therefore, always mandatory when looking for metastases to compare the post-contrast T1-weighted images with the pre-contrast images. MRI is otherwise the best modality for assessing epidural extension of a vertebral metastasis and the presence of spinal cord compression. Currently, it is difficult to define precisely the respective indications for MRI, CT and scintigraphy in the study of vertebral metastases. MRI is a more sensitive technique than scintigraphy [11, 22], resulting in an earlier diagnosis. However, scintigraphy remains an excellent technique for the detection of metastases. At the present moment, it is difficult to propose that MRI should be used routinely in the search for vertebral metastases for all osteophylic cancers (due to the difficulty in performing an MRI examination of the whole spine both with and without gadolinium). However, an MRI examination should be performed as the examination of choice if their is any suspicion of spinal cord compression by epidural metastasis.

MRI should also be considered when there is difficulty in differentiating osteoporotic from metastatic vertebral collapse in an elderly patient [16]. There are certain features on MRI that favor the diagnosis of osteoporotic collapse: (1) posterior displacement of the posterior border of the vertebral body; (2) normal appearances of the spinous processes and soft tissues; (3) normal signal of the vertebra 6 months or more after the initial collapse or residual fatty islands; (4) abnormal bands of signal for the vertebral collapse in less than 6 months old (hypointense on T1-weighted imaging and iso- or hyperintense on T2-weighted imaging).

On the other hand, the following features are more in favor of a vertebral collapse of metastatic origin:
- convex posterior bulging of the vertebral body;
- involvement of the posterior neural arch and soft tissue;
- the signal intensity of the vertebra containing the metastasis is always abnormal.

There is either hypointensity on T1-weighted imaging and hyperintensity on T2-weighted imaging of the whole vertebra or rounded areas of abnormal signal intensity. Following gadolinium injection, there is always abnormal enhancement in the cases of metastatic collapse. In cases of osteoporotic collapse, the contrast enhancement disappears following the acute episode.

Finally, MRI should be mandatory in cases of metastatic disease. In fact, MRI is particularly valuable to the surgeon in cases of spinal metastasis. The radiologist must be sure not only to study the level of the compression but also to perform a sagittal sequence of the whole of the spine to confirm that the neurological symptoms are related to the level of compression rather than other lesions elsewhere in the spine which have been missed on standard radiographs.

Myeloma

Myeloma is a malignant tumor occurring in the elderly (50 to 70 years). It is a malignant proliferation of plasma cells, usually within the bone marrow of the spine. This neoplasm represents 35% of malignant bone tumors. Bone rarefaction due to replacement by tumor can result in pathological fractures which may be complicated by neurological signs. Solitary myelomas or plasmocytomas occur in the same age group and have identical pathological characteristic as the multifocal form of the disease.

CT is able to define discrete abnormalities in bone density which are imperceptible on standard radiographs. These appear as a rounded area of osteolysis within the vertebral body without any peripheral reactive osteosclerosis. The bone destruction may lead to a vertebral collapse.

On MRI [11], the signal intensity of untreated myelomatous vertebral deposits is identical to that of spinal metastasis due to the replacement of the normal vertebral marrow by neoplastic tissues. Involvement, however, is usually more diffuse than with metastasis. The areas of tumor infiltration are hypointense on T1-weighted imaging and hyperintense on T2-weighted imaging. There is diffuse displacement of the vertebral marrow by pathological tissue with the presence of multiple well defined lesions. Associated vertebral collapse is easily visualized on the sagittal T1-weighted images.

Lymphoma and leukemia

Lymphoma is a systemic malignant disease and involvement of the spine is not uncommon. Spinal involvement is most frequently by direct contiguous spread from disease of the paraspinal lymph node chains [18]. However, it is equally common to see direct involvement of the vertebrae without an associated paraspinal mass. CT is of little value in the early stage of tumor infiltration. On the other hand, at a later stage, CT demonstrates diffuse reduction in the bony trabecular pattern.

MRI is the examination of choice for detecting tumor deposits which appear hypointense on T1-weighted imaging and hyperintense on T2-weighted imaging. This technique also identifies paraspinal tumor masses and infiltration of the epidural spaces.

Leukemic infiltration of the spine is not rare and occurs particularly in children [20]. Standard radiographs and CT show a diffuse osteoporosis of the vertebrae. MRI demonstrates abnormal areas within the vertebral body appearing hypointense on T1-weighted imaging and hyperintense on T2-weighted imaging. In addition MRI is able to follow the progress of the tumor deposits on treatment.

Intraspinal tumors

Epidural tumors, carcinomatous epiduritis

The majority of the lesions of the epidural space are malignant tumors, generally secondaries which most commonly arise from primary cancers of the lung, breast, prostate and kidney. There are two mechanisms to explain the invasion of the epidural space:

- direct contiguous extension from a spinal metastasis (the commonest);
- direct involvement of the epidural space by hematogenous spread.

CT is useful in the evaluation of vertebral lesions when the examination is targeted to the suspected level based on the standard radiographs or bone scintigraphy.

Carcinomatous epiduritis is occasionally demonstrated following intravenous contrast injection as abnormally enhancing tissue within the spinal canal displacing the spinal cord.

MRI is the examination of choice for the investigation of a patient with suspected spinal cord compression due to carcinomatous epiduritis [3, 7, 14, 32] and should be performed as an emergency. MRI clearly demonstrates the juxtadural intracanalicular tumor proliferation, the degree of associated spinal cord compression, as well as the superior and inferior limits of the compression (fig. 7.6). The pathological tissue in the epidural space contiguous with the pathological vertebra is clearly demonstrated on T1-weighted imaging (iso- or hyperintense relative to the cord) and on T2-weighted imaging (usually hyperintense relative to the cord). It is useful to use two orthogonal scan planes, particularly sagittal and axial, to improve delineation of the spinal cord compression. On the post-gadolinium T1-weighted images, carcinomatous epiduritis shows an enhancement.

Epidural extension causing spinal cord compression may equally be seen in primary vertebral tumors (giant cell tumor and active hemangioma, osteosarcoma, aneurysmal bone cyst, multiple myeloma, chordoma and osteochondroma) or in lymphomas, sarcomas or neuroblastomas.

Intradural extramedullary tumors

Intradural extramedullary tumors are usually benign, the commonest lesions being meningiomas and neurinomas (90%). The other tumors are much rare and essentially comprise of intradural metastasis and lipomas which may be extradural particularly in the lumbar region.

Meningiomas

These are slowly growing benign tumors, commonest in elderly females (over 50 years old), and occur in the postero-lateral aspect of the thoracic spine in 80% of cases. They are sometimes visible on contrast enhanced CT, but are much more clearly identified and analyzed on MRI. On T1-weighted sagittal images, the mass is isointense to the spinal cord and is essen-

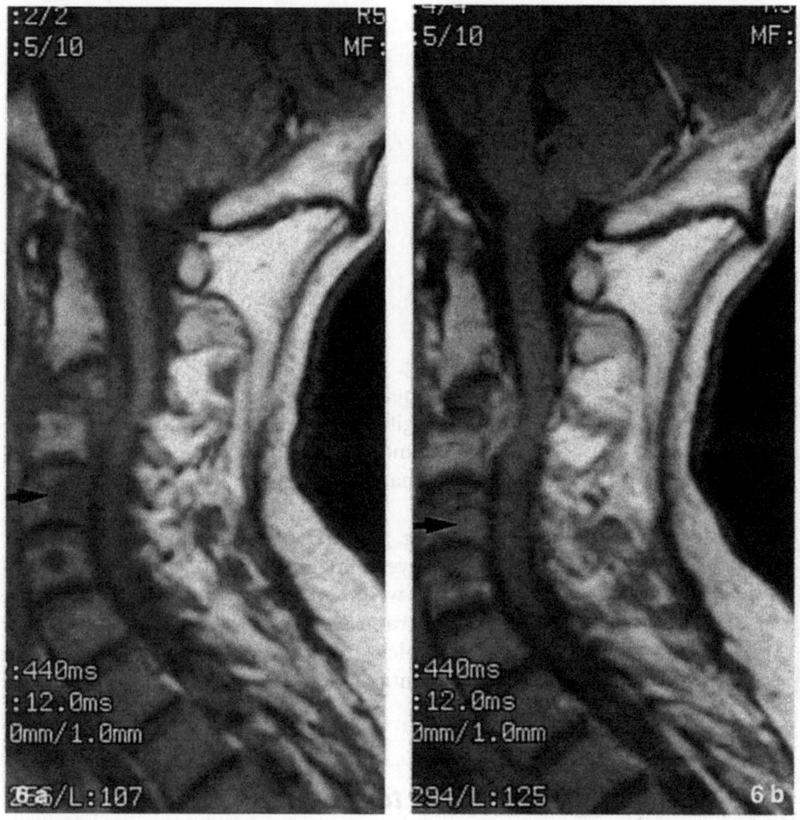

Fig. 7.6 a, b. Cervical vertebral metastasis from primary lung cancer with early metastatic epidural involvement in a 50 year old male. MRI scan (sagittal T1-weighted images pre- (**a**) and post- (**b**) gadolinium injection). There are metastases in the C3 and C5 level. At the C3 level, there is vertebral collapse with pathological tissue invading the prevertebral soft tissues anteriorly and the epidural space posteriorly. Early spinal cord compression. Following gadolinium injection (**b**), the metastatic epidural involvement is seen more clearly due to enhancement. Note the disappearance of the C5 metastasis following contrast since it has become isointense with the signal of the normal vertebra due to enhancement *(arrows)*

tially oval in shape with its long axis vertical. Meningiomas have a large fixed base and displace and compress the cord. The mass also appears isointense to the cord on the T2-weighted images. Following injection of gadolinium, there is intense homogeneous enhancement of the lesion [21, 26, 30]. There may sometimes be difficulties differentiating meningioma from neurinoma. The following features are more in favor of the diagnosis of a meningioma: the presence of calcification within the tumor, absence of tumor extension into the neuroforamina and the site of the lesion (in a female over 50 years old).

Neurinomas

Two distinct anatomic-pathological entities are often grouped together under the term neurinomas: schwannomas and neurofibromas. These lesions represent a half of all extramedullary intradural tumors. Neurofibromas occur in von Recklinhausen's disease and are often multiple. Malignant degeneration into a neurofibrosarcoma can occur but is very rare without previous therapeutic intervention. Neurinomas occur in the cervico-dorsal region in 60% of cases. Their slow growth pattern explains the bony changes which are changes seen on CT: enlargement of the neuroforamina ("dumbbell neurinoma"), widening of the interpedicular distance or rib erosion. There is usually an intense and homogeneous enhancement of the tumor following contrast injection although in 15% of cases they remain isodense. On MRI, the lesion appears iso- or hypointense on T1-weighted imaging relative to the cord and slightly hyperintense on T2-weighted imaging. The marked enhancement of the tumor following gadolinium injection gives a better assessment of its relationship to the spinal cord and demonstrates any extracanalicular extension [21, 26, 30]. Surgery is indicated irrespective of whether the tumor is a neurinoma or meningioma.

Intradural metastases or "drop metastases"

Dissemination of metastasis within the meningeal spaces occurs particularly from primary brain tumors: glioblastomas, ependymomas, pinealoblastomas (fig. 7.7) and especially medulloblastomas. This latter neoplasm occurs principally in children [5]. Carcinoma of the breast and bronchus, as well as melanomas may also present with meningeal secondaries.

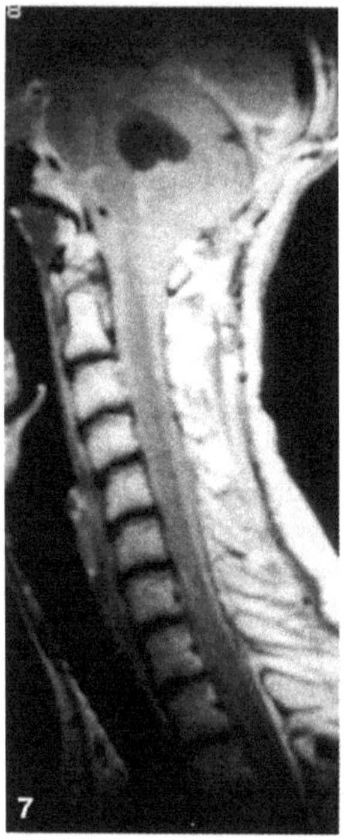

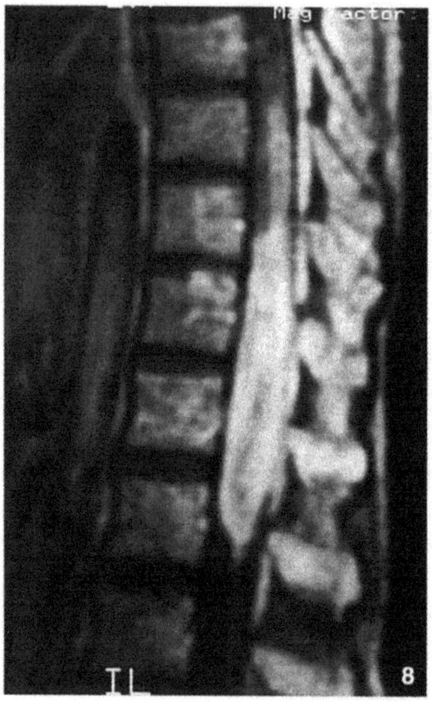

Fig. 7.7. Subarachnoid dissemination of a pinealoblastoma in a 26 year old patient. Sagittal post-gadolinium T1-weighted image demonstrating diffuse enhancement of the subarachnoid space due to tumor

Fig. 7.8. Intramedullary ependymoma in a 39 year old female. Sagittal post-gadolinium T1-weighted image demonstrating a large intramedullary space occupying lesion which become enhanced intensely with contrast

Post-gadolinium MRI is the best method of detecting these secondary deposits, even when they are small. Tumor infiltration appears as a thin perimedullary or periradicular enhancement. True tumor nodules may also be seen, particularly in the dependent regions of the spine.

Lipomas

These are benign tumors composed of fat cells, often occurring in the region of the filum terminale and frequently associated with spinal malformations: sacral agenesis, tethered cord, meningocele [23]. Lipomas have a characteristic negative density on CT and cause cord compression to a lesser or greater extent.

On MRI, the signal intensity of these lesions is equally characteristic: hyperintense on T1-weighted imaging and hypointense on T2-weighted imaging. It may be useful to perform specific sequences for imaging fat in order to confirm the diagnosis in difficult cases.

Other intradural extramedullary tumors

The other intradural extramedullary lesions are very rare, and include teratomas, dermoid or epidermoid cysts and neuroenteric cysts.

Intramedullary tumors

Ependymomas

These represent 60 to 70% of intramedullary tumors and occur predominantly between the ages of 30 and 60 years. They arise from the ependymal cells of the central canal or from embryonic rests in the filum terminale. Due to a greater concentration of ependymal cells, the sites of predilection are the conus of the cord and the filum, but the tumors may occur anywhere, including in an extracanalicular location, particularly in the sacrum. The myxo-papillary form is the commonest histological type. Due to the slow progression of these lesions, there are often associated bone changes seen on CT (widening of the diameter of the spinal canal, scalloping of the vertebrae).

MRI nowadays should be used for the diagnosis and pre-treatment assessment of these lesions and demonstrates enlargement of the cord which is often very extensive (fig. 7.8). MRI is also able to differentiate the various components of the lesion. The soft tissue tumor component appears iso- or hypointense on T1-weighted imaging and moderately hyperintense on T2-weighted imaging. Cystic areas are very hypointense on T1-weighted imaging and hyperintense on T2-weighted imaging. Perilesional edema appears equally hyperintense on T2-weighted imaging.

Hemorrhagic areas with hemosiderin deposition are sometimes visible at the inferior and superior limits of the tumor. Chronic bleeding appears slightly hypointense on T1-weighted imaging and markedly hypointense on T2-weighted imaging. The soft tissue component of the tumor enhances in a relatively homogeneous fashion following the injection of gadolinium thus differentiating it from perilesional edema and cyst formation [1, 3, 31].

Astrocytomas

These represent 40% of intramedullary tumors, 75 to 90% are low grade lesions. The peak age incidence is between 30 and 40 years, but the lesions may also occur in children. Pain is the commonest presenting symptom. The tumors have a predilection for the cervico-dorsal region.

MRI demonstrates irregular enlargement of the cord which appears hypointense on T1-weighted imaging and hyperintense on T2-weighted imaging. The tumor is surrounded by a zone of peripheral edema appearing very hyperintense on T2-weighted imaging. The soft tissue areas of the tumor become enhanced inhomogeneously following gadolinium injection. The soft tissue component may be associated with non-neoplastic cysts (signal intensity identical to CSF) or neoplastic cysts, more hypointense than CSF (more proteinaceous or hemorrhagic contents) [1, 3, 9]. These latter lesions contain tumor tissue in their walls and become enhanced following injection of contrast.

Hemangioblastoma

This is a benign tumor arising from endothelial cells and is composed of a dense capillary network and small venous lakes separated by a fibrous stroma. It represents 2 to 4% of intramedullary tumors. The tumor may be solitary, but multiple hemangioblastomas are seen in cases of von Hippel-Lindau disease. Radiologically, these lesions are characterized by the presence of cystic masses containing markedly hypervascular mural nodules.

CT is of little value but may sometimes demonstrate intense enhancement of the mural nodule.

On MRI, there is often extensive enlargement of the cord, hypointense on T1-weighted imaging due to the cysts which may be large and sometimes multiple. The mural nodule becomes enhanced very intensely in a homogeneous fashion following the injection of gadolinium (fig. 7.9) [3, 15, 33]. Dilated, serpiginous, pathological vessels may be seen in the subarachnoid space which increase the diagnostic confidence level (dilated vessels are never seen in other medullary tumors).

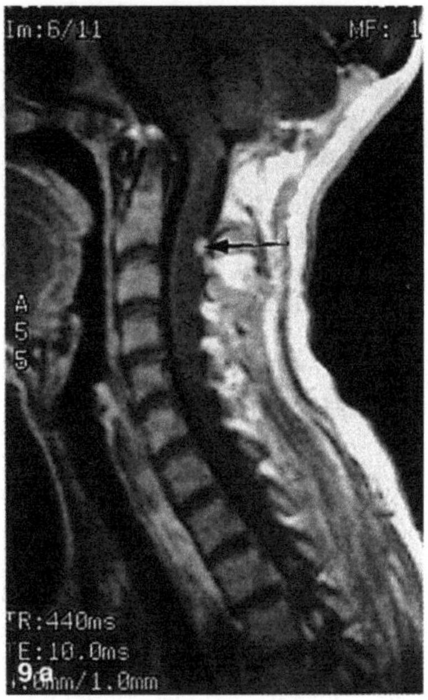

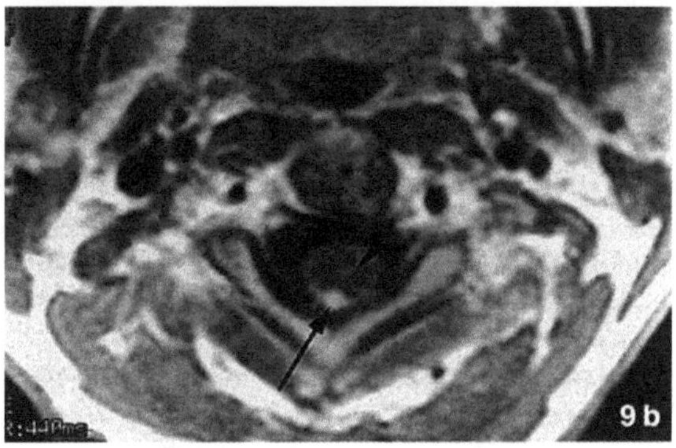

Fig. 7.9 a, b. Cervical intramedullary hemangioblastoma in a 32 year old female with von Hippel-Lindau disease. **a** Sagittal post-gadolinium T1-weighted image showing enlargement of the cervical cord due to the presence of an intramedullary cyst. In addition, there is enhancement of the posterior aspect of the cord at the C2-C3 level corresponding to the tumor nodule of the hemangioblastoma *(arrow)*; **b** this axial post-gadolinium T1-weighted images at the level of the lesion differentiates the two components of the lesion, cystic *(arrow head)* and soft tissue *(arrow)*

Intramedullary metastases

Intramedullary metastases are very rare. The primary neoplasms may be outside the central nervous system (lung, breast, melanoma), or occur within the brain (glioblastoma, ependymoma, medulloblastoma).

Dissemination of the tumor may occur by hematogenous spread or direct secondary spread from leptomeningeal involvement [5].

MRI demonstrates single or multiple secondary deposits which are often small and well defined within an enlarged cord. Edema around the metastasis is usually very extensive, and its high signal intensity contrasts with the lower signal intensity of the tumor. The lesion becomes enhanced intensely following the injection of gadolinium.

CT density and MRI signal characteristics of an intramedullary lipoma should be remembered.

In conclusion, MRI is currently the investigation of choice in the investigation of vertebral and spinal cord tumors. The sagittal sequences allow assessment of the length of the lesion. A study of the thoracic region should always include either the cervico-dorsal junction including C2, or the dorso-lumbar junction including L5, which are the accurate preoperative landmarks. The axial sections are also indispensable for planning the surgical approach. If a lateral approach is planned, the identification of the spinal artery by arteriography may also be necessary depending on the level of the lesion.

Post-treatment appearances

MRI is the examination of choice for post-treatment follow-up (post-surgical and/or radiotherapy) of vertebral and spinal cord tumors. It is almost always necessary to perform the examination with and without gadolinium injection. However, the performance and interpretation of these examinations require attention to detail and it is not always easy to differentiate recurrent tumor from post-operative changes. The performance of a baseline MRI examination, however, is made difficult by the presence of metallic material causing artefacts and hence the value of using titanium instruments and performing spin echo sequences (less ferromagnetic artefact than the gradient echo sequences). There is often distortion of the anatomy due to the surgical approach (removal of the spinous processes for a laminectomy, presence of a post-operative pseudomeningocele). Radiotherapy treatment causes equally significant alterations in the morphology and appearances of the spine. Ionising radiation induces destruction of the different cellular components of the bone marrow with subsequent replacement by fat cells [11]. This may be observed three months following irradiation of the spine resulting in a high signal intensity on T1-weighted imaging of the vertebral bodies in the irradiated field.

Conclusion

CT and particularly MRI are able to localize very accurately vertebral and spinal cord tumors and act as a guide for surgical biopsy or excision which remains the methods of obtaining a histological diagnosis although the diagnosis on imaging alone is becoming more and more accurate with the technological improvements of the scanners.

References

1. Andrew MC, Goy AMC, Pinto RS, Ragavendra BN, Epstein JF, Kricheff II (1986) Intramedullary Spinal Cord Tumors: MR Imaging, With emphasis on associated Cysts. Radiology 161: 381-385
2. Aoki J, Yamamoto I, Hino M, Shigero C, Kitamaru N, Itoh H, Torizuka K (1986) Sclerotic Bone Metastasis: Radiologic-Pathologic Correlation. Radiology 159: 127-132
3. Balériaux D, Parizel P, Segebarth C. Pathologie intra-rachidienne et médullaire. In: Manelfe C (1989) Imagerie du Rachis et de la Moelle. Vigot, Paris
4. Beltran J, Simon DC, Leroy M, Herman L, Weis L, Mueller CF (1986) Aneuvrysmal Bone Cysts: MR Imaging at 1,5 T. Radiology: 158: 689-690
5. Blows DE, Wang H, Kumar AJ, Robb PA, Phillips PC, Bryan RN (1990) Intradural Spinal Metastases in Pediatric Patients with Primary Intracranial Neoplasms: Gd-DTPA Enhanced MR CT myelography. J Comput Assist Tomogr 14: 730-735
6. Brady TJ, Gelbhardt MC, Pickett IL (1982) NMR Imaging of forearms in healthy volunteers and patients with giant cell tumor. Radiology 144: 549-552
7. Chadwick DJ, Gillott DA, Mukejee A, Penry JB (1991) Magnetic Resonnance Imaging of Spinal Metastases. J Royal Society of Medicine 84: 196-199
8. Dahlin DC (1978) Bone tumors. Charles C. Thomas, Springfield, Illinois
9. Dillon WP, Norman D, Newton TH. Bolla K, Mark A (1989) Intradural Spinal Cord Lesions : Gd-DTPA enhanced MRI. Radiology 170: 229-237
10. Dorwart RH, La Masters DL, Watanabe JJ (1983) Tumors. In: Newton TH and Potts DG (eds) Computed Tomography of the Spinal Cord. Clavadel Press

11. Enzmann DR, Delapaz RL (1990) Tumor. In: Enzmann DR, Delapaz RL, Rubin JB (eds) Magnetic Resonance of The Spine. Mosby, Baltimore, pp 301-422
12. Gilbert RW, Kim JH, Posner JB (1978) Epidural Spinal Cord Compression from Metastatic Tumor: Diagnostic and Treatment. Ann Neurol 3: 40-51
13. Hajek PC, Baker LL, Goodbar JE, Sartoris DJ, Hesselink JR, Haghighi P, Resnick D (1987) Focal Fat Depositon in Axial Bone Marrow: MR Characteristics. Radiology 162: 245-249
14. Harnsberger HR, Dillon WP (1989) The Radiologic Role in Diagnosis Staging and Follow-up of Neoplasia of the Brain, Spine and Head and Neck. Semin Ultrasound CT MR 10:431-452
15. Kaffenberger DA. Sach CP, Mortagh FR, Wilson C, Silbiger ML (1988) MR Imaging of Spinal Cord Hemangioblastoma associated with Syringomyelia. J Comput Assist Tomogr 12: 495-498
16. Lafforgue P, Bayle O, Massoumat J, Cournelle JM, Schiano A, Kasharian M, Acquaviva PC (1991) L'IRM au cours des tassements vertébraux ostéoporotiques et métastatiques à propos de 60 cas. Annal de Radiologie 34: 157-165
17. Laredo JD, Reitine D, Bard M, Merland JJ (1986) Vertebral Hemangiomas: Radiologic Evaluation. Radiology 161: 183-189
18. Linden A. Zankivich R, Theissen P, Diehl V, Schidra H (1989) Malignant Lymphoma: Bone Marrow Imaging 28 Versus Biopsy. Radiology 173: 335-339
19. Mc Inerney DP, Middlemiss JH (1978) Giant Cell Tumor of Bone. Skeletal Radiol 2: 195-204
20. Moore SG, Gooding CA, Brasch RC, Ehman RL, Ringertz HG, Ablin AR, Matthay KK, Zoger S (1986) Bone Marrow in Children.with Acute Lymphocytic Lenkemia: MR relaxation Times. Radiology 160: 237-240
21. Parizel PM, Baleriaux D, Rodesch G, et al (1989) GdDTPA Enhanced MR Imaging of Spinal Tumors. AJNR 10: 249-258
22. Petren-Hallmin M, Nordstrom B, Andresson I, Nyman R, Johsson H, Ranschning W, Hemmingsson A (1992) MRI with Histopathological Correlation in Vertebral Metastases of Breast Cancer. Acta Radiol 33: 213-220
23. Roos RAC, Vielvoye GJ, Voormolen JHC (1986) Magnetic Resonnance Imaging in Occult Spinal dysraphism. Pediatr Radiol 16: 412-416
24. Ross JS, Masaryk TJ, Modic MT, Carter JR, Mapstone T, Dengel FH (1987) Vertebral Hemangiomas: MR Imaging. Radiology 165: 165-169
25. Schey WL, Shkolnik A, White H (1979) Clinical and Radiographic Considerations of Sacrococcygeal teratomas: an analysis of 26 new cases and review of the litterature. Radiology 125: 189-195
26. Schroth G, Thron A, Guhl L, et al (1987) Magnetic resonance imaging of spinal meningiomas and neurinomas: improvement of imaging by paramagnetic contrast enhancement. J Neurosurg 66: 695-699
27. Sugimura K, Yamasaki K, Kitagaki H, Tanaka Y, Kono M (1987) Bone Marrow Diseases of the Spine: Differentiation with T1 and T2 Relaxation Times in MR Imaging. Radiology 165: 541-544
28. Sze G, Vichanco LS, Brant-Zawadzki M (1988) Chordomas MR Imaging. Radiology 166: 187-191
29. Sze G, Twohig M (1991) Neoplasic diseases of the spine and spinal cord. In: Atlas SW (ed) Magnetic Resonance Imaging of the Brain and Spine. Raven Press, New York, pp 921-966
30. Sze G, Bravo S, Krol G (1989) Spinal lesions: Quantitative and Qualitative Temporal Evolution of Gadopentate Dimeglumine Enhancement in MR Imaging. Radiology 170: 849-856
31. Sze G, Krol G, Zimmerman RD, Deck MDF (1988) Intramedullary Disease of the Spine: Diagnosis using Gd-DTPA Enhanced MR Imaging. AJR 151: 1193-1204
32. Tassel PV, Leeds NE (1991) Diagnostic Imaging Advances in Neurooncology. Current Science: 439-448

CHAPTER 8

Imaging of malignant head and neck tumors (cervico-facial)

Clinicians
O. Laccourreye, D. Brasnu, J. Zerbib, S. Bobin, D. Nizri, N. Renody, F. Assadian, H. Szpirglas, A. Thomas, H. Laccourreye

Radiologists
J.-L. Bensimon, D. Buthiau

Malignant cervico-facial tumors consist of lesions of the paranasal sinuses or cancers of the upper aerodigestive tracts. These require a precise therapeutic approach to achieve the best chance of cure, minimize disfigurement and maintain function. Tumor extension of few millimeters in a critical zone will radically change the treatment, prognosis of these lesions and the quality of life of the patients. Close collaboration [43] between the surgeon, pathologist, radiotherapist, chemotherapist and radiologist will achieve the best result for the patient. Imaging is the indispensable complement of clinical endoscopic examination [36]. The use of ultrasound, CT and MRI [64] provides essential information about the localization, size and extent of these tumors. Technological improvements such as high resolution ultrasound with color doppler imaging, ultra high definition CT [59], improvement in contrast agents, use of automatic injection devices and progress in image reconstruction in 2 or 3 dimensions [50] have resulted in an extremely accurate assessment of tumor volume and spread. Magnetic resonance imaging has further transformed the diagnostic algorithm by its high sensitivity in the assessment of normal and pathological soft tissues. In France, access to MRI is still very limited and the resultant delays for an appointment are incompatible with the provision of fast, efficient treatment in oncological practice. MRI has an increasingly important role in the investigation of malignant lesions in the field of otorhinolaryngology.

Despite the high sensitivity of MRI, the specificity does not yet reach the cellular level and therefore the histological diagnosis depends on biopsy. Tissue characterization is still inadequate to evaluate with certainty the histological nature of the lesion [68].

Endoscopy with multiple biopsies, particularly at the edges of the lesion and at the likely excision boundaries, is the key examination for determining the nature and superficial spread of the lesion. In our practice, this often precedes imaging, contrary to the opinion of other authors [17] who advise against biopsy before any imaging. Undoubtedly biopsies artificially alter the imaging findings and extent of the pathological appearances, but we believe that the endoscopic findings should be available to the radiologist in order to have a better idea of the depth of extension within the areas with positive or suspicious biopsies. The local changes resulting from the biopsy can be interpreted more easily if the radiologist is aware of the biopsy site and, if necessary, the imaging can be delayed for a few days to allow for healing to occur.

It is important to indicate the overall volume of the lesion on imaging for both the surgical and radiotherapy treatment. In addition, it is vital to determine the locoregional extent of the tumor, particularly deep extension to the muscles, ligaments, cartilage and bone which are the key determinants of treatment choice. The superficial mucosal extent of the lesion must be noted although this is much more difficult to appreciate on imaging.

Imaging should also help in the assessment of distant spread of a tumor to the draining lymph node chains [39] (see later, fig. 13.2) and other possible metastatic sites. A coexistent second tumor is common in otorhinolaryngological cancers.

In the case of primary lymphadenopathy [55], imaging is of value in the search for the primary tumor.

In order to make any useful contribution, the radiologist must have an excellent knowledge of the regional anatomy, natural history of the disease and routes of tumor spread.

Imaging can also improve the TNM classification and have a direct [25] influence on the treatment [2].

It is also invaluable in the early or late follow-up of patients who have undergone surgery, radiotherapy or chemotherapy in whom clinical examination is difficult and the anatomy has been altered by the treatment. Imaging contributes to the post-treatment follow-up of these lesions either in the detection of local recurrence, lymph node involvement or metastasis. Interpretation of the images is not always obvious partly because scarring following surgery causes asymmetry of the anatomy in this region. In general, surgical scars have clear borders, and radiotherapy causes muscular atrophy and has a tendency to enlarge the perimuscular fat spaces. Fibrotic scar tissue may considerably complicate interpretation.

It is for this reason that comparison of successive examinations is often invaluable to confirm the presence of recurrent disease. A baseline CT or MRI examination should ideally be performed during the 6th to 12th week following treatment [19].

The improvements in imaging techniques have resulted in a much more accurate assessment of the extent of these tumors. Imaging is indispensable and complementary to clinical and endoscopic examination. However, although the sensitivity approaches 100% with the exception of microscopic lesions, the specificity is much less, particularly in the following three areas: histology, differentiation of tumor/edema, early infiltration of lymph nodes and cartilage. The three principle techniques currently used in the assessment of malignant cervico-facial tumors are ultrasound, CT [45], and MRI [32].

Ultrasound

Ultrasound should today be considered as a direct extension of the clinical examination in the assessment of lymph node involvement (see fig. 13.2). It increases the detection rate compared to palpation and is able to evaluate the blood flow in the major blood vessels of the neck. Currently the role of simple ultrasound is restricted to the examination of the latero-cervical region and complements clinical examination of the lymph node chains. Color doppler and duplex ultrasound have a role in the assessment of the relationship of large lesions with the major vessels of the neck, in the study of blood flow and extension of tumor into the vessels in the latero-cervical gutters.

A high frequency multidirectional probe of 7.5 MHz is used to obtain axial and longitudinal sections relative to the long axis of vessels. The size and internal echo pattern of the lymph nodes are assessed.

CT

The principal aim of imaging by CT or MRI is to determine the depth of locoregional spread and to detect lymph node involvement.

In this chapter we describe the general principles of the CT technique. Specific details applicable to each anatomical site will be described in the relevant paragraphs dedicated to each region.

Coronal sections may be performed either in the supine or the prone position, the head in hyperextension. The sections are usually obtained with a breath hold technique and, if possible, without swallowing.

The examination always commences with a lateral scanogram from which the sections can be prescribed by defining the plane of section, thickness, position and number of slices. The scan must include the whole of the lesion and all the draining lymph node chains which may be involved by the tumor.

Once the first section has been obtained, the field of view can be precisely modified if required. The scan data is stored if either multiplanar reconstructions or reconstructions with different filters, for the bony structures for example, are required.

Contrast injection is necessary to distinguish pathological lymph nodes, define the extent of the primary lesion, demonstrate intracranial spread and define the boundaries of extension into the surrounding fat. Similarly, contrast will help differentiate an enhancing tumor opacity from a non-enhancing retention opacity and delineate the blood vessels and their relationships to the lesion.

Automatic injection pumps are indispensable for continuous rotation scanners and for spiral acquisitions which are capable of acquiring all the sections of the larynx in a single breath hold and requiring only a single contrast injection. The excellent vascular enhancement obtained using this technique allows reconstruction of the major neck vessels in different planes. The 3-dimensional vascular reconstruction demonstrates the relationship of the vessels to the lesion.

Table 8.1. Table of the different tissues encountered: CT densities and MRI signal intensities with and without contrast

Tissues	CT	Iodine	MRI -T1	Gd	MRI- T2
Fat	low	no	hyper	no	iso
Bone	high	no	void	no	void
Bone marrow	low	no	hyper	slight	iso
Cartilage	medium	no	hypo/iso	no	hypo/iso
Muscle	medium	medium	iso	yes(medium)	iso
Liquid	medium	no	hypo	no	hyper
Vessels	medium	marked	hypo	yes(veins)	hypo
Mucus	medium	no	iso/hyper	no	iso/hyper
Tumor	medium	marked	iso	yes	iso/hyper

iso: signal intensity equal to that of muscles or cerebral tissue
hypo: signal intensity less than muscles, appears greyer on the image
hyper: signal intensity greater than muscles, appears whiter on the image
void: absence of signal, appears black on the image

For a manual injection [17], having first inserted a 19 or 20 gauge intravenous cannula and given any anti-allergic premedication if necessary, an initial bolus of 40 ml non-ionic (usually) contrast with an iodine concentration of 60% is injected in about 2 to 3 minutes. The first section is commenced at the middle or end of the bolus. The rest of the contrast dose is either given by slow continuous injection or by fractionated 20 ml bolus injections up to a total dose of 2 ml per kg of weight.

With an automatic injector, having first inserted a 19 gauge or preferably larger venous cannula (cathlon), the contrast agent is initially injected at a rate on 0.5-1 ml per second followed by a bolus of 30 ml and subsequent other bolus injections of 10 to 15 ml in order to obtain dynamic images in the arterial phase. Alternatively, a larger injection volume of 60 ml can be given using a slower flow rate to obtain continuous contrast penetration. Although the use of an automatic injection pump results in excellent, sometimes spectacular enhancement of the tumor tissues or blood vessels, there is a not insignificant risk of extravasation of contrast agent at the injection site. These different methods take approximately 8 to 10 minutes to acquire the high quality images with enhancement of the mucosa, tumor, lymph nodes and blood vessels.

MRI

MRI is at least as informative as CT, and much of what has been said for CT is equally as applicable to MR. It has an intrinsically higher sensitivity in differentiating soft tissues and is more versatile in the manipulation of the various tissue contrasts. Unfortunately, there are too few machines available resulting in significant delays for scans in France, and this is often incompatible with effective cancer treatment. This therefore limits the use of this technique leaving CT as the examination of choice.

Images can be acquired in any plane without having to move the patient and are prescribed from an initial quick localizing sequence. The plane of section is chosen, and the number of slices of predetermined thickness (thin from 3 to 5 mm) and position are selected. The saturation bands are placed in position in order to eliminate a number of artefacts of vascular origin. The tissue contrasts are very variable, with the T1 and proton density contrasts giving good anatomical detail and the T2 contrasts being more specific in the differentiation of healthy and pathological tissue, and edema and tumor. The number of acquisition sequences available are numerous, and the most commonly used sequences in our experience are the spin echo, gradient echo and "time of flight" angiographic sequences [24] (see table 8.1 listing the different tissue contrasts on CT and MRI).

There are different respective advantages for both CT and MRI. The advantages for CT are rapid access, reduced cost, ease of use, good spatial resolution, excellent visualization of bony and vascular structures, reduced susceptibility to movement artefacts and the ease of identifying lymph node structures following contrast injection. The advantages of MRI are the absence of ionizing radiation, the ease of multiplanar acquisition, the multiplicity of sequences and different tissue contrasts, the good visibility of blood vessels without contrast injection and the ability to assess flow, the high sensitivity in differentiating tissues from fluids or hemorrhagic effusions. Constant advances recently in this technique with both the use of contrast agents (gadolinium) whose effects on tissues [31] are comparable to those seen with the CT iodinated contrast agents, and the development of new imaging sequences such as MR angiography and rapid imaging sequences which reduce the scan time, allow more complete examinations be performed in scan times that are acceptable to the patient.

The malignant centro-facial granuloma presents its own specific problems:

a clinical syndrome of malignant centro-facial granuloma may arise from multiple etiologies of which the neoplastic causes are: metastasis, sarcoma, melanoma, spino- and basocellular tumors, accessory salivary glands. The plane radiograph demonstrates an abnormality of the sinus but is inadequate for a precise diagnosis; CT shows early bony lesions, MRI assesses the soft tissues and differentiates tumor from reactive inflammatory changes and defines the extent and post-radiotherapy changes of the disease.

References

See page 125

CHAPTER 9

Cancer of the pharynx and larynx

Clinicians
F. Assadian, N. Renody, H. Laccourreye, D. Brasnu, J. Zerbib, S. Bobin

Radiologists
J.-L. Bensimon, D. Buthiau

The diagnosis, pre-treatment assessment and follow-up of malignant tumors of the pharyngo-larynx require a close collaboration between the surgeon, pathologist, radiotherapist, chemotherapist and radiologist because determination of the exact nature of the lesion and its extension, particularly into the anatomical boundaries such as the cartilage, conus elasticus or lymph node chains will determine the prognosis of these lesions and the patients' quality of life.

CT [17] is still currently the principle examination [26] for the diagnostic assessment. Magnetic resonance imaging (MRI) [11] is complementary with its ability to perform coronal sections. It can demonstrate minimal disease of the paralaryngeal spaces and cartilages and assess peritumoral edema.

Review of anatomy

See figure 9.1 a - c

Techniques for examination of the pharyngo-larynx

CT [38]

The examination commences with a lateral scanogram in arrested respiration in order to demonstrate the vocal cords and ventricular opening.

The axial sections are prescribed from the scanogram [17] in a plane parallel to the vocal cords or "vocal plane".

Contiguous 3 mm thickness sections are acquired on a 512 x 512 matrix using a 16 cm field of view covering the glottic and superior portion of the subglottic regions.

We prefer to perform the whole examination in arrested respiration for each section and ask the patient to refrain from swallowing. At the end of the examination it is also possible to perform a few slices of about 1 mm thickness through the vocal cords on inspiration and phonation "O" [14] in order to assess the mobility of the medial borders of the vocal cords.

Sagittal and coronal reconstructions are performed in the majority of cases. Injection of an adequate dose of contrast agent is essential to identify correctly the arteries and veins [34]. This can be achieved by a manual injection of 20 ml boluses of contrast agent for every three sections, giving a total dose of 80 to 100 ml for a complete examination of the larynx in 3 mm sections. A better alternative is to use an automatic angiographic-type injection pump with boluses of 10 ml at a rate of 2 to 3 ml per second every three sections. This gives a better visualization of the vessels and reduces the dose of contrast agent used by half.

CT examination preferably should be performed before any surgical intervention and biopsy or alternatively perhaps after a few days of anti-inflammatory treatment so as not to overestimate the extent of the lesion due to edema resulting from the surgery.

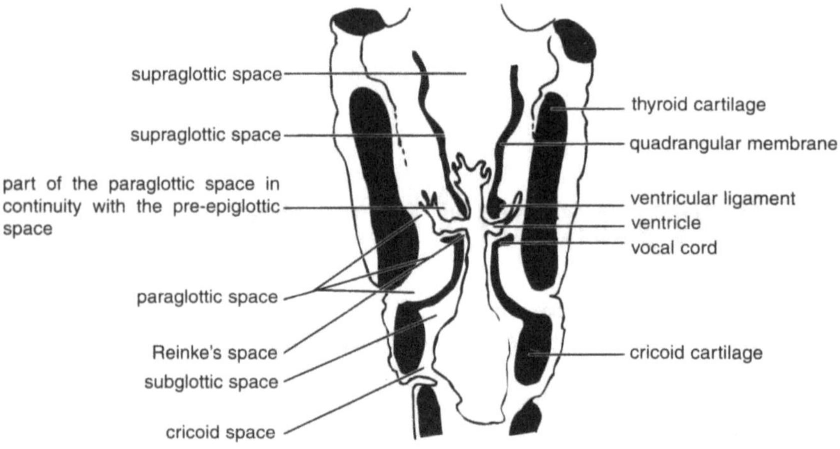

1 a

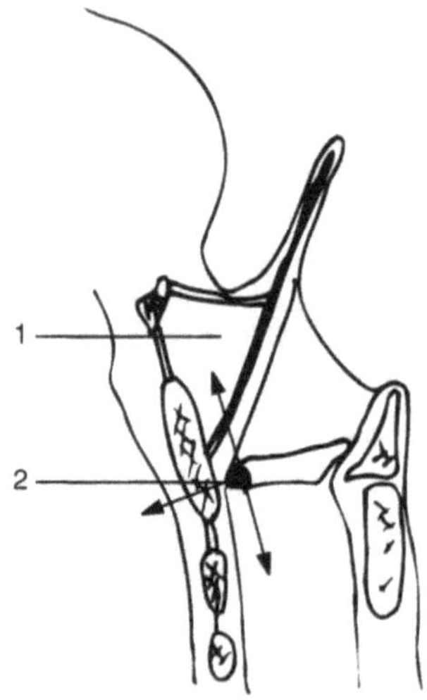

1 b

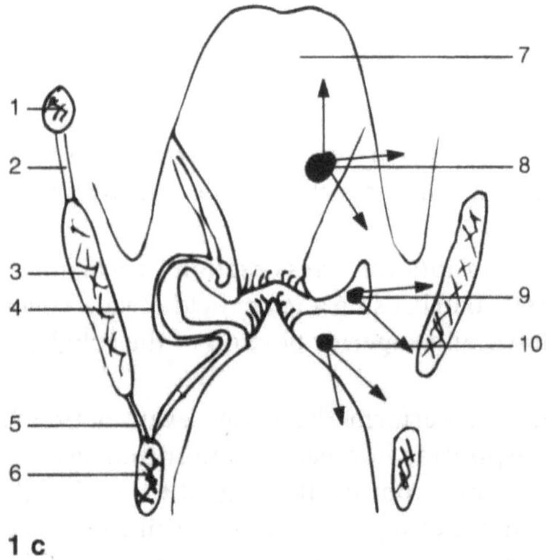

1 c

Fig. 9.1. a Compartments which form the boundaries of the larynx (modified from Silver CE "Surgery for cancer of the larynx and related structures", Churchill Livingstone, New York, 1984). **b** Diagram of the pathways for spread of cancers of the larynx. Lateral section of the larynx demonstrating the pathways of spread for lesions of the anterior commissure; *1* hypo-thyro-epiglottic space; *2* anterior commissure. **c** Coronal section of the larynx; *1* hyoid bone; *2* cricohyoid membrane; *3* thyroid cartilage; *4* conus elasticus; *5* cricothyroid membrane; *6* cricoid cartilage; *7* epiglottis; *8* epiglottic tumor; *9* tumor of the ventricles; *10* tumor of the vocal cord

MRI [51]

Its fundamental value and superiority over CT are linked to its multiplanar capability and ability to perform not only axial but also coronal and sagittal sections. The potential to image different contrasts, particularly on the spin echo T1, spin echo T2 and proton density weighted sequences, provide more accurate information than CT on local tumor invasion.

The injection of gadolinium, a paramagnetic element which essentially shortens the T1 relaxation time of tissue, gives similar information to that obtained on contrast enhanced CT. The comparison of identical T1-weighted sequences both with and without gadolinium is still essential to evaluate enhancement patterns.

Gradient echo T1-weighted sequences with fat suppression and gadolinium injection have a significant role in the differentiation of enhancing hyperintense tissue from intrinsically hyperintense fatty spaces.

The low signal intensity or signal void within the vessels with high flow is useful in differentiating cervical lymph nodes from vessels.

The T2 weighted sequences are essential in assessing infiltration of muscle and can differentiate the tumors from adjacent muscle masses.

Currently, however, due to some of the inconveniences associated with MRI, CT still has an important role in the assessment of cancers of the pharyngo-larynx. First, the slice thickness on the spin echo sequences is limited to 3 mm in order to obtain a satisfactory signal to noise ratio. This can be compensated by using 3DFT gradient echo sequences, but the acquisition time is a little too long and particularly sensitive to movement or vascular artefacts.

The spin echo T1- and T2-weighted sequences cannot yet be acquired on a single breath hold due to the fairly long acquisition times (at least two minutes), even for the fast sequences [11] and are therefore performed with slow and regular respiration. The examination may be uninterpretable due to movement artefacts which are dependent on patient cooperation, the patient's respiratory state and problems caused by the tumor itself. The advent of fast turbo spin echo sequences has not yet overcome these difficulties.

Currently, a 190 × 254 matrix is used, but matrices of 340 × 512 which improve spatial resolution are being employed with increasing frequency.

The field of view must be as small as possible and adapted to the area under investigation. It varies from 160 to 200 mm.

An initial sagittal T1-weighted echo sequence is performed with 5 mm thickness sections either contiguous or with an interslice spacing of 0.1 mm. This sequence acts as a localizer. Axial T1-weighted spin echo images with the 3 mm thickness and interslice gap of 0,1 or, if possible, contiguous sections both with and without gadolinium are obtained and followed by a dual asymmetrical echo T2-weighted spin echo sequence (proton density and T2 contrast).

The final sequence is a coronal T1-weighted spin echo sequence with thin 3 mm thickness slices.

This protocol may be modified if there is the need to obtain thin sections of a mm or less on a T1-weighted gradient echo sequence. The selected plane of section depends on the exact information which is required, i.e. axial for assessment of cartilaginous invasion [8], coronal for assessment of the glottic/subglottic junction. Axial fat saturated sequences and fast gradient echo sequences may be usefully added to this protocol, as well as MR angiography.

Cancers of the endolarynx [47]

In France, these make up 25% of cancers of the aerodigestive tract and 4 to 5% of all cancers. The overall 5 year survival rate is 50%. They occur between the ages of 45 and 70 years with a peak incidence at about 59 years in males and 62 years in females. There are several predisposing etiologic factors: cigarettes, alcohol, irradiation of the neck and other irritants: asbestos, chromium and nickel. This list is not exhaustive.

The existence of certain precancerous lesions is well known, for example planar keratoses (leucoplasias) and hypertrophic keratoses (villous keratosis, papillomas).

Pathological anatomy

The classification system is still based on the Klienssasser classification:
- stage I: epithelial hyperplasia with or without keratinization;
- stage II: epithelial hyperplasia with or without keratinization and dysplasia;
- stage III: carcinoma in situ with intact basement membrane;
- stage IV: invasive carcinoma with breach of the basement membrane.

Invasive carcinoma is infiltrative, vegetative or nodular; all these different forms can be of interest.

It is the infiltrative part of the tumor which must be assessed the most accurately by imaging.

The verrucose forms pose a differential diagnostic problem with a papilloma and is much more difficult to image.

Most of these tumors (98%) are epidermoid carcinomas, but adenocarcinomas, cylindromas and sarcomas may also be encountered. The prognosis is dependent on the degree of differentiation.

The anatomical position of the tumor can be classified into three distinct levels:
- supraglottic level,
- glottic level,
- subglottic level.

The supraglottic level is further subdivided into two parts: the epilarynx (including the margin) and subglottic level minus the epilarynx.

The epilarynx comprises:
- the laryngeal surface of the suprahyoid epiglottis,
- the free border of the epiglottis,
- the aryepiglottic folds,
- the arytenoid cartilage.

The subglottic level minus the epilarynx includes:
- the subhyoid epiglottis,
- the ventricular band,
- the ventricular cavity.

The glottic level includes:
- the vocal cords,
- the anterior commissures,
- the posterior commissures,
- the subglottic level.

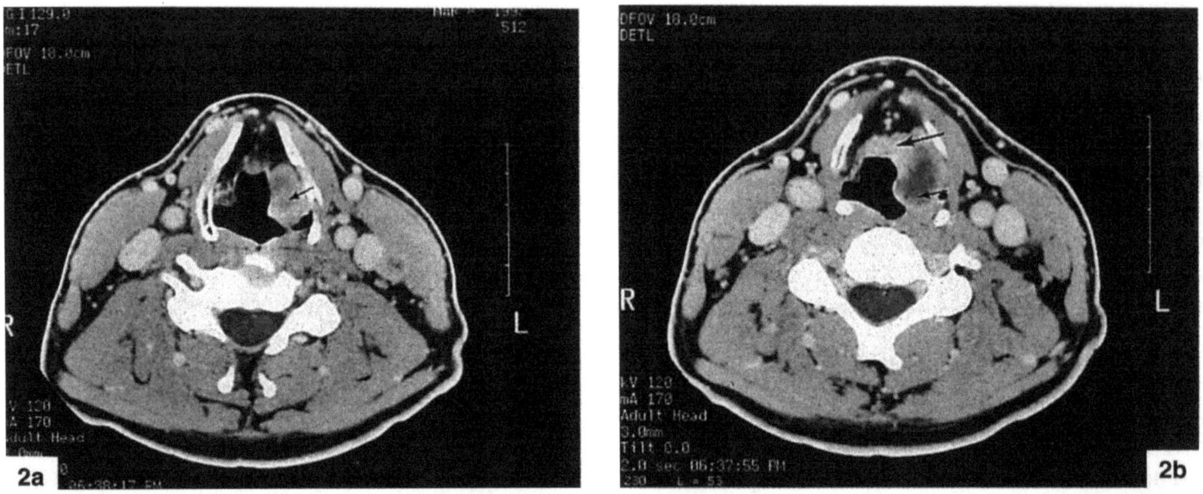

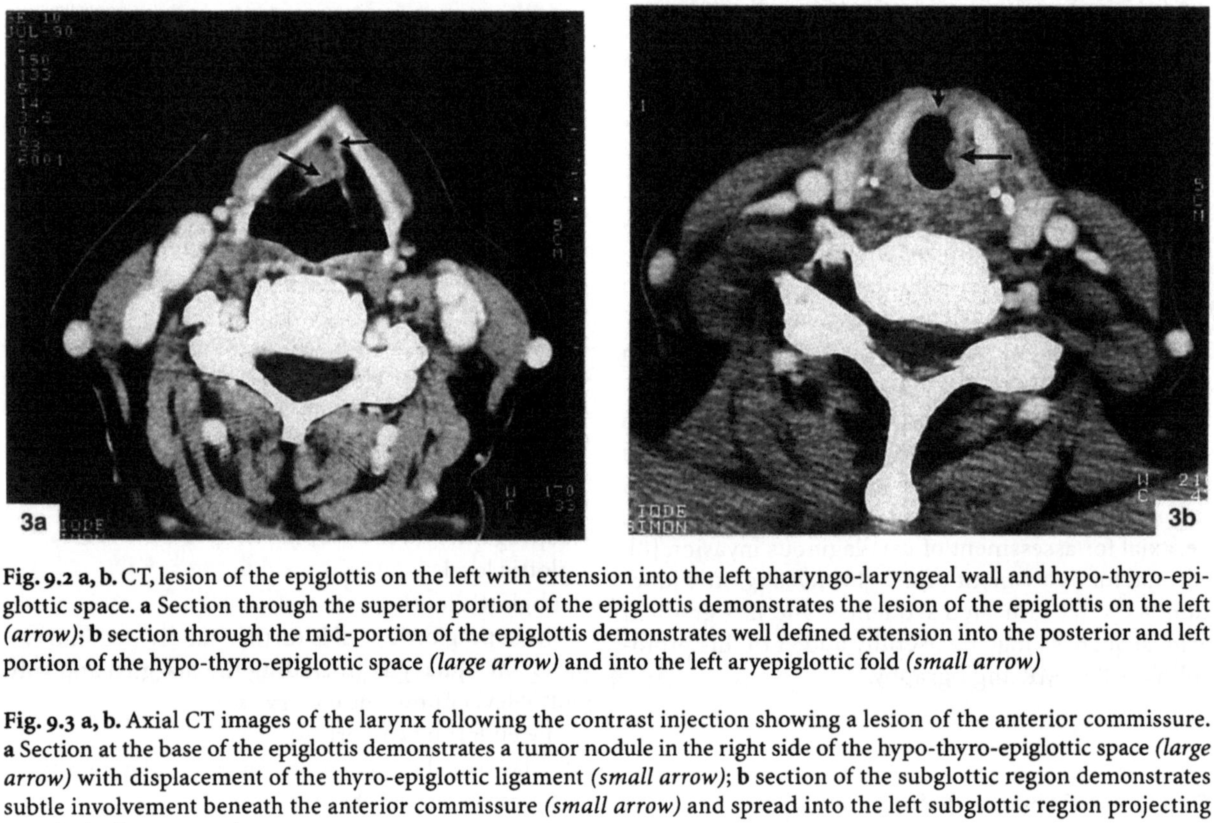

Fig. 9.2 a, b. CT, lesion of the epiglottis on the left with extension into the left pharyngo-laryngeal wall and hypo-thyro-epiglottic space. **a** Section through the superior portion of the epiglottis demonstrates the lesion of the epiglottis on the left *(arrow)*; **b** section through the mid-portion of the epiglottis demonstrates well defined extension into the posterior and left portion of the hypo-thyro-epiglottic space *(large arrow)* and into the left aryepiglottic fold *(small arrow)*

Fig. 9.3 a, b. Axial CT images of the larynx following the contrast injection showing a lesion of the anterior commissure. **a** Section at the base of the epiglottis demonstrates a tumor nodule in the right side of the hypo-thyro-epiglottic space *(large arrow)* with displacement of the thyro-epiglottic ligament *(small arrow)*; **b** section of the subglottic region demonstrates subtle involvement beneath the anterior commissure *(small arrow)* and spread into the left subglottic region projecting anteriorly *(large arrow)*

The possibility of multiple lesions in cancers of the aerodigestive tract must be emphasized.

The three principle clinical symptoms [5] of laryngeal pathology are:

- dysphonia: any persistent dysphonia in an adult, particularly in a smoker, requires investigation of the larynx;
- dyspnea: in the form of inspiratory bradypnoea with drawing in which is often progressive and only rarely an isolated symptom;
- dysphagia: typically, simple difficulty in swallowing for supraglottic and ulcerated lesions, or complete dysphagia for larger tumors.

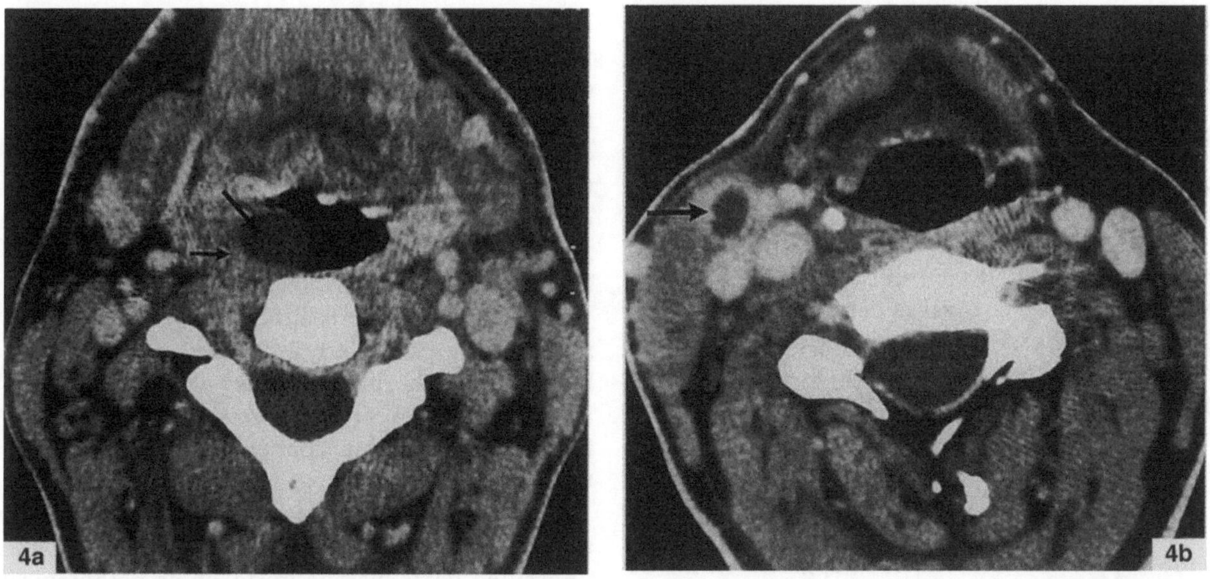

Fig. 9.4 a, b. Malignant cystic-looking lesion in the wall of the right laryngo-pharynx with an associated metastatic right supra-omohyoid lymph node measuring 17 mm in diameter. **a** Axial CT image of the superior part of the hypopharynx demonstrates the deceivingly cystic appearance of the lesion *(large arrow)*; no deep extension but there is thickening of the lateral wall *(small arrow)*; **b** more caudal section demonstrating the metastatic lymph node on the right *(arrow)*

Indirect laryngoscopy demonstrates the site of the lesion and has an essential role in determining laryngeal motility.

Endoscopy under general anesthetic by direct laryngoscopy in suspended respiration and hypopharyngoscopy precisely determine the spread, particularly at the level of the glottis, ventricle and ventricular bands and enable biopsies to be performed.

Imaging should be performed before biopsy so as not to overestimate the extent of the lesion. Imaging defines the extension and infiltration of the tumor, and detects extralaryngeal spread and metastasis to the lymph nodes or elsewhere.

Supraglottic lesions

These are detected later than the other laryngeal tumors because of the minimal associated symptomatology. They arise in the epiglottis (fig. 9.2), aryepiglottic folds, ventricular bands and ventricles. Spread of these lesions is anteriorly into the pre-epiglottic space or hypo-thyro-epiglottic region, superiorly towards the base of the tongue, inferiorly towards the anterior commissure and glottic region, posteriorly towards the posterior wall and laterally towards the aryepiglottic folds.

Lymph node involvement is commoner than for the other laryngeal locations.

Involvement of the pre-epiglottic space is easily recognized on CT [17] or MRI, because this region contains fatty and fibrous tissue which appears hypodense on CT (fig. 9.3) and markedly hyperintense on all T1-weighted sequences on MRI, in marked contrast to the tumor which appears dense on CT and iso- or relatively hypointense on MRI. The axial sections for both techniques are very accurate in demonstrating pathology except at the limits of this region due to the interpretation difficulties caused by partial volume effects, notably superiorly in the floor of the valleculae and inferiorly at the base of the epiglottis and anterior commissure. In these areas, MRI seems to be superior to CT due to the possibility of performing sagittal sections which demonstrate well the base of the epiglottis and the valleculae.

Spread towards the base of the tongue is often more difficult to recognize on CT due to the presence of the lingual tonsil which develops to a variable extent and has a CT density or MRI signal intensity which is very similar to a tumor, resulting in overestimation of tumors. MRI is slightly more accurate. Spread into the intrinsic muscle of the tongue is easier to detect on MRI. The signal intensity of the muscle is similar to that of tumor on T1-weighted imaging. Loss of the normal fatty fascia which separates the muscles is an indirect sign of tumor invasion. However, the T2 sequences particularly show the high signal intensity of the tumor-associated edema adjacent to the muscle fibres which remain iso- or relatively hypointense. The base of the tongue is particularly well shown on the sagittal sections.

Clinical assessment of tumor involvement of the aryepiglottic folds is far from accuracy [29]. CT or MRI demonstrate changes in density or signal of the pharyngolaryngeal wall involved by tumor as well as morphologic changes, thickening or deformity. Theoretically MRI should be slightly superior to CT, but in practice the movements artefacts resulting from swallowing and respiration often degrade MR images. CT is still the examination of choice.

Assessment of mucosal spread [37] is accessible to endoscopy; it may sometimes be apparent on the CT images as mucosal thickening which is well seen on MRI. This localized or irregular mucosal thickening adjacent to or in continuity with the tumor, must be compared with the endoscopy findings when it becomes contrast-enhanced.

Involvement of the posterior wall is well seen by both techniques on the posterior muscle masses and inferiorly towards the retro-arytenoid region. CT and MRI are equally accurate in diagnosing lymph node involvement. The lymphatic drainage of these lesions is superiorly and posteriorly towards the subdigastric nodes and is often bilateral.

On CT, nodes are considered to be highly suspicious if they are greater than 15 mm in diameter and situated in the drainage pathways of the tumor, even if they appear regular and homogeneous, isolated or multiple; or smaller lymph nodes which are multiple and asymmetrical also occurring in the drainage territory of the lesion.

Lymph nodes which contain hypodense necrotic areas on CT or marked hyperintensity on the T2-weighted MRI sequences should equally be considered as pathological nodes.

Capsular break [39] is common in lymph nodes greater than 3 cm in diameter. This break may be detected on CT as a lymph node having indistinct and irregular contours with poor visualization of the boundaries of structures adjacent to the node. Muscular infiltration is, on the other hand, more difficult to confirm, the muscle having the same density as the lesion. MRI is more accurate due to the hyperintensity of the pathological tissue on T2-weighted imaging which is easily differentiated from the hypointensity of the muscles and vessels. The diagnosis of capsular rupture can be made earlier on MRI. Involvement of lymph nodes adjacent to the major vessels, particularly the carotid arteries, should be demonstrated with MRI being slightly more accurate than CT. It is extremely important to demonstrate encasement of the carotid arteries by lymph nodes or the lesion itself and to try to assess involvement of the arterial wall.

Assessment of tumor spread by vascular emboli is beyond the scope of imaging.

Invasion of cartilage is difficult to appreciate unless it is extensive, particularly if the cartilage is transfixed by the tumor. The difficulty arises with hyaline cartilage because the cartilages ossify with age in an inhomogeneous fashion, particularly the thyroid cartilage.

On CT, the ossified portion has a very dense cortex and a less dense medullary bone. Conversely, the unossified parts may be mistaken as pathological areas of osteolysis. The distinction between this pathological and physiological ossification of cartilage is sometimes impossible on CT. Cartilaginous involvement is therefore very often underestimated on CT.

MRI is more accurate in the assessment of cartilaginous invasion. The T1-weighted sequences differentiate the isointense tumor tissue from the hyperintense medullary bone. However, the hypointensity of the cortical bone poses the same problems as CT in the detection of minimal infiltration of cortical bone and is underestimated by both techniques. The T2-weighted or fat suppression (fat sat) sequences are more useful in the assessment of the involvement of hyaline cartilage, the signal intensity of the tumor tissue being greater than that of the normal cartilage.

Imaging, therefore, has a role in the classification of the tumor, detecting the degree of spread in the deep impalpable regions and assessing involvement of subclinical or clinically unsuspected lymph nodes.

Glottic tumors

This is the commonest site for malignant laryngeal tumors and presents at the earliest stage due to dysphonia. With glottic lesions, one usually hears about involvement of the vocal cords, the anterior and posterior commissures. Lesions of the anterior commissure are a special case because these lesions often involve all three levels of the larynx.

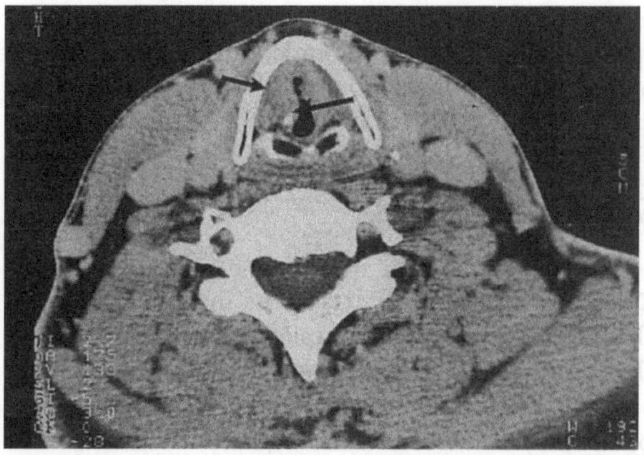

Fig. 9.5. Axial contrast enhanced CT image in the plane of the vocal cord of the glottic and subglottic regions of the larynx: nodular lesion of the mid third of the right vocal cord *(large arrow)* without involvement of the paraglottic space *(small arrow)* or alteration in the calcified arytenoid cartilage

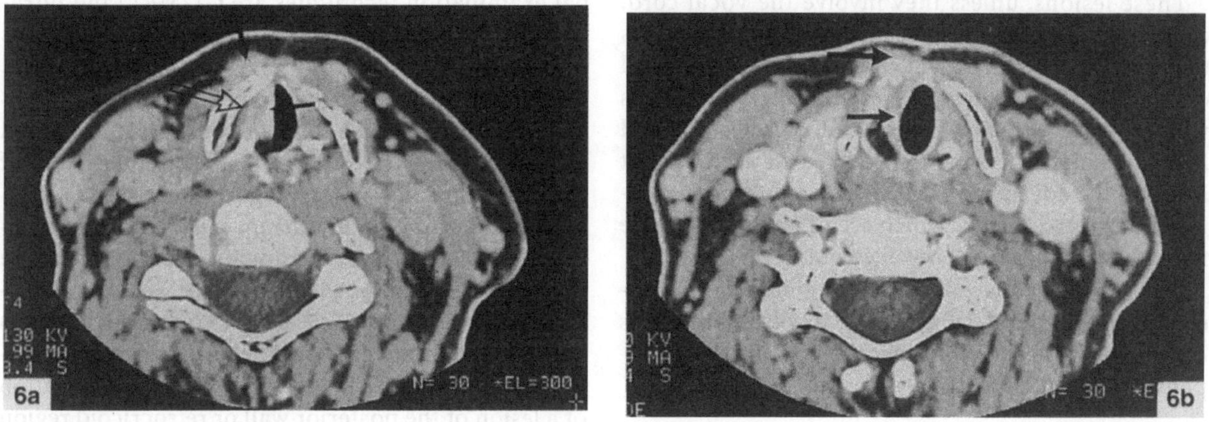

Fig. 9.6 a, b. Contrast enhanced axial CT images of the glottic region. **a** Section of the glottis in inspiration with immobility and infiltrative fixation of the right vocal cord *(small arrow)* without involvement of the paraglottic space *(hollow arrow)*. Note the asymmetry of the prethyroid region, thickened on the right *(large arrow)*. **b** Section of the subglottic region demonstrates subglottic involvement on the right *(small arrow)* and involvement of the cricothyroid membrane; condensation of the superior border of the anterior arch of the cricoid ring indicating full thickness involvement *(large arrow)*

Lesions of the middle third of the vocal cord (fig. 9.5) extend superficially and deeply towards the paraglottic space and it is particularly at this level that imaging has an important role. Thin sections and a bolus injection of contrast agent are essential for CT. The examination is looking for the loss of the paraglottic fatty space. MRI and CT are equally accurate. In thin subjects, the visualization of this space is difficult in the physiological state.

Coronal MRI sections give a better assessment of the subglottic region and ventricles.

Spread to the anterior commissure and anterior subcommissure is visualized on axial and sagittal sections.

The difficulty in assessing the degree of subglottic spread on axial sections alone must be stressed. However, at the level of the cricoid cartilage ring, any mucosal thickening should be considered as pathological.

Lesions of the anterior commissure are occurring in a weak area of the larynx, and thus there is often a thickening of the pre-epiglottic region, dislocation of the base of the epiglottis and transfixation by tumor spread anteriorly (fig. 9.6).

Imaging helps in the assessment of tumor involvement of the thyrocricoid membrane and spread of tumors anteriorly into the prethyroid muscle planes.

The problem of cartilaginous involvement again arises, and it must be remembered that CT underestimates whereas MRI tends to overestimate. Tumor invades the medullary cavity of the ossified cartilage without causing destruction or deformity of the bone trabeculae, explaining one of the difficulties in detection (advantage of CT). Lesions of the posterior commissure are rare (1% of glottic lesions) and tend to spread towards the arytenoids and posterior tissue planes.

Subglottic lesions

The subglottic space starts at the inferior surface of the vocal cord and comprises of the medial surface of the cricothyroid membrane and cricoid cartilage. Pure subglottic lesions are rare and represent 4% of cancers of the larynx. More commonly, they are due to subglottic spread of glottic lesions.

These lesions, unless they involve the vocal cord, cause few symptoms, and the main value of imaging is the ability to visualize them and assess the height and depth of spread as these are often infiltrative lesions which invade the membranes and muscles. CT and MRI give similar information on the axial sections, but MRI has the advantage of being able to perform sagittal and coronal images which are of particular value for assessing vocal cord involvement.

Any subglottic mucosal thickening must be considered as pathological. Lymph node involvement is less common for these lesions, but there is a greater propensity for distant metastases.

Lesions of the hypopharynx

Tumors of the hypopharynx are dealt with similar diagnostic and therapeutic problems as those of the larynx. In the presence of an extensive lesion, it is difficult to determine the exact site of origin of the tumor. These lesions involve the piriform fossa, the posterior wall and retro-arytenoid region. There is a significant risk of lymph node and metastatic spread. At the time of the initial examination, a lymph node metastasis is present in more than 50% of cases.

These tumors essentially occur in males who drink and smoke heavily, and are often in a mediocre general physical condition, aggravated by feeding problems related to the tumor. The prognosis is poor.

They represent 10-15% of tumors of the aerodigestive tract with a similar epidemiology to the rest. The exception is the retrocricoid lesions which occur more commonly in women. Macroscopically, the lesions are usually nodular in the superior half of the hypopharynx and more ulcero-infiltrative in the inferior half. Spread is usually to the jugulo-digastric and supra-omohyoid lymph node groups, and the more inferior lesions spread into the cervical and mediastinal nodes (see later fig. 13.2).

Locoregional spread is medially towards the pharyngo-laryngeal wall, anteriorly towards the hypo-thyro-epiglottic region, laterally towards the lateral wall and wing of the thyroid cartilage, superiorly towards the subtonsillar region and antero-inferiorly towards the Killian opening and prevertebral muscles.

Investigation by imaging should include an assessment of the corresponding lymph node chains and a search for distant metastasis (bone, lung, liver and brain).

The common association of a coexistent lesion must always be borne in mind. As for the larynx, the principal examination techniques are CT, MRI (and ultrasound). The same problems arise for the radiologist as in the subglottic lesion.

There are two particular points of note. Firstly, lateral spread at the level of the cricothyroid muscle and extension of the lesion towards the lateral surface of the wing of the thyroid cartilage between the constrictor muscles and perichondrium causes more destruction of the lateral surface and posterior border of the thyroid wing than the medial surface which is in contact with the tumor. The lesion commonly spreads along the pathway of the vessels and nerve, particularly if the thyroid is involved. Secondly, investigation of a lesion of the posterior wall or retrocricoid region is more difficult due to movements from swallowing and the presence of secretions. In addition, some pedunculated lesions, which rest against the posterior wall in the supine position, are well known traps for imaging. Certain authors, therefore, have suggested that the examination should be performed with the patient prone [1].

The classical imaging protocols for the laryngopharynx need to be modified as these lesions have a tendency to spread to the esophagus and mediastinal lymph node chains necessitating examination of the thoracic and celiac regions.

The radiologist must recognize that, although mucosal spread is poorly demonstrated, deep spread of the tumor to the fascia, prevertebral muscles, the presence of impalpable enlarged posterior lymph nodes, and spread superiorly into the retropharyngeal region are only visible on imaging. Fat saturation T2-weighted sequences on MRI are more sensitive in detecting muscle involvement.

References

See page 125

CHAPTER 10

Cancer of the oropharynx and buccal cavity

Clinicians
N. Renody, J. Zerbib, F. Assadian, S. Bobin, O. Laccourreye, D. Brasnu, H. Laccourreye

Radiologists
J.-L. Bensimon, D. Buthiau

Tumors of the buccal cavity can arise at several sites:
- the buccal floor,
- the mobile portion of the tongue (anterior two thirds),
- cheek,
- retromolar trigone (limited medially by the intermaxillary commissure and laterally by the ascending branch of the inferior maxillary artery,
- medial surface of the ramus of the mandible,
- junction of the fauces and tongue,
- gingival crest,
- intermaxillary commissure,
- vault of the bony palate.

Lesions of the oropharynx arise in the:
- lateral wall:
  - tonsillar fossa (including the supratonsillar fossa),
  - anterior and posterior fauces,
  - palatine tonsil,
  - glosso-palatine sulcus;
- anterior wall:
  - glosso-epiglottic sulcus (valleculae),
  - base of the tongue;
- superior wall:
  - antero-inferior surface of the soft palate,
  - free edge of the palate and uvula;
- posterior wall.

The majority of lesions are epidermoid (squamous) carcinomas of varying degrees of differentiation, more rarely muco-epidermoid carcinomas, adenoid cystic carcinomas, adenocarcinomas or non-Hodgkin's lymphomas. Exceptionally, malignant melanomas of the tonsil or its fossa may occur. Tumors of bony origin arising from the mandible will not be discussed here [6].

Although the clinical examination of these two regions is easy, these tumors are often diagnosed relatively late for several reasons: on the one hand, self neglect of the patients due to chronic alcoholism; on the other hand, particularly relevant for the oropharynx, there are no real anatomical barriers to the spread of these lesions.

The degree of infiltration can be appreciated by clinical palpation, but this is no substitute for accurate imaging.

In fact, the development of the new radiological techniques, particularly CT and MRI, has provided details of tumor size and extension into adjacent structures. These tumors are extremely lymphophilic and it is not uncommon for patients to present initially with apparently primary lymph node enlargement.

It is therefore imperative to assess the cervical lymph node chains and treat them in the same way as the primary tumor.

Review of anatomy

See figure 10.1

Clinical features

Oropharynx

The clinical signs of tumors in the oropharynx are non specific and include intermittent unilateral pain-

1

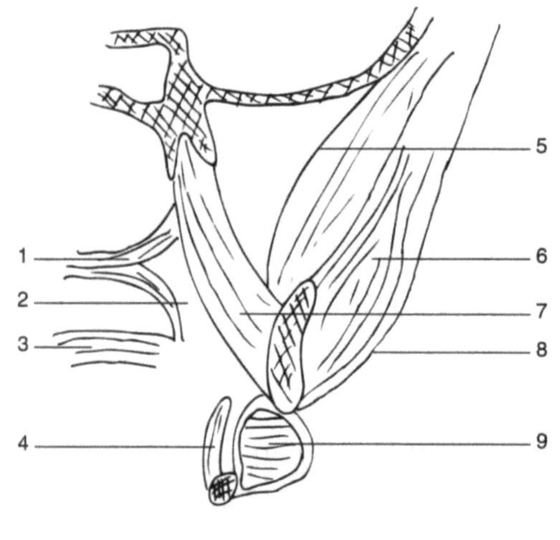

Fig. 10.1. Diagram of the lateral spaces of the buccal cavity on a coronal section. *1* Soft palate; *2* parapharyngeal space; *3* tongue; *4* mylohyoid muscle; *5* masticatory space; *6* masseter; *7* medial pterygoid; *8* aponeurosis; *9* submandibular gland

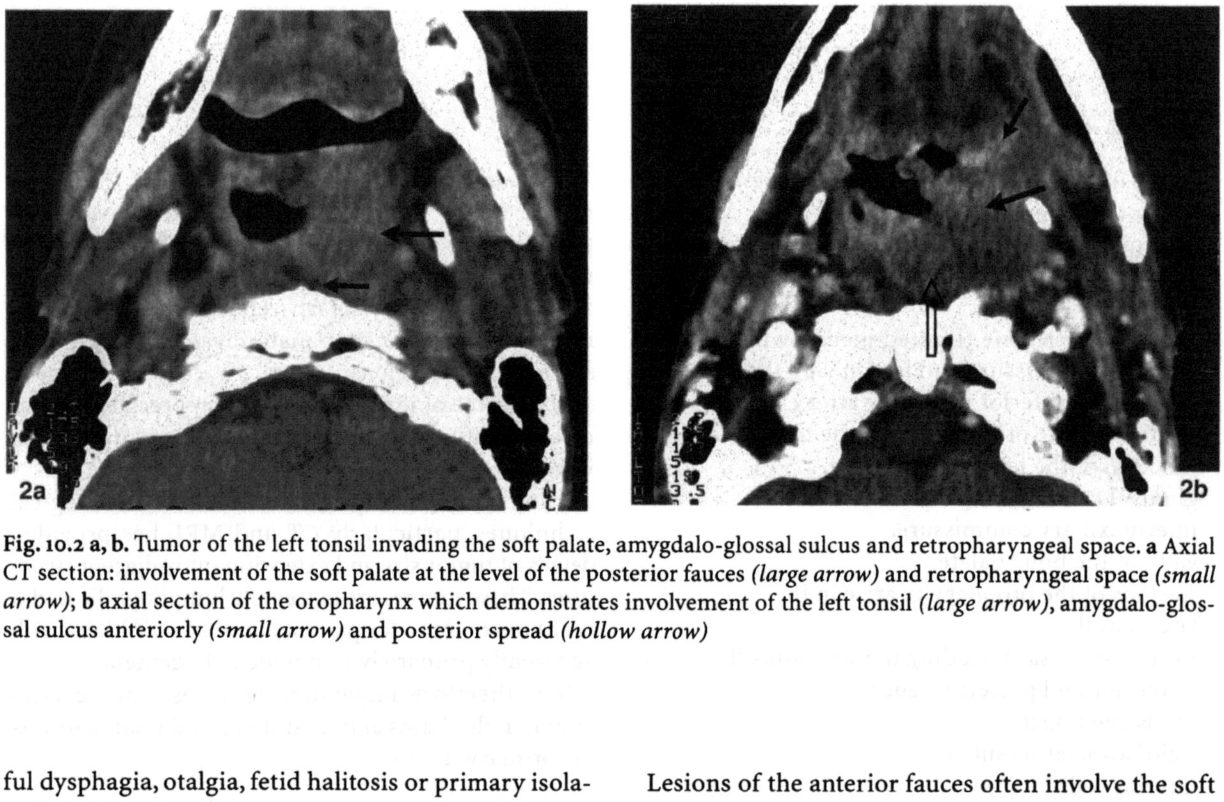

Fig. 10.2 a, b. Tumor of the left tonsil invading the soft palate, amygdalo-glossal sulcus and retropharyngeal space. **a** Axial CT section: involvement of the soft palate at the level of the posterior fauces *(large arrow)* and retropharyngeal space *(small arrow)*; **b** axial section of the oropharynx which demonstrates involvement of the left tonsil *(large arrow)*, amygdalo-glossal sulcus anteriorly *(small arrow)* and posterior spread *(hollow arrow)*

ful dysphagia, otalgia, fetid halitosis or primary isolated lymph node enlargement. The macroscopic appearances of the lesion determine its imaging appearance; it may be nodular or ulcero-vegetative and more rarely infiltrative. Locoregional and lymph node spread depend on the site of origin. Lesions of the palatine tonsil (fig. 10.2) arise in contact with lymphoid tissue and are particularly lymphophilic [42]; they are rather ulcerative and nodular, sometimes difficult to detect if they arise in a cryptic tonsil. Spread is towards the fauces, the tonsillo-glossal sulcus with deep spread towards the constrictor muscles, fat spaces and the muscles of mastication explaining the late occurrence of trismus.

Lesions of the anterior fauces often involve the soft palate and intermaxillary commissure anteriorly, the tonsil posteriorly, the palatoglossus muscle and particularly the mandible laterally and the junctional zone of the tongue. Lesions of the posterior fauces invade deeply to the palatopharyngeal and pterygoid muscles superiorly. They extend anteriorly towards the soft palate and inferiorly towards the hypopharynx.

Lesions of the tonsillo-glottic sulcus extend towards the base of the tongue, and the prognosis is the same as for tumors of the tongue base.

Lymphatic drainage is to the subdigastric, superior spinal, jugulo-carotid and transverse cervical groups and more rarely to the submental or submaxillary

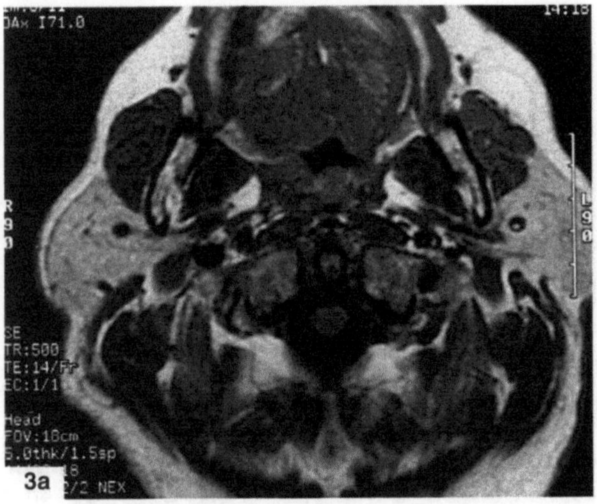

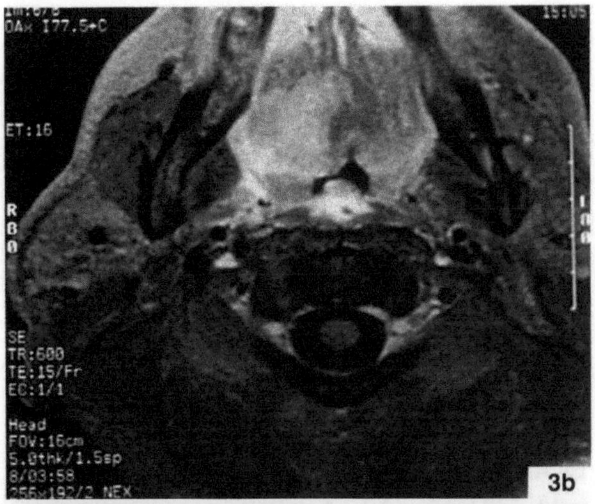

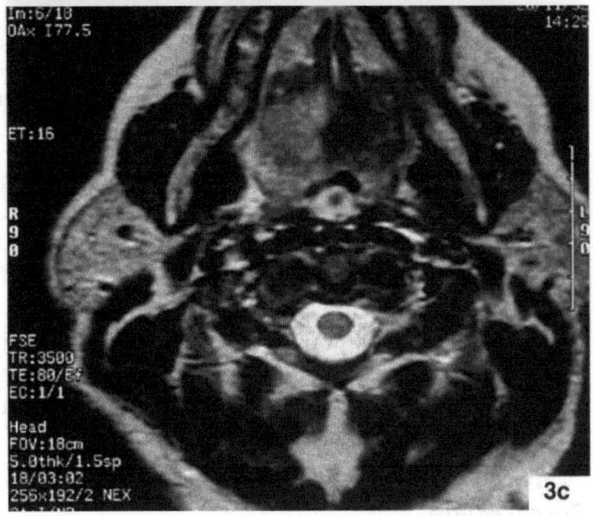

Fig. 10.3 a-c. Lesion of the tongue base on the right, T3N2; necrotic epidermoid carcinoma on MRI. **a** T1 spin echo sequence; the lesion is difficult to distinguish from the normal intrinsic muscles of the tongue; **b** same sequence with gadolinium; the tumor enhancement is apparent; **c** axial T2 spin echo sequence differentiates the tumor contours from the surrounding inflammation

lymph node chains. Lymph node involvement is common, and 70% of patients present with lymphadenopathy at the initial examination, 15% have bilateral lymphadenopathy.

Lesions of the posterior wall tend to be ulcerative and nodular, and clinically apparent. Generally, they remain separate from the posterior fauces. The superior and inferior limits of the tumor are well appreciated clinically and imaging should be used to define deep extension, particularly posteriorly towards the prevertebral space. These lesions are very lymphophilic (60% have lymph node involvement at the initial examination).

In the field of otorhinolaryngology, cancer of the base of the tongue (fig. 10.3.) is the one with the worst prognosis (5 year survival around 17%). Unfortunately it is often detected late because the clinical symptoms are fairly minor. Only deviation and reduced protraction of the tongue alert the clinician to a tumor at this site, but these symptoms signify that the lesion is already very advanced. There is often associated lymphadenopathy, uni- or bilateral, and usually fixed.

Palpation and examination with a mirror will give the diagnosis but underestimate the depth of infiltration. The lesion extends anteriorly towards the mobile portion of the tongue, posteriorly to the valleculae and epiglottis, laterally to the glosso-tonsillar sulcus and tonsil. Imaging, particularly MRI and if necessary CT, accurately defines the depth of infiltration into the intrinsic musculature and buccal floor.

Lymphadenopathy is very common, notably in the subdigastric, mid jugulo-carotid and supra-omohyoid lymph node groups.

Lesions of the soft palate (fig. 10.4) also cause a few symptoms, usually the sensation of a foreign body, and are seldom painful. Lymphadenopathy is often the

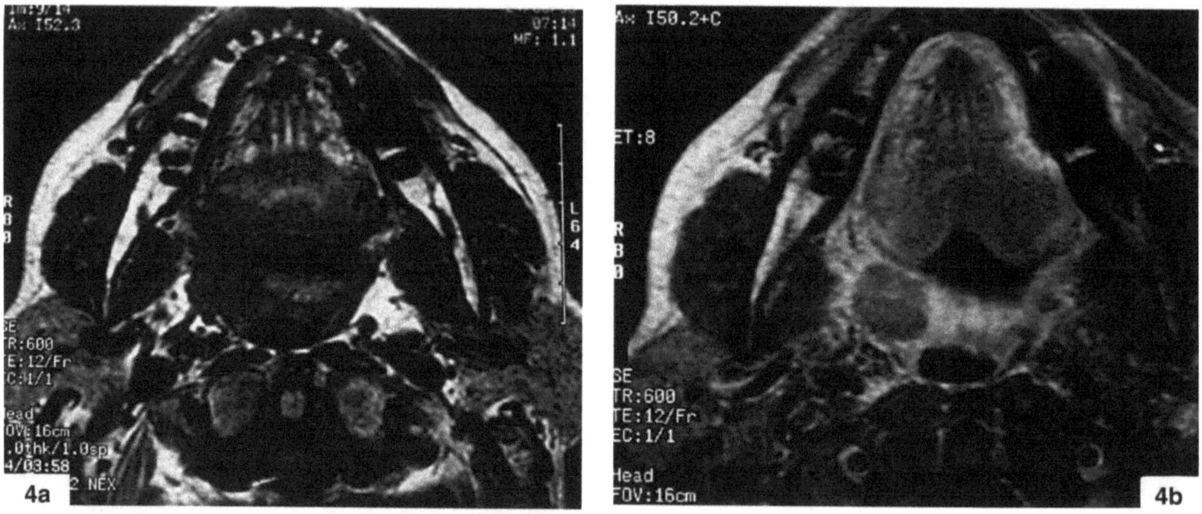

Fig. 10.4 a, b. Epidermoid carcinoma of the right side of the soft palate. Well defined nodular lesions on MRI. **a** Axial T1 image without gadolinium. The tumor is well defined with preservation of the fat plane separating the tongue base and the pterygoid muscles; **b** axial T1 image with gadolinium. Moderate enhancement of the tumor, less than that of the normal soft palate

presenting feature. These lesions are frequently nodular or nodular with ulceration, serpiginous, diffuse, poorly defined and bleed on contact. Superficial spread is via the mucosa, and deep spread by multidirectional infiltration towards the tonsillar region, vault of the bony palate and skull base following the course of the maxillary nerve (V2). Lymph node involvement is usually in the subdigastric group.

Buccal cavity

Superficial spread of lesions of the gingival sulcus is anteriorly towards the mandible, posteriorly towards the area of the anterior fauces, and medially towards the base of the tongue. Deep spread is to the mandible [66].

Lesions of the retromolar trigone involve the anterior fauces and tonsil posteriorly, the gingival sulcus anteriorly and the pterygo-mandibular space deeply. Bone involvement is at a later stage.

Lesions of the vault of the palate extend towards the nasal fossae, maxilla and muscles of mastication.

Imaging techniques

CT

Axial and coronal sections are performed which are always prescribed from a lateral scanogram with the patient supine and the head in extension without the headrest so that the examination can be extended to the inferior cervical region if necessary. Each section is performed in arrested respiration and without the patient swallowing.

The plane of the axial sections is parallel to the inferior border of the mandible. Only a study of the vault of the palate, soft palate or a search for extension into the cavum require sections parallel to the plane of the hard palate.

The plane of the coronal sections should be perpendicular to the hard palate whenever possible.

The axial sections are often degraded by artefacts caused by permanent dental prostheses, particularly at the level of the tonsil and intermaxillary commissure. This problem can be partially overcome by performing the first two or three sections with the mouth open and the rest of the examination continued in the normal fashion with the mouth closed.

The images are acquired using a 512 × 512 matrix. Subsequent image reconstructions are performed with both a soft tissue and bone filter to look for bone involvement.

The thickness of section varies from 1 to 5 mm. We prefer sections of around 1 mm thickness which may either be contiguous or have an interslice gap of 3 mm depending on the organ under investigation. For example, early bone involvement will only be detected using sections of the order of 1 mm thickness

A bolus contrast injection of 10 to 25 ml is indispensable.

The examination should include the whole of the lesion and its local spread, as well as the draining lymph node chains.

MRI

These section are acquired in three orthogonal planes.

Slice thickness is 3 to 5 mm, either contiguous or with an interslice gap of 0.1 mm. The examination should include identical comparative T1-weighted sequences with and without gadolinium, as well as proton density and truly T2-weighted sequences. Some authors suggest that the turbo spin echo sequences can replace the classical T2-weighted sequences.

The examination may be complemented by supplementary fat saturated sequences with gadolinium which give a better appreciation of tumor infiltration into the fat spaces and medullary bone and improve the detection of early lymph node metastasis.

Time of flight MR angiogram sequences may provide useful information in terms of the relationship of the vessels to the lesion. One may also see invasion of the carotid artery or jugular vein by tumor, or a lymph node mass. Lymph node assessment can equally well be performed by MRI.

Advantages and disadvantages of the two techniques

CT has significant advantages due to the rapid image acquisition with resultant absence of artefacts from respiration or swallowing. It is also superior in the detection of early invasion of cortical bone. However, artefacts caused by dental prostheses are unavoidable. CT requires contrast injection, often at a dose of 2 ml per kg of body weight. Compared to MRI, CT has a moderate accuracy in assessing infiltration of muscles. Assessment of the deep fat planes is difficult on CT in thin patients. Visualization of the mucosa is difficult, and the distinction between lymphoid tissue and muscle is often subtle.

MRI, on the other hand, is more sensitive in differentiating the tumor from inflammatory tissue on the T2-weighted sequence. Involvement of muscle is better demonstrated on the T2- or post-gadolinium T1-weighted sequences.

MRI also gives a more accurate assessment in different anatomical planes of patients following treatment, particularly post-irradiation. It is sometimes possible to differentiate fibrosis from recurrent tumor. The extent of the lesion is more accurately assessed in 72% of cases, and there is better visualization of deep infiltration to the base of the tongue and the buccal floor.

Demonstration of the vessels does not require a contrast injection.

MRI is definitely the best examination for this region but currently has the disadvantage of being susceptible to motion artefacts caused by respiration and deglutition which degrade the image quality. This may be overcome with the arrival of the new rapid sequences. Another disadvantage still present in France is the delay in the appointment times due to an inadequate number of scanners which is often unacceptable for a patient requiring prompt treatment for a carcinoma.

Within the buccal cavity, the assessment of a tumor and its extension are well demonstrated both by CT and MRI, the latter being more sensitive at the level of the tongue, buccal floor and for spread into the bony medulla. CT is superior for the detection of cortical bone involvement.

MRI is particularly useful in the post-treatment follow-up and provides early information on recurrent tumors or fibrotic scar tissue.

MRI and CT are equivalent in the assessment of the deep fat spaces although the sagittal MRI images are often indispensable for lesions of the tongue, soft and hard palate and posterior wall of the oropharynx.

Coronal sections are useful for studying the gingival sulcus which along with the intermaxillary commissure is often a difficult region to assess.

Early bone involvement must be recognized. Early involvement of cortical bone may only appear as area of bone condensation in contact with the lesion without any evidence of osteolysis. These appearances are only visible on CT. It must also be remembered that infiltration of the bony medulla may occur without involvement of the cortical bone, and this will only be demonstrated by MRI, particularly on the fat saturated sequences which render fat hypointense relative to the relatively hyperintense enhancing tumor following the contrast injection.

Both CT and MRI may be used for assessment of the base of the tongue. MRI is preferable due to the images in the sagittal plane and the better visualization of muscles, aponeuroses, intermuscular fat planes and lymphoid tissue. Both techniques are used for looking at the tonsillar lesion, again with a preference for MRI due to the better visualization of submucosal involvement and the good differentiation between lymphoid tissue and muscle.

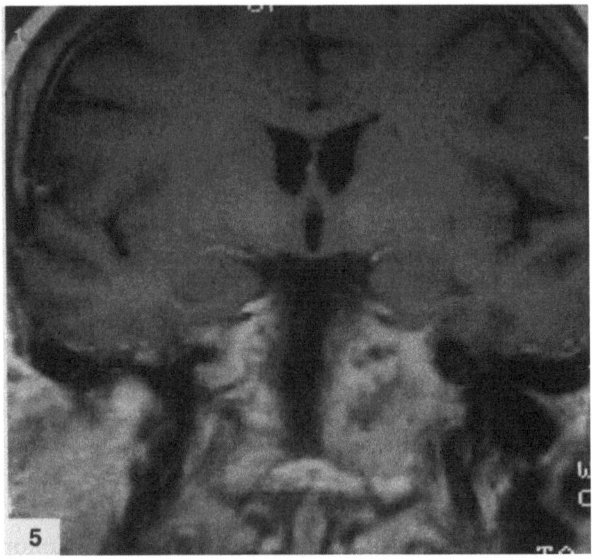

Fig. 10.5. MRI: second tumor at the level of the left superior portion of the cavum and the skull base with involvement of the pterygo-palatine region; initial tumor occurring at the base of the tongue. Coronal image following gadolinium demonstrating enhancement of the tumor mass; the necrotic center is relatively hypointense; note erosion of the skull base without extension into the cavernous region or intracranial cavity

There are also advantages in replacing CT by MRI for the detection of locoregional spread from tonsillar lesions.

The lymph node assessment for these lesions must cover from the retropharyngeal and the jugulocarotid lymph node chains as far as the mid-cervical region (see later fig. 13.2). The assessment of the tumor requires the injection of gadolinium on MRI (fig. 10.4), and examinations performed without gadolinium injection underestimate the volume of the tumor.

Follow-up and detection of recurrences

Recurrence of tonsillar lesions [55] is a particular problem which occurs in 80% within the first 2 years following treatment. According to some authors, this may be linked to an erroneous assessment of the size of the lesion, particularly in cases undergoing surgery for the reduction in tumor size after chemotherapy. The clinical signs are usually pain or trismus at a later stage, particularly for disease of the tonsil and retromolar trigone. Imaging can detect subclinical recurrences and provides important information in the search for these recurrent lesions (fig. 10.5).

The clinical symptoms may be due to a local complication rather than a recurrence, such as an abscess, necrosis or radionecrosis of bone. It is advisable to perform a CT or MRI examination 6 to 8 weeks following treatment to act as a reference for subsequent follow-up.

References

See page 125

CHAPTER 11

Cancer of the nasopharynx

Clinicians
N. Renody, D. Nizri, F. Assadian, O. Laccourreye, D. Brasnu, H. Laccourreye, J. Zerbib, S. Bobin, A. Thomas, H. Szpirglas, D. Khayat

Radiologists
J.-L. Bensimon, D. Buthiau, D. Herbreteau

The clinical history, epidemiology and evolution of cancers of the nasopharynx differ from the other cancers of the aerodigestive tract.

The most commonly encountered tumors are of epithelial origin, of which the common form is the undifferentiated epidermoid carcinoma (UCNT: undifferentiated carcinoma nasopharyngeal type). This tumor arises in the lympho-epithelial tissues, and there is a strong association with the the Epstein Barr virus (EBV). However, other connected tumors may also be seen such as non-Hodgkin lymphomas, embryonic rhabdomyosarcomas, achromatic melanomas and sarcomas.

Unlike other tumors of the aerodigestive tract, there is no association with alcoholism or smoking. These tumors affect young subjects and females in a frequency unusual for a cancer of the aerodigestive tract.

There is a specific geographic distribution, the tumors being uncommon in Europe or the USA, approximately 1-5% of cancers of the aerodigestive tract, occurring at a rate of 5-7 cases per 100,000 in the North African countries and becoming exceptionally common in the countries of Southern Asia, in the order of a 100 cases per 100,000.

Predisposing etiologic factors include genetic, environmental and viral factors. The association of this cancer with the Epstein Barr virus (EBV) is easily demonstrated using immunological studies. However, this does not prove the causative role of the virus in the development of the disease. The EBV appears to be a major epidemiological influence, but is not definitely a direct causative factor for the lesion. The genetic factors are linked to the leukocyte histocompatibility antigens (HLA) which result in a marked predisposition to the development of cancers of the nasal cavity.

Studies of different ethnic groups suffering from malignant lesions of the cavum have clearly demonstrated the variable incidence of the lesion between the same groups living within and outside the endemic areas. This has lead to a search for etiologic factors linked to the environment, and resulted in the discovery of inhaled carcinogenic agents contained in Chinese medicines or the action of nitrosamine present in salted fish in South China.

Review of anatomy

See figure 11.1

Clinical features

Lesions of the rhinopharynx are often detected late, and the average delay from the onset of symptoms is 8 to 10 months. This is due to the deep seated position of the rhinopharynx, the difficulty of clinical examination and the deceptive symptomatology caused by the tumor.

These lesions present with three major types of symptoms; otological, rhinological and neurological symptoms.

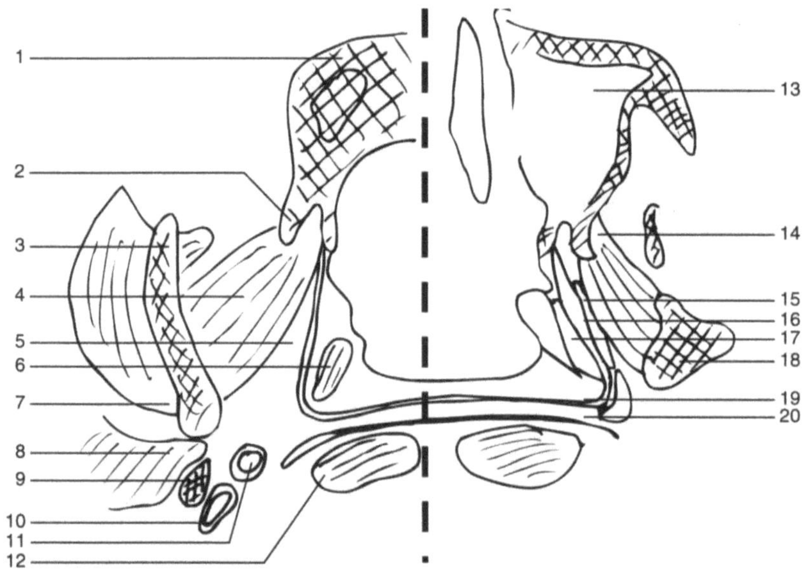

1

Fig. 11.1. Diagram of the superficial and deep spaces of the nasal cavity (cavum) on axial sections at two levels: the section on the right is inferior to the section on the left. *1* Hard palate; *2* lateral pterygoid plate; *3* mandible; *4* lateral pterygoid muscle; *5* parapharyngeal space; *6* levator veli palatini and salpingopharyngeus muscles; *7* pharyngobasilar fascia; *8* deep lobe of the parotid; *9* styloid process; *10* jugular vein; *11* carotid artery; *12* longus colli muscle; *13* maxillary sinus; *14* lateral pterygoid muscle; *15* tensor veli palatini muscle; *16* pharyngobasilar fascia; *17* levator veli palatini muscle and cartilaginous part of the auditory (pharyngotympanic) tube; *18* mandible; *19* superior constrictor of the pharynx; *20* prevertebral space

The otological symptoms are essentially signs of airway obstruction which raise concern when they are unilateral and of a particularly painful nature.

The rhinological symptoms are nasal obstruction, unilateral epistaxis, rhinorrhoea and rarely a nasal speech.

The neurological signs are related to involvement of the cranial nerves, superior maxillary or mandibular pain, diplopia (VI) or trismus (V).

In nearly 50% of cases, the tumor presents with lymphadenopathy of the superior and posterior groups, notably the superior supradigastric and superior spinal groups.

Metastases are common and directly related to initial lymph node involvement. The commonest sites for metastases are bone, lung, liver and axillary or inguinal lymph nodes.

Imaging techniques

CT

Initially a lateral scout view is performed with the patient supine and the head semiflexed. The axial sections are prescribed in a plane parallel to the hard palate, and coronal sections perpendicular to this. Each scan is performed in arrested respiration and without swallowing.

The slice thickness is comprised between 1-3 mm with a 2-5 mm interslice gap, and a bolus contrast injection is used. The acquired data is reconstructed using soft tissue and bone filters. The examination is completed by axial sections of the oropharynx and neck to assess the draining lymph node chains.

The coronal sections are essential and only capable of confirming tumor spread into the infratemporal fossa, skull base or cavernous sinus region.

Involvement of the pterygopalatine fossa is better shown on the axial sections.

Assessment of the deep regions may be more sensitive using a continuous infusion of contrast agent in association with parotid sialography.

MRI

This is performed using a head coil. It is the best examination for assessing involvement of the superficial and deep soft tissues of the cavum, but is still inferior to CT for early bone involvement.

The axial and coronal sections are performed in the same planes as CT, and the examination should always

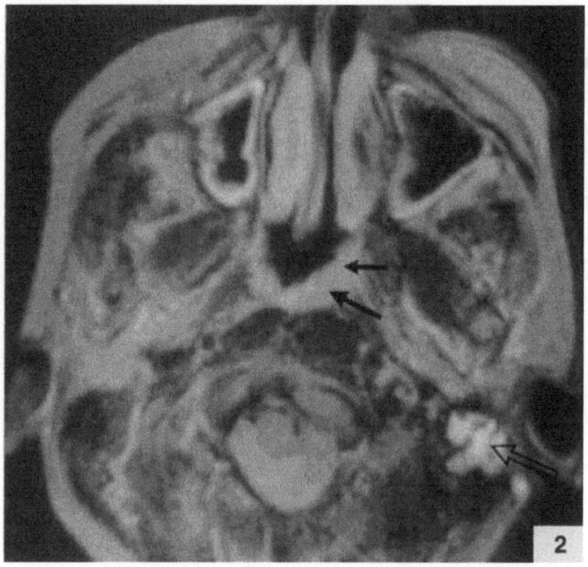

Fig. 11.2. Axial T2-weighted MRI image at the level of the cavum which demonstrates thickening and inflammation (hyperintense) of the posterior recess on the left *(large arrow)* extending anteriorly through the torus tuber *(small arrow)* without involvement of the deep spaces; note the serous reaction in the left middle ear *(hollow arrow)* from this small lesion of the cavum

include sagittal sections. Thin slices, 3-5 mm, with an interslice gap of 0 or 0.1 mm are acquired using spin echo sequences. The examination comprises of exactly comparable T1-weighted sequences with and without gadolinium followed by T2 sequences usually using a spin echo technique. Gradient echo T2-weighted sequences may be useful for the assessment of lymphadenopathy.

Time of flight MR angiogram sequences essentially give useful information about the carotid artery and cavernous sinuses.

Fat saturation sequences with gadolinium are useful for detecting minimal involvement of the deep fatty spaces.

A field of view of a 160-200 mm is used preferably with a 512 × 512 matrix.

For two main reasons CT currently remains the routine examination. One is a matter of practicality, as there is only a limited access to MRI; the other is due to the better visualization of bone involvement on CT. MRI is used as complementary technique, particularly for detecting extension of tumor along the course of nerves, into the submucosal spaces, for involvement of the bony medulla without a significant lesion of the cortical bone, for involvement of the cavernous sinuses and intracranial spread and early muscle infiltration.

It is certain that, in the near future, the respective roles of these two techniques will be reversed, and that MRI will be the initial examination of choice for assessment of lesions of the nasal cavity, with CT being used for detection of bone involvement.

Certain anatomical structures offer minimal resistance to tumor spread. Such is the case, for example, for the fasciae and aponeuroses.

The development of tumors is easily detected by noting displacement of the deep fatty spaces and, in particular, the parapharyngeal space following break of the pharyngobasilar fascia. Once into the deep spaces, the lesion can spread within this space which extends from the skull base to the cephalic region either superiorly towards the skull base or inferiorly towards the oropharynx.

It is possible on CT to detect early lesions by the indirect signs, but MRI is much more accurate and, in particular, is the only technique which can demonstrate invasion of the pharyngobasilar fascia.

Early perineural spread is directly demonstrated by MRI. Later stages are demonstrated if there is enlargement of the exit foramina of the skull base (foramen ovale) or atrophy of the muscles innervated by the involved nerve.

Detection of bony involvement requires highly symmetrical axial and coronal sections. Asymmetrical positioning of the patient may result in misdiagnosis of osteolysis.

In general, the lymph nodes are hard, multiple and measure more than 20 mm. They usually occur in the intermasto-mandibular region and are fixed to the vascular axis in half of the cases. Lymphadenopathy is found in 75% of patients (see fig. 13.2).

The internal jugular and spinal veins are also considered to be principal drainage pathways. It should be remembered that sometimes there is a direct drainage to the middle internal jugular node. Lymph node enlargement is bilateral in 50% of cases at the initial examination. Involvement of the retropharyngeal lymph nodes is common.

Imaging also has a role in post-treatment follow-up. Image interpretation can be extremely challenging in patients following radiotherapy in whom clinical examination is difficult. It is for this reason that some authors have suggested that the imaging examination (CT or MR) should be performed in the first 6 to 12 weeks following treatment to act as a reference scan for subsequent follow-up.

References

See page 125

CHAPTER 12

Cancer of the paranasal sinuses

Clinicians
J. Zerbib, D. Nizri, G. Michaux, N. Renody, F. Assadian, A. Thomas, H. Szpirglas, S. Bobin

Radiologists
J.-L. Bensimon, D. Buthiau, D. Herbreteau

Cancers of the paranasal sinuses exhibit particular characteristics which distinguish them from other cancers of the upper aerodigestive tract. These characteristics include their great histological variability, epidemiology, the severity of a local disease, the rarity of metastases or lymphadenopathy and the infrequent presence of a second coexistent lesion.

Their development in natural anatomical cavities explains the often late diagnosis and fundamental role of the imaging techniques, either CT [6] or magnetic resonance imaging [5, 7, 10]. The severity of the disease is related to the local spread towards the skull base, brain, orbits and pterygomaxillary fossa.

Recent surgical advances, particularly techniques using a combined dual approach by the otolaryngologist and neurosurgeon, have provided access to extensive lesions and improved the terrible prognosis of intracranial spread. Bone involvement is unfortunately common and explains the low 5 year survival rate.

Clinical features

These are rare tumors representing only 0.2 to 0.8% of all cancers and 3 to 5% of cancers of the aerodigestive tract specifically.

80% of cancers occur in the ethmoidomaxillary sinuses, and pure ethmoidal and sphenoidal tumors are rare and lesions of the frontal sinuses exceptional.

The tumor predominantly affects men, rarely before the age of 40, the average age being between 40 and 70 years. Adenocarcinomas are common from the age 40, and carcinomas as well as adenoid cystic carcinomas are the rule in elderly patients between the ages of 50 and 70. Sarcomas are more often encountered in younger patients.

The etiologic role of infection or chronic inflammation is still controversial. There is certainly an associated chronic inflammation in the majority of epidermoid carcinomas, but its precise role, as for polyposis, is difficult to determine. Bucco-sinus fistulae of dental origin have also been implicated, but as yet there is no definite proof.

More certain are the malignant degeneration of papillomas and mostly the toxic effects of sawdust from hard or exotic woods which explains the increased incidence of ethmoidal adenocarcinomas in wood workers.

These cases are recognized as occupational diseases. Tannins in the sawdust are the responsible toxic agents. There is a long latent period of up to 30 years before the onset of these tumors. Other toxic industrial agents have been incriminated such as isopropanolol, asbestos, uranium and thorotrast. The histological appearances are diverse and are listed in order of frequency:

- epidermoid (60 to 65%), glandular or undifferentiated carcinomas (28%) [10],
- malignant lymphomas (10%),
- sarcomas of the soft tissues, bone or hemopoietic origin,
- melanomas,
- esthesio-neuroblastomas (neuroblastomas of the olfactory nerve) [20].

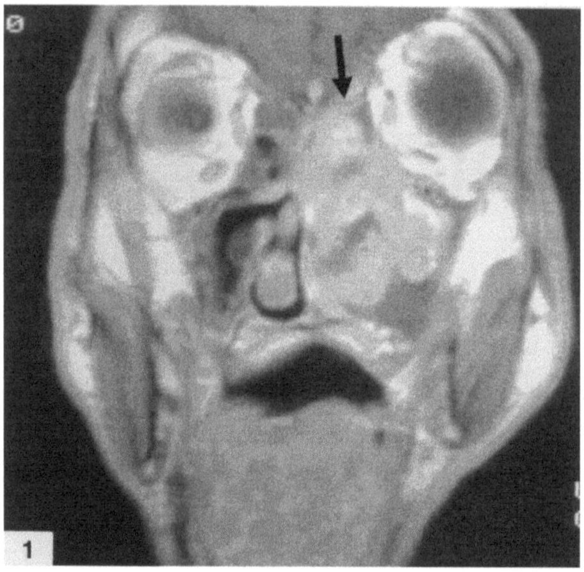

Fig. 12.1. MRI, coronal T1-weighted image of a cancer of the left ethmoido-maxillary sinuses showing enhancement of the tumor and inflammatory tissue, with intracranial extension *(arrow)*, but no enhancement of the retained secretions in the inferior half of the maxillary sinus

Carcinomas

These arise in the respiratory mucosa secondary to a metaplasia. Macroscopically the tumors are ulcerative, infiltrative, nodular or mixed and of a variable degree of differentiation. The undifferentiated form is the commonest and is associated with the highest incidence of lymph node involvement.

The adenocarcinomas are classified as well differentiated, papillary or trabecular, colloid or poorly differentiated adenocarcinomas.

The adenoid cystic carcinomas (cylindromas) are considered to be malignant tumors but are slow growing. They usually arise in the vault of the palate.

The sarcomas, hematosarcomas, fibro- or osteosarcomas, chondrosarcomas or angiosarcomas, depending on their cell of origin, have a very poor prognosis.

The malignant melanomas are rare and often achromatic, they frequently metastasize.

Esthesio-neuroblastomas are tumors which arise from the olfactory bulb. They are peculiar due to their localization on the cribriform plate and their early attachment to the anterior aspect of the skull base. They extend inferiorly towards the nasal fossae.

Other tumors are rare but gliomas, meningiomas, sympathomas, schwannomas, plasmocytomas and oncocytic tumors may all be encountered [1]. The presenting signs are very variable, nasal symptoms predominate, and patients often present with recurrent minimal epistaxis, chronic mucopurulent rhinorrhoea and progressive nasal obstruction. Unilateral involvement is extremely suggestive.

Deformities occur later and indicate tumor extension to the bony walls of the sinus.

Neurological symptoms occur late and are due to invasion of the nerves with resultant anesthesia or paresthesia of the territory supplied by the nerve, particularly the maxillary nerves. Pain is often an indication of skull base involvement. The signs of orbital involvement are unilateral disease with diplopia, reduced visual acuity, lid edema and exophthalmos. These are only present in 50% of cases. The buccodental signs are not rare, with deformity or abnormal mobility of a tooth, poor healing following extraction or the formation of a fistula. Trismus is a later sign due to involvement of the pterygo-maxillary fossa and muscles of mastication. Lymphadenopathy is rarely the presenting feature.

Imaging techniques

The imaging is indicated only after a careful clinical examination, including a full neurological and general examination and endoscopy of the otorhinolaryngological system. Standard radiographs of the sinuses in the frontonasal, Blondeau (water), Hirtz and lateral projections may give clues to the diagnosis of fully developed tumors, but are totally insufficient for assessing tumor spread. Tomograms [35] have been completely replaced by CT [18] which remains the examination of choice for all sinus pathology [36].

The classical CT technique [6, 36, 65] is a series of axial sections in the plane of the hard palate and coronal sections perpendicular to the axial plane. The slices must be thin, in the order of 1 to 2 mm, as sections with any thicker than this may suffer from partial volume effects which cause interpretation difficulties, particularly in the assessment of early bone extension [22]. The use of contrast agent [45] is imperative as assessment of enhancement degree may help in diagnosing the nature of the lesion and improve the definition of the tumor contours and visualization of spread [35]. Reconstructions in the sagittal and other planes are less widely used at the moment, but will become more and more popular with the increasing computing power available on the scanners [50].

Complementary magnetic resonance imaging [32, 33, 36, 57, 64] has become almost indispensable for the assessment of tumor extension into the soft tissues, such as the pterygomaxillary fossa and orbits [7], or intracranial spread with involvement of the dura mater. Currently it is the best technique for post-operative follow-up.

Thin slices of 3-5 mm thickness are acquired using a head coil in 3 planes, axial, coronal and sagittal. The axial plane is the same as that for CT, i.e. parallel to the plane of the hard palate, and the coronal plane is perpendicular to the latter.

The examination comprises always of T1-weighted spin echo sequences (fig. 12.1), with and without gadolinium [31], which assess the tumor volume and diagnose and differentiate intrasinus fluid retentions [33] due to blockage of the ostia by tumor from true intratumoral extensions. The coronal sections demonstrate extension into the infratemporal fossa, towards the skull base, and intracranially, the axial sections demonstrate spread into the pterygomaxillary fossa. The examination should also include T2-weighted spin echo sequences which may also differentiate inflammatory changes or retained secretions from true tumor extension.

There is also interest in the 3DFT gradient echo sequences due to the image reconstruction capabilities and the thinness of slices, often less than 1 mm, which are often useful for detecting minimal bone involvement [24]. The MR angiogram sequences are used to study the carotid arteries and region of the cavernous sinuses. Fat saturated (fat sat) spin echo sequences are useful for assessing intraorbital tumor extension [12]. The interpretation of the MR images requires a meticulous attention to detail. The intrasinus bony septa appear as signal voids (i.e. black) unless they are thick enough to contain bone marrow which appears hyperintense on the T1-weighted sequences (e.g. the sphenoid sinus) and is difficult to differentiate from pathological mucosa. Precise determination of the degree of edema and inflammation around a tumor mass is sometimes more difficult in practice than in theory. The classical signal intensity of retained secretions on T1- or T2-weighted imaging may be modified by the presence of a recent of old hemorrhage and hemosiderin (due to its ferromagnetic properties). On the other hand, the chemical composition of the fluids within the retained secretions as a function of the mucoprotein content may cause complete reversal of the classical signal intensity making interpretation extremely difficult without the use of gadolinium [33, 36].

The signal of a small tumor within a large sinus full of inflammatory tissue may be completely masked.

On CT, the tumor appears as a soft tissue opacity mixed with peritumoral inflammation and intracavity retained secretions. The injection of a bolus of contrast agent may help differentiate the non-enhancing retained fluids from the tumor and peritumoral inflammatory tissue which take up the contrast agent. However, this distinction is often equivocal, and MRI is definitely much more accurate. Nonetheless, CT still remains irreplaceable for the detection of bone involvement [45], intrasinus lysis or invasion of the pterygomaxillary fossa, infratemporal fossa and cribriform plate. CT and MRI are equivalent for the assessment of intraorbital spread, particularly if fat saturated sequences with gadolinium are used for intraconal spread [7].

Perineural tumor extension is often difficult to detect with either technique. It requires a detailed assessment of the different cranial nerves in the proximity of the lesion and thin sections along the course of the nerve as far as its passage through the skull base. On MRI, using T1-weighted sequences, the cellular tumors appear hypo- or iso-intense with areas of high signal intensity due to recent intratumoral hemorrhage. They enhance strongly following the injection of gadolinium, becoming hyperintense relative to all the other normal tissues. On T1-weighted imaging, inflammatory tissue may be slightly more hypointense than the tumor and enhances to the same extent following gadolinium. Fluid retentions are usually hypointense if composed of non-hemorrhagic fluid or have a low protein content. They follow the whole spectrum from grey to white depending on the mucoprotein content, and this can be deceptive. Gadolinium is therefore essential due to the absence of enhancement

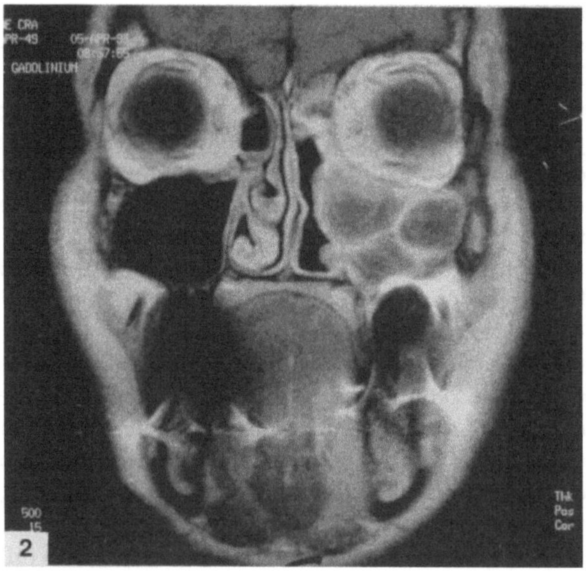

Fig. 12.2. MRI, T1-weighted sequence following gadolinium. Follow-up of a post-operative cavity in the left ethmoido-maxillary sinus. Note the particular appearance of the edematous mucosa and inflammation of the maxillary sinus with no sign of recurrent tumor

within the areas of retained fluid. On T2-weighted images, the signal intensity of the tumor alters little, remaining iso- or slightly hyperintense relative to the muscle apart from certain tumors of the salivary glands and lymphomas [42] in whom the signal is higher.

Peritumoral inflammatory tissue has higher signal intensity and can therefore be differentiated from the tumor itself giving a more accurate localization. Retained secretions are more hyperintense than the tumor, sometimes concealing inflammatory tissue. Some lesions have imaging characteristics which may give clues to the histology or particular routes of spread which need highlighting. The rare chondrosarcomas have a predilection for the walls of the ethmoids and nasal septum; on CT, the presence of intralesional calcification is suggestive of a tumor of bony or cartilaginous origin.

MRI is the examination of choice for assessing intracranial spread and can confirm the invasion or integrity of the meninges.

In conclusion, CT and MRI are complementary techniques in the assessment of malignant lesions of the paranasal sinuses. They should provide the most accurate localization of the tumor itself, evaluate peritumoral inflammation and associated intrasinus retained secretions, and detect invasion into the infratemporal fossa, pterygo-palatine fossa and intracranial cavity. Imaging sometimes also detects more distant spread via the perineural route, assesses intraorbital invasion and much rare lymph node involvement. The exact histology cannot be determined by imaging.

Imaging has an important role in the post-therapeutic follow-up (fig. 12.2), particularly MRI due to its clear superiority over CT in the differentiation of tumor and fibrosis.

References

See page 125

CHAPTER 13

Malignant tumors of the salivary glands

Clinicians
J. Zerbib, D. Nizri, F. Assadian, N. Renody, S. Bobin, A. Thomas, H. Szpirglas, O. Laccourreye, D. Brasnu, H. Laccourreye

Radiologists
D. Buthiau, J.-L. Bensimon, D. Herbreteau

Malignant tumors of the salivary glands [4, 16] may arise in the parotid, submandibular, sublingual glands or accessory glands which are scattered throughout the buccal cavity and pharyngo-larynx.

Parotid gland tumors are the commonest and 80% are benign. Malignant tumors [27] are therefore relatively uncommon, 2/3 of which are primary lesions and 1/3 are secondary lesions [30], lymph node [52] or parenchymal metastasis.

The histology is variable [15], and treatment is dependent on the tumor localization in either the superficial or deep lobes, and involvement of the facial nerve.

Imaging complements the clinical examination; ultrasound, CT, MRI (fig. 13.1) and CT or MR sialography provide a more accurate assessment of the lesion.

Clinical and anatamopathological review

The histology of malignant salivary gland tumors [40, 54] is variable. Tumors of the main salivary glands are cylindromas or adenoid cystic carcinomas [41, 53] which represent 2-4% of malignant parotid tumors and 15-18% of submandibular gland tumors. This is a very infiltrative tumor which spreads along the nerve pathways. Adenocarcinomas involve the parotid and submandibular glands, and present a problem when associated with pleomorphic adenomas. It is important to recognize if an adenocarcinoma occurs in a pleomorphic adenoma or if there is an area of malignant degeneration within one.

Nowadays, it seems that the majority of authors prefer to describe a carcinoma developing within a pleomorphic adenoma, replacing the previous terminology of mixed malignant tumors. Epidermoid carcinomas are commoner in elderly subjects and occur particularly in the submandibular glands. Undifferentiated carcinomas arise in the elderly as well as children and may simulate a lymphoma. Muco-epidermoid carcinomas represent 5% of salivary tumors and may occur at any age. The grade of malignancy is variable depending on the degree of cellular differentiation. Tumors of the acinar cells arise in young adults, predominantly females and are less malignant, but lymph node involvement and distant metastasis can occur.

Secondary tumors may be lymph node or parenchymal metastases either from cutaneous lesions of the face or oropharynx, or from visceral lesions (especially lung, kidney, pancreas and stomach). It should be noted that lymphoma, as well as the rare rhabdomyosarcomas, liposarcomas, angiosarcomas, malignant hemangioendotheliomas and neuroepitheliomas may also be encountered occasionally.

Malignant tumors are more common in the accessory salivary glands than the main glands (35-58%). The adenoid cystic and muco-epidermoid carcinomas are commoner. Adenocarcinomas represent 5-29% of malignant tumors of the accessory glands. The following lesions are also encountered and listed in decreasing order of frequency, tumors of the acinar cells, carcinomas within pleomorphic adenomas, undifferentiated carcinomas and epidermoid carcinomas.

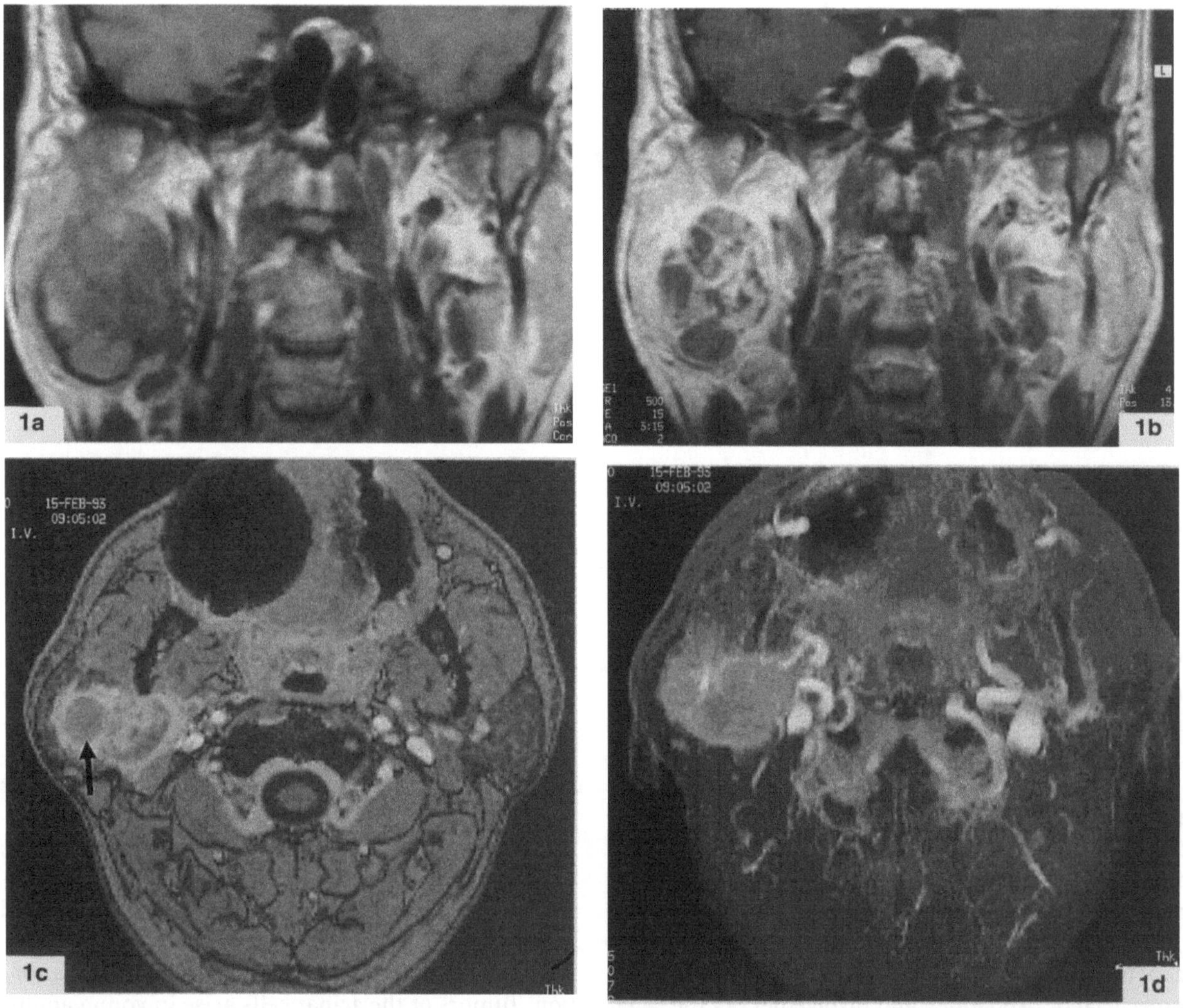

Fig. 13.1 a-d. Tumor of the parotid on MRI. **a** Coronal T1-weighted image without gadolinium: the tumor in the deep lobe of the right parotid appears heterogeneous and isointense relative to the normal parotid parenchyme. Note the visualization of the carotid artery. **b** Same section following gadolinium demonstrating enhancement of the tumor. Note that the tumor contours are less obvious due to parenchymal enhancement. **c** Gradient echo axial section, submillimetre thickness, clearly showing the necrotic areas *(arrow)*. **d** Post-gadolinium MR angiography with 3-dimensional reconstruction demonstrating the relationships of the lesion with the vessels

Parotid gland

Tumors of the parotid are the commonest salivary gland tumors [63] and are unique because of the risk of facial nerve involvement, the frequency of surgical intervention for recurrence (20-40% of patients), and the increased risk of malignant degeneration within these recurrences. Malignant tumors represent about 20-30% of parotid tumors of which 5% are secondary lymph node or parenchymal deposits (this percentage being higher in some series).

In the majority of cases, it is the presence of a parotid mass (which may have been apparent for anything from a few weeks to 20 years) which leads patients to seek medical advice. Less frequent symptom are a pain or a progressive facial paralysis. The age of the patient is a very important feature, but the male/female distribution is less significant. Clinical examination confirms the presence of a mass, assesses facial nerve function and detects lymphadenopathy. This is followed by imaging and subsequently biopsy. It should be remembered at this point that parotid lesions with pharyngeal extension may present clinically as parapharyngeal lesions. In addition, there are difficulties with the clinical examination for small recurrences in patients who have undergone previous surgery.

Submandibular glands

The presenting feature is usually that of a mass in the submandibular region of variable mobility, with or without associated lymphadenopathy. The patient is alerted by the progressive nature of the lesion and the mandibular pain in cases of bone involvement.

Accessory salivary glands

The clinical picture depends on the site of the lesion and may present as masses of the soft palate, parapharyngeal space, pharynx, larynx or cervical region.

Imaging techniques

Scintigraphic examination of the salivary glands will not be described here.

Ultrasound [3, 21]

This is the easiest examination to perform for all these lesions. It requires a multidirectional examination using a high frequency probe (7.5 MHz), sometimes with a water bath stand-off for the more superficial tissue planes. Color doppler is a useful adjunct for the recognition of the vascular structures within the parotid and submandibular regions.

Ultrasonically, the tumor appears as a mass, usually well defined and rather hypoechoic and heterogeneous. It is difficult to determine the benign or malignant nature of a tumor. It is possible to localize a tumor as either intra- or extraglandular, to demonstrate associated lymphadenopathy and determine the size, structure, tumor invasion and state of the parenchyme adjacent to the lesion. Cystic or necrotic areas may be seen within the tumor, and percutaneous biopsy should be guided to the soft tissue areas.

Certain features are suggestive of malignancy, namely a hyperechoic tumor with poorly defined boundaries of the tumor or gland indicating an infiltrative lesion, associated lymph nodes of greater than 1.5 cm diameter with loss of the normal echostructure and loss of the adjacent muscle plane, particularly in the floor of the mouth and boundaries of the submandibular region.

Sialography

This used to form the basis for the investigation of the main salivary glands prior to CT and MRI. It could only demonstrate displacement of the intraparenchymal duct by the tumor and in the majority of cases gave no indication as to the malignant or benign nature of the tumor. Rarely, abrupt amputation and significant irregularity of the ducts suggested a malignant tumor.

In our experience, the best results are achieved by routinely combining sialography with ultrasound. This combination results in an accurate tumor localization relative to the gland and rules out inflammatory disease or ductal pathology. Its use has reduced since the advent of CT and particularly MRI. It is still very useful for localizing small lesions when coupled with CT [58].

CT

Fine sections of 1 to 4 mm are performed in an axial plane prescribed from a lateral scanogram to avoid dental artefacts which are a problem particularly in the investigation of the parotid region. Coronal sections are more useful for the investigation of the buccal floor and submandibular region or for lesions located in the buccal or soft palate accessory salivary glands. It is imperative to perform a scan both with and without contrast which may be complemented by a sialographic injection of a water soluble contrast agent for the main salivary glands involved by the lesion. Image reconstructions are performed using the soft tissue and subsequently bone algorithms to look for any associated bone involvement.

The examination comprises of an initial axial series without contrast through the gland and tumor. A second series is subsequently performed using a bolus injection of 150 ml of a contrast agent with an iodine concentration of 60%, followed by a few delayed scans through the tumor. The examination is completed by sections following sialography. The examination assesses not only the salivary gland in question but also all the other neighboring anatomical structures and the draining lymph node chains.

Despite the good definition, CT is unable to determine the malignant nature of a lesion by a morphological analysis but can often localize tumor within the deep or superficial lobes and assess its relationship to the intraparotid portion of the facial nerve.

The morphological assessment of the tumor should include its shape, clarity of contours, lobulation or irregularity of the lesion and enhancement pattern (homogeneous or heterogeneous).

Tumors of the deep lobe of the parotid constitute 11 to 12% of the parotid tumors and are often difficult to evaluate clinically because the deep lobe comprises only 10% of the total volume of the parotid gland. The parapharyngeal fat space and particularly any displacement of it help to localize the tumor. A fat plane separates the deep lobe of the parotid from the mucosal structures and parapharyngeal space. A tumor arising in the deep lobe of the parotid or spreading to the pharynx pushes the parapharyngeal fat plane anteromedially. A lesion of an accessory salivary gland displaces the fat space laterally, and a hypodense fatty sheet separates the lesion from the deep lobe of the parotid.

Precise localization of the tumor relative to the plane of the facial nerve is, on the other hand, more difficult. The plane of the facial nerve, which artificially divides the parotid into a superficial and deep lobe, is only visible if the fat content is sufficiently abundant, but unfortunately this is often not the case.

The characteristics of malignant lesions of the salivary glands on CT are non-specific, particularly when they are associated with inflammatory changes and signs of obstruction of the secretory ducts. The commonest signs encountered are: poorly defined margins of the lesion and increased density relative to the normal glandular parenchyma; the presence of a central fluid zone indicating necrosis; associated pathological lymphadenopathy and the presence of significant and irregular ductal obstruction without associated lithiasis. It must be underlined that small malignant lesions often appear identical to benign lesions on CT, and this explains the difficulty in diagnosis.

Small cystic adenocarcinomas and mucoepidermoid carcinomas have a tendency to be perfectly well defined and round. When they enlarge, the parenchymal reaction at the periphery of the lesion causes a blurring of the boundaries of the lesion and ductal obstruction due to compression. The peritumoral reaction may appear as an increase in the density of the periphery of the lesion.

Microscopic invasion cannot be detected by CT. Invasion of the stylomastoid foramen and the third part of the facial canal is only visible at a late stage.

Lymphomas are characterized by the infiltration of almost whole gland by dense lymphomatous tissue which is strongly enhanced. They are associated with lymph node involvement. The lymph nodes are homo-

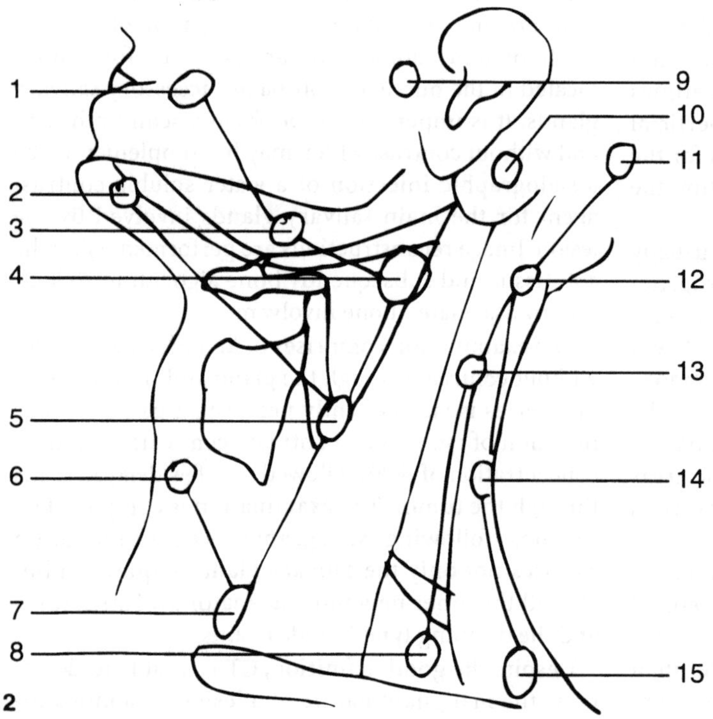

2

Fig. 13.2. Diagram of the principal cervico-facial lymph node groups: *1* facial; *2* submental; *3* submandibular; *4* subdigastric; *5* middle jugular; *6* anterior and recurrent jugular; *7* inferior jugular; *8* supraclavicular; *9* pre-auricular; *10* mastoid; *11* occipital; *12* superior spinal; *13* posterior jugular; *14* mid-spinal; *15* spinal accessory geneous without central necrosis. Nonetheless, these signs are not pathognomonic.

The secondary tumors invading the gland by direct contiguous spread are visible at the same time as involvement of the gland. Lymphatic spread is another mode of invasion (fig. 13.2)

MRI

This is now the most accurate technique for assessing malignant lesions of the salivary glands, in particular the parotid.

Sections are performed in the axial plane and complemented as required by coronal or sagittal images. We use an axial plane parallel to the inferior border of the mandible. This is very close to the plane recommended by some authors to obtain optimal visualization of the facial nerve or a plane at -35° to the orbitomeatal plane.

The sequences used T1 and T2 spin echo sequences complemented, if necessary, by time of flight angiographic sequences. Thin sections of 3 to 5 mm thickness and an interspace of 0.1 mm are obtained. Unlike CT, the images are rarely degraded by dental prostheses, but they may be of mediocre quality if there are numerous movement artefacts (swallowing or movements of the mandible).

T1-weighted spin echo sequences demonstrate that the salivary glands which are rich in fatty tissue have a higher signal intensity than that of the surrounding musculo-aponeuroses, and the course of the facial nerve, which is relatively hypointense, is often visible within the parotid gland. Its visualization requires a careful study of its course from its exit from the stylomastoid foramen to its intraparotid portion. The use of a 512×512 matrix improves its definition.

For tumors (fig. 13.1), the intermediate signal intensity (isointense) on T1-weighted imaging and hyperintensity on T2-weighted imaging are not specific for the histology or malignancy.

Like CT, the most suggestive signs of malignancy of a lesion are morphological, namely indistinct, poorly defined contours of the tumor and associated pathological lymph nodes. Assessment of the tumor margins is easier on MRI. The differential diagnosis with lesions extrinsic to the parotid is also easier than on CT and depends on the same criteria, particularly the displacement of the parapharyngeal fat space. It should be noted that this fatty sheet narrowed by tumor compression is better visualized on MRI than on CT.

MRI is superior to CT for the detection of small intraglandular lesions and for accurate localization relative to the intraparotid portion of the facial nerve. The use of surface coils does not achieve all the desired improvement in image quality. In fact, the signal intensity from the deep spaces of the parotid region is often inadequate, and there are no comparative images of the opposite side.

The detection of fluid containing cystic areas of the tumor is superior to CT and helps guide the site for cytological sampling.

Assessment of the infiltration by malignant tumors, especially the intraparotid portion of the facial nerve or infratemporal region, is also of higher quality. MRI is the examination of choice for the detection of recurrent tumors in patients who have previously undergone radiotherapy or surgery.

References of pages 95-125

1. André P, Laccourreye H (1964) Oncocytome des fosses nasales. Ann Otolaryngol (Paris) 81: 281-185
2. Apestrand F, Kolbenstvedt A, Boysen M (1990) Carcinoma of the hypopharynx CT staging. J Comput Assist Tomogr 11: 72-76
3. Baker S, Ossoinig KG (1977) Ultrasonic evaluation of the salivary glands. Trans Am Ophtalmol Soc 84: 755-762
4. Batsakis JG, Regezi JA, Bloch D (1979) The pathology of head and neck tumors: Salivary glands. In: Head and Neck Surgery, part 3, 1: 260-273
5. Batsakis JG (1979) Tumors of the head and neck. 2nd edn, Williams & Wilkins, Baltimore
6. Bourjat P, Veillon F (1990) Le massif facial normal. Tomodensitométrie et IRM. Masson Paris
7. Cabanis EA et coll (1992) IRM en ophtalmologie: résultats et indications de l'IRM dans les principales situations pathologiques rencontrées. Bull Soc Ophtalmol Fr 162-177
8. Casteljins JA, Geerten J and all (1988) Invasion of laryngeal cartilage by cancer: comparison of CT and MR Imaging. Radiology 296: 199-205
9. Chabolle F, Hagege E, Rassi B, Marsot-Dupuch K, Meyer B, Chouard CH (1990) Adénomes pléiomorphes de l'espace sous-parotidien antérieur. A propos de 5 cas. In: Tumeurs des glandes salivaires. Masson, Paris, pp 99-105
10. Chow JM, Leonetti JP, Mafee MF (1993) Epithelial tumors of the paranasal sinuses and nasal cavity. Radiol Clin North Am 31:61-73
11. Foster DW (1988) Le larynx en imagerie par résonance magnétique: technique et résultats normaux. Thèse de médecine, Paris
12. Fulbright RK, Panush D (1992) Applications of IR Fast se (a fat suppression technic) in head and neck disorders. 78th Meeting Chicago. Radiology (suppl) 185
13. Furusawa M, et al (1992) Cavernous sinus invasion in malignant head and neck tumors: role of the dynamic

MRimaging (se) 78th Meeting Chicago. Radiology (suppl) 185
14. Gamsu G, Webb WR, Shallit JB, Moss AA (1981) Computed tomography in carcinoma of the larynx and pyriform sinus - the value of phonation CT. AJR 136: 577-584
15. Gorguet B, Brousset P, Mazerolles C, Duga I, Alard C (1990) Histopathologie des tumeurs des glandes salivaires principales. Actualités de Carcinologie Cervico-faciale. Masson, Paris, pp 1-6
16. Goudot P, Payement G, Chomette G, Guilbert F, Vaillant JM, Thomas A (1990) Tumeurs des glandes salivaires principales et accessoires. Etude statistique sur 1038 tumeurs. Actualités de Carcinologie Cervico-faciale. Masson, Paris, pp: 43-48
17. Hanafee WN, Ward PH (1990) The larynx, radiology, surgery, pathology.In: Clinical Correlations in the Head and Neck. Thieme, Stuttgart, pp 64 65
18. Hansberger HR, Osborn AG, Smoker WRK (1986) CT in evaluation of the normal and disease paranasal sinuses. Semin Ultrasound CT MRI 7: 68
19. Harnsberger HR, Mancuso AA, Muraki AS, Parkin JL (1983) The upper aerodigestive tract and neck: CT evaluation of recurrent tumor. Radiology 149: 503-510
20. Jugie M, et al (1992) Localisation exceptionnelle d'un esthésioneurome olfactif. Ann Radiol 35:477-482
21. Kaneko T, Kobayashi N, Miura T, Asano H, Kitamura T (1975) L'échographie ultrasonique pour l'exploration des tumeurs parotidiennes. Ann ORL 92: 685-690
22. Kopp W, Stanberger H, Fotter R (1987) Special radiologic imaging of the paranasal sinuses, a prequisite for functionnal endoscopic sinus surgery. Eur J Radiol 165-195
23. Korentager R, Noyk A, Chapnik J, et al (1988) Lipoma and liposarcoma of the parotide gland: High resolution per operative imaging diagnosis. Laryngoscope 98: 967-971
24. Kubal WS, et al (1992) Rapid echo gradient MR imaging for patients with head and nock carcinoma. 78th Meeting Chicago. Radiology (suppl) 185
25. Laccourreye H (1991) La chirurgie partielle des épithéliomas du pharyngo-larynx. In: Les monographies du CC Wagram, Paris
26. Laccourreye H, Beutter P, Brasnu D, Lacau St Guilly J, Candau P, Laval-Jeantet M, Buy JN (1983) Intérêt de la tomodensitométrie dans les tumeurs du pharyngo-larynx. Ann Otolaryngol Chir Cervicofac 100: 341-345
27. Lacomme Y, Leroux-Robert J (1990) Actualités de carcinologie cervico-faciale. Tumeurs des glandes salivaires. Masson, Paris
28. Lallemant JG, Roumieux JL, Leguillette JL, Abbou S, Chapon C, Amadeo F, Guerrier B, Guerrier Y (1990) Carcinomes adénoïdes kystiques (cylindromes) de la parotide. A propos de 27 cas. In: Tumeurs des glandes salivaires. Masson, Paris, pp 188-195
29. Larsson S, Mancuso AA, Hoover L, Hanafee WN (1981) Differentiation of pyriform sinus cancer from supraglottic laryngeal cancer by computed tomography. Radiology 141: 427-432
30. Le Clech G, Le Gland C, Rivron A, Demoulin PY, Maréchal V, Bourdinière J (1990) Tumeurs parotidiennes secondaires. Actualités en Carcinologie Cervico-faciale, Masson, Paris,pp 156 - 161
31. Lloyd GAS, Barqker PG, Phelps PD (1993) Substraction gadolinium enhanced magnetic resonance for head and neck imaging. Br J Radiol 66: 12-16
32. Lufkin RB, Hanafee WN (1991) MRI of the head and neck. In: The Raven MRI teaching file. Raven Press, New York
33. Mafee MF (1993) Non epithelial tumors of the paranasal sinuses and nasal cavity. Role of CT and MR imaging. Radiol Clin North Am 31: 75-90
34. Mafee MF, Schild JA,Valvassori GE, Capek V (1983) Computed tomography of the larynx: correlation with anatomic and pathologic studies in cases of laryngeal carcinoma. Radiology 147: 123-128
35. Mancuso AA. Hanafee WN, Winter J, Ward P (1978) Extensions of the paranasal sinus tumors and inflammatory disease as evaluated by CT and pluridirectionnal tomography. Neuroradiology 16: 449-453
36. Mancuso AA, Hanafee WN (1985) Computed tomography and resonance imaging of the head and neck, 2nd edn. Williams and Wilkins, Baltimore
37. Mancuso AA, Hanafee WN (1983) Exlusive head and neck carcinoma beneath intact mucosa. Laryngoscope 93: 133-139
38. Mancuso AA, Hanafee WN, Juliard GJF, et al (1977) The role of computed tomography in the management of cancer of the larynx. Radiology,124: 243-244
39. Mancuso AA, Harnsberger HR, Muraki AS, Stevens MH (1983) Computed tomography of cervical and retropharyngeal lymph nodes: normal anatomy, variant of normal and applications in staging head and neck cancer. Radiology 148: 715-723
40. Marandas P, Janot F, Schwaab G, Martinez F, et al (1990) Tumeurs malignes de la glande parotide. A propos de 69 cas traités à l'Institut Gustave Roussy. Actualités de Carcinologie Cervico-faciale. Masson, Paris, pp 147-155
41. Marie JP, Trotoux J (1989) Tumeurs parotidiennes à malignité intermédiaire. Appréciation pronostique. Mise au point bibliographique. Société de Laryngologie des Hôpitaux de Paris
42. Mastumoto S, et al (1992) Comparison of the CT findings in non Hodgkin's lymphoma and squamous cell carcinoma of the maxillary sinus. Acta Radiol 33: 523-527
43. Million RR, Cassissi NJ (1984) Management of head and neck cancer: a multidisciplinary approach. Lippincott, Philadelphia
44. Muraki AS, Mancuso AA, Harnsberger HR (1984) Metastatic cervical adenopathy from tumor of unknown origin: the role of CT. Radiology 152: 749-753
45. Newton T, Haso A, Dillon W (1988) Computed tomography of the head and neck. Raven Press, New York
46. Perlemuter L, Waligora J (1971) Cahiers d'anatomie, tête et cou. Masson, Paris

47. Pinel J, Cachin Y, Laccourreye H, et al (1980) Cancers du larynx. Rapport de la Société d'Otorhino Laryngologie et de Pathologie Cervico-faciale. Arnette, Paris
48. Piquet JJ, Onimus G, Chevalier D, Malard T, Piedor P, Vanecloo FM (1988) Les cylindromes de l'extrémité céphalique. Rev Laryngol 109: 25-27
49. Raveau V (1992) Espace masticateux: radio-anatomie et pathologie. Ann Radiol,35: 416-423
50. Ray CE, Mafee MF, Friedman M, Tahmoressi CN (1993) Applications of the three dimensional CT imaging in the head and neck pathology. Radiol Clin North Am 31: 181-194
51. Sakai F, Gamsu G, Dillon WP, Lynch DA, Gilbert TJ (1990) MR imaging of the larynx at 1.5 T. J Comput Assist Tomogr 11: 60-71
52. Seifert G, Heinnings K, Caselitz J (1986) Metastatic tumors to the parotid and submandibular glands. Analysis and differential diagnosis of 108 cases. Path Mes Pract 181: 684-692
53. Sénechaut JP (1982) Tumeurs parotidiennes. A propos de 363 cas. Thèse, Paris
54. Sharkey FE (1977) Systematic evaluation of the WHO. Classification of the salivary gland tumors. Am J Clin Pathol 67: 272-278
55. Som P, Biller HF (1983) Computed tomography of the neck in the post-operative patient: radical neck dissection and the myocutaneous flap. Radiology 148: 157-160
56 Som PM, Biller HF (1979) The combined computerized tomography scialogram. Ann Otol Rhinol Laryngol 88: 590-595
57. Som P, Dillon W (1989) Benignant and malignant sinusonasal lesions with intra-cranial extensions, differentiation with MR imaging. Radiology 172: 763- 766
58. Stone DN, Mancuso AA, Rice D, Hanafee WN (1981) Parotis CT scialography. Radiology 138: 393-397
59. Suojanen JN, Muikherji SK, Duput DE, Takahasi JH, Costello P (1992) Spiral CT in evaluation of the head and neck lesions: work in progress. Radiology 183: 281-283
60. Szpirglas H, Goudot P, Thomas A, Payement G, Guilbert F, Vaillant JM (1990) Cancers muco-épidermoïdes des glandes salivaires (1969-1989: 73 cas). In: Tumeurs des glandes salivaires. Masson, Paris, pp 212-217
61. Tabor EK, Curtin HD (1989) MR of the salivary glands. Radiol Clin 27: 379-391
62. Teresi LM, Lifkin RB, Wortham DG, Abemayor E, Hanafee WN (1987) Parotid masses: MR Imaging. Radiology 163: 405-409
63. Vaillant JM, Laudenhach P (1988) Pathologie des glandes salivaires. Flammarion Médecine-Siences, Paris
64. Vignaud J, Cosnard G (1991) Imagerie par résonance magnétique crânio-encéphalique. Vigot, Paris
65. Vilde F, Arkwright S (1990) Aspects anatomopathologiques des tumeurs des glandes salivaires accessoires. Actualités de Carcinologie Cervico-faciale, Masson, Paris, pp: 6-14
66. Weber AL (1993) Imaging of cyst and odontogenic tumors of the jaw. Definition and classification. Radiol Clin North Am 31: 101-120
67. Yeager VL, Archer CR (1982) Anatomic routes for cancer invasion of laryngeal cartilages. Laryngoscope 92: 449-452
68. Yousem DM (1992) Dashed hopes for MR imaging of the head and neck: the power of the needle. Radiology 84: 25-26

CHAPTER 14

Cancer of the thyroid and parathyroid glands

Clinicians
M. Schlumberger, J.-V. Chantelard, T. Petit, E. Vuillemin

Radiologist
D. Buthiau

Cancer of the thyroid [1, 2, 13]

Indications for CT and MRI

The role of the CT (fig. 14.1) is limited in thyroid cancer and has only a marginal role in the diagnosis and assessment of local extension. Its principal value concerns the assessment of spread to adjacent viscera, and the detection of lymph node or systemic metastasis as for the staging of any carcinoma. It may occasionally be requested to assess a large lesion, for example lymphoma [11], and rarely will demonstrate a primary thyroid carcinoma during the investigation of metastatic disease to lymph nodes, cervical viscera or distal metastasis including bone (fig. 14.3).

MRI also has a very limited role in this pathology even though the non-requirement of an injection may seem an advantage since this is not often advisable in these patients. In practice, its role is limited by its failure to provide any further information concerning the tissue characterization of tumors, its inability to distinguish benign from malignant tumors or functioning and non-functioning nodules (fig. 14.2). Currently there are four areas of possible interest which are limited to:

• 3-dimensional assessment of local tumor spread,

• the detection of muscle invasion,

• the assessment of medullary cancers which are not detected by radioactive iodine; MRI can differentiate a non-fibrous tumor from fibrous tissue,

• in some incidence, MRI is able to differentiate post-therapeutic fibrosis from recurrence. It should be remembered that MRI can complement CT and other techniques in the routine assessment of the spread of a cancer.

Signs

– On CT, thyroid tumors are heterogeneous with localized or diffuse hypertrophy, alteration of the contours, soft tissue and/or cystic changes. The appearances are entirely non-specific (fig. 14.1) [12].

CT can demonstrate local invasion, notably to the trachea and esophagus, extracapsular cervical spread, spread to adjacent or distant lymph nodes (investigation of recurrent laryngeal nerve palsy).

Following treatment the distinction between postoperative fibrous tissue and possible recurrence is very difficult on CT.

On MRI, lesions generally are of high signal on T1- and T2-weighted imaging, which is non-specific. It is impossible to differentiate benign from malignant lesions. Heterogeneous signal changes, particularly blood or colloid may cause a pseudogoiter. There are no specific signal changes on T1- or T2-weighted imaging that can differentiate the follicular or anaplastic forms, or benign lesions. The same applies to lymph nodes.

MRI may be sensitive for the assessment of tracheal, esophageal, vascular and muscular spread by its

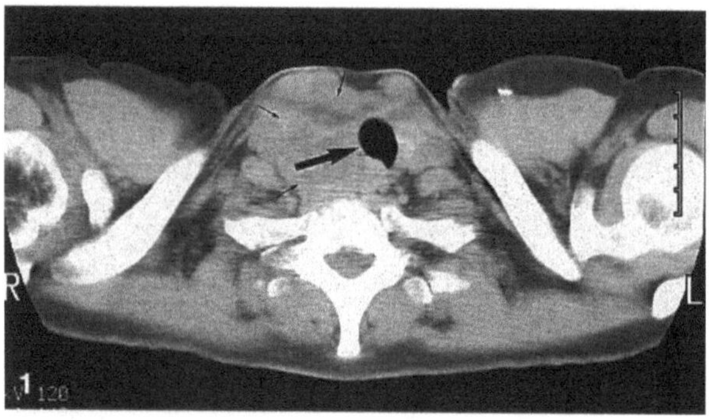

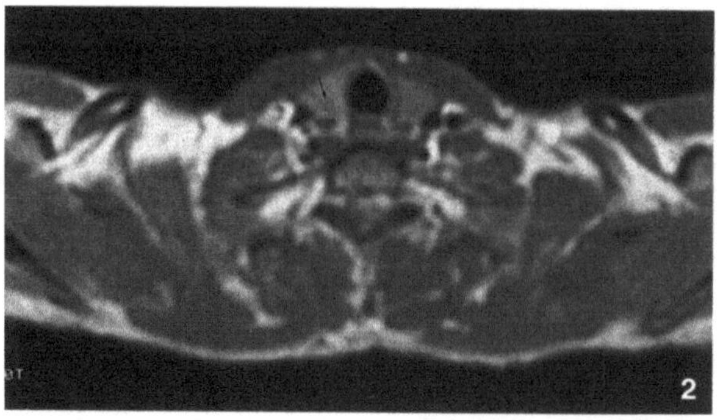

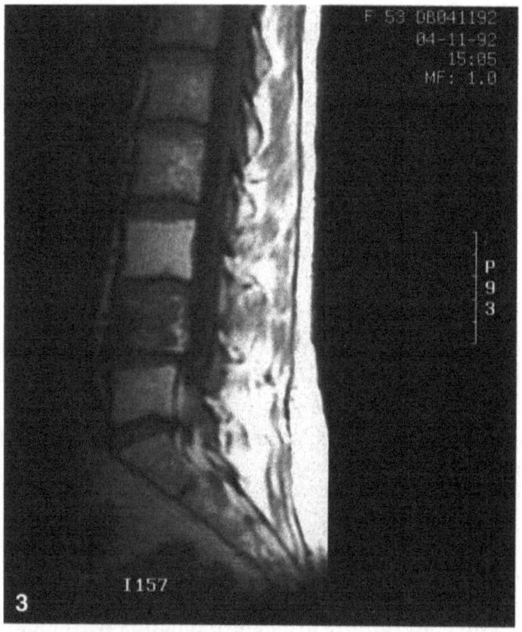

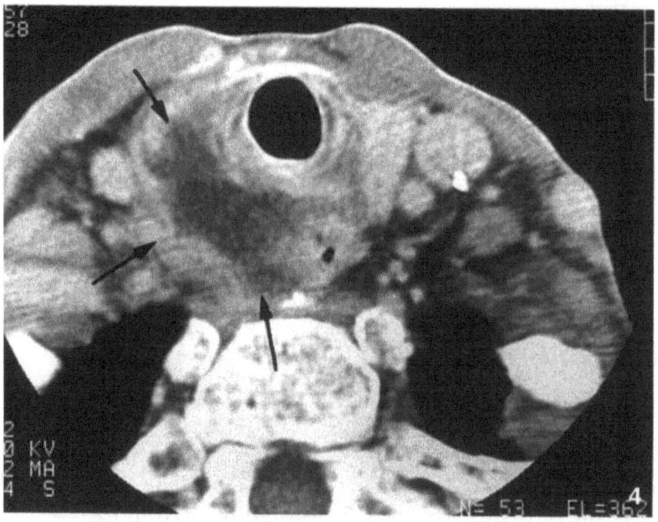

Fig. 14.1. Cancer of the thyroid on CT. The lesion *(small arrows)* involves the right lobe of the thyroid. There is posterior lymph node extension which is inseparable from the mass itself and extrinsic compression with early nodular involvement of the tracheal wall *(large arrow)*

Fig. 14.2. Axial proton density MRI of the thyroid demonstrating a small, non-specific hypointensity in the posterior part of the right lobe of the thyroid *(arrow)* corresponding, in this patient, to an early papillary carcinoma of the thyroid, confirmed histologically

Fig. 14.3. Distant spread of a thyroid cancer. Secondary deposit in the spine from a thyroid cancer (recurrence in a previously irradiated area): MRI demonstrates a clear hypointensity on T1-weighted imaging at the L4 level

Fig. 14.4. Cancer of the parathyroid on post-contrast CT: large necrotic lesion *(arrows)* arising from the right parathyroid with spread into the thyroid lobe and extrinsic compression of the esophagus which is deviated laterally to the left. Note extrinsic compression of the jugular and carotid vessels and trachea with no evidence of direct spread into these structures

multiplanar capability and T2-weighted sequences. The high signal intensity on T2-weighted imaging within adjacent muscles which is well contrasted with the normal signals of muscles is a significant sign of involvement by contiguous spread, particularly if there is loss of visualization of the normal tissue plane between the thyroid and muscle itself.

Post-treatment fibrous tissue can be distinguished from a residual or recurrent lesion after an interval of at least 5-6 months following completion of all treatment by demonstrating an increase in signal of a nodule or infiltrative process whereas simple fibrosis is low signal on T2-weighted imaging.

Otherwise CT and MRI have no place in the assessment of thyroid tumors.

Their main role is:

• to define the spread of the thyroid tumor into the neighboring cervical structures and demonstrate systemic metastasis (fig. 14.3);

• to detect lymph node extension (particularly mediastinal) either prior to the initial surgery if the tumor is large and extensive, or more often before the surgery looking for recurrent disease.

Cancer of the parathyroid glands

[1, 2, 7-10, 12, 13]

Indications for CT and MRI

CT is limited by artefacts arising from the scapula at the cervico-thoracic junction, lower cervical level and thoracic apex, and by its spatial resolution (even using fine sections and repeated bolus injections, the distinction between a parathyroid tumor and a tortuous vessel in the apex is often difficult). On the other hand, it is useful because of its ability to cover a large area of the cervical region and mediastinum. The indications are concerned mainly with the general investigation of cancer, particularly the visceral and lymphatic metastases. The diagnosis of a parathyroid tumor by CT is rare (usually detected fortuitously). Assessment of local spread is relatively limited for the reasons previously described.

MRI does not appear to have a role for this pathology even if its 3D capability is well suited to the cervico-thoracic region. It can demonstrate 75% of parathyroid carcinomas [10], particularly with the use of a surface coil and axial scans. There is absolutely no specificity in terms of relaxation times for differentiating a carcinoma, adenoma or even a lymph node. Lesions with a signal intensity different from that of the vessels, muscles and fat planes are well demonstrated. Its role is limited, although well recognized in cases where other techniques have failed, in the recognition of recurrent tumor. MRI, unlike CT, is not significantly affected by artefacts from clips and can differentiate fairly well fibrosis from tumor.

Signs

A lesion may be small, or larger, necrotic and extensive, and therefore detected on CT (fig. 14.4). Local spread is similar to that of thyroid cancers (cf see above). Lesions frequently contain microcalcifications.

On MRI , the T1-weighted image distinguishes vessels and fat; on T2-weighted imaging, the hyperintensity of the tumor differentiates it from the muscles and fat planes. There is no specific signal intensity for benign and malignant lesions or even lymphadenopathy, the latter nevertheless being well demonstrated. Similarly, perivascular infiltration or spread along the cervical fascial planes is well shown on T1- and T2-weighted sequences but is non-specific, inflammatory changes giving similar appearances on T2-weighted imaging.

For recurrent tumors, MRI is minimally or not at all affected by artefacts from clips, and the differentiation between hypointense fibrosis and hyperintense active tumor tissue on T2-weighted imaging may help in the diagnosis.

References

1. Bourjat P, Kahn JL, Roy C, et al (1988) Thyroide et parathyroides. In: Tomodensitométrie cervico-faciale. Masson, Paris, pp 123-128
2. Buthiau D, Ducobu J, Chigot JP (1991) Thyroïde et parathyroïdes. In: D. Buthiau (ed) TDM et IRM Cliniques. Frison-Roche, Paris, pp 489-500
3. Clark OH, Duh QY (1989) Primary hyperparathyroidism. Endocrinol Metab Clin North Am 18: 701-714
4. Eisenberg H, Pallotta J, Sacks B, et al (1989) Parathyroid localization, three dimensional modeling and percutaneous ablation techniques. Endocrinol Metab Clin North Am 18: 659-699
5. Glazer GM, Axel L, Moss AA (1982) CT diagnosis of mediastinal thyroid. AJR 138: 495-498
6. Glinoer D, Verelst A, Ermans A (1987) Place et utilité de la ponction à l'aiguille fine dans l'évaluation clinique du nodule froid de la thyroide. Revue Médicale de Bruxelles 8: 10-16
7. Hamilton R, Greenberg BM, Gefterw, et al (1988) Successful localization of parathyroid adenomas by magnetic resonance imaging. Am J Surg 155: 370-373
8. Krubsack AJ, Wilson SD, Lawson TL, et al (1989) Prospective comparison of radionuclide, computed tomographic, sonographic, and magnetic resonance. Localization of parathyroid tumors. 46th Annual Meeting of the Central Surgical Association
9. Reede DL (1989) The neck, thyroid and parathyroid glands. In: Computed tomography of the head and neck. Churchill Livingstone, Edinburgh, pp 31-57

10. Stark DD, Clark OH, Moss AA (1984) Magnetic resonance imaging of the thyroid, thymus and parathyroïd glands. Surgery 96: 1083-1090

11. Takashima S, et al (1990) Primary thyroid lymphoma: comparison of CT and US assessment. Radiology 171: 439-443

12. Takashima S, et al (1990) CT evaluation of anaplastic thyroid carcinoma. AJR 154: 1079-1085

13. Zerhouni EA, Herold CJ, Hahn D (1992) Mediastinum and lung. In: DD Stark, WG Bradley (eds) Magnetic resonance imaging. Mosby-Year Book, St Louis, pp 1429-1489

CHAPTER 15

Breast cancer

Clinicians
E.-Ch. Antoine, O. Rixe, P. Pouillart, N. Renody, J.-V. Chantelard, T. Petit, M. Weil, J.-P. Lefranc, E. Vuillemin, A. Benhammouda, D. Khayat

Radiologist
D. Buthiau

In France, as in the majority of industrialized countries, cancer of the breast is the commonest cancer in women. There has been a constant increase in its incidence over last 30 years, and it is the major cause of death from malignant disease in females. It affects about one woman in ten.

The risk factors are poorly understood or unavoidable. Clinical examination and early identification of asymptomatic lesions by mammography are currently the only preventative measures available. It is clear that the prognosis for these tumors depends on the stage at the time of detection.

One study has shown that mass screening by mammography of women aged between 50 and 69 years reduced the mortality rate by 30 to 40% with an acceptance rate of 60% (the best cost effectiveness being achieved with a single lateral oblique view for each breast every 2 years). On the other hand, the benefit of screening all women aged between 40 and 49 years has not been proven. The funding for these screening programs poses inevitable problems in the knowledge that quality is the principal determining factor of the cost/benefit ratio.

Clinical examination, mammography and fine needle aspiration give the diagnosis of breast cancer in 98% of cases when the results are concordant. Cytology is only of value when positive.

Applications of CT and MRI

CT and MRI have had no effect on these statistics for two reasons:

- first, the reliability of the combination of clinical examination, mammography and fine needle aspiration leaves little place for these new investigations;
- second, there is an absence of natural contrast between the different elements which make up the glandular tissue of the breast.

CT

There is no indication for CT in the diagnosis of the lesion itself due to its complete absence of specificity. Its role is limited to the rare cases of chest wall involvement when the lesion arises in the submammary tissue. 3D helical mode is of particular value in this instance.

However, *CT should be routinely used in the search for visceral metastasis* if there are clinical, radiological or biochemical indications, and for *lymph node involvement* (e.g. internal mammary chains and axillary nodes).

In theory, CT could be used in the follow-up of treated breasts, but there is no significant feature which can differentiate recurrence from post-radiation fibrosis (current interest in helical CT).

It is of value for radiotherapists who can calculate pre-treatment dosimetries (helical CT and 3D reconstructions under assessment).

MRI (fig. 15.1, tables 15.1 & 15.2)

This has no place in screening because it does not demonstrate the microcalcifications (absence of signal and too small size).

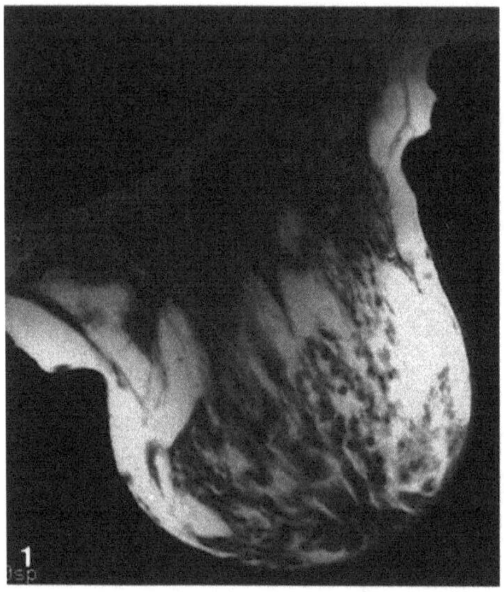

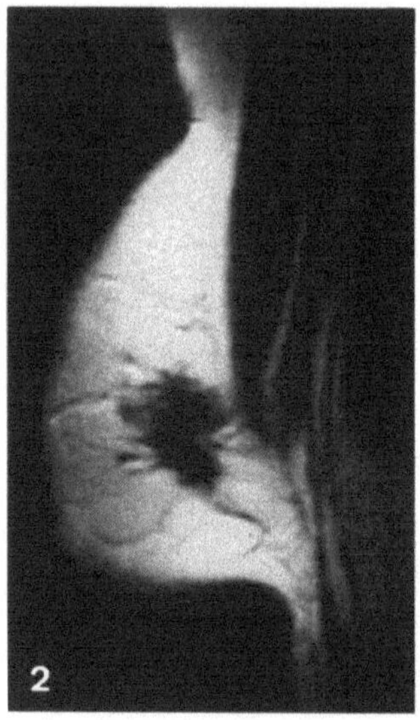

Fig. 15.1. MRI, axial T1-weighted image: normal appearance of the mammary gland in a female of 35 years showing good detail of the subcutaneous fat, glandular parenchyme, muscles, vessels and connective tissues with early fatty replacement. The relationship between the mammary gland and the chest wall is well demonstrated

Fig. 15.2. MRI, sagittal proton density weighted image: invasive carcinoma in a 65 year old female. The lesion is almost completely of low signal with peripheral intermediate signal intensity antero-superiorly and postero-superiorly associated with thin hypointense umbilicated strands extending towards the deep tissue planes. There is no skin retraction. On the histological specimen there was a dense central collagen zone surrounded by a cellular zone corresponding to the slightly higher peripheral signal intensity

Table 15.1. MRI: review of anatomy

- The identification of the normal tissues of the breast on MRI correlates well with mammography and xerography.
- On T1- and T2-weighted imaging, the connective tissue, blood vessels, glandular elements and lactiferous tubules appear of low signal, contrasting with the surrounding fat; on the other hand, the signal intensity of these structures is higher than muscle. Changes in the signal intensity of the breast are dependent on the relative proportions of fat, water and collagen.
- It is not possible to distinguish glandular tissue from the adjacent fibrous elements.
- The axillary or subcutaneous blood vessels and their branches appear regular unlike the excretory ducts converging towards the nipple.
- Cooper's ligament is rarely visible.
- Although this is not apparent, the signal intensity of the parenchyma on T1-weighted imaging varies throughout the menstrual cycle but not on T2-weighted imaging.

In practice, MRI is of most value in the assessment of local recurrence. However, it may be useful in the assessment of locoregional spread (deep planes), rarely in the analysis of a mammographically poorly demonstrated mass, to ensure assessment of dense or mastitic breasts using gadolinium injections and in the unarguably improved follow-up of patients with breast implants. Essentially an examination with and without gadolinium injection can differentiate fibrosis from recurrent tumors. The assessment of lymph nodes has not benefited from MRI which is unable to appreciate the internal structure of the node and, like CT, depends on size criteria (see later and conclusion).

Signs

CT

The lesion shows the same density as the normal glandular tissue but will always be well highlighted. This absence of specificity is one of the main limiting factors in the detection of recurrences. The microcalcifications can be recognized, but their morphology is poorly appreciated in the axial plane.

In cases of locoregional tumor recurrences (see fig. 15.5), the differentiation between the post-radiation fibrotic changes and the deep tumor mass is not easy.

Table 15.2. MRI techniques [6]

- Surface coil
  By using specific surface coils, single or double allowing investigation of one or both breasts, one can obtain a better signal to noise ratio although the examination can be performed either with a classical surface coil or a coil specifically designed for other regions (e.g. shoulder coil). The use of the body coil does not give good results. The patient is placed prone with the breast surrounded by the surface coil to avoid respiration and movement artefacts. Cardiac motion artefacts are avoided by the correct direction for phase encodings.

- Sequences
  - Spin echo technique
  - Gradient echo sequences

- Assessment of contrast enhancement [11]
  - Subtraction techniques (see fig. 15.6 c, d)
  - Mathematical analysis of dynamic structures
  - Region of interest (ROI)

- MRI angiography
  Flow phenomena and flow rates are no longer sources of artefact using this technique but become factors determining contrast. There are two separate techniques:
  - time of flight MR angiography,
  - phase contrast MR angiography: for breast pathology, it seems that the time of flight technique using 3D acquisition is the most useful, particularly due to its speed.

- CT reconstructions
  These are obtained from a helical acquisition during which there is a constant rotation of the X-ray tubes and detectors with advancement of the table top at a constant speed.

However, CT can act as a guide for fine needle aspirations of a suspicious area. The distinction between recurrence and post-radiation or post-surgical fibrosis is not facilitated by the injection of iodinated contrast.

MRI (table 15.3)

The microcalcifications are either invisible or appear as a low signal intensity (fig. 15.3) or a signal void. This represents a significant drawback of the technique.

The lesion itself often has poorly defined irregular contours and may appear as multiple rings, umbilicated nodules (fig. 15.2) or spicules.

On T1-weighted imaging, the signal intensity of the lesion is identical to that of the adjacent glandular elements but is contrasted well with the fat tissues.

Various *signal* intensities of the tumor are encountered on T2-weighted imaging [16]: either hypointense (fig. 15.2) in the infiltrative spiculated forms, or higher signal intensity in the nodular forms (sometimes close to the fat signal intensity), or even more hyperintense in the cystic forms, but often less than the signal of a benign cyst, fibroadenoma or papilloma. These variations in signal are associated with hemorrhage, necrosis, the degree of water content, the cellularity and edema. Spread into the deep tissue planes is well demonstrated by MRI, sometimes better with a body coil rather than a specific breast surface coil.

Table 15.3. Mammographic and breast MR evaluation [10]

	Mammography	MRI
Study in sections	-	+++
3D analysis	-	+++
Connective tissue	+	++
Epithelium	-	-
Fibrosis	++	+++
Water	++	+++
Fat	+++	+++
Calcium	+++	-

This causes problems in the differential diagnosis; in the stellate, infiltrative and spiculated forms (fig. 15.2), it may be difficult to exclude sclerosing adenosis or cystic fat necrosis (this lesion is often associated with trauma and may be deceptive on mammography). Areas of fat necrosis have signal intensities identical to fibrous tissue on T1- and T2-weighted imaging

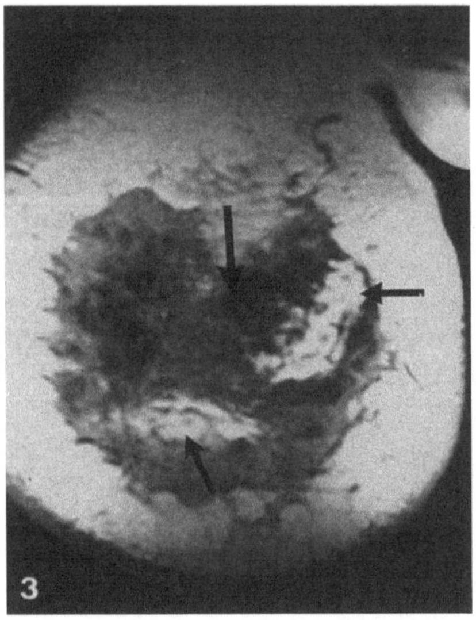

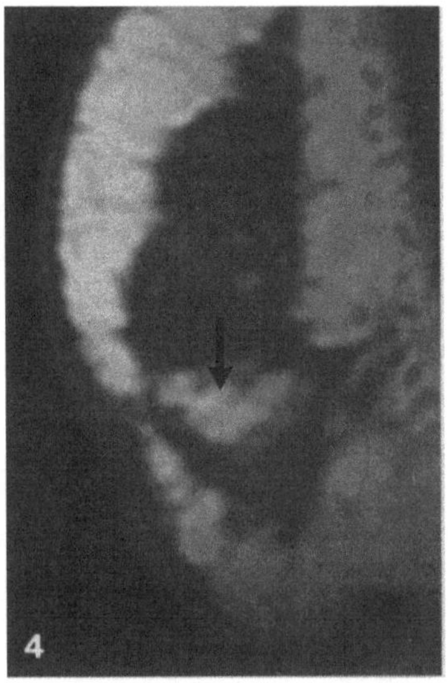

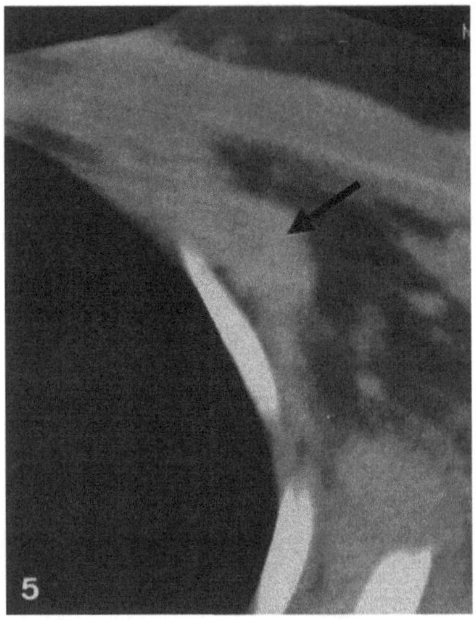

Fig. 15.3. Area of focal proliferative dysplasia on post-gadolinium T1-weighted MRI coronal image. MRI demonstrates relatively irregular areas of enhancement but not with a stellate appearance *(small arrows)*, corresponding to areas of cellular atypia at biopsy. Note the hypointensities are more or less grouped together close to the largest lesion corresponding to the calcification seen in "negative" on MRI as a non-specific hypointensity *(large arrow)*, well demonstrated by mammography

Fig. 15.4. Sagittal post-gadolinium T1-weighted MRI image of a carcinoma with early enhancement (in the first two minutes) of the lesion itself *(arrow)*, with retraction and thinning of the overlying skin and fat planes

Fig. 15.5. Deep recurrence close to the chest wall of a breast cancer following previous surgery and radiotherapy; post-contrast CT demonstrates arching of the medial aspect of the axillary fold *(arrow)* which shows the same density as the muscle wall. Only the expansive nature of the lesion suggests the diagnosis

with the peripheral edema appearing more hyperintense.

As a general rule, when carcinomas have a high signal intensity on T2-weighted imaging, it is less than that seen in fibroadenomas and papillomas. Poorly defined borders are unusual in lobular or canalicular hyperplasia, even if the signal intensity may be equally increased.

Appearances after injection of a contrast agent [16]. In animals, there is an increase in the signal in carcinomas on the post-gadolinium T1-weighted sequence after about 10 minutes. The tumor is clearly differentiated from necrosis. The increase in signal is greater for a malignant lesion than for benign pathologies.

In humans, the enhancement of a breast carcinoma (figs 15.3 & 15.4) is more intense than for benign lesions or fibrosis by way of composition of the tissues. However, this enhancement may be identical to fibroadenomas and inflammatory conditions resulting in an absence in the specificity of the technique. Contrast injection improves the detection of lesions situated in dense breasts (fig. 15.3), thus avoiding mammography. Rapid imaging after the injection of a contrast agent can demonstrate intense enhancement in the first 2 minutes followed by a plateau up to the 10th minute. This pattern distinguishes it from the less obvious enhancement of the benign and fibrous lesions and the slow progressive enhancement of normal parenchyma. However, there is some overlap between the behavior of some necrotic or poorly vascularized carcinomas and hypervascular benign lesions. There are therefore no specific appearances but simply mechanisms of hypervascularization which are independent of the composition of the tissue.

In the study of recurrent disease (figs 15.5-15.7), the use of a gadolinium contrast agent enables MRI to play a role in the follow-up of breasts by differentiating the non-enhancing zones of post-radiation or post-surgical fibrotic scarring (fig. 15.6 a, b) from the enhancing areas of presumed recurrence (figs 15.6 c, d & 15.7 a, b)

In the evaluation of lymph node involvement, CT criteria are always based on the size of the node and not

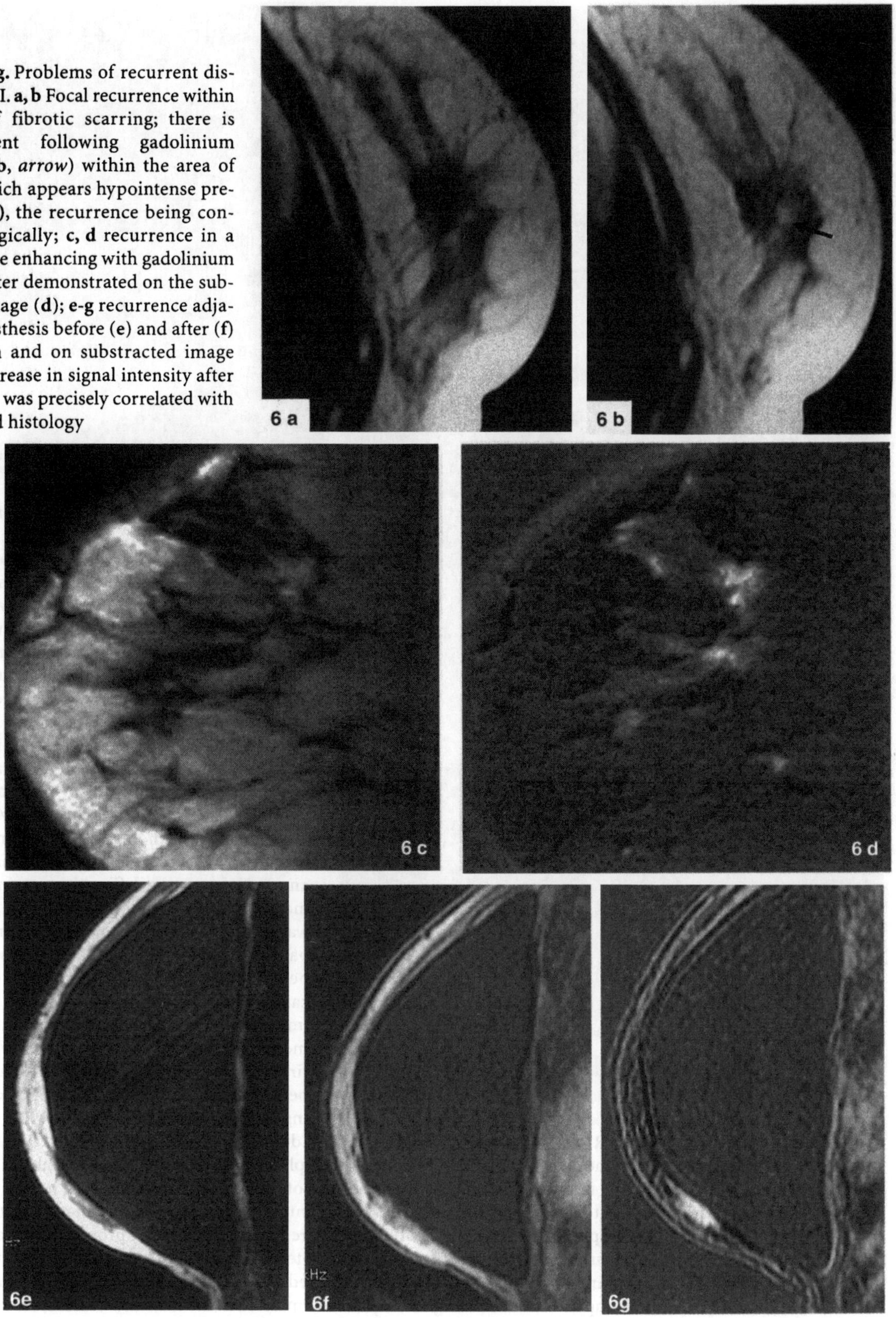

Fig. 15.6 a-g. Problems of recurrent disease on MRI. **a, b** Focal recurrence within an area of fibrotic scarring; there is enhancement following gadolinium injection (**b**, *arrow*) within the area of fibrosis which appears hypointense precontrast (**a**), the recurrence being confirmed surgically; **c, d** recurrence in a fibrotic zone enhancing with gadolinium (**c**) and better demonstrated on the subtraction image (**d**); **e-g** recurrence adjacent to prosthesis before (**e**) and after (**f**) gadolinium and on substracted image (**g**). The increase in signal intensity after gadolinium was precisely correlated with surgery and histology

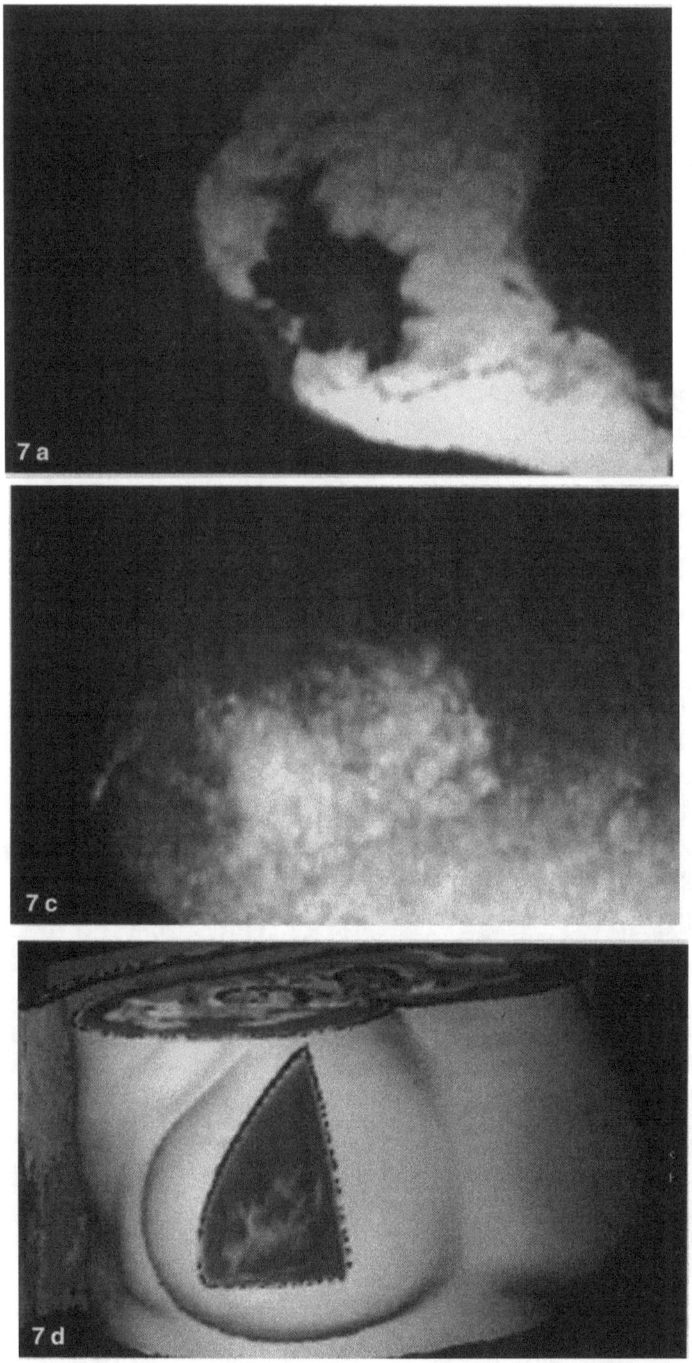

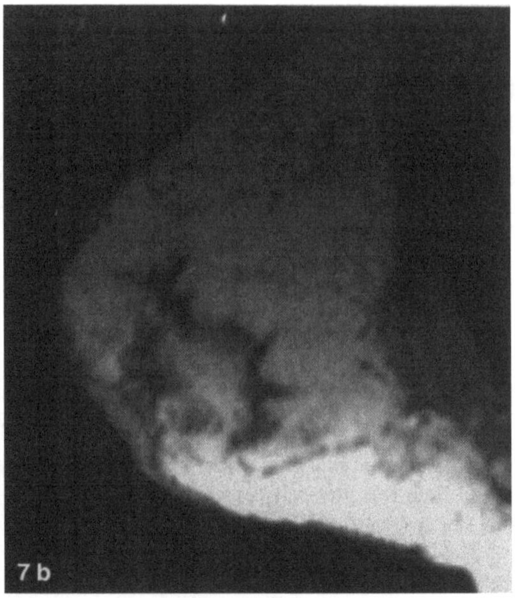

Fig. 15.7 a-d. *The diagnostic problem of treated breast cancer* [3]. There has been a trend over the last few years for conservative treatment of small breast tumors; however, the changes resulting from radiotherapy and chemotherapy make clinical examination and mammography difficult or sometimes even impossible. Even the comparison of successive mammograms does not routinely solve this problem. **a, b** Example of tumor recurrence on MRI, pre- (**a**) and post-gadolinium (**b**) images through the region of recurrence. Our initial study on 17 patients following radiotherapy and chemotherapy has shown a 90% histo-radiological correlation [2, 4]: on the post-gadolinium MRI, in cases of simple fibrosis there is never any enhancement demonstrated. If there is early enhancement within an area of presumed fibrotic scarring, approximately 30 seconds following injection, recurrence was always proven at histology. If the enhancement pattern was nodular, then the lesion was likely to be an invasive and linear carcinoma or an intracanalicular carcinoma. Subtraction techniques improves the sensitivity in detecting this enhancement (fig. 15.6 c, d). These results have been confirmed by previous studies [6,12]; **c** MRA performed in the same patient clearly demonstrating the boundaries of the lesion. MRA is a complementary technique to standard MRI and subtraction imaging. It should not be requested in isolation as it is unable to analyze the glandular structure of the breast; on the other hand, as a complementary technique it only slightly increases the examination time without any cost implications (the examination cannot be disassociated from MRI itself). It should be considered in the follow-up of treated breasts: **d** 3D helical CT reconstruction provides a representation of the lesion in space. The 3D helical CT cannot improve the distinction between recurrence and fibrosis but provides accurate information on the spread of lesions, particularly posteriorly to the chest wall, internal mammary chain and axilla. It can also provide better pre-radiotherapy planning when this can still be administered. However, given the frequency of mastectomies for recurrent tumors and radiotherapy treatment having already been completed in the majority of cases, the role of 3D CT is more limited in this setting unless the recurrence is separated from the initial primary site (images courtesy of Dr D Buthiau, Scanner Paris 14, General Electric, High Speed Advantage)

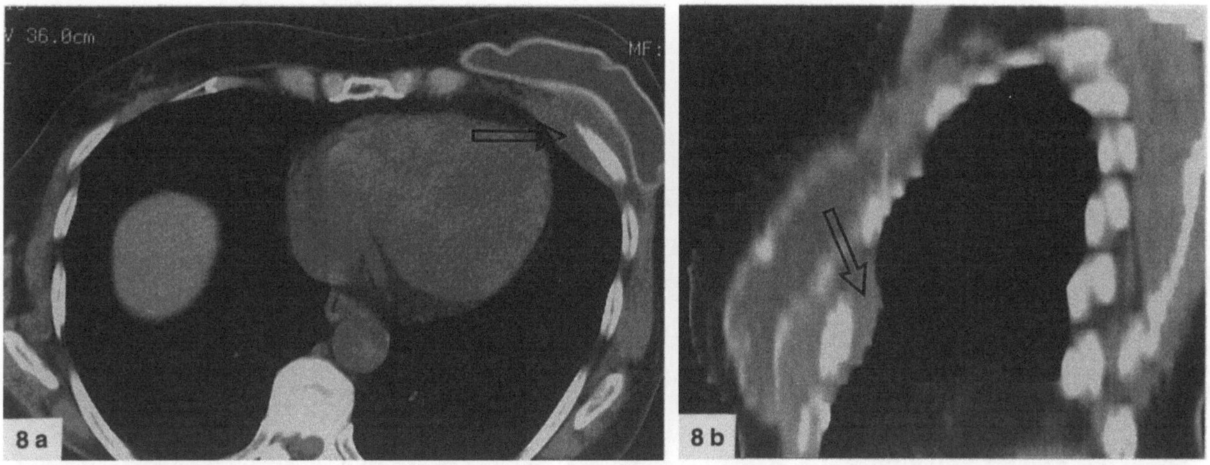

Fig. 15.8 a, b. Subprosthetic recurrence of breast carcinoma on axial CT: (**a**) following contrast injection, (**b**) sagittal reconstruction. CT demonstrates the soft tissue lesion deep to the prosthesis with thickening of the chest wall on both sides of the ribs, this lesion is causing extrinsic compression of the deep surface of the prosthesis. There is associated pleural spread *(arrows)*

the internal structure. There is no specific appearance on MRI even if an increase in signal following gadolinium in lymph node recurrences has been described (not confirmed by any major series). In the absence of any specific signal changes, the same size criteria as CT are used.

In the follow-up of breast implants (figs 15.8 & 15.9), MRI has an important role. It should be remembered that mammography is of very limited value following the insertion of a prosthesis for breast reconstruction following total mastectomy if there is no residual normal glandular tissue. Digitalization has not altered this situation. Ultrasound is undoubtedly limited by the reverberation echoes from the prosthesis. Post-contrast MRI can assess the subprosthetic deep tissue planes and show enhancement of a suspicious area following gadolinium injection on T1-weighted imaging [5, 6]. These findings have also been confirmed in our study [2]. The complications of silicon implant (intra- or extracapsular rupture) are also visualized [3]. 3D helical CT may also be a contributive technique for demonstrating the morphology of the prosthesis and the deep retroprosthetic tissue planes [2, 3].

Conclusion [2-4, 6] (table 15.4)

Concordance between the results of clinical examination, mammography and fine needle aspiration provides an accurate diagnosis in almost every case. In cases of discordance in those patients with ambiguous mammographic results in whom fine needle aspiration is not possible due, for example, to the absence of a clinically palpable mass, histological examination by guided biopsy will be necessary. As soon as more reliable imaging has been validated, some biopsies may be avoidable, particularly in women with fibroadenomas.

In the breast treated conservatively (fig. 15.7) by radiotherapy alone or lumpectomy followed by radiotherapy, mammography becomes less reliable, and interpretation is complicated by the disorganization of the breast architecture and iatrogenic fibrosis. Similarly, following mastectomy, chest wall relapses occurring deep to the breast prosthesis are missed by mammography. Therefore, the other imaging techniques would have a place alongside mammography if they were able to overcome the deficiencies of mammography which are particularly evident in previously treated women.

MRI of the breast with gadolinium, MR angiography and 3D helical CT (fig. 15.7) are only considered to be complementary in those cases where clinical examination and the classical imaging methods have failed. These are non-invasive, atraumatic techniques which will address all the following equivocal situations (after R Gilles et al [6]):

- the dense breasts of young women,
- post-treatment appearances, particularly post-radiation and post-tumorectomy as well as the follow-up of breast prostheses,

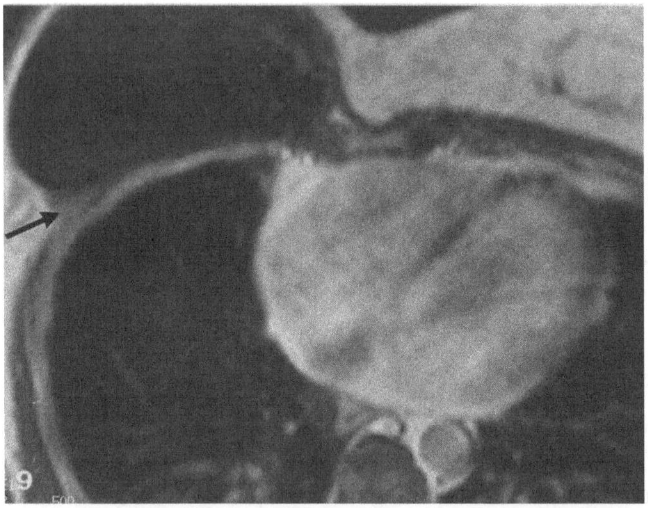

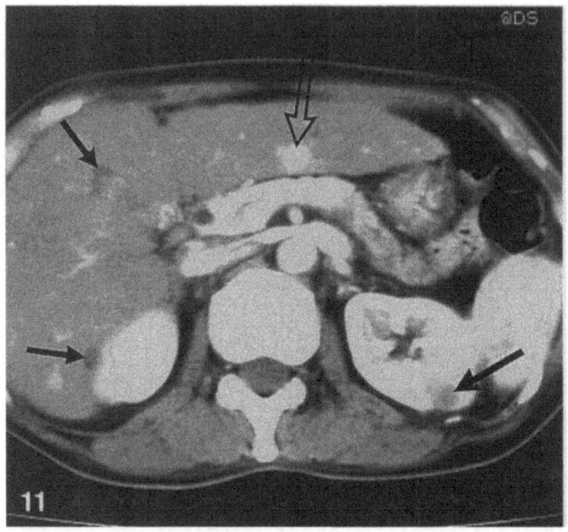

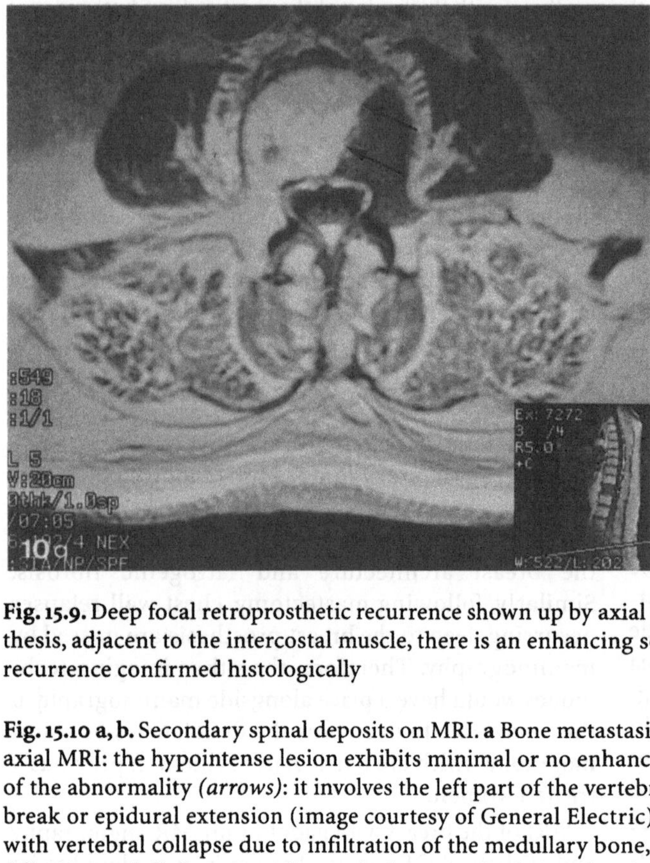

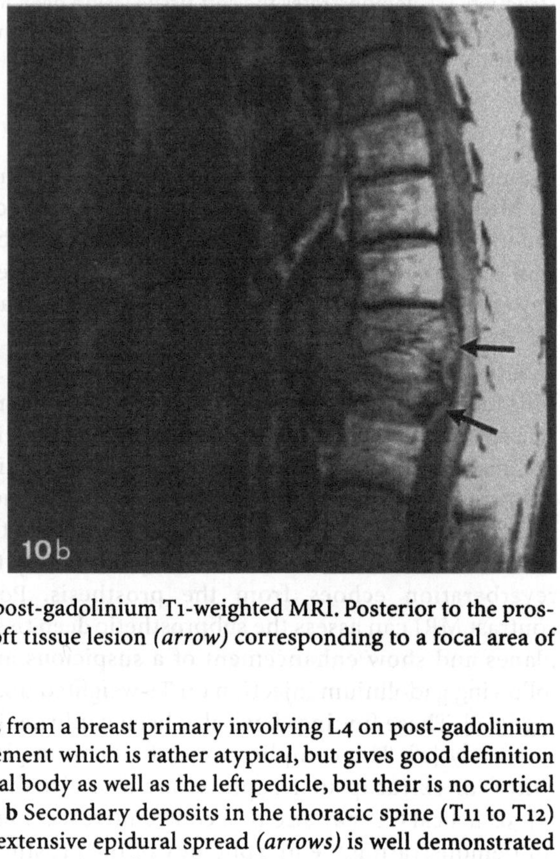

Fig. 15.9. Deep focal retroprosthetic recurrence shown up by axial post-gadolinium T1-weighted MRI. Posterior to the prosthesis, adjacent to the intercostal muscle, there is an enhancing soft tissue lesion *(arrow)* corresponding to a focal area of recurrence confirmed histologically

Fig. 15.10 a, b. Secondary spinal deposits on MRI. **a** Bone metastasis from a breast primary involving L4 on post-gadolinium axial MRI: the hypointense lesion exhibits minimal or no enhancement which is rather atypical, but gives good definition of the abnormality *(arrows)*: it involves the left part of the vertebral body as well as the left pedicle, but their is no cortical break or epidural extension (image courtesy of General Electric). **b** Secondary deposits in the thoracic spine (T11 to T12) with vertebral collapse due to infiltration of the medullary bone, extensive epidural spread *(arrows)* is well demonstrated following gadolinium. Note the marked prevertebral spread and compression of the conus of the cord by epidural disease

Fig. 15.11. Hepatic metastases on CT at a very early stage (Helical CT). The secondary deposits *(small black arrows)* are hypodense in the hepatic arterial phase, in contrast to the adenoma of segment 3 which is of high density at the time of the contrast injection *(hollow arrow)*. Note the similar appearance of a rare secondary renal deposit *(large black arrow)*

- atypical radiological appearances, suspicious or simply equivocal:
  • asymmetry of the breast density,
  • isolated disorganization of the breast architecture,
  • regular solid soft tissue lesions on ultrasound.

It has been shown in a study by ourselves and R Gilles et al, as well as in numerous other published studies, that there is a higher sensitivity following gadolinium injection in these different circumstances, greater than 90% and even approaching 100% according to some teams [12].

The limitations of gadolinium enhanced MRI are the differentiation of benign and malignant microcalcifications, the assessment of well circumscribed lesions and the distinction of inflammatory pathology. It is therefore advisable to perform the examination at least 6 months to one year after the completion of all treatments. The theoretical but nevertheless real risk of missing a small intracanalicular carcinoma on MRI must be remembered.

MR angiography (MRA) (fig. 15.7 c) increases the potential of MRI with gadolinium and may be a complementary method, particularly in recurrent disease. MRA clearly localizes the recurrence within an area of fibrosis and provides, after gadolinium injection, better definition than conventional MRI, even after subtraction, and in certain cases can give information on the tumor vascularization which may have prognostic implications (unpublished data).

Three-dimensional helical CT (fig. 15.7 d) also seems to be a useful complementary technique for the diagnosis and initial assessment of the patient by its ability to appreciate deep tumor extension , spread to the chest wall and axillae, and to provide a quality pre-therapeutic map prior to surgery and particularly to radiotherapy. In the follow-up of prostheses, its multiplanar capability is useful. In cases of recurrent disease in a conserved breast, 3D CT is of more limited value as it does not differentiate reliably recurrence from fibrosis, and its pre-therapeutic role is more limited due to the rarity of complementary radiotherapy treatments at this stage apart from cases with the site of the recurrence separated from the initial primary.

The applications of these techniques are restricted to situations where clinical and radiological investigations are unreliable in the search for recurrences and reduction of the number of patients undergoing unnecessary surgery in the investigation of the mass. The development of rapid sequences and simultaneous acquisition from both breasts may change this situation which will essentially remain valid for the foreseeable future due to health cost constraints [6]. CT for visceral (fig. 15.11) and lymph node spread, and

Table 15.4. A decision pathway for suspected breast carcinoma [1]

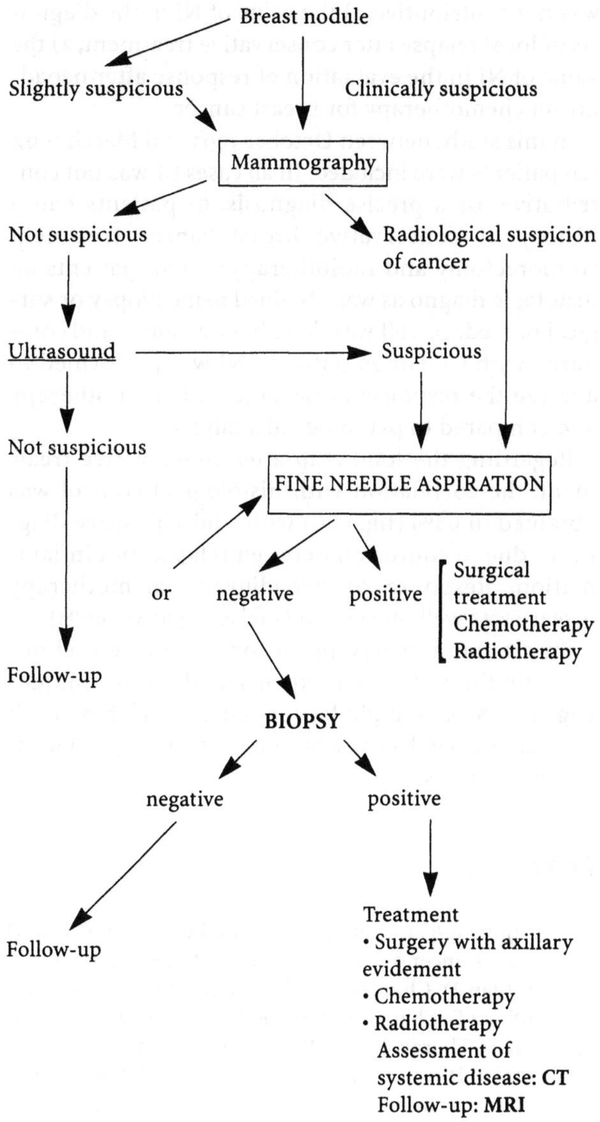

MRI of the spine (fig. 15.10) are, however, routine indications for scanning. MRA and helical CT are still under evaluation.

In conclusion, and in accordance with a new communication [D. Buthiau, E-Ch. Antoine, D. Khayat (1997) Potential Interest of MRI in the follow-up after breast Cancer Treatment; 15th Annual Symposium of the ECPO, Bruges] we can say: Conventional imaging (CI) after conservative treatment for breast cancer (which includes mammography and ultrasound) have demonstrated limited efficiency. Recently, new imaging (NI) techniques such as post-contrast MRI and MR angiography, realized in one examination, have been developed. The purpose was to evaluate, when CI was not contributive: 1) the value of NI in the diagnosis of local relapse after conservative treatment, 2) the value of NI in the evaluation of response after neoadjuvant chemotherapy for breast cancer.

In this study, between October 1993 and March 1997, 120 patients were included. In all cases CI was not contributive for a precise diagnosis. 91 patients had a history of conservative breast cancer treatment (tumorectomy and radiotherapy). In all patients an histologic diagnosis was obtained using biopsy or surgical procedures. NI was done before biopsy and compared with CI. For 29 patients, NI was performed to analyze the response to neoadjuvant chemotherapy and compared to pathological analysis.

Regarding the follow-up after conservative treatment, the correlation with histological control was obtained in 94% (fig. 15.6) with 7 false positive diagnoses due to confusion between relapse and inflammation. Response to neoadjuvant chemotherapy disease was well objectived (1 false negative: 96%).

Studies are undergoing to confirm those preliminary findings. Though expensive, these techniques (figs 15.6 & 15.7) might be cost-effective if they result in a substantial decrease of unnecessary surgical invasive procedures.

References

1. Antoine E.-Ch, Coeffic D, Saglier J, Buthiau D, Khayat D (1998) Cancer du sein. CD Rom FMC, Le Généraliste
2. Buthiau D, Chantelard JV, Lefranc JP (1992) Sein. In: Buthiau D, Chaumier P, Piette JC (eds) TDM et IRM cliniques, Thorax. Frison-Roche, Paris, pp 125-132
3. Buthiau D, Antoine E.-Ch, Khayat D (1997) MRI of treated breast cancer. Breast, San Antonio, dec 1997
4. Buthiau D, Rixe O, Petit T, Nizri D, Weil M, Piette JC, Khayat D (1994) Cancer du sein. In: Buthiau D et coll (eds) Progrès en scanner et IRM. Perspectives cliniques. Vigot, Paris
5. Buthiau D, Antoine E-Ch, Khayat D (1994) Nouvelle imagerie du cancer du sein. Cahiers d'Oncologie. Springer-Verlag, Paris, vol 3, n°4
6. Gilles R, Guinebretière JM, Shapeero LG, Lesnik A, Contesso G, Sarrazin D, Masselot J, Vanel D (1993) Assessment of breast cancer recurrence with contrastenhanced substraction MR imaging: preliminary results in 26 patients. Radiology 188: 473-478
7. Heywang SH, Basserman R, Fenzl G, Nathrath W, Hahan D, Beck R, et al (1987) MRI of the breast-histopathologic correlation. Eur J Radiol 7: 175-182
8. Heywang SH, Hilbertz T, Beck R, Bauer WM, Eiermann, Permanetter W (1990) Gd-DTPA enhanced MR imaging of the breast in patients with postoperative scarring and silicone implants. J Comput Assist Tomogr 14: 348-356
9. Kaiser WA, Zeitler E (1989) MR imaging of the breast: tast imaging sequences with and without Gd-DTPA. Preliminary observations. Radiology 170: 681-686
10. Lamarque JL, Rodière MJ, Salicru B, Boyer L (1989) Fédération Nationale des Collèges de Gynécologie Médicale. 4ème Journées Scientifiques, pp 79-82
11. Lewi-Jones HG, Whitehouse GH, Leinster SJ (1991) The role of MRI in the assessment of local recurrent breast carcinoma. Clin Radiol 43: 197-204
12. Megido-Ravid M, Itzchak Y, Kopolovic J (1993) MR imaging for evaluation of breast scar tissue. 79th Scientific assembly and annual meeting RSNA, Chicago
13. Nyman RS, Rehn SM, Glimelius BLG, Hayberg HE, Hemmingsson AL, Sundstrom CJ (1989) Residual mediastinal masses in Hodgkin disease: prediction of size with MR imaging. Radiology 170: 435-440
14. Ross RJ, Thompson JS, Kim K, Bailey RA (1982) Nuclear magnetic resonance imaging and evaluation of human breast tissue: preliminary clinical trials. Radiology 143: 195-205
15. Stack J, Redmond O, Codd S, et al (1988) Tissue enhancement profiles with Gd-DTPA in breast carcinoma. Radiology 169:22
16. Stark DD, Bradley WG (1988) Magnetic Resonance Imaging. Mosby, St Louis, pp 861-885
17. Stelling B, Powell DE, Mattingly SS (1987) Fibroadenomas: histopathologic and MR imaging features. Radiology 162: 399-407
18. Turner DA, Alcorn FS, Shorey WD, Stelling CB, Mategrano VC, Mertern CW, et al (1988) Carcinoma of the breast: detection with MR imaging versus xerography. Radiology 168: 49-58
19. Weiner JI, Chako AC, Merten CW, Gross S, Coffey EL, Stein HL (1986) Breast and axillar tissue MR imaging: correlation of signal intensities and relaxation times with pathologic findings. Radiology 16: 299-305

CHAPTER 16

Bronchopulmonary cancer

Clinicians
E.-Ch. Antoine, T. Le Chevalier, J.-C. Piette, P. Chaumier, P. Baldeyrou, O. Rixe, E. Vuillemin, D. Khayat

Radiologists
D. Buthiau, C. Yana

The main role of CT and MRI in bronchopulmonary cancer is to determine operability and monitor progress following treatment. We will see to what extent they achieve this and what are their relative roles. In terms of diagnosis, they form part of an overall assessment which also includes clinical examination, the endoscopic and scintigraphic findings, surgery and histology.

Diagnosis and pretherapeutic assessment of bronchial cancers

Indications for CT and MRI

See table 16.1.

Signs

Bronchopulmonary cancers (other than small-cell variety) [1, 7, 14, 16, 19-21, 32, 34, 35, 37].

CT

It must be remembered straight away that CT examination includes the whole of the thorax and upper abdomen as far as the adrenals and is able to appreciate within the thorax the tumor volume, local invasion, particularly the relationship of the lesion with the chest wall and/or mediastinum, and mediastinal lymph node involvement. Contiguous sections are performed following injection preferably in the left arm in order to obtain good opacification of the innominate vein.

Table 16.1. The indications for CT and MRI in bronchopulmonary cancers [37]

Bronchopulmonary cancers

a) In the presence of a known tumor

- CT
  - staging
  - follow-up
  - radiotherapy planning (field, dosimetry)
- MRI reserved for specific problems
  - vascular (e.g. superior vena cava, pericardial or cardiac spread)
  - Pancoast-Tobias syndrome
  - spread of peripheral cancer
  - spinal spread (paramedullary, dural)
  - post-therapeutic follow-up in the presence of suggestive signs
  - hilar lymph nodes (rare)

b) In the absence of a known tumor

- CT
  - diagnostic role (lesion not apparent on standard radiographs)
  - mediastinal evaluation
  - guidance for percutaneous biopsy
  - detection of metastases

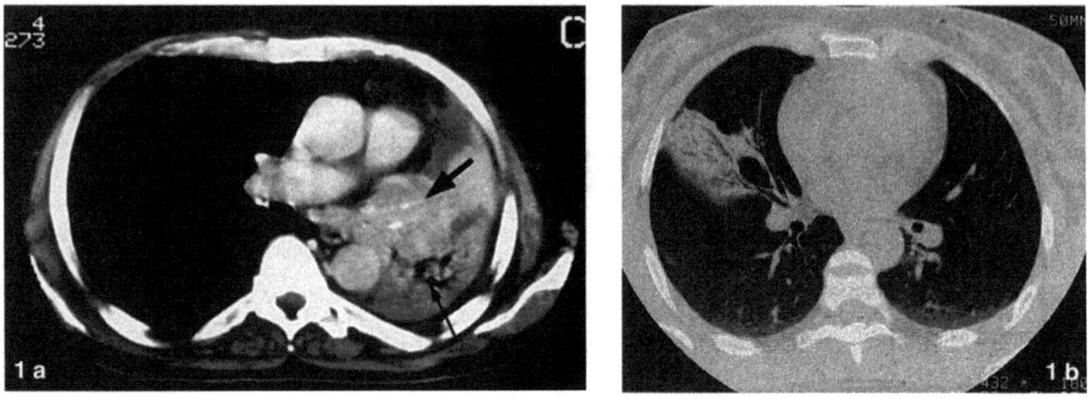

Fig. 16.1 a, b. Non-small-cell bronchopulmonary cancer on post-contrast CT. **a** Tumor obstructing the left lower lobe bronchus with compression of the pulmonary vessels *(thick arrow)*. This lesion is responsible for partial collapse *(thin arrow)* of the left lower lobe. In this case the tumor is easily differentiated from the obstructive sequelae, but this is not always the case on CT. **b** Collapse due to obstruction of the right middle lobe as the result of an endobronchial lesion which is not readily apparent. The unusual configuration of this middle lobe is due to pleural adhesions laterally

Table 16.2. TNM classification (1986)

T0	No primary tumor found
T1	Solitary tumor less than 3 cm located in a lobar or segmental bronchus
T2	Tumor greater than or equal to 3 cm located more than 2 cm from the carina, or involvement of the visceral pleura, or atelectasis of less than a whole lung
T3	Tumor extending beyond the lung (chest wall, diaphragm, mediastinum, supraclavicular region, mediastinal pleura, pericardium) or tumor located less than 2 cm from the trachea but sparing it
T4	Tumor invading the mediastinum, or heart, or great vessels, or trachea or esophagus, or vertebral bodies, or carina or associated neoplastic effusion
N0	No histologically involved lymph nodes
N1	Peribronchial or ipsilateral hilar lymphadenopathy, including direct spread
N2	Metastasis to the ipsilateral mediastinal nodes or subcarinal nodes
N3	Metastasis to the contralateral mediastinal lymph nodes, scalene or supraclavicular nodes
M0	No distant metastasis
M1	Distant metastasis present

The tumor itself

• Tumor volume

CT can assess the volume of peripheral tumors using a sufficiently wide window so as not to artificially increase the size of the lesion. The volume is more difficult to assess for the proximal and perihilar cancers (fig. 16.1) due to the frequency of associated respiratory problems [33] and the difficulty in distinguishing satellite lymph node involvement. The injection of contrast agent may in some but not all cases help in the differentiation of the tumor from associated atelectasis.

When the Golden's sign is present, the size of the lesion is determined by measuring the diameter of the tumor projection.

Measurement of the tumor diameter by CT is relatively accurate but often slightly overestimated due to the frequently associated inflammatory and infective components. The size is reported according to the TNM classification (table 16.2).

Classically the epidermoid or squamous cancers are usually central, sometimes cavitating (fig. 16.2), whereas the adenocarcinomas are more frequently peripheral and develop more slowly. However, in practice the histology cannot be determined from the CT appearances.

• Appearances of the tumor

The lesion is usually rounded or oval, but this is variable. The outlines are sometimes regular or conversely spiculated or radiating. The presence of pleural umbil-

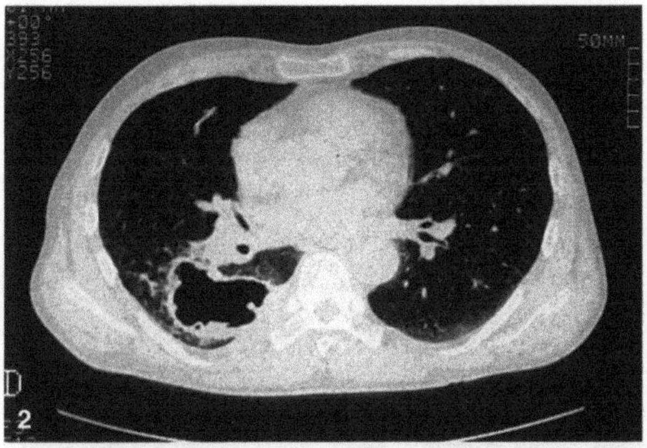

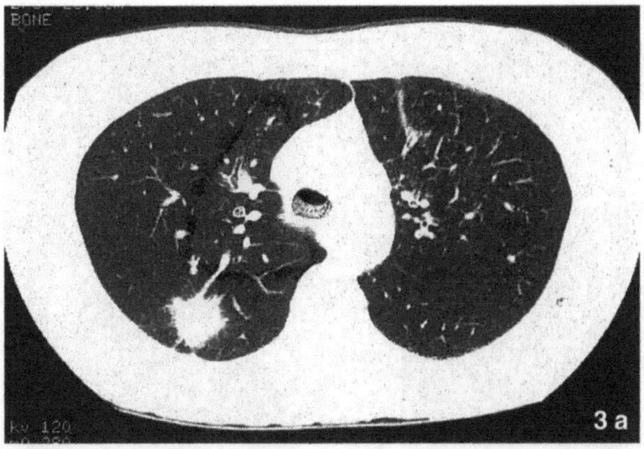

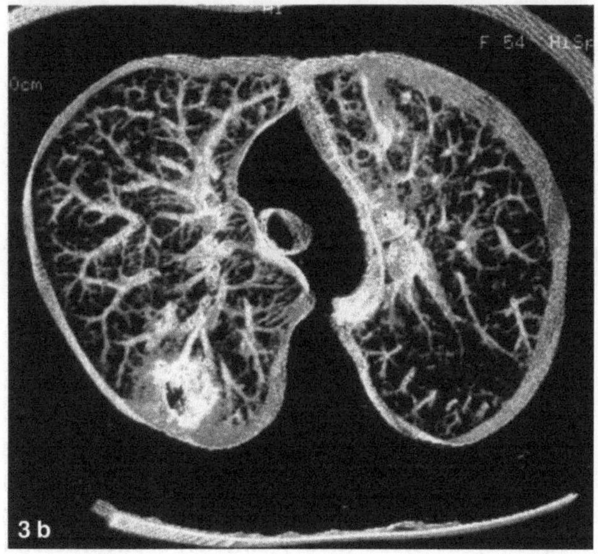

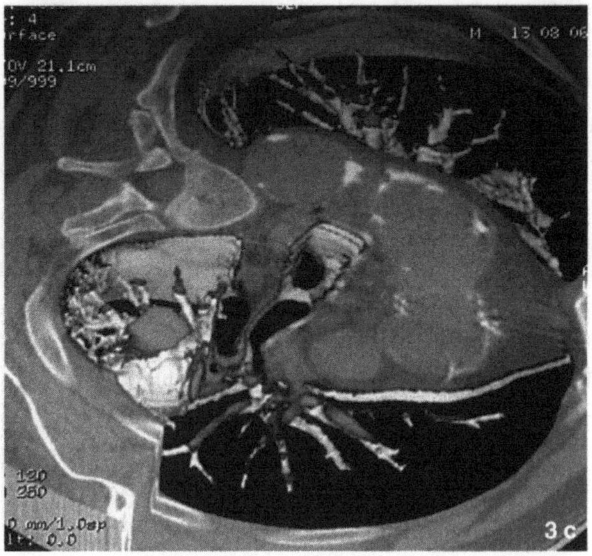

Fig. 16.2. Cavitating peripheral tumor in the apical segment of the right lower lobe: irregular thick walled cavity. The presence of intratumoral cavitation shown on CT does not seem to influence the progression or prognosis of pulmonary tumors

Fig. 16.3 a-c. Peripheral tumor on CT. **a** CT section with 1mm thickness demonstrating a spiculated lesion in the apico-dorsal segment of the right upper lobe. **b** Three dimensional evaluation shows a cavitation within this lesion with improved demonstration of the adjacent interstitial stasis. Another volumetric CT study (**c**) in a different patient demonstrates well the peripheral lesion and the stasis with retrograde lymphatic permeation between the lesion and pleura (**a, b** images courtesy of General Electric; **c** Dr D Buthiau, Scanner Paris 14)

ications, particularly for peripheral tumors, does not necessarily signify spread to the parietal pleura.

- Internal structure of the tumor

The larger the lesion the more likely it is to be heterogeneous, often hypodense, poorly vascularized centrally and vascularized peripherally. When performing percutaneous biopsies, the needle must be placed accurately into the periphery of the lesion. Cavitating lesions (figs 16.2 & 16.3) usually have a thick wall peripherally suitable for biopsy, and the outer borders are more regular than the internal borders.

The presence of calcification does not exclude the diagnosis of a bronchial tumor since a lung cancer may arise within a previously calcified area (e.g. old TB granuloma).

Lymphatic spread [12, 13, 23, 26, 37]
(tables 16.4-16.8, fig. 16.4)

In terms of pathology, the mediastinal lymph node chains are comprised of (from Ph Grenier, table 16.4 [13]):

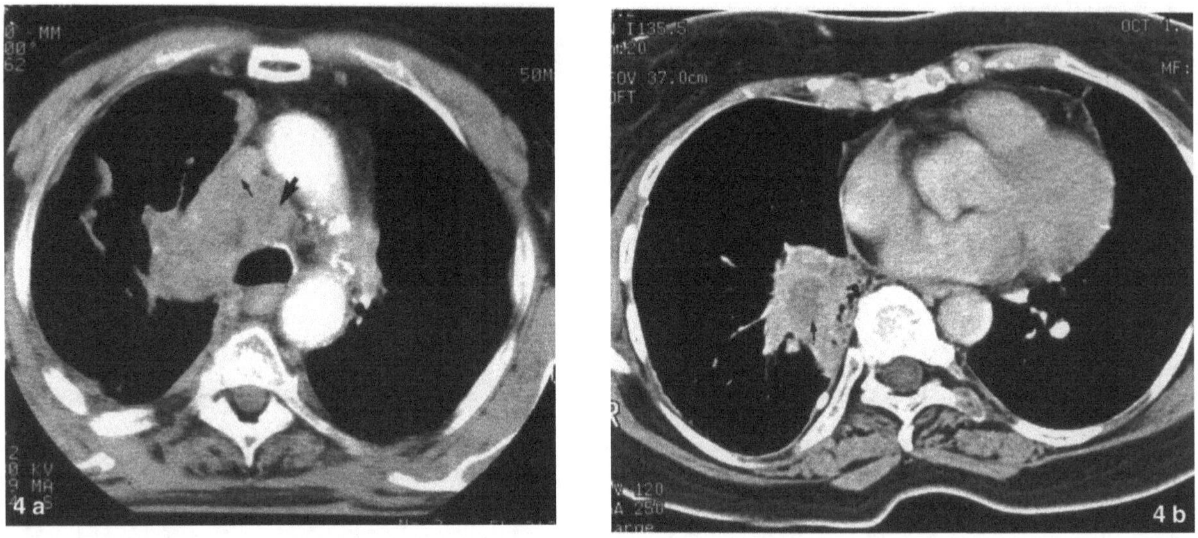

Fig. 16.4 a, b. Lymphatic spread from bronchopulmonary cancers on CT. **a** Peribronchial lymphatic spread from a right hilar tumor *(arrow heads)* with subsequent spread to the principal drainage areas, namely the right middle mediastinal and paratracheal lymph node chains (Barety's region: *large arrow*). Direct contiguous spread into the mediastinum with definite lymphatic middle mediastinitis, extrinsic compression of the trachea and superior vena cava with an endoluminal vascular nodule *(small arrow)*. **b** Peri- and right sub-bronchial lymph node involvement *(arrow)* distinguished from the tumor itself on contrast enhanced angio-CT using continuous rotation

Table 16.3. Role of CT in mediastinal lymph node pathology [37]

• High sensitivity
• Poor specificity
• Important role in the topographic assessment
• Guided biopsy: confirms or excludes the need for mediastinoscopy before deciding treatment
• Post-treatment follow-up

- the visceral chains, in other words, right paratracheal (region of Barėty), left paratracheal (recurrent, aorto-pulmonary window), subcarinal, anterior, middle and posterior mediastinal;

- the chest wall lymph node chains are comprised of the internal mammary, diaphragmatic, posterior parietal and inframediastinal lymph node chains.

Enlarged lymph nodes are rounded or oval, often well defined unless they are confluent, occurring particularly in mediastinal carcinomatosis (fig. 16.4 a); they are homogeneous with soft tissue density, occasionally calcified and little altered by the injection of contrast. The differential diagnosis is with a major vessel (importance of the contrast injection), a thymic remnant, intrathoracic thyroid goiter, a pericardial recess or inflammatory sequelae.

Although CT is highly sensitive (table 16.3), the evaluation is limited by its poor specificity. Bronchial carcinomas are often associated with large reactive inflammatory lymph nodes ("sarcoid-like"), and this is explained by the type of patient in whom the tumor frequently develops (heavy smoker, bronchitic and often with chronic superadded infection, occupational disease).

The size criteria are:

- lymph nodes less than 1 cm are benign in 80-90% of cases;

- nodes greater than 1.5 cm are malignant in 70-80% of cases;

- nodes greater than 2 cm are malignant in 90% of cases;

- the nodes between 1 and 1.5 cm inclusively have no specific figures in terms of pathology.

The threshold diameter is considered to be 10 mm, but may prove to be less for certain lymph node chains: 8 mm for the anterior prevascular mediastinal chains, 7 mm for the superior paratracheal, paraesophageal and left peribronchial chain, 6 mm for the internal mammary chains and 5 mm for the diaphragmatic chains.

Differentiation between the hilar lymph nodes and a central tumor is difficult, and the sensitivity is no greater than 70% but is improved by the newer techniques (fig. 16.4 b). However, it is quite clear that CT is

Table 16.4. Classification of mediastinal lymphadenopathy according to Ph. Grenier. (Tomodensitométrie du thorax. J. Rémy (ed). Vigot, Paris 1987) [13]. Diagram of the topographic classification of mediastinal lymph nodes according to the American Thoracic Society and reviewed by Glazer et al [10]. The lymph nodes numbers 6 and 9 are not included

2D	Right superior paratracheal nodes situated to the right of the trachea and included in a region between the intersection of the brachiocephalic artery with the trachea and the apex of the lung or situated above the arch of the aorta.
2G	Left superior paratracheal nodes located to the left of the midline of the trachea and included area between the top of the aortic arch and lung apex. They correspond to the supra-aortic level of the left paratracheal chain and left anterior mediastinal chain.
4D	Right inferior paratracheal lymph nodes located to the right of the midline of the trachea and area included between the superior border of the azygos vein and the inferior intersection of the brachiocephalic artery with the trachea. They do not include the precarinal nodes.
4G	Left inferior paratracheal nodes located to the left of the midline of the trachea medial to the ligamentum arteriosum and included area between the top of the aortic arch and the carina.
5	Aorto-pulmonary nodes situated lateral to the ligamentum arteriosum, the aorta or left pulmonary artery before the origin of its first branch. They belong to the left anterior mediastinal chain.
6	Anterior mediastinal nodes located anterior to the ascending aorta or brachiocephalic artery. They correspond to the right anterior mediastinal chain.
7	Subcarinal or bifurcation nodes separated from the lobar bronchi and arteries in the lung.
8	Posterior para-esophageal mediastinal nodes located to the right or left of the midline of the esophagus or around the descending aorta and below the level of the subcarinal region.
9	Posterior mediastinal nodes of the right or left triangular ligament.
10D	Right tracheo-bronchial nodes situated to the right of the midline of the trachea and included area between the superior of the azygos vein and origin of the right upper lobe bronchus. They include the precarinal nodes.
10G	Left peribronchial nodes located to the left of the midline of the trachea and medial to the ligamentum arteriosum and included area between the carina and left upper lobe bronchus.
11	Intrapulmonary nodes located in the right or left lung, and nodes situated beyond the major bronchi. There may be subdivided into interlobar (11), lobar (12) and segmental (13).
14	Diaphragmatic or cardiophrenic nodes located at least 2 cm from the diaphragm or pericardium.

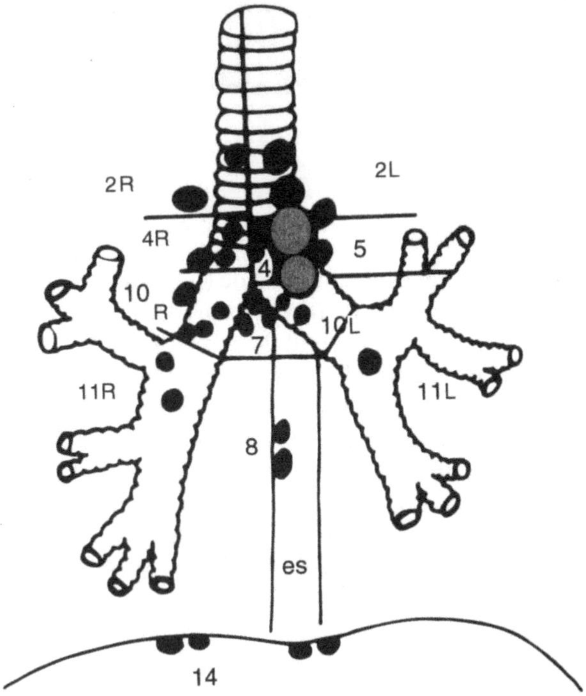

much more accurate than plain radiographs in the lymph node assessment.

In a recent study, B. Dubray et al [4] showed that:

– the accuracy rates for CT and MRI are limited for the different lymph node sites apart from the 4D lymph node. Information on the 4D lymph node provided by these examinations is a sufficient indication for mediastinoscopy. Less information is obtained for the lymph nodes 5 and 6 which are accessible to mediastinotomy, and the data for this examination is nonetheless limited (table 16.4);

– neither CT nor even MRI are able to select the patients at high risk of invasion of the anterior mediastinal, left latero-tracheal lymph node chains in whom the presence of involvement histologically either by mediastinoscopy or percutaneous guided biopsy would have avoided an unnecessary thoracotomy. Similarly, these examinations are unable to select out patients at low risk of nodal invasion.

This study confirms the limited specificity of using size criteria as a sign of involvement. Increa-sing the physiological threshold limit increases the specificity and reduces the sensitivity. The value of this threshold limit is difficult to define.

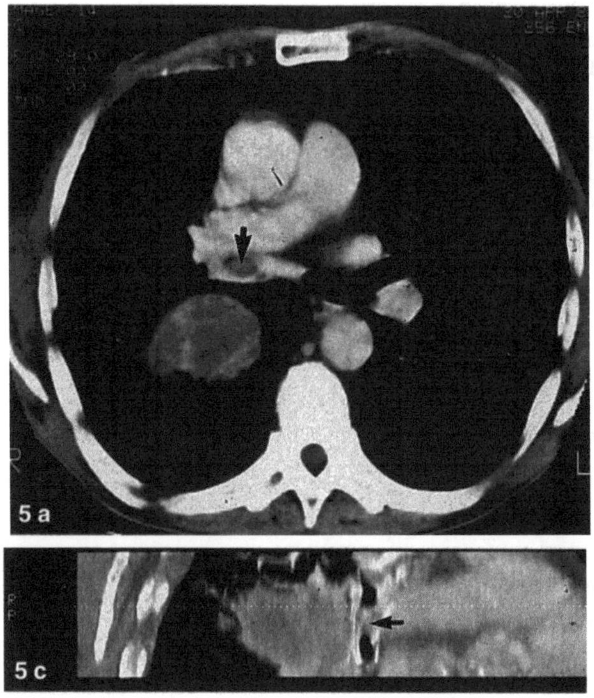

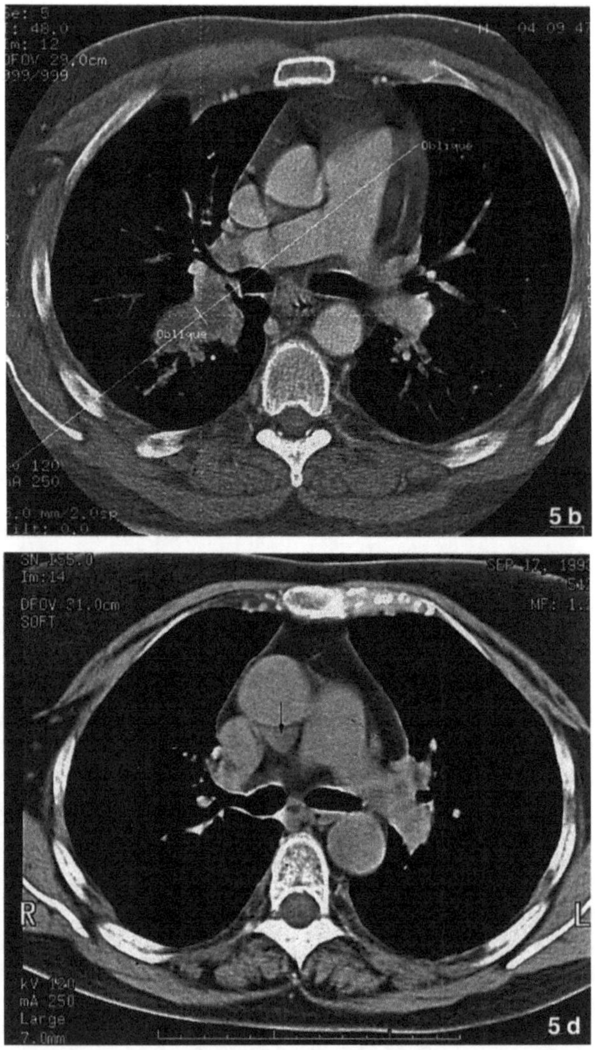

Fig. 16.5 a-d. Bronchial spread on post-contrast CT. **a** Direct visualization of the endoluminal nodule in the right upper lobe bronchus *(arrow)*; **b, c** sagittal oblique reconstruction of a proximal right hilar lesion (**b**) demonstrating endobronchial spread *(arrow)* (**c**); **d** pericardial effusion on continuous rotation CT: the presence of a localized effusion (superior pericardial recess) does not necessarily indicate pericardial involvement, particularly as there is no irregularity or nodularity of the pericardium

Neither CT nor MRI seem able to reduce the indications for histological examination essentially by mediastinoscopy prior to thoracotomy so long as the clinical examination, radiographs, bronchoscopy and respiratory function tests have not detected any contraindications for surgery. The determination of the false positive rate is limited by the need for histological confirmation of mediastinal lymphadenopathy. CT can also act as a guide towards the lymph node chains not routinely explored due to a difficult surgical approach (classification of mediastinal lymphadenopathy: table 16.4). It is worth reemphasizing that a normal size lymph node does not exclude involvement by tumor (table 16.5).

CT only assesses the volume and not the internal structure, even if there are some features which help in the differential diagnosis: tables 16.6-16.8.

Locoregional spread [37]

- Bronchial spread

The endoluminal bronchial nodule (fig. 16.5) is sometimes demonstrated on CT, but it is predominantly the peribronchial thickening and the reduction of the caliber of the bronchus which can be confirmed by this examination. CT is usually performed after bronchoscopy and not as the primary investigation for making the diagnosis. Regions where the bronchial walls are in direct contact with the lungs are easier to assess: posterior surface of the origin of the right main bronchus, trachea, bronchus intermedius, right upper lobe bronchus and lower lobe bronchi. CT is of value in the assessment of tumor spread towards the carina by measuring the length of healthy tissue between the tumor and carinal apex. It is also important to assess the extraluminal bronchial spread, particularly peri-

Table 16.5. Preoperative staging by CT compared to the histological findings (according to Goldstraw)

T	correct	81.5%
	overestimated	3%
	underestimated	15.5%.
N	correct	55%
	over estimated	7%
	underestimated	38%

Table 16.6. Etiology of mediastinal and hilar lymphadenopathy [37]

Common
- Bronchopulmonary cancers
- Tuberculosis
- Lymph node metastases from extrathoracic cancers
- Lymphomas (Hodgkin's and non-Hodgkin's), CLL
- Sarcoidosis
- Pneumoconiosis
- Non-specific reactive hyperplasia

Rare
- Bacterial and viral pneumonia
- Superinfected bronchiectasis
- Pulmonary abscess, chronic infections
- Histoplasmosis and actinomycosis
- Pulmonary eosinophilia
- Wegener's granulomatosis
- Lymph node metastases from cancers (breast, esophagus, thymus, kidney, or malignant chest wall tumors)
- Castelman's disease and angio-immunoblastic lymphadenopathy
- Histiocytosis X
- Thoracic amyloidosis and light chain diseases

Table 16.8. Guide to etiology of mediastinal lymphadenopathy based on the CT appearances [37]

- Cystic or necrotic lymphadenopathies
  - tuberculosis
  - certain metastases, pre- or post-treatment (particularly cancer of the testis or kidney)

- Hypervascularization
  - inflammatory adenopathy
  - lymph node metastases (sarcoma, cancer of the thyroid and kidney)
  - carcinoid tumors
  - Castelman's disease and angio-immunoblastic lymphadenopathies

- Lymph node calcification
  - sequelae of primary tuberculous infection
  - metastases
  - silicosis
  - sarcoidosis (rare)
  - amyloidosis
  - histoplasmosis
  - lymphoma post-chemotherapy or radiotherapy

Table 16.7. Mediastinal lymphadenopathy: principal causes encountered in malignant disease [37]

- Bronchopulmonary cancers
- Hodgkin's and non-Hodgkin's lymphomas
- Other intrathoracic cancers
- Extrathoracic cancers
  - ORL (ENT)
  - Genito-urinary
  - Kidney
  - GIT
  - Thyroid
  - Melanoma
- Cancer of the breast
- Cancer of the esophagus
- Infectious etiologies secondary to iatrogenic complications

bronchially at the mediastinal level with replacement of the surrounding fat by tumor. These factors may actually alter the proposed surgery: for example, bilobectomy or pneumonectomy instead of lobectomy, especially for lower lobe lesions.

The demonstration of bronchial spread which was missed at the initial bronchoscopy can act as a guide for biopsy at a subsequent bronchoscopy. This will also result in a modification of the treatment.

- Mediastinal spread

– Loss of the fat plane between the lesion and mediastinum does not necessarily signify mediastinal invasion and inoperability, but may simply correspond to mediastinal contiguity with a possible plane of cleavage.

– Similarly, replacement of the mediastinal fat by dense inhomogeneous tissue is suggestive of a mediastinal carcinomatosis (fig. 16.4 a). Despite the accuracy of CT, this appearance alone is not a contraindication to thoracotomy.

- Vascular spread

Extension into the superior vena cava is strongly suspected if the vein is surrounded by a lymph node or tumor mass, confirmed by a contrast injection, with a reduction in the caliber of the vessel and opacification of chest wall and mediastinal collaterals. An endoluminal nodule (fig. 16.4 a) may be seen, but false positives occur due to dilution of the contrast at the level of the confluence of the innominate veins. Simple displacement of the superior vena cava does not necessarily indicate vascular extension.

In cases of tumor adherence to the aorta, the rule of quadrants acts as a guide and is only of theoretical value. It is considered that aortic wall involvement is likely if the contact with the tumor is greater than 90° and rare if it is less than 45°; between 45° and 90°, it is equivocal. Adherence to the aortic wall is not necessarily synonymous with inoperability, and surgery may be performed by the peri-adventitial approach. The same is true for cardiac spread where loss of the fat plane of cleavage does not necessarily indicate cardiac invasion. Left atrial extension which is difficult to diagnose on classical CT, is better seen using cine CT and appears as an endoluminal nodule or, to a lesser degree, as irregularity of the wall with focal thickening. Pericardial effusion does not always indicate involvement of the pericardium (fig. 16.5 d) and is not a contraindication to intrapericardial surgery.

Encasement of the left or right pulmonary arteries, although extremely rare, is very suggestive of vascular spread, particularly when associated with hypovascularization on the ipsilateral side. This is the only indication for pulmonary angiography. Invasion of the pulmonary veins uses the same criteria: it is extremely likely when the lesion encases the vein but equivocal in cases of simple contact with the tumor. Analysis of the pulmonary veins becomes difficult when there is adjacent obstructive atelectasis, and the endoluminal tumor nodule can only be visualized in practice using echocardiography, particularly trans-esophageal one.

• Extension to the pleura (see fig. 19.2)

The composition of a pleural effusion cannot be characterized by CT: CT is also unable to determine whether an effusion is of reactive or neoplastic origin. However, CT demonstrates all effusions regardless of their size, particularly those missed on standard radiographs. Generally speaking, the presence of even a small amount of pleural fluid is an indicator of a worse prognosis;

There is no pathognomonic sign on CT for pleural extension, but there are certain very suggestive signs: thickening of the parietal pleura in contiguity with the lesion; smooth interface between the tumor and pleura; tumor and pleura in contiguity over greater than 3 cm. The tumor may back onto a fissure and follows the orientation of the fissure with a resultant rectilinear shape.

• Extension to the chest wall

See chapter 20, Malignant tumors of the thoracic wall.

Metastases from bronchial cancers

Assessment of the contralateral hemithorax should be performed routinely and may demonstrate other lesions or pathologies.

Adrenal metastases [22] are commonly detected, and their frequency varies between 10 and 25% depending on the series quoted, usually asymptomatic and only painful if large. The demonstration of a pathological adrenal mass is not pathognomonic of a metastasis as 5% of normal subjects may present with non-functioning benign adenomas which cannot be differentiated from metastasis by CT. It should also be remembered that 50% of enlarged adrenals are benign. Routine adrenal biopsy is justified when the adrenal mass is unilateral, solitary and measures more than 2 cm in diameter. The detection of adrenal metastasis in principle is a contraindication to surgery, but there are occasions when excision of an adrenal metastasis is considered at the time of the thoracotomy if it is a solitary secondary deposit in the ipsilateral adrenal. A prerenal position of the adrenal gland may prevent biopsy.

CT is able to look for hepatic or renal metastases.

The indication for abdominal and cerebral CT essentially depends on the clinical presentation. Although these investigations are indicated in the presence of the appropriate suggestive symptoms, their role is more disputable in cases of an inoperable tumor. In fact, in cases of early stage disease (stages I, II) or equivocal operability (stage III), these investigations must not delay the surgery in the first case which should be performed as an emergency, whereas in the second case they should be performed prior to thoracotomy in view of the high risk of metastatic disease. In stage III disease, abdominal ultrasound is arguably indicated initially and cranial CT as a routine. Continuous rotation CT ("spiral CT") has a vital role since the whole liver can be assessed in a single or two breath holds giving contiguous sections through the organ.

Pancoast-Tobias syndrome and chest wall involvement by peripheral tumors

CT (fig. 16.6) is greatly superior to conventional radiography. The volume and the position of the tumor can be defined as well as spread into the cervical and mediastinal soft tissues. For anterior spread, CT demonstrates bone lysis in the chest wall, and encasement of the carotid, jugular and subclavian vessels ipsilateral to the tumor following contrast injection. Vessel encasement should be suspected in the presence of phrenic nerve paralysis (carotid artery) or recurrent laryngeal nerve palsy (right subclavian artery). For medial and inferior spread, CT can detect peri-esophageal or tracheal mediastinal infiltration, perivascular infiltration (common carotid arteries,

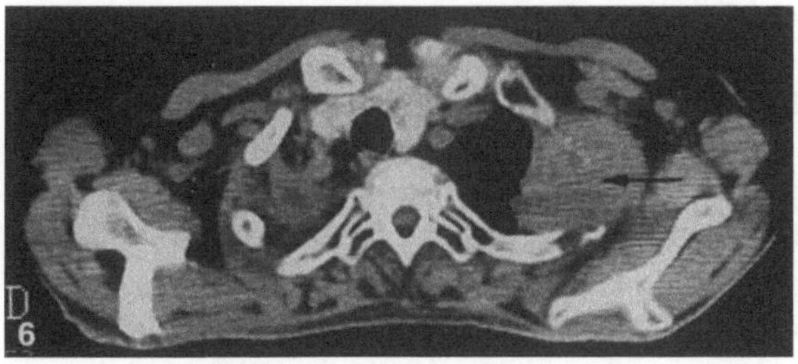

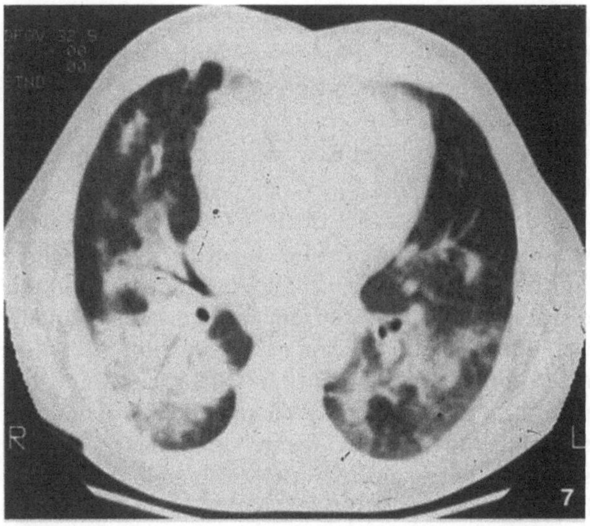

Fig. 16.6. Pancoast-Tobias syndrome on contrast enhanced CT: CT assesses the tumor volume *(arrow)*, position and endo- and extrathoracic spread to the supraclavicular region, as well as bone destruction in the chest wall

Fig. 16.7. Bronchiolo-alveolar cancer during the bronchogenic diffusion phase on post-contrast CT. In the diffuse form, there are multiple peripheral densities which may be confluent giving the appearance of air-space filling associated with linear opacities. Air bronchograms are present but not widespread in this patient

innominate veins) or encasement of the subclavian vessels at the level of the axillary fold. For extension superiorly, CT can detect thyroid involvement. For posterior lesions, CT clearly demonstrates involvement of the chest wall, ribs and vertebrae using thin sections in the order of a millimeter. CT is requested particularly for the Claude-Bernard-Horner syndrome. Intraspinal neuroforaminal spread with epidural infiltration or even spinal cord compression may be demonstrated by CT.

CT assess the general thoracic disease extent, particularly the mediastinal lymph nodes, as for any other pulmonary cancer.

Assessment of the relationship of the tumor with the vessels guides diagnostic percutaneous biopsy, helps define the surgical approach, complemented by angiography, and evaluates the feasibility of extensive surgery with or without vascular replacement.

Bronchiolo-alveolar cancer [6]

This is a non-small-cell bronchial cancer with different radiological appearances. CT, particularly using thin sections, is far superior to radiography;

In the diffuse forms, the CT appearance (fig. 16.7) is one of sometimes confluent nodules which may be uni- or bilateral [6, 10] and even organized, mimicking a pneumonia or alveolar proteinosis. Nonetheless, it is possible to confirm the presence of an intra-alveolar process. CT helps to distinguish the localized forms and is able to demonstrate contralateral involvement, the presence of pleural, pericardial, chest wall, bone, subdiaphragmatic metastases which are contraindications to surgery, or the presence of a pneumothorax.

Certain appearances are highly suggestive of the focal form of bronchiolo-alveolar carcinoma; mass, condensation of tissue, solitary homogenous nodule, poorly defined, sometimes containing the appearances of alveologram or bronchogram on the fine millimetric sections.

MRI [9]

First it should be remembered that bronchial lesions are hypointense on T1-weighted imaging and hyperintense on T2-weighted imaging and that the spin echo T1 sequences with cardiac gating give the best differentiation between tumor and vessels.

MRI does not have any additional specificity compared to CT in the assessment of lymphadenopathy, particularly in the distinction between a malignant and inflammatory node, apart from the assessment of the hilar lymph nodes for which MRI is superior to CT. Conversely, MRI is of limited value in the evaluation of lymph node 11. The combination of CT and MRI does not have any additional advantage compared to CT alone. The diagnosis is made solely on size criteria which are identical to those for CT (see above). The demonstration of mediastinal carcinomatosis is also identical.

MRI has a contributory role in the assessment of tumor extent:

- MRI is more sensitive than CT for the assessment of vascular, pleural, pericardial or cardiac spread which constitute some of the most important features in this disease. Vascular spread from apical masses is equally well appreciated [19]. The demonstration of cardiac extension requires a study in three planes and has proved to be reliable; MRI is mandatory in cases of suspected meningeal or intracerebral spread and should be performed preoperatively to look for cerebral and spinal metastasis;
- chest wall invasion appears hyperintense on T2-weighted imaging, MRI being very sensitive but non-specific (inflammatory changes). It is extremely valuable post-operatively for recurrence;
- two important points must be highlighted: firstly, MRI helps in the differentiation between fibrosis and recurrence on the T2-weighted and post-gadolinium sequences (see later); secondly, it helps to distinguish the tumor itself (particularly central lesions) from the post-obstructive sequelae (distal collapse), but its role is nonetheless limited;
- there is no known indication for MRI in bronchiolo-alveolar cancers; normally the pulmonary parenchyma is composed of air and vessels and of very low signal, and alveolar edema causes a focal or diffuse non-specific increase in this pulmonary signal intensity.

The principal role of MRI is in the assessment of bony or vascular spread in the Pancoast-Tobias syndrome, as well as the appreciation of pleural and chest wall invasion, particularly by apical tumors, and cervico-thoracic paraspinal spread.

Small-cell cancers [37]

There is no recognized indication for surgery in small-cell bronchial cancers (however, the histological diagnosis may only be determined following lobectomy for a peripheral tumor without a known histological diagnosis pre-operatively). The principal role of CT is in the assessment of tumor spread: whole body CT, in other words thoracic, upper abdomen and brain is indicated in this disease as much as for follow-up. Thoracic CT particularly may demonstrate peritracheal, pericarinal, peribronchovascular mediastinal spread and encasement of a vascular pedicle.

CT

The thoracic lesions are often central in the paramediastinal region but a small peripheral tumor associated with relatively large mediastinal lymphadenopathy is suggestive of the diagnosis.

Mediastinal [23] and subdiaphragmatic spread consisting of hepatic, retroperitoneal lymph node, adrenal or bony involvement are better demonstrated than on standard radiography. There should be a routine search for cerebral metastases, given that these are commonly asymptomatic. The detection of a metastatic lesion is sufficient to cancel further investigations.

The presence of bronchial stenosis has no predictive value on the efficacy of treatment.

Overall, CT increases the TNM staging relative to classical radiography.

MRI

MRI has a particular value in the detection of intramedullary metastasis and the extent of cerebral metastasis previously detected by CT.

Other tumors

Primary pulmonary lymphomas [5]

Pulmonary parenchymal involvement in non-Hodgkin's lymphomas may not be associated with lymph node involvement in about 30% of cases [17, 21, 27], whereas in Hodgkin's disease the two are much more frequently encountered in association.

CT can demonstrate the non-specific association of interstitial disease, infiltrate, intra-alveolar disease and subpleural peripheral parenchymal nodules.

Metastases

See chapter 17: diagnosis of a pulmonary nodule.

Lymphangitis carcinomatosa (fig. 16.8)

The diagnosis is made earlier by CT. The most characteristic signs are the presence of septal opacities evolving at a variable rate which may or may not be associated with micronodules (generally less than 5 mm). The intralobular reticular densities are rare.

There is no indication for MRI in this pathology.

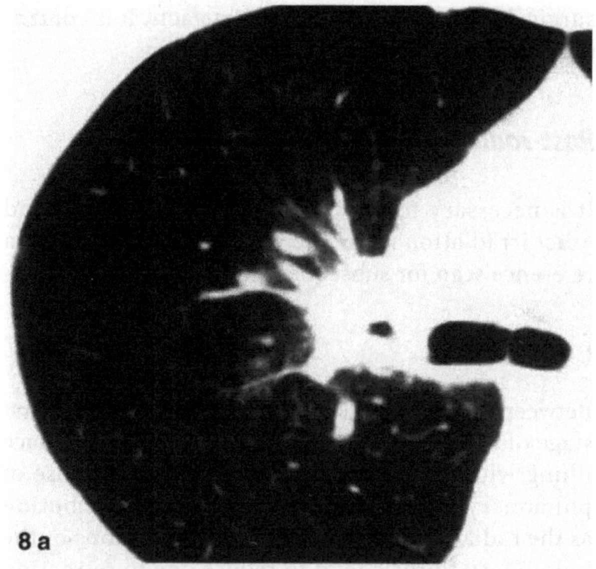

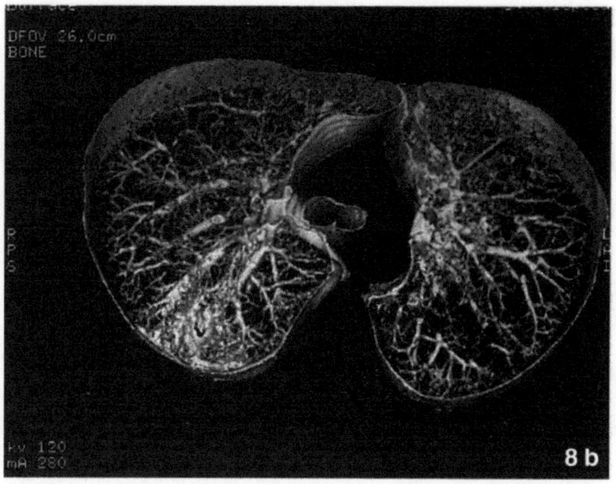

Fig. 16.8 a, b. Lymphangitis carcinomatosa on CT. Standard CT (**a**) and helical study in another patient (**b**) demonstrating the centripetal peribronchial spread of a tumor of the right main bronchus (**a**); early centrifugal disseminated micronodular lymphangitis (**b**)

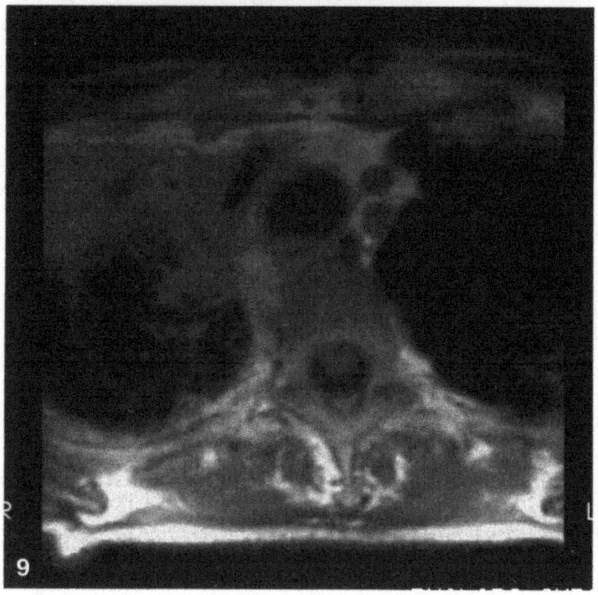

Fig. 16.9. Post-treatment appearance on MR: differentiation of recurrence from fibrosis on post-contrast T1 MRI. Anterior apical heterogeneous zone, fibrotic appearance exhibiting no or minimal contrast enhancement with septal and non-septal thickening, linear collapse and infolding. No evidence of recurrence confirmed by the evolution clinically

Carcinoid tumors

These highly vascular enhancing tumors are located centrally, either endo- or transbronchially.

Cylindromas

These may involve the major bronchi or trachea.

Pulmonary involvement in AIDS [18, 28, 36]

CT

Its main role is:
- the detection of early disease, sometimes occult to standard radiology;
- the assessment of interstitial lesion using thin section (around 1 mm) (e.g. "ground glass" interstitial involvement in pneumocystis);
- the very accurate assessment of the extent of the disease:
  - lymphadenopathy (lymphomas),
  - pulmonary and mediastinal Kaposi sarcomas,
  - mycobacterial infections;
- guidance of percutaneous biopsies (bacteriological and histological analysis).

MRI

No known application in this disease.

Primary sarcomas, melanomas or pneumoblastomas have no specific macroscopic appearances.

Post-therapeutic appearances [37]

(fig. 16.9)

Post-operative

CT [2, 25]

CT is probably the best imaging modality for the thorax following pneumonectomy due to its axial plane of section.

Following pneumonectomy there is ipsilateral mediastinal shift. The structures are analyzed as in a normal thorax, apart from the deceptive appearances suggestive of previsceral anterior mediastinal lymph node enlargement following a left pneumonectomy due to the juxta-aortic position of the pulmonary artery.

The residual cavity generally contains fluid or fibrous tissue and is delineated by the parietal pleura which is more obviously thickened at the level of the axilla and posteriorly than on its mediastinal surface. There is compensatory hyperinflation of the contralateral hemithorax with herniation of the anterior mediastinum, herniation of the posterior mediastinum being rare. The diaphragm is depressed on this side and elevated on the side of the pneumonectomy. Following lobectomy, the fissures are visible and allow localization of any pulmonary lesion. CT is able to demonstrate early complications and detect any recurrences which are equivocal on the standard radiographs. Mediastinal lymphadenopathy, chest wall involvement and recurrence very close to the bronchial sutures are detectable on CT.

CT is indicated when there are clinical signs of compression: pain, dysphagia, superior vena cava syndrome, recurrent laryngeal nerve palsy, and intractable cough. Similarly, it is indicated if there is a change in the general health of the patient, for routine regular follow-up of the post-operative patient in order to demonstrate any recurrence, and for the pre-radiotherapy planning.

MRI [15]

This provides similar information to CT, demonstrating particularly the heterogeneous appearance of the fluid and/or fibrous tissue in the residual cavity. The surgical clips sometimes cause artefacts. It is contraindicated in the presence of vascular clips.

Post-radiotherapy

It is necessary to know the dose, fractionation and exact irradiation field. The value of CT is to obtain a reference scan for subsequent follow-up.

CT

Between the third week and third month [24], the first stage of radiation pneumonitis manifests as air space filling within the irradiated area; then the phase of pulmonary fibrosis appears in the same distribution as the radiation pneumonitis. The dimensions of the pulmonary fibrosis tend to reduce due to retraction and may contain air bronchograms or alveolograms (which may or may not be constant), areas of linear, triangular or round pulmonary thickening and bronchiectasis. Recurrent disease is difficult to demonstrate within the radiation pneumonopathy, comparison of the reference examination with successive examinations helps make the diagnosis in conjunction with the associated endoscopic findings. Contrast enhancement of the recurrence is more intense than the fibrosis.

MRI

Differentiation between fibrosis and recurrence (fig. 16.9) is possible on T2-weighted imaging by the hypointensity of the fibrosis and hyperintensity of the active area. This may be detected relatively early, and it should be known that it is necessary to delay the MRI examination for at least 4-6 months after the last treatment to avoid any confusion with inflammatory changes [11, 30].

Conclusion

In patients considered to be operable after clinical, radiological, endoscopic and functional evaluation, the role of CT is relatively limited to the investigation of direct spread to the mediastinum or chest wall. It can give some indication of resectability. However, it is the method of choice for the assessment of mediastinal lymph nodes, despite its limitations, and guides histological confirmation to the hypertrophied nodes.

In addition, CT helps in the follow-up of post-operative and post-radiotherapy thoraces and is the key examination for detecting generalized spread (brain, abdomen...).

The accuracy of MRI is similar to CT; nonetheless there are certain complementary features in the evaluation of the cardiac wall and major vessels, as well as the assessment of apical tumors (sagittal plane) for posterior spinal extension and spread to vessels and nerves (subclavian origin, brachial plexus). Similarly it seems to be useful in the assessment of the aorto-pulmonary window and in the differentiation of pericardial from cardiac involvement. These indications are not routine, but are dependent on each individual case. Its use in the follow-up of residual masses is more justified.

There is no longer any indication for angiography to assess the origin of the left pulmonary artery. Endo-esophageal ultrasonogram studies the peri-esophageal mediastinum, left atrium, termination of the pulmonary vein and posterior mediastinal lymph nodes. Isotope perfusion scintigraphy evaluates the perfusion of the contralateral lung and the uninvolved lobes, and can predict the functional sequelae of surgery, complemented by VEMS.

References

1. Baron RL, Levit RG, Sagel SS, et al (1982) Computed tomography in the preoperative evaluation of bronchogenic carcinoma. Radiology 145: 727-732
2. Biodetti PR, Fiore D, Sartori F, et al (1982) Evaluation of the post-pneumonoctomy space by computed tomography. J Comput Assist Tomogr 6: 238-242
3. Buthiau D, Gardeur D (1987) Protocoles des examens tomodensitométriques. Schering Diffusion
4. Dubray B, Grenier Ph, Carette MF, Frija G, Musset D, Chastang C (1991) Extension ganglionnaire médiastinale des cancers broncho-pulmonaires: comparaison de la TDM et de l'IRM par méthodologie ROC. Rev Imaging Med 3 : 249-256
5. Devita VT, Jaffe ES, Hellman S (1985) Hodgkin's disease and the non-Hodgkin's lymphomas. In: De Vita VT, Hellman S and Rosenberg SA (eds) Cancer: principles and practice of oncology. JB Lippincott, Philadelphia
6. Epstein DM, Gefter WB, Miller W (1982) Bronchio-alveolar cell carcinoma. AJR 139: 463-468
7. Gamsu G (1983) Computed tomography of the mediastinum. In: A Moss, G Gamsu and H Genant (eds) Computerized tomography of the body. WB Saunders, Philadelphia
8. Gamsu G, de Geer, Cann C, et al (1987) A preliminary study of MRI quantification of simulated calcified pulmonary nodules. Invest Radiol 22: 853-858
9. Gefter WB (1990) Magnetic resonance imaging in the evaluation of lung cancer (review) Semin Roentgenol 25: 73-84
10. Glazer GM, Gross BH, Quint LE, Francis IR, Bookstein FL, Orringer MB (1985) Normal mediastinal lymph nodes: number and size according to American Thoracic Society Mapping. AJR 144: 261-265
11. Glazer HS, Lee JK, Levitt RG, et al (1985) Radiation fibrosis: differentiation from recurrent tumor by MR imaging. Radiology 156: 7216
12. Glazer GM, Orringer MB, Chenevert TL, et al (1988) Mediastinal lymph nodes: relaxation time/pathologic correlation and implications in staging of lung cancer with MR imaging. Radiology 168: 429-431
13. Grenier Ph (1987) Les adénopathies médiastinales. In: J Rémy (ed) Tomodensitométrie du Thorax. Vigot, Paris, pp 90-100
14. Grenier Ph, Dubray B, Carette MF, Frija G, Musset D, Chastang Cl (1989) Preoperative thoracic staging of lung cancer: CT and MR evaluation. Diagn Interv Radiol 1: 23-28
15. Laissy JP, Rebibo G, Trotot PM, et al (1989) Post- pneumonectomy evaluation of the chest: a prospective comparative study of MRI with CT. Magn Reson Imaging 7: 55-60
16. Laurent F, Drouillard J, E)orcier F, et al (1988) Bronchogenic carcinoma staging: CT versus MR imaging, assessement with surgery. Eur J Cardiothorac Surg 2: 31-36
17. Lewis ER, Caskey Cl, Fishman EK (1991) Lymphoma of the lung: CT findings in 31 patients. AJR 156: 711-714
18. Marciano S, Chaumier P, Buthiau D, Guillevin L, Raphael M (1992) Manifestations thoraciques du SIDA. In: D Buthiau (ed) TDM et IRM Cliniques - Pneumologie et Cardiologie. Frison-Roche, Paris, pp 230-234
19. Musset D, Grenier Ph, Carette MF, et al (1986) Primary lung cancer staging: prospective comparative study of MR imaging with CT. Radiology 160: 607-611
20. Mintzer RA, Malave SR, Neiman HL, et al (1979) Computed vs conventional tomography in evaluation of primary and secondary neoplasms. Radiology 132: 653-659
21. Negendank WG, al Katib AM, Karanes C, Smith MR (1990) Lymphomas: MR imaging contrast characteristics with clinical-pathologic correlations. Radiology 177: 209-216
22. Nielsen ME, Heaston DK, Dunnick NR (1982) Preoperative CT evaluation of adrenal glands in non-small cell bronchogenic carcinoma. AJR 139: 317-320
23. Osborne DR, Korobkin R, Ravin CE, et al (1982) Comparison of plain radiography, conventional tomography and computed tomography in detecting intrathoracic lymph node metastases from lung carcinoma. Radiology 142: 157-161
24. Pagani JJ, Libshitz HI (1982) CT manifestations of radiation- induced change in chest tissue. J Comput Assist Tomogr 6: 243-248

25. Peters JC, Desai KK (1983) CT demonstration of postpneumonectomy tumor recurrence. AJR 141: 259-262
26. Poon PY, Bronskill MJ, Henkelman RM, et al (1987) Mediastinal lymph node metastases from bronchogenic carcinoma: detection with MR imaging and CT. Radiology 162: 651-656
27. Rahmouni AD, Zerhouni EA (1990) Role of MRI in the management of thoracic lymphoma. Contemp Issues CT 11: 23-33
28. Servois V, Tudoret L, Laissy JP, Sibert A, Thomas E, et Menu Y (1993) Sarcome de Kaposi pulmonaire: aspects tomodensitométriques chez 43 patients atteints du SIDA. Rev Imaging Med 5: 611-617
29. Stark DD, Higgins CB, Langer P, et al (1989) Magnetic resonance imaging of the pericardium normal and pathologic findings. Radiology 469-474
30. Surbone A, Longo DL, De Vita VT, et al (1988) Residual abdominal masses in aggressive non-Hodgkin's; lymphoma after combinationchemotherapy: significance and management. J Clin Oncol 6: 1832-1837
31. Templeton PA, Caskey Cl, Zerhouni EA (1990) Current uses of CT and MR imaging in the staging of lung cancer. Radiol Clin North Am 28: 631-646
32. Tisi GM, Friedman PJ, Peters RM, et al (1983) Clinical staging of primary lung cancer. Am Rev Respir Dis 127: 659
33. Tobler J, Levitt RG, Glazet HS, et al (1987) Differentiation of proximal bronchogenic carcinoma from postobstructive lobar collapse by magnetic resonance imaging. Comparison with computed tomography. Invest Radiol 22: 538-543
34. Webb WR (1988) MR imaging in the evaluation and staging of lung cancer (review). Semin ultrasound CT MR 9: 53-66
35. Webb WR, Gatsonis CA, Zerhouni EA, et al (1989) Comparison of CT and MR imaging in lung cancer staging: preliminary results of the RDOG study. Radiological Society of North America, November 89
36. White DA, Matthay RA (1989) Non infectious pulmonary complications of infection with the human immunodeficiency virus. Am Rev Respir Dis 140: 1763-1787
37. Yana C, Chaumier P, Buthiau D, et al (1992) Pathologie thoracique. In; D Buthiau (ed) TDM et IRM Cliniques - Pneumologie - Cardiologie. Frison-Roche, Paris, pp 78-124

CHAPTER 17

Pulmonary metastases

Clinicians
J.-L. Breau, J.-C. Piette, O. Rixe, F. Guinet, P. Chaumier, P. Baldeyrou

Radiologist
D. Buthiau

Any tumor, apart from cerebral tumors, can metastasize to the lung parenchyma which acts as a filter for tumor cells carried in the blood stream (and also in the lymphatic system). The radiological and CT appearances depend on the mode of metastatic spread. Hematogenous metastases are usually nodular (micronodular, sometimes with a miliary or macronodular appearance). They may be solitary or multiple with the typical appearance of cannon balls of almost equal or variable sizes, the dissemination being probably due to successive waves. This appearance of a rounded hematogenous metastasis is usually seen in sarcomas (the lung is the site of predilection), and testicular, renal, thyroid cancers, choriocarcinoma... They may also occur in cancers of the breast, esophagus and bladder, and otorhinolaryngological squamous cancers, and primary bronchial cancers in which the risk of metastatic spread to the pulmonary parenchyma away from the site of the primary tumor is underestimated.

On the other hand, dissemination via the lymphatic system appears as interstitial type shadowing (invasion of the lymphatics at the level of the inter-alveolo-capillary spaces). These appearances are better assessed on high resolution CT and are encountered in the lymphophilic cancers: breast, pancreas, stomach, thyroid, prostate... Lymphatic involvement may be associated with pleural changes due to involvement of the pleural lymphatics, mediastinal lymph node enlargement or even nodules.

In the context of the follow-up after treatment of a known primary cancer by routine chest radiographs at regular intervals, the appearance of abnormal pulmonary lesions is highly suggestive of metastatic disease (table 17.1).

The diagnosis of metastasis is supported by:

- simultaneous elevation of tumor markers which may or may not be specific to the previously known primary tumor. Only the PSA, b-HCG and calcitonin levels have a significantly specific value for cancer of the prostate, choriocarcinoma and medullary carcinoma of the thyroid, respectively;
- the rapid progression of the initial pulmonary lesion or the appearance of new lesions on subsequent comparative examinations.

These appearances are usually sufficient to confirm the presence of metastatic disease and to justify antitumor treatment. The choice of treatment depends on the primary tumor, the time lapsed before the appearance of metastases, the clinical context, and the solitary or multiple metastases. Possible treatments include systemic chemotherapy, hormone therapy or surgical excision.

All others are detected accidentally on a routine examination or during the investigation of bronchopulmonary symptoms, any abnormal pulmonary nodules or interstitial shadowing being suspicious of metastatic disease without a known primary cancer. The radiological appearances of multiple nodular opacities, the clinical context and tumor marker levels may point

Table 17.1. Follow-up of a known primary cancer with a risk of pulmonary metastasis. Standard PA (frontal) and left lateral chest radiography (*). Every 4 months for the first two years, every 6 months up to the 5th year

Suspicious image

↓

CT

↙ ↘

1 No metastases		2 Metastases Number, uni- or bilateral	
↙	↘	↙	↘
A- Normal serum tumor markers	B- Elevated serum tumor markers	A- If systemic treatment decided: CT every 3 months ± serum markers	B- if surgical treatment faced: • exclude other metastatic sites. Cerebral, abdominal CT, bone scintigraphy, other examinations depending on the primary cancer
↓	↓	↓	
Follow up	Look for another metastatic site or progressive locoregional recurrence *Examinations depend on primary cancers;*	Assessment of treatment efficacy and detection of locoregional recurrence. If surgery for residual tumor faced → 2B	• exclude locoregional recurrences; investigations depend on site of primary tumor: endoscopy • assessment of respiratory function

(*) an initial thoracic CT (reference examination) is justified in sarcomas, placental choriocarcinoma and testicular tumors

towards a neoplastic pathology. Alternatively, the abnormality may be a solitary nodule. In both cases, histological confirmation of cancer is essential before any therapeutic decision is made.

The diagnosis may also be obtained by:

- bronchoscopic examination in cases of endobronchial lesions accessible to biopsy (lymphangitis of the bronchial submucosa);
- biopsy from another directly accessible metastatic site: lymph nodes, pleura, skin...;
- CT guided percutaneous pulmonary biopsy or even surgical biopsy by thoracotomy or thoracoscopy may be the only way of confirming the neoplastic and probably metastatic nature of the radiological pulmonary abnormality. The histological appearance and immunomarkers help direct the search for the primary cancer and decide on treatment. The hunt for the primary cancer should be non-invasive, mainly clinical and biochemical, and must not delay treatment.

Indications for CT and MRI

CT

CT detects more pulmonary metastases than tomography in both adults and children [1,4].

CT is indicated in the presence of any pulmonary nodule, irrespective of whether it is cavitating, seen on a standard radiograph and is essential for:

- the detection of other nodules;
- the detection of calcification or cavitation, a drainage bronchus;
- the follow-up;
- guiding percutaneous biopsy (see chapter 36).

However, the indications for CT in the search for pulmonary metastases depend of the type of cancer, its propensity to metastasize to the lung, the stage of the disease, the efficacy of treatment, and the prognosis subsequent to the detection of pulmonary metastases. The appearance of a pulmonary nodule in a

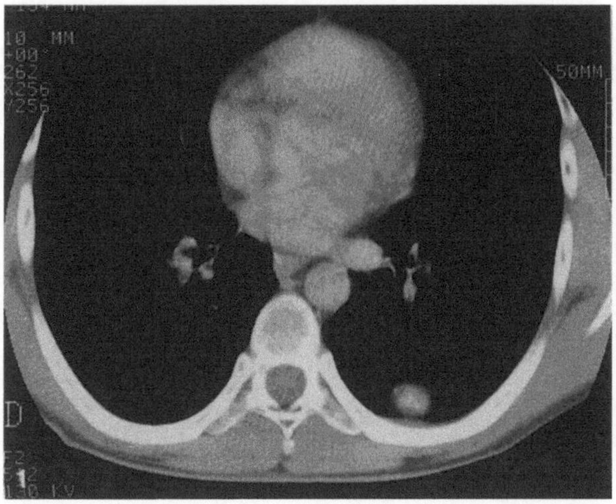

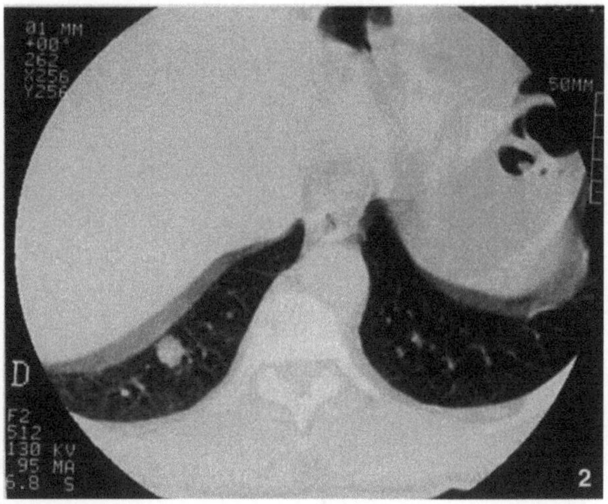

Fig. 17.1. Pulmonary nodule in the left lower lobe: subpleural position measuring 12 mm in diameter on post-contrast CT. Presence of microcalcifications, perinodular fibrosis and slight thickening of the adjacent visceral pleura; the contours are regular. These are non-specific criteria of a benign lesion (hamartoma)

Fig. 17.2. Secondary pulmonary nodule in the right posterior costophrenic recess on CT. There is a 11 mm diameter lesion of low density less than 100 HU (NB difficulty in measurement)

patient with a known malignant tumor does not necessarily indicate a metastasis [1].

Two particular problems are difficult to resolve:

- Firstly, a pulmonary nodule persists unchanged despite chemotherapy which appears to have been otherwise successful: this may represent a persistent benign nodule, a metastasis, or scar which does not contain any malignant cells. This latter phenomenon is well recognized in Ewing's sarcoma and non-seminomatous cancers of the testis. Biological tumor markers are therefore very useful to help make the therapeutic decision: cessation of treatment with careful follow-up and/or thoracotomy. Thoracotomy can often detect a benign cellular transformation in the form of mature teratomas at the site of previous metastases from testiculo-choriocarcinoma.

- The second problem concerns patients who have had one or several metastases surgically resected: pulmonary scars retract, remain stable over several months and commonly persist at follow-up examinations. Any change or subsequent enlargement must raise the suspicion of local recurrence within a previously resected area.

MRI

MRI is inferior to CT [2, 3, 5] in the detection of pulmonary nodules, and it is therefore not indicated.

It has a theoretical value distinguishing a pulmonary nodule from an adjacent hilar blood vessel.

Signs

Pulmonary nodules [1-5]

CT

Definition

The definition of a pulmonary nodule is fairly vague: an intraparenchymal opacity which may or may not be well circumscribed;

- clinically the lesion is asymptomatic;
- there are a number of possible causes, and the diagnosis requires the combination of the clinical and paraclinical findings;
- CT is approximately 20 times more sensitive than radiography in appreciating the density difference (figs 17.1-17.3);
- however, the nature of the nodule is equally difficult to define as on conventional radiography; the following features favor a benign process but are not specific:
  - calcifications (fig. 17.1),
  - perinodular fibrosis,

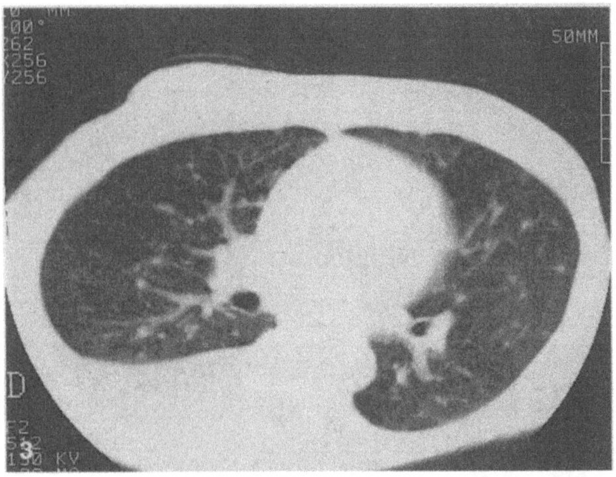

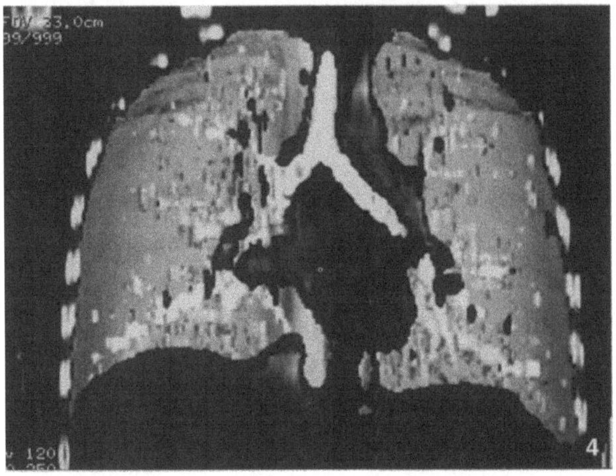

Fig. 17.3. Multiple micronodular hematogenous spread on post-contrast CT; there are multiple micronodules within both hemithoraces almost imperceptible on the standard radiograph. Note the large pleural effusion on the right

Fig. 17.4. Coronal reformat of a volumetric helical 3D CT showing multiple secondary pulmonary nodules; the nodules appear black and are easily distinguished from the vascular and bronchial structures. The value of this technique is essentially due to the strictly contiguous nature of the sections and not related to this reformat (technique still under study) (image courtesy of Dr D Buthiau, Scanner Paris 14)

• other satellite nodules,
• stability or progressive calcification of the nodule on follow-up examinations,
• regular contours but this is not a pathognomonic feature;
– it is not possible to differentiate a peripheral cancer, solitary metastasis or non-calcified granuloma [1, 2, 4];
– measurement of the absorption coefficient may be useful in theory to increase the sensitivity for the detection of diffuse calcification within nodules:
– a density of less than 164 HU is sufficient indication to allow simple follow-up of the patient by chest X-rays every 6 months;
– a solitary nodule whose density is less than 146 HU may be benign or malignant, and should be presumed to be malignant until histological confirmation is obtained;
– between 147 and 163 HU, the situation is unclear, and closer follow-up or percutaneous biopsy will be necessary;
– in fact, the density measurement of a pulmonary nodule is very difficult (fig. 17.2), particularly when it is small, because the proximity of air within the lung causes a partial volume effect responsible for negative measurement even on the high resolution thin sections. This effect may even arise in nodules shown to be calcified in standard radiographs [2]. If there is any diagnostic doubt, a percutaneous biopsy should be considered.

Differential diagnosis
(table 17.2)

In practice, any dense non-calcified nodule of less than a centimeter in diameter requires regular follow-up to confirm its stability. Examinations are repeated every 3-4 months, particularly if the lesion is peripheral (92% of metastases occur in the peripheral third of the lung fields). Any suspect nodule of greater than

Table 17.2. Differential diagnosis of pulmonary metastases

- Transversally sectionned vessels (but surrounded by little linear radiated artefacts due to vascular beat); their size is always equivalent to the size of the neighbouring vessels
- Bone structure in partial volume
- Loculated pleural effusion in the large pleural cavity or in the fissures
- Pleural fibrin clot
- Chronic parenchymatous atelectasis or round atelectasis
- Sequestration (angioscan of great value)
- Bronchiectasis, bronchioceles
- Mucoid impactions
- Hydatid cysts (without visible wall and without enhancement after contrast injection)
- Bronchogenic cysts
- Hamartomas or hamartochondromas
- Neurinomas mostly when intercostal or intervertebral

1 cm in diameter which is accessible to biopsy or any change in the size of a nodule requires the performance of a percutaneous biopsy.

In the majority of cases, a primary bronchial carcinoma can be differentiated from a metastatic deposit by the appearance of its outline. The primary cancer usually has an irregular border with extensions into healthy tissue and does not have the well defined rounded appearance of a metastasis. However, a solitary large metastasis can resemble a primary tumor.

Number of lesions

CT can detect more nodules than standard radiographs or tomography.

Nodules of 2-3 mm in diameter can be detected by CT (fig. 17.4).

Due to its high sensitivity, CT can also act as a control for follow-up of these lesions: increase in volume, appearance of new lesions...

Size of lesions

Pulmonary nodules of greater than 3 cm are usually malignant whereas those of less than 2 cm are usually benign.

A recently appearing solitary nodule of 3 cm requires percutaneous biopsy in order to obtain the diagnosis if bronchoscopy is negative.

Inflammatory nodules are, as a rule, smaller and do not tend to increase in size on follow-up. However, a trial of antibiotic treatment should be considered before biopsy for any recently appearing rounded opacity on the presumption that it is due to simple infection.

It should be remembered that pulmonary metastases may appear not only as parenchymal nodules but also as an interstitial process.

Cavitating lesions

These are defined as an air-filled or air/fluid cavity situated in an area of parenchymal condensation. The diagnosis of the etiology is extremely important and is helped by the combination of the clinical, biochemical, radiological and percutaneous biopsy findings.

CT

CT readily detects one or several air-filled cavities, even if they are small, within a nodule.

The clinical context, topography and evolution of the lesion can sometimes suggest the cause, particularly tuberculosis and hydatid cysts (the latter contraindicating biopsy). However, the CT appearances are not specific.

In the case of diagnostic uncertainty, CT guided percutaneous biopsy can be performed for bacteriological, mycological and cytological analysis.

References

1. Dondelinger RF, Kurdziel JC (1987) Nodules pulmonaires solitaires et multiples. In: J. Rémy (ed) Tomodensitométrie du thorax. Vigot, Paris, pp 271-280
2. Gamsu G, de Geer G, Cann C, et al (1987) A preliminary study of MRI quantification of simulatod calcified pulmonary nodules. Invest Radiol 22: 853-858
3. Muller NL, Gamsu G, Webb WR (1985) Pulmonary nodules: detection using magnetic resonance and computed tomography. Radiology 155: 687-690
4. Yana C, Chaumier P, Buthiau D, et al (1992) Pathologie thoracique. In: Buthiau D (ed) TDM et IRM Cliniques - Pneumologie, Cardiologie. Frison-Roche, Paris, pp 78-124
5. Zerhouni EA, Herold CJ, Dietbert Hahn (1992) Mediastinum and lung. In: DD Stark, WG Bradley Jr (eds) Magnetic Resonance Imaging. Mosby-Year Book, St Louis, pp 1429-1489

CHAPTER 18

Mediastinal tumors

Clinicians
J.-C. Piette, P. Chaumier, D. Khayat

Radiologists
D. Buthiau, C. Yana

CT is indicated in any clinical and/or radiological mediastinal syndrome even if the radiological investigation is normal (tables 16.1 and 16.3, chapter "Bronchopulmonary cancer").

MRI may be contributory in the diagnosis of the nature, topography, spread of the lesion and for follow-up but in practice is only indicated in certain specific circumstances (table 18.2).

The diagnostic, etiologic and topographic signs of mediastinal tumors are summarized in tables 18.3-18.5 and in the tables 16.3, 16.4, 16.6-16.8 of chapter "Bronchopulmonary cancer" (figs 18.1-18.4 and see fig. 16.4).

Table 18.1. Indications for CT in mediastinal disease [7]

• Mediastinal syndrome suggested clinically and/or radiologically.
• Mass not detectable on standard radiographs or tomography, a search for which is motivated by the clinical and/or biochemical findings
• Etiologic approach based on densitometry may help determine the nature of the lesion (benign versus malignant) but with well recognized reservations.
• Assessment of morphology and particularly spread (to any adjacent viscera, lymph nodes, chest wall, subdiaphragmatic - particularly adrenals).
• Follow-up of known pathologies, usually post-therapeutic (differentiation of post-radiation fibrosis from recurrent tumor).

References

1. Bergh N, Gatzinsky P, Larson S, et al (1978) Tumors of the thymus and thymic regions: I. Clinicopathological studie on thymomas. Ann Thorac Surg 25: 91-98
2. Kholl KS, Levitt RG, Glazer HS (1985) Magnetic resonance imaging of fibrosing medistinite. AJR 145: 255-259
3. von Schulthess GK, Mac Murdok T, Scholakoff D, et al (1986) Mediastinal masssses. MT imaging. Radiology 158: 289-296
4. Webb WR, Gamsu G, Stark DD, et al (1984) Magnetic resonance imaging of the normal and abnormal pulmonary hila. Radiology 152: 89-94
5. Webb WR, Gamsu G, Stark DD, et al (1984) Evaluation of magnetic resonance sequences in imaging mediastinal tumors. AJR 143: 723-727
6. Wescott JL, Henschke Cl, Berkmaen Y (1985) MR imaging of the hilum and mediastinum: effects of cardiac gating. J Comput Assist Tomogr 9: 1073-1078
7. Yana C, Chaumier P, Buthiau D, et al (1992) Pathologie thoracique. In: Buthiau D (ed) TDM et IRM Cliniques - Pneumologie, Cardiologie. Frison-Roche, Paris, pp 78-124
8. Zerhouni EA, Scott WW, Baker RR, et al (1982) Invasive thymomas: diagnosis and evaluation by computed tomography. J Comput Assist Tomogr 6: 92-100

Table 18.2. Indications for MRI in mediastinal disease [5, 7].

MRI
Specific indications
– Cervico-thoracic mass
– Paracardiac mass (pericardial or intracardiac invasion)
– Cardiac tumor
– Posterior mediastinal tumors (e.g. neurogenic tumor, spondylodiscitis or meningocele)
– Residual mediastinal post-treatment mass

Table 18.3. Tumors of the anterior mediastinum [7]

1. Superior level
- Thyroid (e.g. retrosternal goiter)
- Thymus
  - cysts
  - circumscribed or infiltrative thymomas, benign or malignant (figs 18.1 & 18.2)
  - routinely looked for in the presence of myasthenia, even with normal standard radiographs,
  - embryonic tumors of the thymus
  - benign or malignant teratomas (fig. 18.3)
  - malignant embryonic tumors
- Vascular tumors

CT has a significant role in the malignant forms in the search for secondary pleural or concomitant lesions which would indicate malignancy but is not always confirmed histologically [1, 8].

Differential diagnosis
Vascular lesions
- Aneurysm of the aorta or dissection
- Unfolding of the aorta
- Dilatation of the superior vena cava
- Unfolding of the brachiocephalic arterial trunk

2. Middle level
- Lymphadenopathy (fig. 18.4)
- Bronchogenic cyst

Differential diagnosis
- Dilatation of the pulmonary artery
- Left sided superior vena cava
- Ectopic thyroid

3. Inferior level
- Cardiac tumors
- Pericardial tumors:
- Pleural tumors

Differential diagnosis
- Pleuro-pericardial cysts
- Pericardial diverticula
- Retro-costo-xyphoid hernia
- Fatty superficial fascia or pericardial fat pad
- Dilatation of the inferior vena cava

Principal causes of blunting of the cardiophrenic angles
- Pericardial fat pad
- Pleuro-pericardial cysts
- Diaphragmatic hernias through Larrey's fissure (subperitoneal fat or occasionally a loop of small bowel or colon)
- Ectopic thymomas

4. All three levels
- Ectopic thymic tumors
- Teratomas (fig. 18.3)
- Dermoid cysts
- Lipomas
- Hemolymphangiomas
- Prevascular anterior mediastinal lymphadenopathy (e.g. enlargement of the internal mammary lymph node chain in Hodgkin's disease)

Differential diagnosis
- Retrosternal collections
- Sternal lesions

Table 18.4. Tumors of the middle mediastinum [7]

1. Superior level
- Lymphadenopathy
- Thyroid
- Esophagus (leiomyoma)

Differential diagnosis
- Unfolding of the aorta
- Aortic aneurysm
- Aneurysm of the great vessels
- Anomalies of the aortic arch
- Coarctation and pseudo-coarctation of the aorta
- Esophageal diverticula
- Granulomas of diverse etiologies

2. Middle level (fig. 18.4)
- Tracheal tumors
- Esophageal tumors

Differential diagnosis
- Large azygos vein
- Retrotracheal left pulmonary artery
- (Granulomas)

3. All three levels
- Bronchogenic cysts (sometimes multiple: Recklinghausen)
- Enterogenic cysts
- Neurinomas (of the phrenic or pneumogastric nerves)
- Esophageal tumors (see specific chapter)

Differential diagnosis
- Mega-esophagus
- Esophageal duplication
- Esophageal diverticula
- Esophageal varices, hematomas of the esophagus

Table 18.5. Tumors of the posterior mediastinum [7]

- Neurogenic tumors
- Meningoceles (sometimes isolated lesions in the paravertebral gutter without communication with the spine)
- Neuroenteric cysts
- Lymphadenopathy
- Cysts of the thoracic canal
- Bronchogenic cysts
- Hemangiomas
- Extramedullary hemopoiesis
- Pleural tumors
- Thyroid goiter
- Tumors of the posterior ribs
- Ectopic thymic lesions
- Pheochromocytoma

Differential diagnosis
- Unfolding of the aorta
- Aneurysm of the descending aorta
- Vertebral lesions
- Paravertebral abscess
- Pancreatic pseudocysts (rarely of the superior mediastinum)
- Continuation of the azygos or hemi-azygos veins
- Intrathoracic kidney
- Intrathoracic or accessory spleen

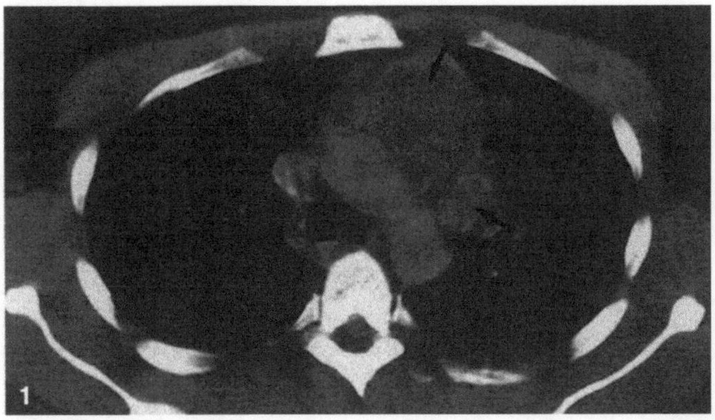

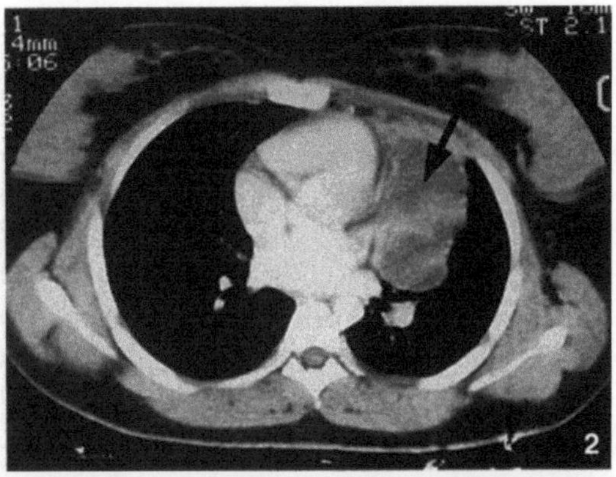

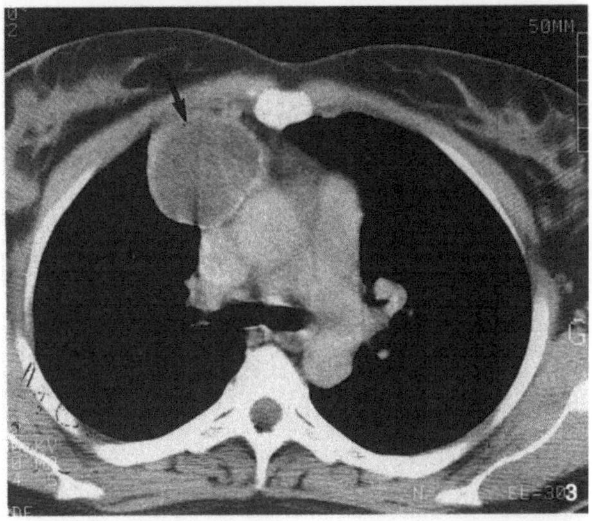

Fig. 18.1. Invasive lympho-epithelial thymoma in a 44 year old man; CT examination showing the extent of the left anterior mediastinal mass *(arrows)* with compression of the pulmonary parenchyma. Differentiation from lymphadenopathy is not possible on CT

Fig. 18.2. Lymphoma of the thymus and lymph nodes, mainly in the anterior mediastinum *(arrow)* with a predominantly cystic composition. The nature of the lesion can only be determined histologically, the CT appearances are entirely non-specific

Fig. 18.3. Malignant teratoma of the anterior mediastinum *(arrow)* on post-contrast CT. The lesion has irregular contours and compresses the ascending aorta and superior vena cava. Thin peripheral microcalcifications are suggestive of a benign lesion such as a dermoid cyst

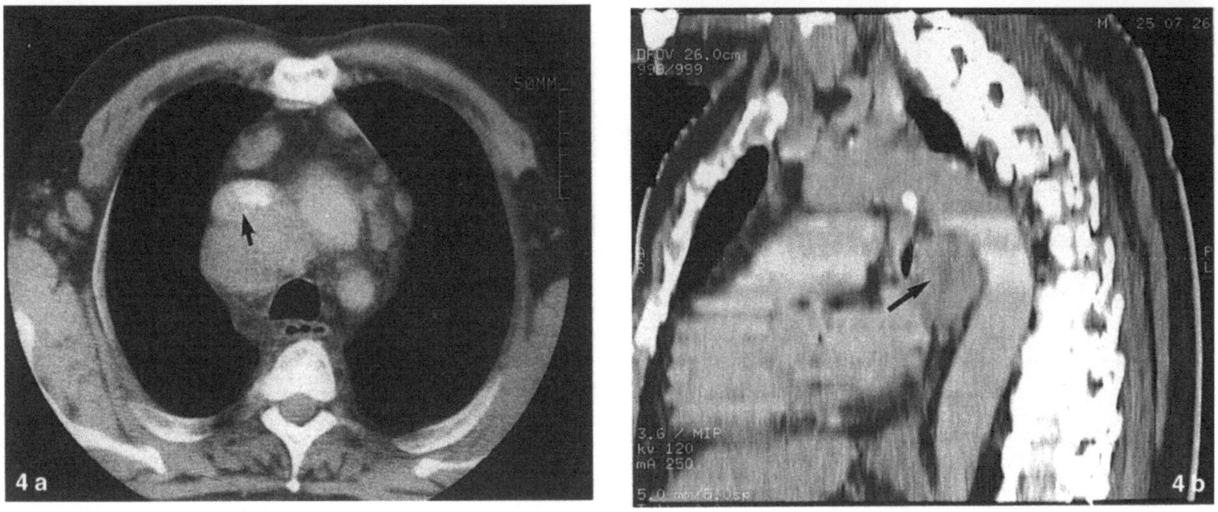

Fig. 18.4 a, b. a Right paratracheal mediastinal lymphomatous lymphadenopathy on post-contrast CT with invasion of the superior vena cava *(arrow)*. Note the multiple small anterior mediastinal lymph nodes on the right and left; **b** lymph node enlargement in the aorto-pulmonary window and retro- and subcarinal region on the sagittal reconstruction of a helical CT acquisition (courtesy of Dr D. Buthiau, Scanner Paris 14)

CHAPTER 19

Malignant tumors of the pleura

Clinicians
J.-C. Piette, P. Chaumier, P. Baldeyrou,
E. Vuillemin, D. Khayat

Radiologist
D. Buthiau

Imaging plays a major role in the diagnosis and management of pleural disease. Standard radiographs remain the initial examination of choice for making the diagnosis. Depending on the clinical context, these radiographs are complemented by ultrasound, CT and occasionally MRI.

Focal pleural thickening

Malignant mesothelioma and metastases may initially be focal lesions (fig. 19.1) but usually present with extensive invasion of the pleura. The commonest other focal malignant pleural lesions are primary tumors of the pleura (liposarcoma) and local spread from a bronchial carcinoma.

CT is clearly superior to plain radiographs for the demonstration of pleural tumors and their spread to the lungs or chest wall.

Focal fibrous tumor

This is a separate entity, representing less than 5% of pleural tumors [3]; more common in men over the age of 50, and not associated with asbestos exposure. The malignant forms (fibrosarcomas) are often large (greater than 10 cm diameter) with associated central necrosis [13]. There are, however, no specific signs to indicate malignancy.

Liposarcoma

This is an extremely rare tumor containing soft tissue and fatty elements and appears heterogeneous on CT.

Spread of a bronchial carcinoma

See chapter 16: Bronchopulmonary cancer.

Diffuse pleural thickening

The commonest causes are mesothelioma and pleural metastases (fig. 19.2).

On a standard radiograph, diffuse thickening is visible when there is significant pleural opacification involving at least 25% of the hemithorax with or without obliteration of the costophrenic angle [11].
The diagnosis is suggested on CT by a pleural lesion extending over a length of 8 cm, a width greater than 5 cm and thickening of the pleura being more than 3 mm [10].

Malignant mesothelioma (fig. 19.3)

60-70% of lesions occur in patients with a history of asbestos exposure.

Radiologically, mesothelioma appears in the form of irregular or nodular thickening with or without an

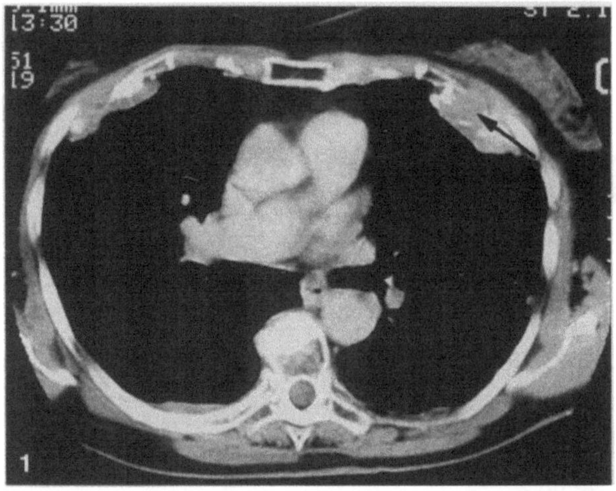

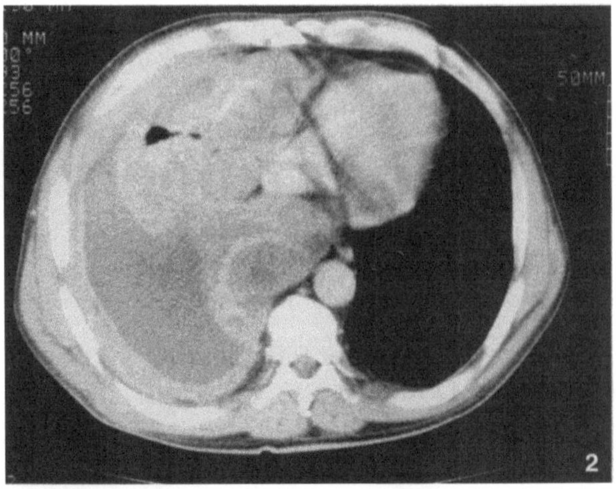

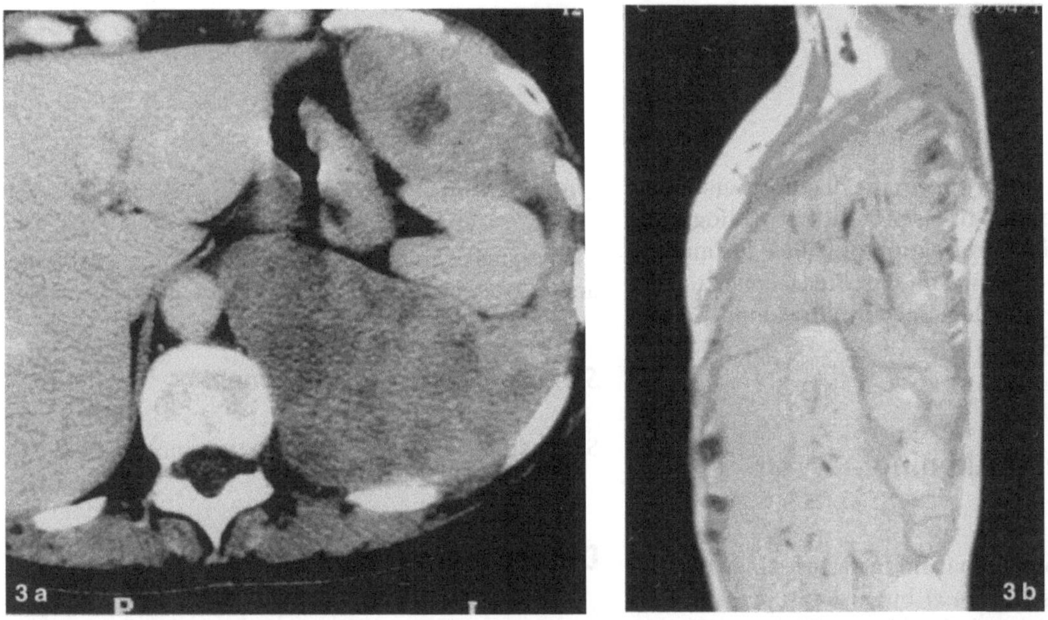

Fig. 19.1. Focal malignant mesothelioma on post-contrast CT: presence of a left anterior axillary pleural plaque *(arrow)* with rapid increase in size and considered to be suspicious by its thickness without spread into the adjacent chest wall

Fig. 19.2. Diffuse pleural metastases of the right hemithorax from a bronchial carcinoma. On post-contrast CT, there is smooth thickening of the visceral pleura but irregular exuberant thickening of the mediastinal pleura with a large pleural effusion

Fig. 19.3 a, b. Malignant mesothelioma on CT (**a**) and MRI (**b**): very markedly irregular, necrotic thickening of the visceral pleura extending to the most dependent part of the anterior and posterior costophrenic recesses on the left for the patient **a** and on the right for the patient **b**

associated pleural effusion. The diagnosis is greatly facilitated by CT which demonstrates:
- homolateral pleural thickening, often on the same side as the pulmonary involvement with associated reduction in the volume of the hemithorax;
- there is often associated contralateral pleural thickening which is not due to mesothelioma;
- pleural calcifications, rare but possible, particularly in cases of asbestosis.

In addition, CT can demonstrate:
- extension to different areas of pleura which are poorly analyzed on standard radiographs (mediastinal pleura, costovertebral gutter) or surgically inaccessible (posterior costophrenic recess);

- pericardial and chest wall involvement;
- mediastinal lymphadenopathy is rare;
- peritoneal involvement results in peritoneal thickening, ascites, mesenteric involvement and a peritoneal mass;
- retroperitoneal lymph node metastases occur late, and hepatic metastases are rare.

MRI [8] is useful in the assessment of apical, diaphragmatic and subphrenic lesions and defining the relationships of the tumor with the mediastinum.

Pleural metastases (fig. 19.2)

These are common in patients with intra- or extrathoracic primary lesions; the commonest underlying tumor is a bronchial carcinoma.

There is usually an associated pleural effusion.

CT demonstrates associated pleural thickening which may be nodular or lobulated; nodular masses have an obtuse entry angle of contact with the chest wall and are easier to detect in the absence of an effusion.

Lymphoma [3, 14]

Subpleural permeation is one of the modes of spread of lymphoma and may simulate a pleural effusion.

This appearance is sometimes seen adjacent to chest wall involvement (e.g. late recurrence of Hodgkin's disease).

Involvement may occur from extension of a mediastinal lesion in the initial stage of Hodgkin's disease.

The appearances may persist after treatment despite a good overall therapeutic response and become heterogeneous.

More sensitive criteria which would indicate a malignant etiology of diffuse pleural thickening have recently been described: circumferential pleural thickening, nodular pleural thickening, thickening of the parietal pleura greater than 1 cm, invasion of the mediastinal pleura.

Conclusion

CT is the examination of choice for the diagnosis and assessment of the extent of malignant lesions of the pleura. It also acts as a guide for percutaneous or surgical biopsies.

MRI (fig. 19.3 b) seems to be useful to define lesions in the apical and diaphragmatic regions.

References

1. Boutin C, Rey F (1993) Thoracoscopy in pleural malignant mesothelioma: a prospective study of 198 consecutive patients. Part 1: diagnosis. Cancer 72: 389-393
2. Edelstein G, Levitt RG, Slaker DP, et al (1984) Computed tomography of Tietze syndrome. J Comput Assist Tomogr 8: 20-23
3. England DM, Hochholzer L, Mc Carthy MJ (1989) Localized benign and malignant fibrous tumor of the pleura; a clinicopathologic review of 223 cases. Am J Surg Pathol 13: 640-658
4. Glazer HS, Ducan-Meyer J, Aronberg DJ, et al (1985) Pleural and chest wall inversion in bronchogenic carcinoma: CT evalution. Radiology 157: 191-194
5. Grant DC, Seltzer SE, Antman KH, et al (1983) Computed tomography of malignant pleural mesothelioma. J Comput Assist Tomogr 7: 626-632
6. Griffin DJ, Gross BH, Mc Cracken S, et al (1984) Observations on CT differentiation of pleural and peritoneal fluid. J Comput Assist Tomogr 8: 24-28
7. Heelan RT, Demas BE, Caraveli JF, et al (1989) Superior salcus tumors: CT and MR imaging. Radiology 170: 637-641
8. Lorigan JG, Libshitz HI. MR imaging of malignant pleural effusions (1990) J Comput Assist Tomogr 14: 192-198
9. Lorigan JG, Libshitz HI (1989) MR imaging of malignant pleural mesothelioma. J Comput Assist Tomogr 13: 617-620
10. Lynch DA, Gamsu G, Abere DR (1989) Conventional and high resolution computed tomography in the diagnosis of asbestos related disease. Radiographics 9: 523-551
11. Mc Loud TC, Woods BO, Carrinston CB, et al (1985) Diffuse pleural thickening in an asbestos exposed population: prevalence and causes. AJR 144: 9-18
12. Mirvis S, Dutcher JP, Haney PJ, et al (1983) CT of malignant pleural mesothelioma. AJR 140: 665-670
13. Saifuddin A, Da Costa P, Chalmers AG, et al (1992) Primary malignant localized fibrous tumors of the pleura; clinical, radiological and pathological features. Clin Radiol 45: 13-17
14. Situman LS, Libshitz HI (1984) Solid pleural manifestates of lymphoma. AJR 142: 269-273
15. Stavas J, Van Sonnenberg E, Casola G, et al (1987) Percutaneous drainage of infected and manifested thoracic fluid collection. J Thorac Imaging 2: 80-87
16. Teplick JG, Teplick SK, Goodman L, et al (1982) The interface sign: a computed tomographic sign for distinguishing pleural and intraabdominal fluid. Radiology 144: 359-362

CHAPTER 20

Malignant tumors of the chest wall

Clinicians
D. Coeffic, E. Vuillemin, P. Chaumier,
J.-C. Piette, P. Baldeyrou, D. Khayat

Radiologist
D. Buthiau

Classification of tumors of the chest wall is difficult due to their great diversity. CT [3] is more accurate than clinical or standard radiological assessment of tumor size which is often underestimated, and determines the degree of local invasion. CT is particularly useful for detecting rib or vertebral destruction, sometimes not visible on the standard radiograph.

It is the best method for appreciating the relationships of the tumor with the muscle planes, mediastinal, supraclavicular and axillary contents (see fig. 20.4). Intercostal ultrasound may act as a guide in operable conditions.

Primary tumors of the sternum and ribs

Malignant sternal tumors [11]

These are primarily chondrosarcomas, osteosarcomas and plasmocytomas. CT is particularly sensitive in detecting calcification within cartilaginous tumors (chondrosarcoma).

Rib tumors (fig. 20.1)

The diagnosis depends on the standard localized radiographs; CT demonstrates the extension into the soft tissues and is able, in certain cases, to characterize the lesion. CT may sometimes detect a rib lesion masked by a pleural effusion or occurring in one of the lower ribs. Ewing's sarcoma is the commonest lesion in a young subject; this appears as an area of osteolysis, sometimes with an associated soft tissue mass.

Soft tissue tumors

The diagnosis is usually clinical, and radiological assessment is essentially by CT. Apart from fatty tissues, CT is rarely able to give a precise diagnosis. The malignant nature of the lesion is suggested by the following characteristics: poor definition and heterogeneity of the lesion, increased density of the subcutaneous fat, involvement of several muscles and, in particular, poorly defined osteolysis of a rib, the sternum or an adjacent vertebra.

Any of the soft tissue sarcomas can involve the chest wall and have no specific features. Radiation induced chest wall sarcomas following radiotherapy for breast cancer or Hodgkin's disease should not be forgotten [10].

Secondary and hematological tumors

Chest wall metastases (fig. 20.2)

Frequently occurring in ribs, they are usually lytic but sometimes sclerotic (prostate). Detection of these lesions depends on the combination of bone scintigraphy and standard radiographs. CT demonstrates the soft tissue mass which is frequently associated with a rib lesion [2].

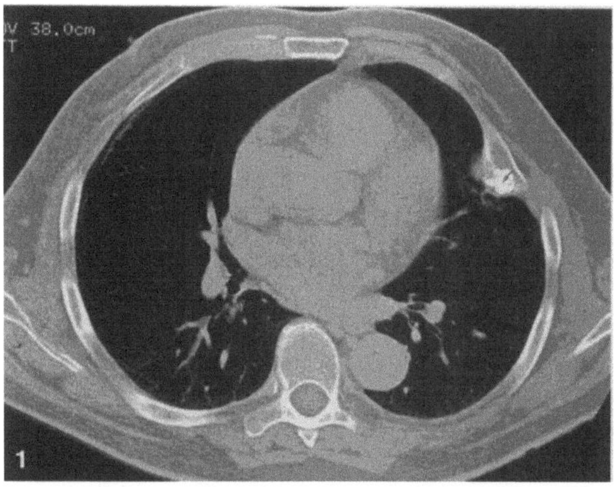

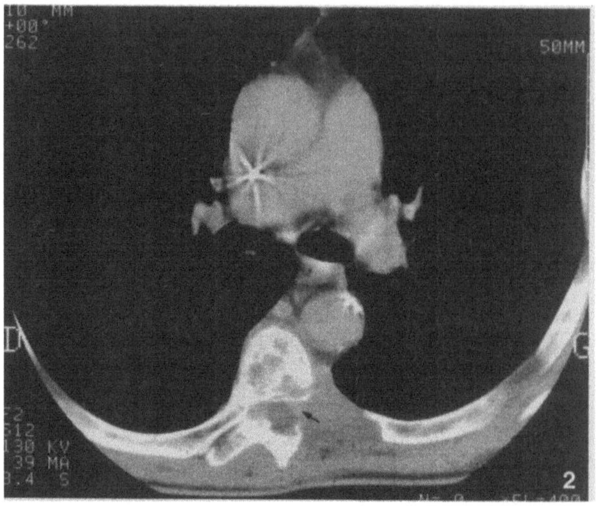

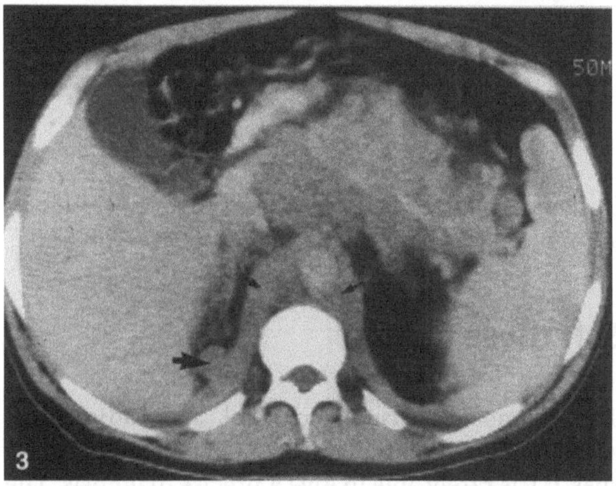

Fig. 20.1. Tumor-like appearance of a rib on CT (3 mm section) giving the false impression of an expansile lesion of the anterior end of the rib corresponding to an old tuberculous pleural granuloma *(arrow)*

Fig. 20.2. Secondary chest wall invasion on post-contrast CT. Extensive chest wall metastasis and lytic change in the left costo-vertebral and costo-transverse junction from a renal carcinoma. Note spread into the left neuroforamen and early epidural infiltration *(arrow)*

Fig. 20.3. Diaphragmatic spread from non-Hodgkin's lymphoma: almost complete obliteration of the posterior retrocrural or posterior inframediastinal space *(small arrows)* and the presence of macronodular direct diaphragmatic involvement *(large arrow)*. Note the diffuse intra-abdominal mesenteric lymph node involvement

Hematological tumors

Myeloma

This appears as well defined lytic lesions within ribs on standard radiographs. If CT is performed, there is rarely an associated soft tissue mass.

Hodgkin's and non-Hodgkin's lymphoma

In both diseases, the development of a chest wall mass is not unusual. The mass may either be isolated, independent of pulmonary or mediastinal involvement developing within or posterior to the pectoral muscles, or arise by direct contiguous spread from a pulmonary or mediastinal lesion. Spread from a mediastinal lesion is generally associated with destructive changes in the sternum [9]. Chest wall lesions may occur either in the initial stages of the disease or following a relapse; following chemotherapy the mass may regress or persist unchanged; it may also be a sterile residual mass, the diagnosis of which requires histological confirmation.

Chest wall invasion by an adjacent malignant lesion

Bronchial cancer

The only definite CT sign of chest wall invasion is bone destruction [8]; a number of other signs on CT are suggestive of chest wall invasion but lack sensitivity or specificity:

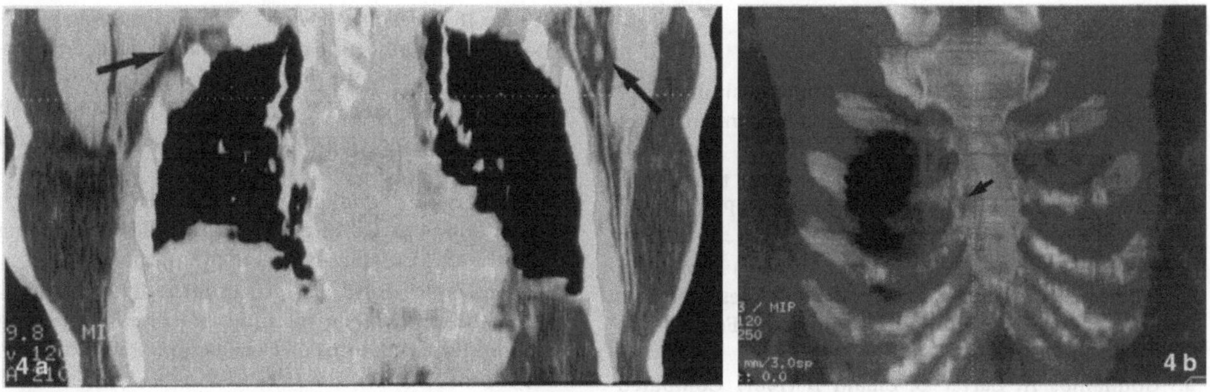

Fig. 20.4 a, b. Coronal reconstructions of 3D CT demonstrating well the axillae (**a**), often difficult in the other planes, and sternum (**b**) in which multiple hypodensities are noted *(arrow)* due to osteolysis from breast cancer metastasis

- pleural thickening adjacent to the lesion [9] is entirely non-specific;
- non-visualization of the extrapleural fat;
- presence of a pericostal mass arising in the fat or muscles of the chest wall.

MRI, on the other hand, is very useful for the demonstration of chest wall invasion. Padovani [7] has reported a sensitivity of 90% and specificity of 86% for chest wall invasion in a series of 34 patients with bronchial cancer. The diagnosis is suggested on T1-weighted imaging by a signal intensity identical to the tumor in the involved area of the chest wall, associated with hyperintensity on T2-weighted imaging and enhancement following gadolinium.

Another advantage of MRI is linked to its 3-dimensional capability which is useful in the assessment of the apical pleural cap. It is able to accurately localize tumors in the Pancoast-Tobias syndrome and demonstrate the relationship with the adjacent cervico-thoracic blood vessels.

Breast cancer

Chest wall changes as a result of surgery and/or radiotherapy are well assessed by CT. Familiarity with these changes results in a more reliable detection of recurrent tumors and chest wall invasion (see chapter 15 "Cancer of the breast").

Pleural tumors

Chest wall invasion from mesotheliomas or secondary pleural tumors is relatively common (cf "Mesothelioma").

Tumors of the diaphragm [1]

Primary tumors of the diaphragm are extremely rare, but invasion of the diaphragm by an adjacent tumor of the liver or gastro-esophageal junction is seen much more frequently. MRI is particularly useful due to its ability to perform coronal and sagittal sections.

Of the primary tumors, fibrosarcoma is the least rare. Secondary tumors are rarely solitary.

Diaphragmatic involvement by lymphoma (fig. 20.3) has been detected more and more frequently since the advent of CT; spread may be contiguous or via integrate or retrograde spread along the lymphatic chains. The two appearances encountered are a localized or diffuse thickening of the diaphragm, or the presence of nodules.

Conclusion

Tumors of the chest wall should be suspected in the presence of local clinical symptoms.

Standard radiographs will visualize only large lesions. Ultrasound is of little value due to its poor assessment of bones but may, however, guide biopsy of a soft tissue mass.

CT (fig. 20.4) is necessary to confirm the diagnosis, assess extent and look for recurrent disease for all chest wall tumors. MRI has some value due to its three dimensional capability and is particularly useful in the assessment of direct contiguous spread from bronchial cancers, and including the upper and lower limits of the chest (apex, diaphragm).

References

1. Coulomb M (1988) Apport de la tomodensitométrie à l'étude du diaphragme et de la région diaphragmatique. Journées Francophones de Radiologie
2. Frija J (1987) Pathologie de la paroi du thorax. In: J Remy (ed) Tomodensitométrie du thorax. Paris, Vigot, pp 419-434
3. Giron J, Senac JP, Chanez P, Mary H (1989) L'imagerie moderne: échographie, TDM et IRM dans les affections de la plèvre et de la paroi thoracique. Feuillets de Radiologie 29: 335-343
4. Gouliamos A, Carter B, Emani B (1981) Computed tomography of the chest wall. Radiology 134: 433-436
5. Haggar AM, Pearlberg JL, Froelich JW, et al (1987) Chest wall invasion by carcinoma of the lung: detection by MR imaging. AJR 148: 1075-1078
6. Paone JF, Spees EK, Newton CG, et al (1982) An appraisal of en bloc resection of peripheral bronchogenic carcinoma involving the thoracic wall. Chest 81: 203
7. Padovani B, Mouroux J, Seksik L, et al (1993) Chest wall invasion by bronchogenic carcinoma: evaluation with MR Imaging. Radiology 187: 33-38
8. Peralberg JL, Sandler MA, Beure GH, et al (1987) Limitations of CT in evaluating ncoplasm involving chest wall. J Comput Assist Tomogr 11: 290-293
9. Press GA, Glazer HS, Wasserman TH, et al (1985) Thoracic wall involvment by Hodgkin's disease and non Hodgkin's lymphoma: CT evaluation. Radiology 157: 195-198
10. Souba WW, Mc Kenna RJ, Meis J (1986) Radiation induced sarcomas of the chest wall. Cancer 57: 610-615
11. Stark P, Jaranillo D (1986) CT of the sternum. AJR 147: 72-77

CHAPTER 21

Tumors of the trachea

Clinicians
J.-C. Piette, E.-Ch. Antoine, D. Nizri, M.A. Rocher, P. Baldeyrou, P. Chaumier, E. Vuillemin, D. Khayat

Radiologist
D. Buthiau

Tumors of the trachea are rare and may be detected on standard radiographs.

CT (fig. 21.1)

CT can appreciate the intraluminal extent of the tumor. It detects thickening of the trachea wall, destruction of the cartilage, infiltration of the mediastinal fat, and displacement or invasion of the mediastinal vessels.

Locoregional lymph node enlargement is also demonstrated when present. CT may demonstrate a possible second tumor, as well as the more unusual secondary pulmonary lesions.

Calcifications are particularly well demonstrated.

CT can accurately assess the degree of tracheal stenosis and the attachment of the base of the endoluminal mass [1].

MRI

MRI is able to appreciate the longitudinal extent of the intra- and extraluminal portions of the tumor due to its ability to perform sagittal and coronal sections orientated parallel to the longitudinal axis of the trachea.

MRI can replace tomograms and CT on the condition that the examination is of high quality; calcifications are often difficult to detect.

It also seems to be valuable in the follow-up of the peritracheal region following surgery, laser treatment, and particularly radiotherapy.

Specific properties of each tumor [3]

Carcinomas (fig. 21.2)

These are the commonest tracheal tumors that represent no more than 1% of cancers of the respiratory tract. The tumor preferentially arises in the inferior segment; mediastinal invasion, lymph node spread and esophageal extension are frequent.

Adenomas

These are classified as malignant tumors due to their potential for local recurrences following excision and the possibility of metastases occurring at a later stage.

The commonest adenoma is the cylindroma or cystic adenoid tumor; this occurs particularly in the middle third of the trachea and represents approximately 40% of tracheal tumors. It has a slow growth rate and metastasizes late, particularly to the lungs and bony skeleton.

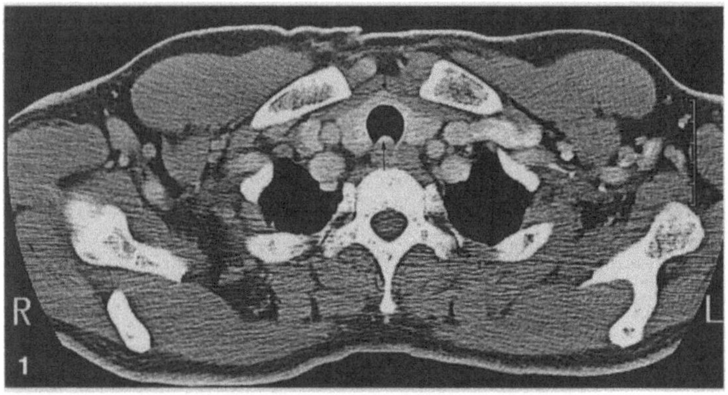

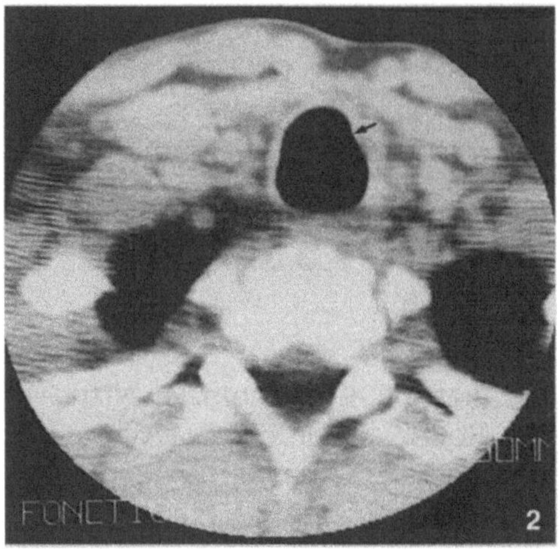

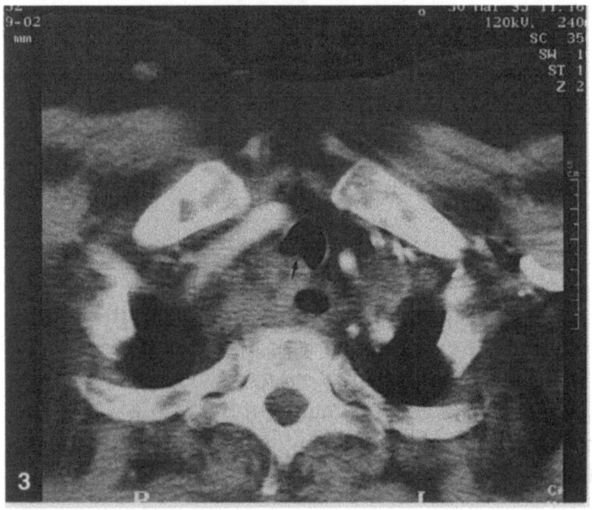

Fig. 21.1. Normal appearances of the trachea on post-contrast CT at the level of the lung apex. Note the physiological convexity of the tracheal lumen posteriorly *(arrow)*

Fig. 21.2. Tracheal carcinoma on post-contrast CT: presence of an early lesion antero-laterally on the left *(arrow)*, initially causing loss of symmetry of the tracheal contours. No evidence of obvious local spread

Fig. 21.3. Tracheal spread *(arrow)* from an esophageal carcinoma with right para-esophageal lymphadenopathy on post-contrast CT

Other malignant tumors

Primary lymphoma of the trachea [4] or involvement as part of a disseminated lymphoma are rare and exhibit no specific radiological features compared to other malignant tumors apart from the sometimes marked lymphadenopathy; spread from lymphomatous nodes into the tracheal lumen may be encountered.

Sarcomas may simulate a benign tumor unless there is mediastinal or distant metastatic spread; chondrosarcoma usually contains abundant tufts of calcifications.

A solitary plasmocytoma is rare and appears as a round or lobulated mass which can invade adjacent structures and metastasize to lymph nodes.

Secondary tumors

Isolated metastases of the trachea are rare and may be solitary or multiple, sessile or pedunculated. The commonest primary tumors are cancers of the kidney, breast, colon or melanoma.

Tracheal spread from an adjacent tumor

Thyroid cancer frequently involves the tracheal wall and may invade its lumen.

Other tumors include cancers of the larynx, esophagus (fig. 21.3) and bronchus.

Tracheal invasion is confirmed by CT by the presence of an intraluminal nodule, but there is a risk of false negative diagnoses concerning involvement of the wall itself.

Conclusion

The detection of tracheal tumors remains the domain of standard radiographs. However, it appears that CT and MRI have a major role in the assessment of spread of malignant tracheal tumors and have replaced standard tomography in this situation [2].

References

1. Gamsu G, Webb WR (1983) Computed tomography of the trachea and main stem bronchi. Semin Roentgenol 18 : 51-60
2. Lemaître L, Rémy J, Saint-Michel J (1987) Masses et pseudo-masses médiastinales. In: J Rémy (ed) Tomodensitométrie du thorax. Vigot, Paris, pp 48-87
3. Pinet F, Loire R, Maret G, et al (1981) Primary tumors of the trachea. A clinical, radiological and pathological evaluation of 12 cases. Eur J Radiol 1: 88-91
4. Pradhan DJ, Rabussi D, Meyer JM (1975) Primary solitary lymphoma of the trachea. J Thorac Cardiovasc Surg 70: 930-940

CHAPTER 22

Tumors of the heart and great vessels

Clinicians
E. Malaurie, C. Petitjean, J. Traversat, C. Chapelon-Abric, A. Vacheron

Radiologist
L. Arrivé

Primary tumors of the heart are very rare [6], the majority being benign. The least rare forms are myxomas (30%) and lipomas (10%) [21]. For this type of pathology, transthoracic and trans-esophageal ultrasound are the examinations of choice [11] and may be complemented by CT and particularly MRI.

Secondary malignant tumors involving the heart are much commoner than the primary tumors (20-40 times). They show rarely the dominant feature and are frequently detected at autopsy. The majority of cases (85%) manifest in the form of pericarditis. In fact, the most important problem concerning neoplastic cardiac disease is the spread of adjacent bronchial carcinomas, mediastinum or the right atrium from renal, hepatocellular or retroperitoneal tumors. It is in these circumstances that CT and MRI are most useful.

Primary tumors of the great vessels are exceptionally unusual and are dominated by sarcomatous lesions (leiomyosarcoma of the inferior vena cava, renal vein, femoral vein, angiosarcoma of the pulmonary artery...) [6]. Spread of malignant tumors to the major arteries and particularly veins is, on the other hand, a common and important problem because tumor extension to a vessel may be a contraindication to surgery or necessitate a change in the operative technique. MRI and CT usefully complement the ultrasound findings since the integrity of the vessel wall beyond the vascular segment of interest and the length of involvement must be defined.

Indications for CT and MRI

The myxoma is the most common the primary tumor of the heart. It is characterized microscopically by a proliferation of ovoid cells within an abundant myxoid stroma. Characteristically the myxoma appears macroscopically as a rounded mass, often large, attached to the interatrial septum close to the fossa ovale [6]. The cardiac lipoma, as a rule, is located on the interatrial septum or the wall of the right atrium. This tumor must be differentiated from simple fatty hypertrophy of the interatrial septum. The other benign tumors are rare and include rhabdomyoma, fibroma and hemangioma. The primary malignant tumors are exceptionally rare: angiosarcoma, rhabdomyosarcoma, lymphoma... The pericardial tumors may be benign (lipoma, hemangioma, lymphangioma, teratoma) or malignant (mesothelioma, lymphoma). Secondary tumors are much more common and may originate from melanoma, choriocarcinoma, embryonic carcinoma, pancreatic, breast or bronchial carcinoma. These metastases, regardless of the cancer origin, most commonly present with pericarditis either by diffuse infiltration of the pericardium, or by multiple pericardial nodules. More rarely, myocardial nodules or endocardial vegetations are seen [6].

Cardiac ultrasound is the examination of choice for primary tumors of the heart. Ultrasound defines the intraluminal or intramural localization of these tumors, the focal or diffuse nature of the tumor, its mobility and anatomical relationships [7]. These findings are complemented by CT and MRI which are particularly useful when technical difficulties interfere with the ultrasound examination (obesity, emphysema). CT is especially well suited for demonstrating endocavitary or pericardial nodular lesions [16]. MRI is equally useful but is of particular value for infiltrative neoplastic processes of the myocardium which do not cause any deformity of the internal or external contours. Definition of the tumor is also facilitated by the intrinsic contrast between the tumor and normal tissue [22].

For the assessment of the spread to the heart or cardiac chambers from adjacent tumors, ultrasound is limited to a study of the cardiac muscles, and it is here where CT and MRI have a role. CT is generally performed initially and is sufficient when it is able to confirm invasion of a cardiac chamber, or the presence of tumor thrombosis of a major vessel. MRI can be performed when the pathology is less obvious, or to differentiate a simple endovascular nodule from invasion of the vessel wall [4].

The common primary tumors of the major vessels is the leiomyosarcoma of the inferior vena cava and presents as a tumor developing at the inter- and subrenal level. The intravascular spread is usually associated with retrograde thrombosis. Ultrasound often demonstrates the intravascular component and involvement of the adjacent organ. CT can be used to define the limits of the lesion. The advantages of MRI are the intrinsic vascular contrast and the ability to perform sections in the three orthogonal planes.

The spread of neighboring tumors into the major vessels is a much more common problem. For the venous system, this is particularly seen in the renal veins and inferior vena cava due to the spread from renal cancers. For the arterial system, this usually concerns involvement of the aorta and the supra-aortic arterial trunks by primary bronchial cancers and mediastinal tumors [10]. In these cases, it is essential to differentiate the endovascular tumor nodule and true neoplastic thrombus from involvement of the vessel wall as these pose different therapeutic problems. MRI is particularly useful as it provides a direct visualization of the vessel wall which is of intermediate signal intensity (grey) relative to the perivascular fat (white) and intravascular flow void (black). Whenever radiotherapy is being considered, CT and MRI enable accurate planning in order to minimize the dose to healthy pulmonary parenchyma, cardiac tissue and spinal cord.

Signs

Technique

The imaging modalities used for examining tumors of the heart and the great vessels must be powerful enough for two main reasons: the tendency for motion artefacts, particularly at the level of the heart, and the necessity to acquire rapid slices following contrast injection in order to obtain optimal contrast between the tumor and normal tissues. For CT, therefore, the gold standard is ultrarapid CT or cine CT [19]. For MRI, it is essential to use cardiac gating. It is also possible to synchronize the gradient echo sequences with the EKG in order to obtain cine MRI.

CT and MRI

Heart

Primary tumors

The myxoma appears as a nodular mass attached to the interatrial septum, bulging towards the left atrium. The myxoma is frequently pedunculated, sometimes with poorly defined boundaries suggesting a friable nature with a risk of embolism by the migration of fragments of the myxoma. On MRI, a myxoma is of intermediate signal intensity in T1-weighted imaging and variable signal intensity on T2-weighted imaging (high signal for tumors with a myxoid stroma, intermediate signal for tumors with a fibrous stroma). The most important problem is to differentiate a myxoma from a possible intracardiac thrombus [14]. On CT, it is the vascular nature of the myxoma which principally differentiates it from thrombus. On MRI, thrombus is initially hyperintense on T1-weighted imaging and hypointense on gradient echo sequences, the contents of the thrombus generally being heterogeneous. However, the best differentiating feature is the attachment of the base of the myxoma onto the interatrial septum on CT or MRI [8].

The lipoma is usually attached to the intraatrial septum and is characterized by a fatty density on CT and hyperintensity on the T1-weighted MRI sequences. A lipoma causes a mass effect on the cardiac chambers whereas fatty hypertrophy of the interatrial septum only causes thickening of the septal wall (fig. 22.1) [20].

Fibromas have a fairly characteristic appearance on MRI, appearing as low signal intensity on the T2-weighted sequences [1].

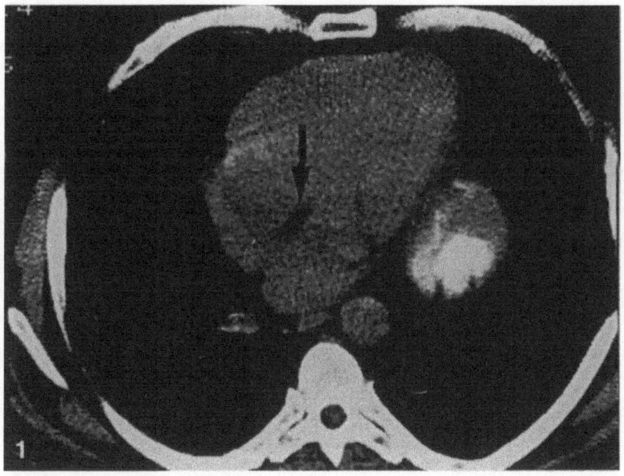

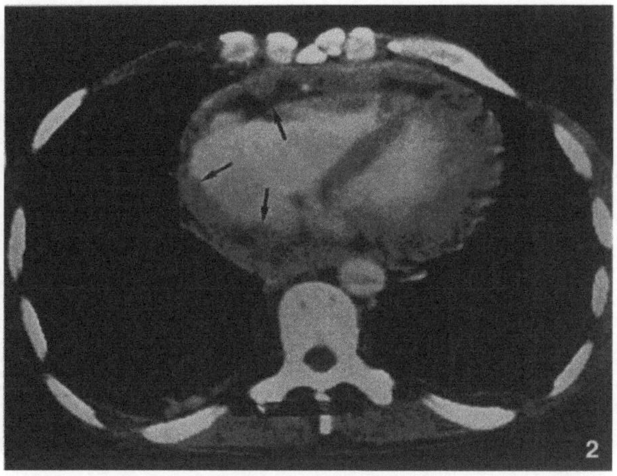

Fig. 22.1. Fatty hypertrophy of the interatrial septum. Pre-contrast CT demonstrating definite thickening of characteristically fatty density of the interatrial septum *(arrow)*

Fig. 22.2. Pericardial lymphoma. Post-contrast CT demonstrating significant nodular thickening of the pericardium *(arrows)*

The pseudotumors due to hydatid cysts appear as cystic lesions of intermediate signal intensity on T1-weighted imaging and high signal intensity on T2-weighted imaging. On CT, the cystic forms are of a fluid density [17].

MRI is probably more accurate for making the positive diagnosis and determining the cause of pericardial tumors. The pericardium appears as a black line on MRI silhouetted by the epicardial and mediastinal fat. The examination is able to appreciate pericardial thickening, the presence of an effusion and nodules. Lipomas or teratomas of the pericardium are characterized by a high signal on the T1-weighted sequences [18].

Secondary tumors

These generally present with secondary pericarditis. The pericardial effusion may be small or large. If the effusion is hemorrhagic, the density may be intrinsically elevated on CT and a heterogeneous signal intensity on MRI. In addition, there is often nodular thickening of the pericardium [12] (fig. 22.2). Much more rarely, cardiac metastases cause a myocardial infiltration, in which case MRI can make the diagnoses due to the intrinsic contrast between the tumor and normal myocardium (fig. 22.3).

The left atrium is the most commonly encountered site for cardiac involvement. Simple contact or even loss of the fat line between the tumor and left atrium are not enough to make the diagnosis of invasion; on the other hand, preservation of the fat line has an excellent negative predictive value. In fact, the only definite signs on CT of tumor involvement of the left atrium are the presence of deformity of the posterior wall of the left atrium, or demonstration of a tumor nodule within the left atrium (fig. 22.4 a). These two signs may be seen on CT, but MRI is better. The diagnostic accuracy is increased by the high intrinsic contrast between circulating blood and cardiac structures and the clear demonstration of the wall of the left atrium (fig. 22.4 b).

MRI is also the best examination to demonstrate the spread to the right atrium from subdiaphragmatic cancers (fig. 22.5).

Great vessels

Primary tumors

Leiomyosarcoma of the inferior vena cava is the common primary tumor of the great vessels and appears as a solid, frequently lobulated, and sometimes large mass. The epicenter of the tumor usually corresponds to the position of the inferior vena cava. There is frequently an associated thrombosis of the inferior vena cava with the demonstration of a collateral circulation. CT can confirm the hypervascular nature of the tumor and assess the upper limits of the tumor and spread to the neighboring organs [15]. MRI is the examination of choice, and performance of coronal and sagittal sections enable accurate definition of the superior extent and spread to adjacent organs.

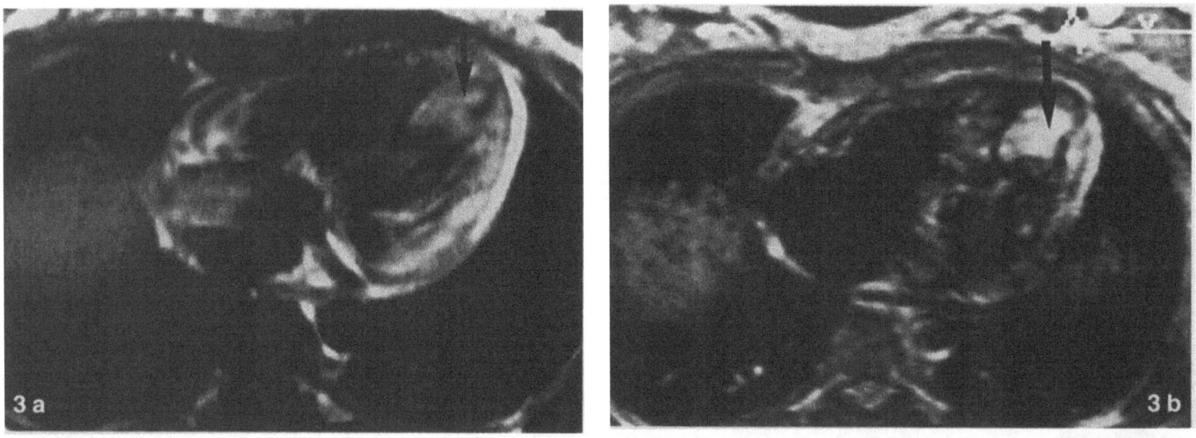

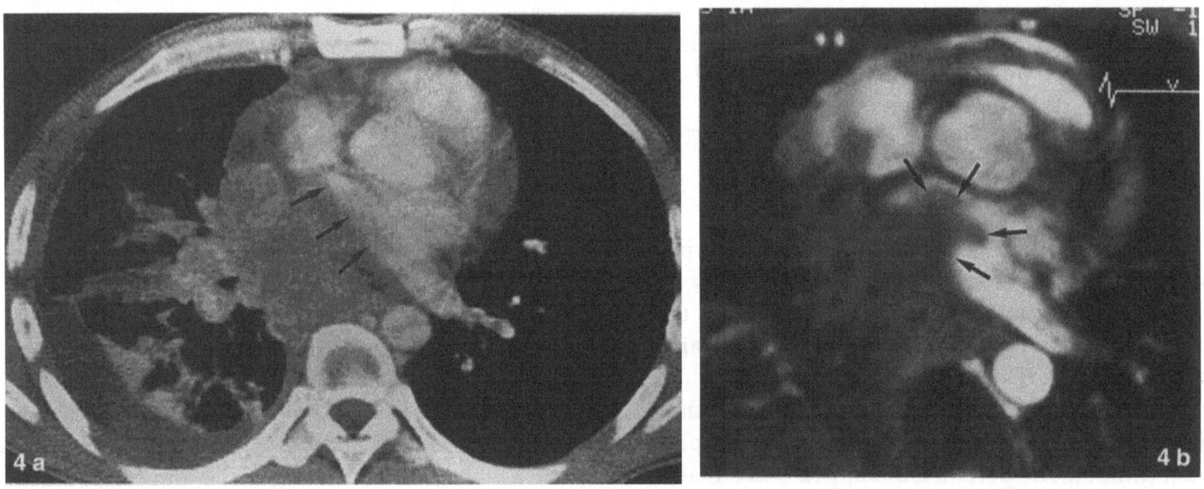

Fig. 22.3 a, b. Myocardial metastases from a pheochromocytoma on MRI. On the T1-weighted post-gadolinium image (**a**), the tumor has the signal intensity of a soft tissue tumor *(arrow)*. On the T2-weighted sequence (**b**), the tumor is hyperintense *(arrow)* differentiating it clearly from the normal myocardium

Fig. 22.4 a, b. Extension into the left atrium from a primary bronchial carcinoma. **a** Post-contrast CT: the posterior wall of the left atrium is poorly defined *(arrows)*; **b** MRI, gradient echo sequence: there is excellent contrast between the tumor *(grey)* and circulating blood *(white)* which enables accurate assessment of the left atrial invasion *(arrows)*

Involvement of major vessels by renal tumors

This concerns the renal vein in 80% of cases; spread to the inferior vena cava occurs in 10% of cases and is much more common in cancers of the right kidney.

On CT [9], endoluminal involvement of the renal veins and inferior vena cava is difficult to diagnose. On the one hand, within the inferior vena cava there is mixing of opacified blood from the renal vein with unopacified blood from the lower limbs which is frequently the cause for the pseudothrombosis appearance. On the other hand, loss of the perivascular fat plane and deformity of the vessels are not in themselves sufficient evidence of invasion of the vessel wall (fig. 22.6). It is for this reason that the majority of experts recommend the performance of MRI for the diagnosis of vascular involvement by tumors. Using a combination of spin echo and gradient echo sequences, MRI has a sensitivity and specificity in the order of 95% for the diagnosis of endoluminal thrombus [3]. MRI is generally able to differentiate tumor thrombi from simple thrombi. The tumor thrombi characteristically have a signal intensity similar to that of the original tumor on all the imaging sequences [3] (fig. 22.7). MRI is particularly useful for assessing vessel wall involvement. The wall of the vessel is usually well visualized on MRI, appearing as intermediate signal intensity (grey) interposed between the low signal

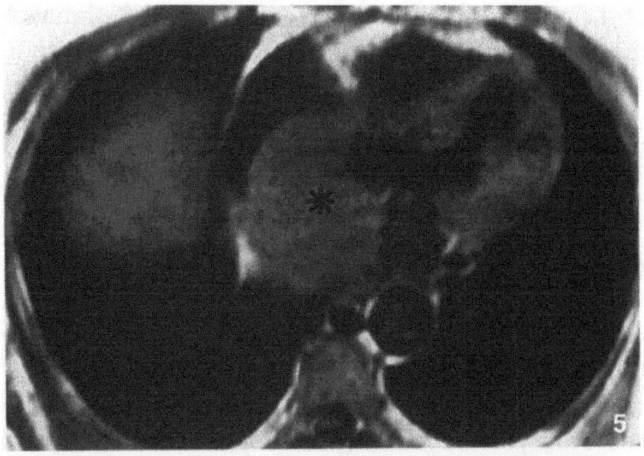

Fig. 22.5. Involvement of the right atrium from a renal carcinoma on MRI. The tumor thrombus (*) expands the right atrium, and its anterior limit is extremely well visualized

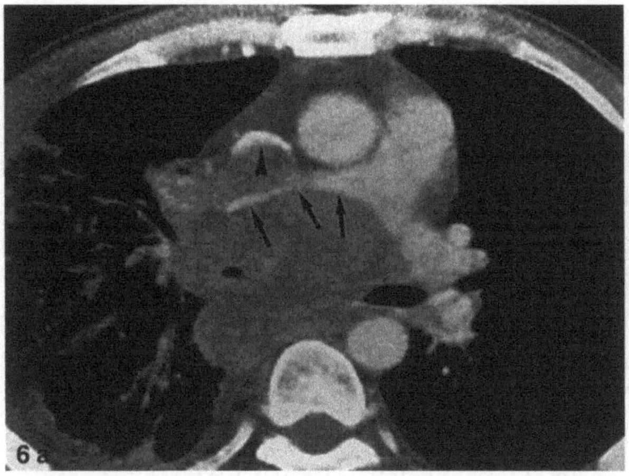

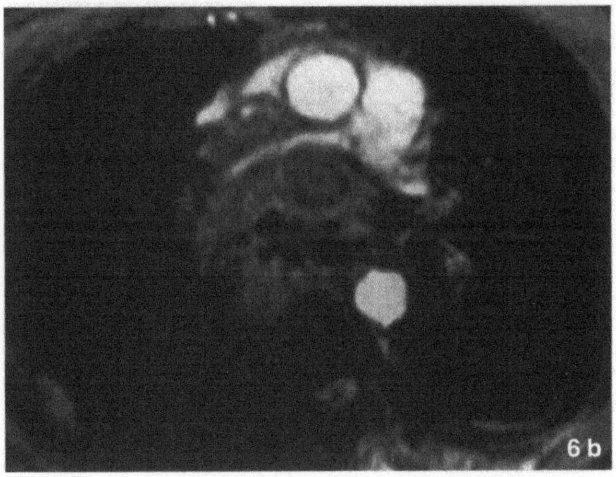

Fig. 22.6 a, b. Invasion of the superior vena cava and right main pulmonary artery by an anaplastic small cell carcinoma. Post-contrast CT (**a**) and gradient echo MRI (**b**). The right main pulmonary artery is encased by tumor *(arrows)*, and the superior vena cava is flattened *(arrow head)*

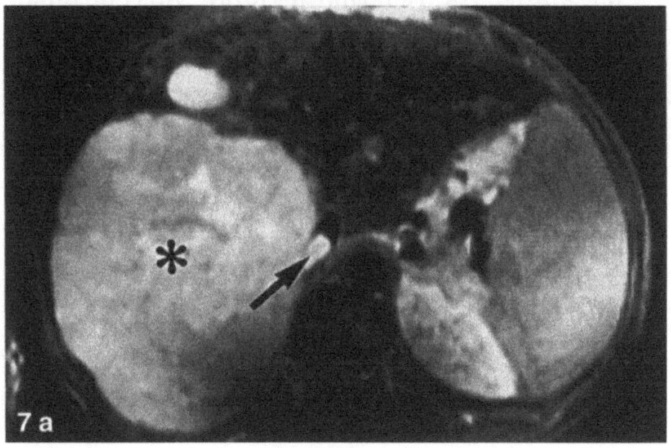

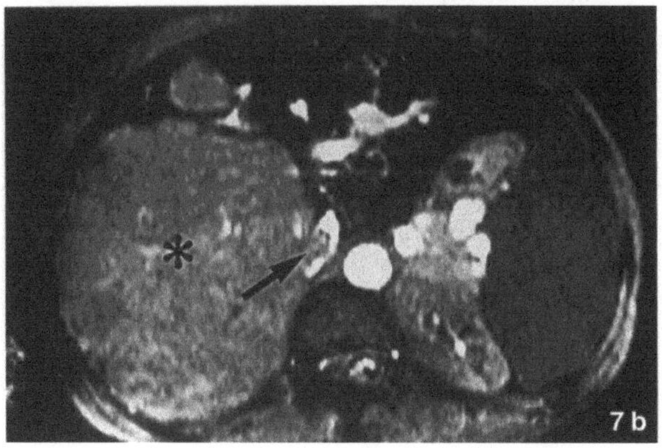

Fig. 22.7 a, b. Involvement of the inferior vena cava by a hepatocellular carcinoma. MRI, spin echo (**a**) and gradient echo (**b**). On both sequences the tumor thrombus *(arrow)* has the same signal as the original tumor (*) (reproduced from reference 3 with permission of the publisher)

of the circulating blood (black) and the high signal of the perivascular fat (white). Loss of this intermediate signal intensity band of the vessel wall and replacement by a tumor mass of characteristic signal intensity is a specific sign of vessel wall involvement.

Conclusion

CT and MRI are often essential in the assessment of malignant tumors of the heart and great vessels due to the ability to assess regional spread. They should always be preceded by an ultrasound examination which may show appearances particularly suggestive of a benign tumor (e.g. myxoma) and thus alter the indication for CT or MRI.

References

1. Amparo EG, Higgins CB, Farmer D, et al (1984) Gated MRI of cardiac and paracardiac masses: initial experience. AJR 143: 1151-1156
2. Arrivé L. Menu Y, Dessarts I, et al (1991) Diagnosis of abdominal venous thrombosis by means of spin-echo and gradient echo MR imaging. Radiology 181: 661-668
3. Barakos JA, Brown JJ, Higgins CB (1989) MR imaging of secondary cardiac and paracardiac lesions. AJR 153: 47-50
4. Bradley WC, Waluch V (1985) Blood flow in magnetic resonance imaging. Radiology 154: 443-450
5. Buthiau D, Chapelon-Abric C, Traversat J (1992) TDM en cardiologie. In: Buthiau D (ed) TDM et IRM cliniques. Frison-Roche, Paris, pp 133-141
6. Cabanne F, Bonenfant JL (1980) Anatomie pathologique. Maloine, Paris
7. Chandraratna PAN, Aronon WS (1981) Detection of pericardial metastases by cross-sectionnal echocardiography. Circulation 63: 197- 199
8. Conces DJ, Vix VA, Klatte EC (1985) Gated MR imaging of left atrial myxomas. Radiology 156: 445-447
9. Didier D, Racle A, Etieven JP, Weill F (1987) Tumour thrombus of the inferior vena cava secondary to malignant abdominal neoplasm: US and CT evaluation. Radiology 162: 83-89
10. Engel IA, Auh YH, Rubenstein WA, et al (1983) CT diagnosis of mediastinal and thoracic inlet venous obstructions. AJR 141: 521-526
11. Fyke FE, Seward JB, Edwards WD, et al (1985) Primary cardiac tumors: experience with 30 consecutive patients since the introduction of two-dimensional echocardiography. JACC 5: 1465-1473
12. Glazer GM, Gross BH, Orringer MB, et al (1984) Computed tomography of pericardial masses. J Comput Assist Tomogr 8: 895-899
13. Godwin JD, Axel L, Adams JR, et al (1981) Computed tomography: a new method for diagnosing tumor of the heart. Circulation 63: 448-451
14. Gomes AS. Lois JF, Child JS, et al (1987) Cardiac tumors and thrombus: evaluation with MR imaging. AJR 149: 895-899
15. Goze A, Bousquet JC, Grellet J, Kieffer E (1986) Les léiomyosarcomes de la veine cave inférieure. J Radiol 67: 897-910
16. Gross BH, Glazer GM, Francis IR (1983) CT of intracardial and intrapericardial masses. AJR 140: 903-907
17. Hernigou A, Plainfossé MC, Merran S, Guermonprez JL (1983) Place de l'échocardiographie dans le diagnostic de cinq kystes hydatiques du cœur. Ann Radiol 26: 648-654
18. Higgins CB (1987) The heart: acquired disease. In: Higgins CB, Hricak H (eds) Magnetic resonance imaging of the body. Raven Press, New York, pp 239-266
19. Lipton MJ, Higgins CB, Farmer DN, et al (1984) Cardiac imaging with a high-speed cine-CT scanner. Radiology 152: 579-582
20. Lund JT, Ehman RL, Julsrud PR, et al (1989) Cardiac masses: assessment by MR imaging. AJR 152: 469-473
21. Mc Allister HA, Fenioglio JJ (1978). Atlas of tumor pathology, Fasc 15, 2nd series. Armed forces Institute of Pathology, Washington
22. Winkler M, Higgins CB (1987) Suspected intracardiac masses: evaluation with MR imaging. Radiology 165: 117-122

CHAPTER 23

Tumors of the liver

Clinicians
O. Blétry, B. Chiche, P. Priollet, D. Nizri,
E. Vuillemin, L. Feuvret, D. Khayat

Radiologist
D. Buthiau

Ultrasound is the initial examination of choice for the demonstration of focal neoplastic lesions of the liver. It is sensitive and accurate, apparently totally non-invasive, inexpensive and widely available. However, this technique is not able routinely to assess the whole of the liver, is relatively non-specific and of limited value for the demonstration of small or diffusely infiltrative lesions. It is also of limited value in the early detection of primary hepatocellular tumors [27]

Both CT and MRI (fig. 23.1 and diagram 23.1) have a practical role to play in the diagnosis and follow-up of focal or diffuse lesions; the indications in each type of pathology will be discussed.

Review of anatomy

See fig. 23.1 and diagram 23.1 [27].

Malignant hepatic tumors

The demonstration of one or several intrahepatic soft tissue abnormalities is suggestive of tumor, once the diagnosis of hepatic abscess has been excluded. Imaging helps in the distinction between primary and secondary lesions and their differentiation from the rare benign pathologies.

Hepatic metastases

The role of imaging in the investigation of hepatic metastases [17, 29]

The search for hepatic metastases continues to be a common problem in the context of a known primary tumor or in the further investigation of clinical symptoms such as right hypochondrial pain, cholestasis or unexplained fever.

A combination of ultrasound, CT and MRI would certainly give the best results. However, this approach is not practicable either for the detection or follow-up of hepatic lesions.

Initial investigations

One approach adopted by a number of experts relates to two particular situations:

– there are no clinical or biochemical (tumor markers) features to suggest the presence of hepatic metastases: if the ultrasound is normal and technically of high quality, no other investigation is necessary. If the examination is technically difficult and unable to examine the whole of the liver (more than 10% of cases), CT is then essential, MRI being preferred to CT if the ultrasound was limited by the presence of steatosis;

– the clinical and particularly biochemical findings are suggestive of hepatic metastases; if ultrasound is abnormal it is usually sufficient to make the diagnosis; if it is normal, CT is necessary, MRI being required

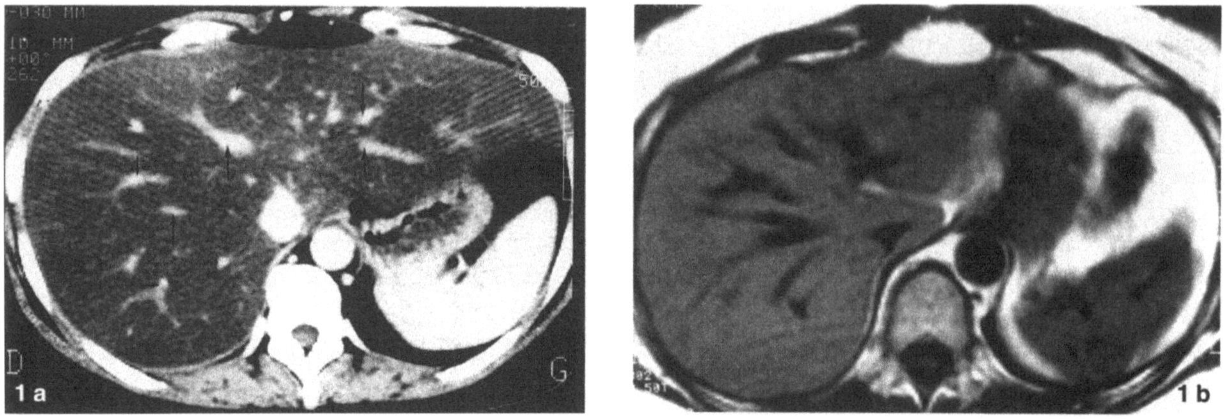

Fig. 23.1 a, b. Normal anatomy of the liver on CT and MRI. **a** Post-contrast hepatic CT: note the excellent visualization of the vessels, particularly in this patient with diffuse steatosis (branches of the hepatic vein: *large arrows*; portal veins: *small arrows*); **b** normal liver on axial T1 MRI: the vessels are well defined and hypointense relative to the hepatic parenchyma. In liver studies, particularly for metastases, the more heavily T1-weighted the sequence (short TR) the better the detection of lesions

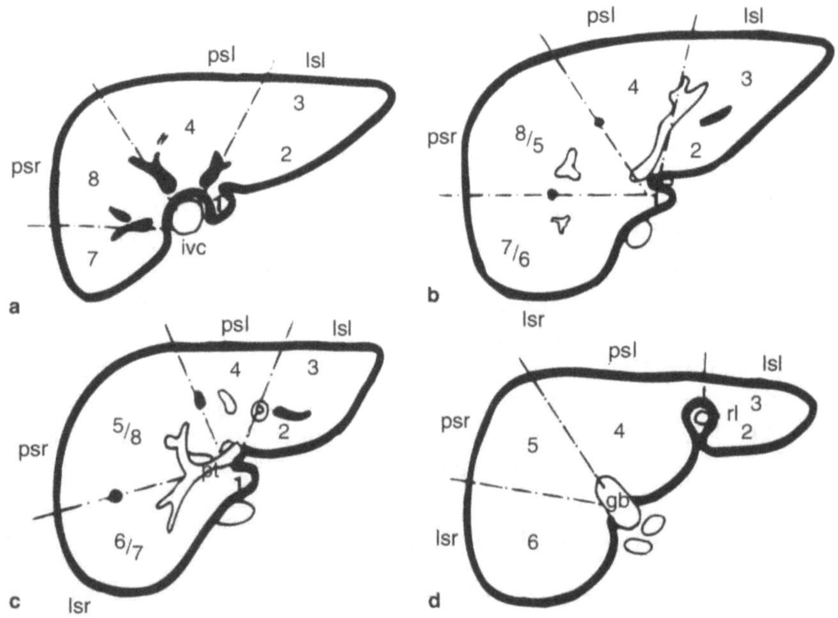

Diagram 23.1 a-d. Diagram of the four principal normal hepatic sections on axial CT and MRI; representation of the sectors and segments of the liver. The vessels are shaded: hepatic veins; *ivc* inferior vena cava; *pt* portal trunk and right main branch; *rl* round ligament; *lsl* lateral sector of the left lobe of the liver; *psl* paramedian sector of the left lobe of the liver; *psr* paramedian sector of the right lobe of the liver; *lsr* lateral sector of the right lobe of the liver. **a** Section passing through the confluence of the hepatic veins; **b** section through the left portal vein; **c** section through the portal trunk and division of the right portal vein; **d** section through the gallbladder (*gb*). The numbers correspond to the segments [7, 27]

if CT is itself normal. A particular case scenario must be remembered: when the biochemical results are unavailable, and the initial investigation demonstrates multiple nodules or particularly a solitary nodule which pose classical differential diagnostic problems. Although the distinction between a metastasis and a biliary cyst is simple on CT and ultrasound (unless the lesion is small), the differentiation between a metastasis and an angioma is difficult, particularly in the presence of a known gastrointestinal cancer (especially colorectal) in which the ultrasonic appearances of the metastases can mimic an angioma. CT is performed for lesions greater than or equal to 2 cm in diameter as it becomes highly sensitive using the bolus contrast and angio-CT techniques. MRI is indicated, and some groups recommend it as the first line examination since it is more able to make the distinction between a metastasis and an angioma on the heavily T2-weighted sequences (increased signal intensity of angiomas on T2-weighted imaging);

- a number of authors currently recommend ultrasound as the principal examination in the investigation of hepatic metastases with complementary CT and MRI being reserved for cases of doubt. Histological confirmation in this instance is rarely required.

An alternative approach consists of performing CT in the first instance and is adopted by a number of important groups who have remarked:

- that the demonstration of metastases alters treatment;
- that, apart from cases of lung and breast cancer, a search simply for hepatic metastases is not adequate: hepatic ultrasound is therefore limited. On the other hand, CT is able on a single examination to assess not only the primary site but also the liver, lymph nodes and bony structures. Conversely, in cases of pulmonary or breast tumors, if CT demonstrates bone metastasis, the demonstration of hepatic lesions does not significantly alter the treatment. Ultrasound is an excellent complementary examination to CT to help in the differential diagnosis and guide biopsy. Recourse to MRI or CT using an angiographic technique via the celiac or mesenteric artery (CT arterioportography or CTAP) are only necessary if there are persistent diagnostic difficulties. The major indication for CT portography [5] is in the preoperative evaluation of hepatic metastases from colorectal cancers and is particularly useful in identifying the inoperable patients. It may also be useful in cases of hepatocellular carcinoma in the absence of cirrhosis, in their classical or fibrolamellar form. 3D reconstructions are possible.

Follow-up [17, 29]

There is undoubtedly less controversy about which examinations to perform in the presence of elevated tumor markers. Ultrasound is inadequate regardless of whether it is normal or abnormal. Even if it demonstrates an hepatic tumor, there is always the problem of the number of lesions and whether or not there is a solitary metastasis. CT can always be performed at this time. It is acceptable practice to perform a CT as the initial study in the presence of elevated tumor markers. Moreover, ultrasound requires a cooperative and mobile patient who is not breathless and able to hold his breath, without painful bony metastasis or interposition of colon. These limitations are less important for CT which does not necessarily require the patient to maintain a breath hold with the modern machines. It is also possible to perform high quality angio-CT on these machines using rapid bolus injections. Finally and most importantly, the measurements are reproducible. The examination using 3D software can measure the tumor volume and accurately locate the lesion. CT can also produce a true representation of the lesions which is even more accurate if the injection is given into a subcutaneous chamber for intrahepatic artery chemotherapy. This technique should, however, be reserved for the evaluation of lesions preoperatively or the assessment of the activity of the lesions for a better understanding of a dissociated response by studying the distribution of the truly perfused areas. The risk of false negative examinations due to liver steatosis is overcome by high quality angio-CT.

CT provides a simultaneous examination of the other regions of the abdomen and pelvis, notably the viscera, lymph nodes and bony structures [29].

Signs

CT

Diagnosis

On the unenhanced scan, metastases are hypodense, related to the frequent partial necrosis and the difference in cellularity compared to normal hepatic tissue. Metastases have irregular borders and are frequently poorly defined, appearing round, oval or of variable shape. They are often heterogeneous, particularly when large.

There is increased discrimination between the hypodense metastasis and healthy tissue in the early phase of angio-CT due to the reduction in the local microcirculation. The tumor itself (fig. 23.2) only enhances in its periphery, the center being typically necrotic and hypodense. There is often a visible hypervascular periphery appearing as a thin hyperdense line corresponding to vascular stasis phenomena. In the later phases of angio-CT, after the first few minutes following bolus injection, there is a reduction in the differentiation between tumor and healthy tissue due to diffusion of contrast agent into the interstitial space of the tumor. This, therefore, contraindicates any slow perfusion injection technique which would result in a uniform uptake of contrast agent by the lesions.

Different appearances may be encountered: calcifications pre- or post-treatment, progressive cyst formation (fig. 23.3) or uniformly hypervascular lesions (fig. 23.4) particularly in metastases from sarcomas. Necrosis is common in adenocarcinoma metastases, and calcifications occur in ovarian tumors, gastrointestinal tumors, sarcomas or melanomas (fig. 23.5 a). In practice, no finding is specific to a primary lesion, hepatic metastases being polymorphic [3, 5]. Fatty

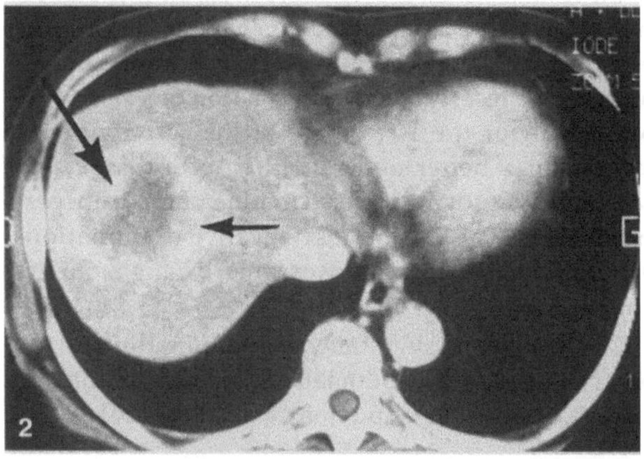

Fig. 23.2. Hepatic metastasis on post-contrast CT: the tumor exhibits slight enhancement *(large arrow)* with a hypodense necrotic center and a thin hyperdense periphery *(small arrow)*, possibly related to vascular stasis

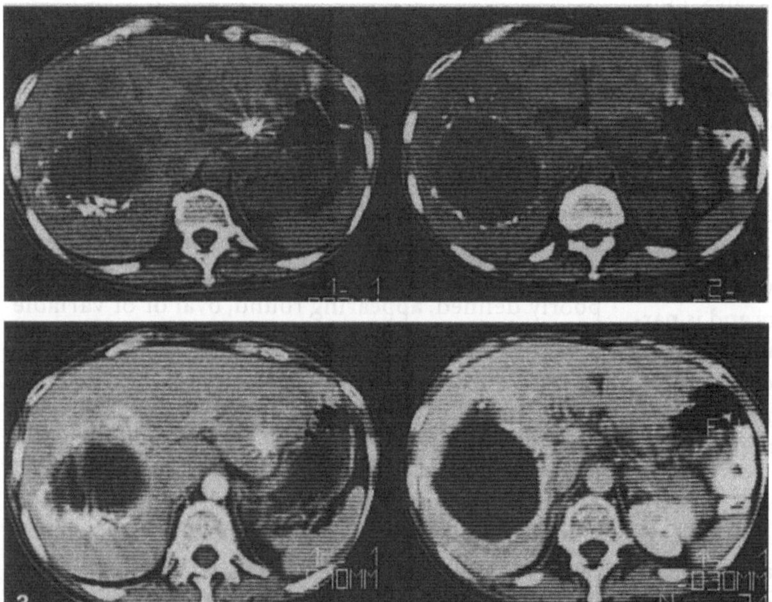

Fig. 23.3. Increasingly cystic metastasis following treatment, on CT pre-contrast *(upper images)* and post-contrast *(lower images)*. Following treatment the lesions become progressively more cystic and calcified giving a pseudo-biliary cyst appearance (primary GIT cancer of origin)

components may be seen in melanoma metastases (fig. 23.5 b).

Even the multifocal nature of metastases is not pathognomonic since any benign or malignant lesion may be multiple, for example angiomas or multifocal primary carcinomas.

Differential diagnosis

Focal fatty change (steatosis) is an easy diagnosis when the hypodensity due to fatty infiltration is localized to a hepatic segment or sector or when the involvement is slightly diffuse. When it is not localized, the differential diagnosis may be resolved by angio-CT which demonstrates a hypodense area of steatosis traversed by portal and intrahepatic vessels with normal caliber following their normal course.

Angiomas can sometimes pose difficulties in the differential diagnosis even though the appearances are usually characteristic when the examination is performed correctly, namely the inclusion of both early and late phase scans. Angiomas exhibit an intense early "blush" with a rounded pseudo-glomerular appearance. The lesion is hypodense or undetectable prior to injection. In the late phase, the small volume lesions fade and become of uniform density. The large lesions (cavernous hemangioma) have an irregular hypervascular periphery with progressive disappearance of the lesion from the periphery to the center, becoming uniform and even homogeneously hyper-

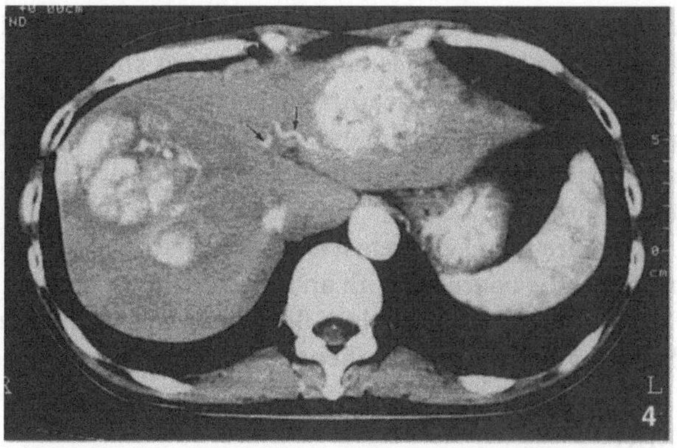

Fig. 23.4. Hypervascular lesions on post-contrast CT (helical angio CT). These metastases from a soft tissue sarcoma are clearly hyperdense at this early phase of the injection. Note that this technique allows assessment during the hepatic arterial phase (visualization of the right and left hepatic arteries at the base of the hepatic fissure: *arrows*; see fig. 23.18)

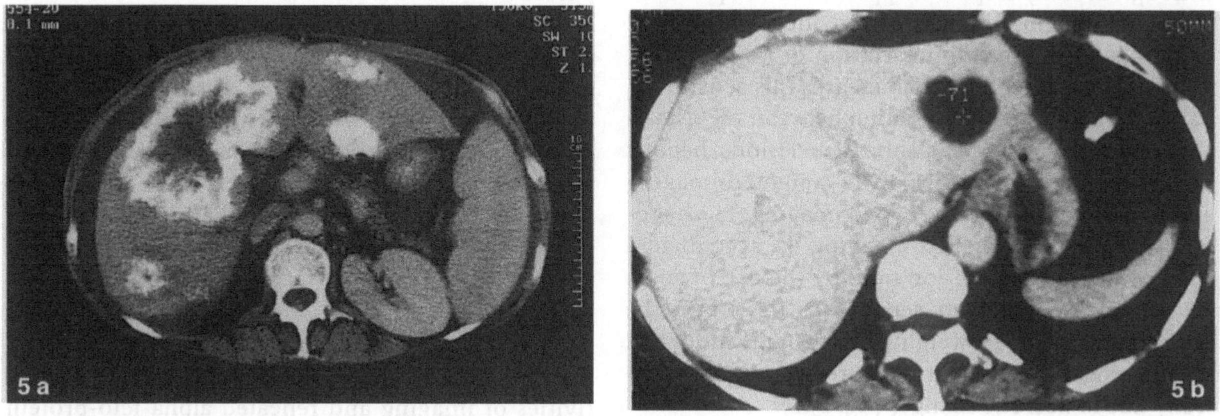

Fig. 23.5 a, b. Variable densities of hepatic metastases on CT. **a** Calcified metastases from a melanoma; **b** negative fatty density (−71 HU) within a fat-containing metastasis from a melanoma

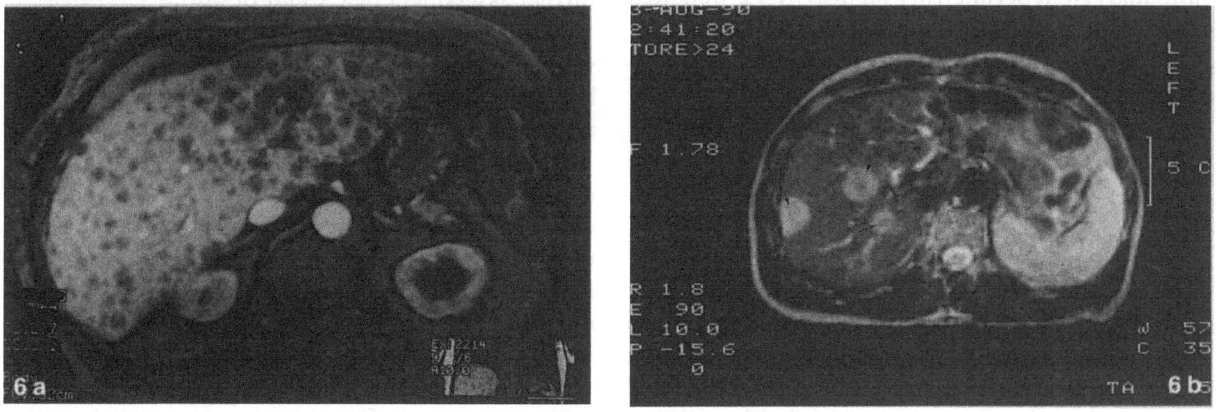

Fig. 23.6 a, b. Hepatic metastases on MRI. **a** This rapid turbo-flash sequence acquired in a single breath hold gives good definition of the lesions; **b** on T2-weighted imaging, the metastases are moderately hyperintense and inhomogeneous *(arrows)*

dense at a late stage. However, the early peripheral hypervascular enhancement at whatever stage is the only characteristic feature of an angioma since necrotic pseudo-angiomatous metastases can exhibit a similar progressive filling in from the periphery to the center.

The rare forms of metastases with a fatty composition may be confused with an intrahepatic lipoma.

It is sometimes difficult to determine whether large lesions are intra- or extrahepatic in nature.

MRI

The sensitivity of MRI without contrast agent, although initially disputed, appears to be superior to the other imaging modalities provided a high field system is used. The administration of a hypermagnetic contrast agent further increases this sensitivity, particularly in the differentiation between metastasis and angioma [20]. Like all soft tissue lesions, hepatic metastasis are hypointense on T1-weighted imaging and hyperintense on T2-weighted imaging. The hypointensity on T1-weighted imaging is accentuated (hence the lesion detection rate) by the use of short TR heavily T1-weighted sequences (fig. 23.1). The hyperintensity on T2-weighted imaging is moderate and heterogeneous, appearing more hyperintense centrally due to necrotic changes (fig. 23.6).

Angiomas represent the most important differential diagnosis. MRI is highly sensitive in the detection of these lesions [27, 48, 62], even achieving a relative specificity by the demonstration within the angiomas of a more marked hyperintensity on heavily T2-weighted images than neoplastic lesions provided they are not cystic or hypervascular [20, 21]. These latter phenomena are, however, rare in metastasis.

Primary cancer of the liver

Hepatocellular carcinoma (HCC) [30-32, 34]

This is the commonest cancer. Usually there is a known history of cirrhosis (figs 23.7 b & 23.8), but it is important not to miss early malignant degeneration because surgical excision may be of value for the small lesions and results in a better prognosis. The risk factors are hepatitis B and C, and the porphyrias (and the association of the latter two).

However, HCC may be detected as a result of complications, usually at a late stage, due to portal thrombosis, abdominal pains or ascites. At this stage, the differential diagnosis may be that of alveolar echinococcosis.

Other types of primary liver cancer

These are much rare. Fibrolamellar HCC only represents 2% of cases of HCC, occurs in children and young adults (50% before the age of 40) and arises in a previously healthy liver. It is generally a small lesion, often with normal tumor markers. At the time of diagnosis, 50-60% of lesions are surgically resectable [22].

The hepatic epithelioid hemangioendothelioma, described by Ichak et al in 1984, is a rare tumor occurring particularly in females, sometimes in children. It is associated with a syndrome of cholestasis, upper abdominal pains and hepatomegaly (often nodular). The tumor is discovered accidentally in more than 1 in 5 cases.

Hepatic angiosarcoma [8] is often associated with an occupational history (polyvinyl chloride poisoning): the early symptoms of the disease are related to portal hypertension without cirrhosis leading to the development of an angiosarcoma in 40% of exposed subjects after a delay of 15-30 years. There are possible iatrogenic causes, resulting from the administration of thorotrast or anabolic androgens.

Indications and signs

Numerous studies have looked at the respective sensitivities of imaging and repeated alpha-feto-protein levels. It is accepted practice and reasonable to perform annual or bi-annual ultrasound examinations coupled with an alpha-feto-protein level in subjects at risk. Any suspicious ultrasonic appearance requires further assessment by CT and/or MRI.

CT is relatively accurate for the demonstration of solitary or multiple nodules (fig. 23.7a). On the other hand, it is disappointing in the diffuse infiltrative form and underestimates the extent of the lesion (fig . 23.7b).

The density of the tumor and the degree of enhancement are non-specific and variable. The presence of a perilesional hypervascular capsule suggests the diagnosis but is not a constant feature (fig. 23.7a) [33]. Tumor extension into the portal vein is better demonstrated by CT than ultrasound, as well as involvement of the intrahepatic veins and inferior vena cava (rare).

The assessment of tumor extent is essential, particularly to appreciate the position of the lesions, because surgery must leave behind a sufficient volume of liver in order to avoid hepatocellular failure post-operatively. CT is sufficient for making this evaluation, but other investigations are sometimes advisable: CT following intra-arterial injection of Lipiodol ultrafluid; a CT examination is performed 7 weeks after the perfor-

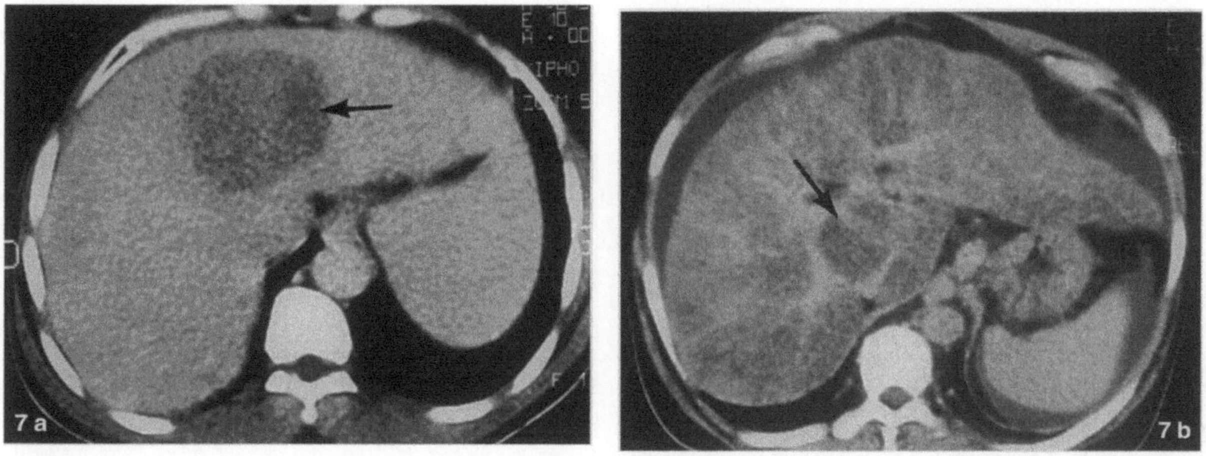

Fig. 23.7 a, b. Hepatocellular carcinoma on post-contrast CT. **a** The solitary nodular lesion has a hypervascular perilesional capsule *(arrow)*; **b** diffuse infiltrative form combining the signs of periportal fibrosis with compression of the intrahepatic portal vein, deformity of the hepatic outline, regenerative nodule, hypertrophy of the paramedian sectors and atrophy of the lateral sectors related to hepatic cirrhosis. There is a nodular area of malignant degeneration *(arrow)* with histological correlation which is extremely difficult to distinguish from the regenerative nodules themselves

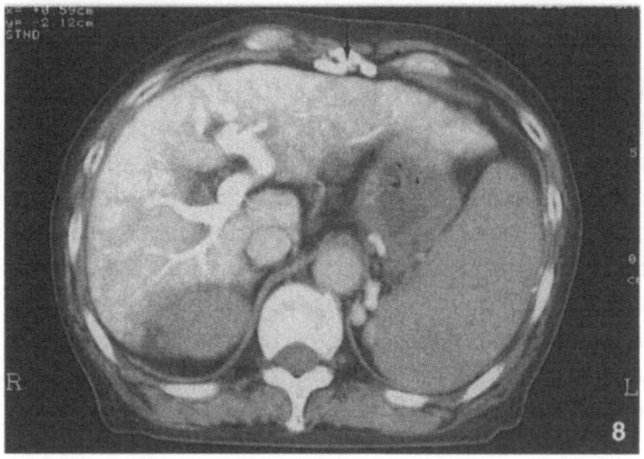

Fig. 23.8. CT portography performed in a case of cirrhosis: direct injection into the superior mesenteric artery combined with helical CT provides a study dependent on the portal blood flow and demonstrates the signs of portal hypertension [enlargement of the portal vessels, recanalisation of the umbilical vein *(arrow)*, collateral vessels and splenomegaly]. There is attenuation of the peripheral vessels and stasis of the contrast related to the periportal fibrosis

mance of selective hepatic arteriography with injection of Lipiodol. This examination is very sensitive but non-specific since an adenoma, angioma or post-biopsy inflammatory changes may also take up the Lipiodol. On the other hand, false negatives occur with poorly vascularized lesions. There is, therefore, currently no single technique which can be performed. CT portography (figs 23.8 & 23.13) [31, 34] may be an alternative but is dependent on the portal blood flow which is often altered in cirrhosis. This investigation should be reserved to the rare cases of HCC occurring in a healthy liver.

As a general rule, on the pre-contrast CT the lesions are hypodense, often multiloculated, causing deformity of the liver outline. These appearances are non-specific, particularly in the presence of regenerative nodules due to cirrhosis (fig. 23.7b).

On angio-CT, there is a combination of inhomogeneous, irregular, hypervascular tumor and hypovascular zones corresponding to necrosis with evidence of endoluminal tumor nodules in the portal system or inferior vena cava in a third of cases. The rapid bolus CT technique is able to demonstrate the vascular anomalies (fig. 23.9 a, b) (cf below), looking particularly for obstruction of the portal vein which results in reduced opacification in liver segments [23], and the presence of shunts or cavernomas.

MRI has an important role [11] because of its ability to differentiate the reactive soft tissue changes from tumor better than ultrasound or CT.

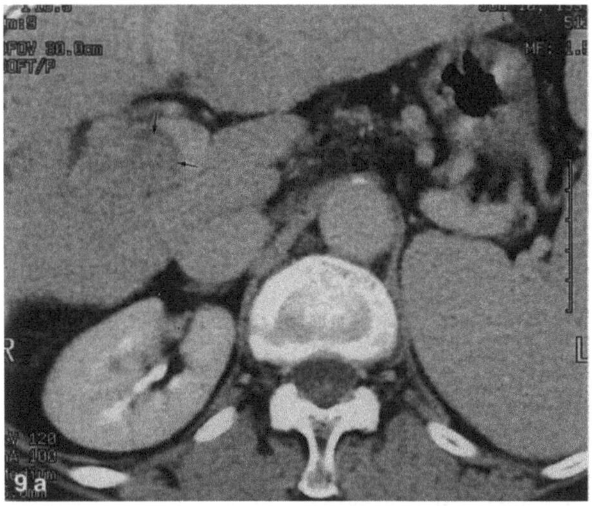

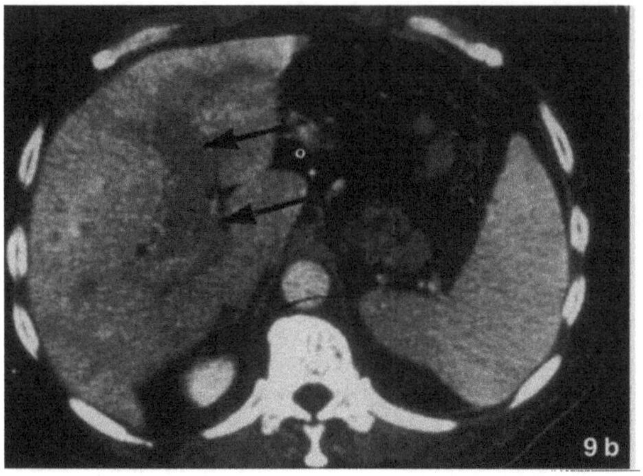

Fig. 23.9 a, b. Atypical vascularization in diffuse hepatocellular carcinoma. **a** Marked portal thrombosis *(small arrows)* with increased caliber of the portal trunks. **b** Note in another patient the marked enlargement of the portal trunk and particularly of the left portal vein *(arrows)*, hypodense following contrast injection due to thrombosis. In the periphery of this thrombus, there are several hyperdensities corresponding to the recanalization of the vasa vasorum

The HCC is hyperintense on T2-weighted imaging (fig. 23.10) but the signal intensity is less than that for angiomas or biliary cysts. MRI demonstrates the peritumoral capsule more reliably than CT, appearing hypointense on T1-weighted imaging and hyperintense on T2-weighted imaging, with enhancement following gadolinium. In almost a third of cases there is hyperintensity on T1-weighted imaging suggesting chronic hemorrhagic changes, fatty infiltration or an accumulation of intralesional copper [33]. The flow sensitive rapid gradient echo sequences help in the evaluation of endoluminal extension into the portal vein (fig. 23.10). The additional injection of gadolinium makes it possible to appreciate the vascular kinetics and to detect atypical areas (cf later). The use of ferrite compounds (fig. 23.11) (AMI 25, Guerbet Laboratories) improves the differentiation between healthy liver and the lesion, particularly when the HCC occurs in a patient with hemochromatosis.

MRI aids in the "histological diagnosis" of particularly the fibrolamellar carcinoma [33]. MRI demonstrates the central, often stellate fibrous zone appearing hypointense on T1- and T2-weighted imaging, providing a better differentiation between a tumor and a regenerative nodule. There are no specific imaging appearances in the other forms of primary cancer.

Arteriography is nowadays rarely performed and is reserved for the so-called diffuse form or for the performance of locoregional treatments. Interventional radiological techniques include percutaneous alcohol injection, chemo-embolization and arterial embolization. These techniques can give good results, sometimes comparable to those of surgery.

Associated vascular anomalies on CT and MRI [27]

Portal hypertension
(figs 23.7 & 23.8)

Obstruction of the portal vein may be due to thrombosis complicating a cirrhosis and/or much more frequently an endoluminal invasion by tumor nodules. Cirrhosis remains the main cause of portal hypertension due to intrahepatic obstruction. The other mechanism of intrahepatic obstruction in neoplastic disease is the presence of a very extensive hepatic infiltration.

CT and MRI demonstrate hepatosplenomegaly, ascites, esophageal varices and collateral vessels (rapid flow appearing hypointense on T1-weighted MRI).

Budd-Chiari syndrome

This is essentially an ultrasonic diagnosis, and doppler ultrasound is complementary and useful, particularly when there is moderate dilatation of the intrahepatic veins proximal to a stenosis. Venography is no longer essential for making the diagnosis. Ultrasound, CT and MRI can give useful information concerning the state of the inferior vena cava prior to treatment.

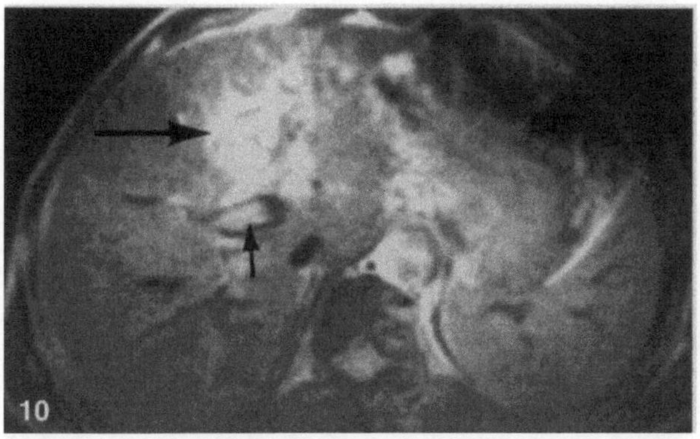

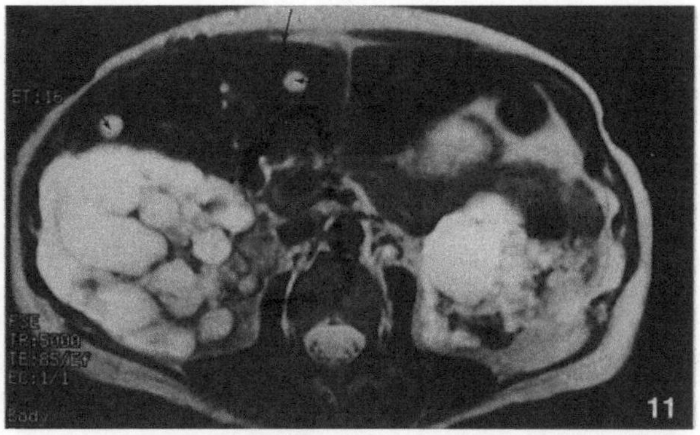

Fig. 23.10. Hepatocellular carcinoma with atypical vessels on MRI: carcinoma invading the portal trunk and left portal vein: the lesion is hyperintense on T2-weighted imaging *(large arrow)* with poorly defined contours. Invasion of the left portal vein with visualization of collateral vessels. There is extension of thrombus into the portal trunk and origin of the right portal vein *(small arrow)*

Fig. 23.11. Use of ferrite contrast on T2-weighted MRI (injection of 20 mmol Fe/kg of ferrite). This technique can demonstrate small lesions *(small arrows)*; the distinction between healthy liver *(large arrow)* and the lesions *(small arrows)* is improved by this technique

However, cavography is still often necessary to demonstrate the caval compression due to hepatomegaly, hypertrophy of the caudate lobe, endoluminal thrombosis or direct spread of the tumor.

CT demonstrates dilatation of the intrahepatic veins proximal to a stenosis, hepatomegaly, ascites, inhomogeneous enhancement around the hepatic artery branches and inferior vena cava, hypodensity of the periphery of liver, and lobulated enhancement in a pericaval distribution.

MRI demonstrates the reduction in flow velocity, enlargement of the intrahepatic veins, and sometimes directly delineates the compression by the hepatomegaly, the endoluminal thrombus or intracaval extension.

Atypical vessels

These represent an important element in the diagnosis of hepatocellular carcinoma and are much rare in diffuse metastatic involvement. Irrespective of portal vein thrombosis due to direct invasion, CT and MRI demonstrate enlargement of the portal vessels, a reduction in the endovascular density on CT, a slow flow velocity giving the appearance of thrombosis on MRI, and segmental changes in the density and signal intensity of the hepatic parenchyma. In the presence of complete thrombosis, these examinations may demonstrate dilatation of the vasa vasorum within the walls of the portal vessels (fig. 23.9 b) and progressive multiplication of locoregional collateral vessels resulting in a "portal cavernoma". It should be remembered that the presence of endoluminal high signal on MRI is not necessarily due to thrombosis and may also be seen in portal hypertension or even be physiological. However, only thrombus remains constantly hyperintense on all sequences and imaging planes, without knowing the presence or absence of persistent flow locally. In cases of complete occlusion, hepatic ischemia appears as a triangular hyperintensity with the base peripherally on the T2-weighted sequence and is due to the edema and ischemia itself.

Occlusion of the hepatic artery trunks or branches results in hepatic infarction. This appears triangular or more often rounded or oval in shape which may or may not be clearly defined and preferentially localized centrally. There may be areas of air density present due to possible communication with the bile duct which can be misleading. The MRI appearances are not well documented.

Arterioportal shunts are demonstrated on angio-CT by the synchronous opacification of the aorta and both the proximal and distal branches of the portal vein.

Hepatic lymphoma [30]

Hepatic lymphoma is generally a complication of Hodgkin's disease which is usually detected at the time of staging and much more rarely during investigation of PUO (pyrexia of unknown origin) or an inflammatory syndrome.

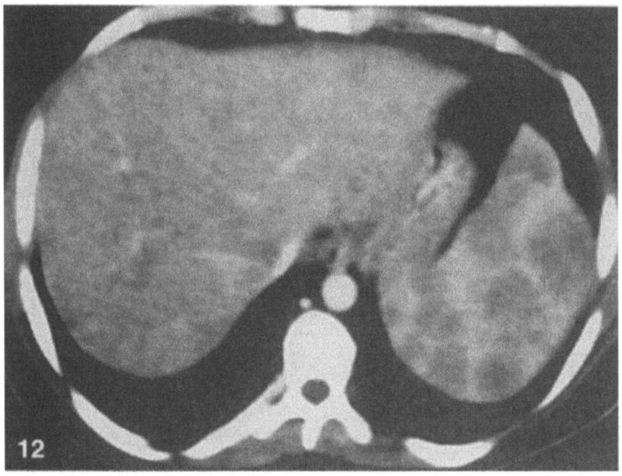

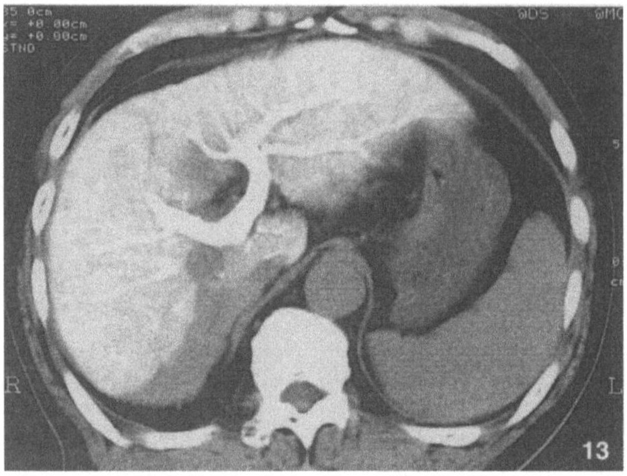

Fig. 23.12. Hepatic and splenic lymphoma on post-contrast CT: note the significant macronodular intrasplenic lesions and diffuse subcapsular micronodular heterogeneity, particularly posteriorly in the liver due to lymphomatous infiltration

Fig. 23.13. Thrombosis of the right portal segment with an avascular zone in the medial portion of the lateral sector of the right lobe of the liver (posterior branch of the right portal vein) on CT portography (courtesy of General Electric)

Indications

Even though CT only demonstrates lymphomatous infiltration in barely 50% of cases [30], it remains the initial investigation of choice due to its ability to simultaneously demonstrate possible lymphadenopathy. Experience with MRI remains limited, especially in its ability to detect hepatic infiltration or lymphomatous nodules.

Signs (fig. 23.12)

Usually the lesions are focal and of small or intermediate size with similar appearances to those of other solid tumors.

The diagnosis of the diffuse forms becomes very difficult on CT which shows only a non-specific heterogeneity and a moderate diminution in the homogeneity of the hepatic density which is also non-specific.

Conclusion

The initial ultrasound examination usually confirms the diagnosis and the subsequent follow-up can also be performed by ultrasound (e.g. chronic viral hepatitis, metastases).

Angio-CT with rapid scanning of the whole liver is a highly accurate technique in the demonstration of focal lesions of greater than or equal to 8 mm. The diagnosis of the specific nature of the lesion remains relatively limited, particularly for small lesions. However, the advent of spiral and helical CT may noticeably reduce these limitations (see fig. 23.4) with the application of 3D imaging of atypical vascularization and the vessels themselves. CT is usually performed as a second line investigation and can confirm the ultrasound findings. CT, however, is the main examination for the follow-up of primary and particularly secondary hepatic tumors, especially with the advantages of the new techniques. As with ultrasound, CT can be used to guide percutaneous biopsy or fine needle aspiration for cytology. CT portography (figs 23.8 & 23.13) is essential in the preoperative evaluation of metastases, especially of colo-rectal origin [31]. The direct injection of contrast agent into chemotherapy chambers may prove to be a useful technique for assessing the efficacy of treatment and for appreciating possible asymmetrical perfusion (fig. 23.14 a, b) [7].

MRI is more sensitive in the detection of small lesion, can help determine the nature of the lesion, and already represents an extremely valuable gold standard in certain situations: the differentiation between angioma and metastasis, the diagnosis of hepatocellular carcinomas, particularly at an early stage, and fibrolamellar carcinomas. It is possible that eventually, with the development of diffusion techniques and the

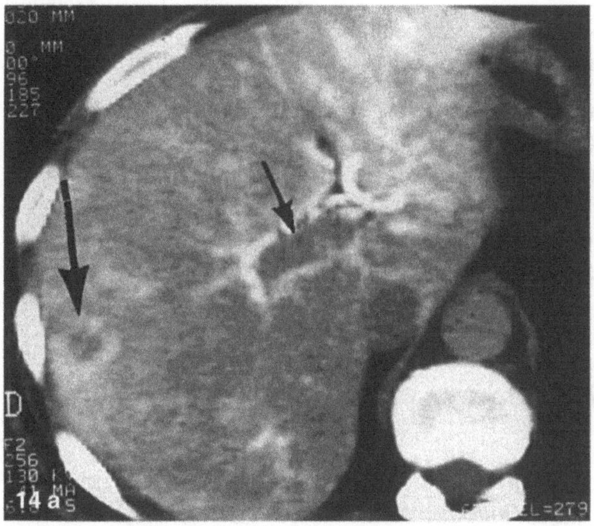

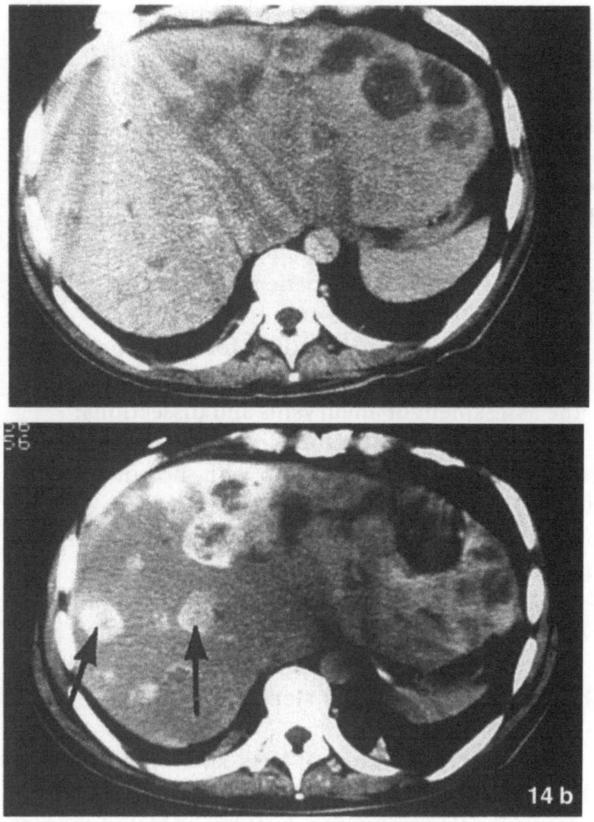

Fig. 23.14 a, b. CT performed following direct injection into the subcutaneous chemotherapy chamber. This method is used for the follow-up of treated hepatic metastases and for aiding preoperative evaluation. It can demonstrate lesions missed on standard CT examinations in 10-12% of cases. **a** Note, after intra-arterial injection via the chemotherapy chamber, the demonstration of a subcapsular lesion in the lateral part of segment VI *(large arrow)*. This technique can result in the false appearance of portal thrombosis at a very early stage of the injection when the vasa vasorum in the walls of the portal trunk are still well seen *(small arrow)*. **b** Comparison between CT following intravenous injection *(above)* and intra-arterial injection via a chemotherapy chamber *(lower figure)*; demonstration of two lesions by the intra-arterial technique which are poorly or not visualized at all on the standard CT technique (technique by D. Buthiau et al [7])

use of new contrast agents (fig. 23.11), MRI may take its place alongside ultrasound in certain specific circumstances. Peroperative ultrasound has an important role in the diagnosis of deep lesions and in demonstrating the relationship of the tumor to vessels depending on the plane of section.

Future prospects of helical CT

(see also last chapters on Helical CT)

P. Priollet, D. Buthiau

Three-dimensional hepatic imaging is able to calculate the hepatic volume and detect congenital morphological anomalies prior to partial hepatectomy. This volumetric study could have other further indications:
- during a course of chemotherapy, the 3-D volumetric study can provide a measurement of tumor volume to assess the efficacy of the treatment;
- an accurate segmental localization of hepatic tumors which determines the type of resection to be performed, and an assessment of the vascular relationships;
- an aid for pre-transplant assessment.

Angiography performed using helical CT joins a group of non- or minimally invasive investigations of the blood vessels such as color doppler ultrasound and MR angiography. It would seem to have the following advantages which are yet to be confirmed:
- due to its speed (section in less than 1 second), it is possible to obtain images of mobile structures such as the abdominal vessels;
- demonstration of the endoluminal vascular contents, intimal or vessel wall calcification and the structure of the vessel wall itself (submural thrombus);
- reduced radiation dose and the use of smaller volumes of contrast;
- continuous acquisition over a large volume in a single breath hold with homogeneous and increased opacification of vessels allowing subsequent high quality multiplanar reconstructions in three dimensions.

Its main limitations are:
- the difficulty in analyzing the vessels parallel to the plane of section is reduced by the improvements in image reconstruction;
- circumferential vascular calcifications, particularly when they are regular, result in underestimating the degree of a stenosis. They are best demonstrated on the axial sections. A good understanding of the cardiovascular function of the patient is necessary for optimal vessel opacification.

There are certain applications for which helical CT may become a new method for vascular investigation:
- the assessment of aneurysms and dissections;
- the detection of thrombosis of the inferior vena cava, portal vein or any deep vein, not in order to determine the surgical technique but to exclude patients from surgery and to monitor post-operative progress;
- the assessment of the relationships between the vessels and tumors;
- the investigation of reno-vascular hypertension (detection of renal artery stenosis);
- mesenteric ischemia;
- to monitor the patency of intra-abdominal vascular shunts post-operatively.

However, this technique must be evaluated according to the following usual criteria:
- comparative accuracy with preexisting techniques;
- the ease of access to the technique which depends mainly on the number and geographical distribution of the machines;
- the cost of the examination (there is no additional cost to the patient for helical CT);
- the constraints for the patient, in other words the necessity or otherwise for a contrast injection;
- the limitations of feasibility, for example the requirement for an extended breath hold.

Taking into account all these parameters, it still has to be proven that helical CT has a major advantage over the traditional combined imaging approach in the investigation of a vascular abnormality which is currently based on doppler ultrasound, CT and transarterial arteriography.

There are few areas of vascular pathology for which imaging is currently found needed, the most important being imaging of the aortic arch and thoracic aorta in suspected embolic disease. The development of this helical method in this application is under evaluation.

In a more general sense, in order to validate helical CT, it will undoubtedly be necessary to compare it with the more traditional approach of ultrasound-doppler-CT-arteriography and not with MR angiography which is not yet a reference technique for vascular examination and is still itself under evaluation.

In summary, the role of helical CT seems to be particularly important in the investigation of cancer spread due to its speed, and ability to acquire contiguous or even overlapping sections resulting in the complete continuity of organs or whole anatomical regions. This is all still under evaluation.

References

1. Araki T, Itai Y, Furui S, et al (1980) Dynamic CT densitometryofhepatictumors. AJR 135: 1037-1043
2. Baum JK, Holtz T, Bookstein JJ, et al (1973) Possible association between benign hopatomas and oral contraceptives. Lancet 2: 926-929
3. Bernardino ME, Erwin BC, et al (1986) Delayed hepatic CT scanning: increased confidence and improved detection of hepatic metastasis. Radiology 159: 71-74
4. Berland LL, Lawson TL, Foley WD, et al (1982) Comparison of pre and post contrast CT in hepatic masses. AJR 138: 853-858
5. Bressler LL, Alpern MB, Glazer GM, et al (1987) Hypervascular hepatic metastases: CT evaluation. Radiology 162: 49-51
6. Burgener FA, Hamlin DJ (1983) Contrast enhancement of hepatic tumors in CT: comparison between bolus and infusion techniques. AJR 140: 291-295
7. Buthiau D (1992) Apport de la TDM et de 1'IRM dans la surveillance de la réponse des métastases hépatiques à la chimiothérapie. Recherche Servier en Cancérologie. Paris, novembre 1992
8. Closuit B, Micléa JM, Frija J, Laval-Jeantet M (1991) Angiosarcome hépatique splénique et médullaire. Revue Imagerie Médicale 3: 559-561
9. Dahan H, Vilgrain V, Belghiti J, Fléjou JF, Menu Y, Nahum H (1991) Imagerie du carcinome fibrolamellaire. Revue Imagerie Médicale 3: 503-507
10. Dunninck NR, Ihde DC, Doppman JL, et al (1980) Computed tomography in primary hepatocellular carcinoma. J Comput Assist Tomogr 4: 59-62
11. Ebara M, Ohto M, Watanabe Y, et al (1986) Diagnosis of small hepatocellular carcinoma: correlation of MR imaging and tumor histologic studies. Radiology 159: 371 -377
12. Ferucci JT (1986). MR imaging of the liver. AJR 147: 1103-1116
13. Foley WD (1989). Dynamic hepatic CT. Radiology 170: 617
14. Henderson JM, Campbell JD, Olson R, et al (1988) Role of computed tomography in screening for hepatocellular carcinoma in patients with cirrhosis. Gastrointest Radiol 13: 129

15. Herrero C, Vicente A, Bruguera M, et al (1993) L'infection par le virus de l'hépatite C est-elle un facteur déclenchant de la porphyrie cutanée tardive ? Lancet 341: 788-789
16. Itai Y, Ohtomo K, Furui S, et al (1986) MR imaging of hepatocellular carcinoma. J Comput Assist Tomogr 10: 963-968
17. Kunstlinger F (1992) Recherche de métastases hépatiques: faut-il utiliser l'échographie, l'IRM ou le scanner? Revue Imagerie Médicale 4: 569-572
18. Legmann Ph (1993) Valeur diagnostique du porto-scanner. Revue Imagerie Médicale 5: 199-200
19. L'Herminé C, Lescanne D: Bonodeau F, Delesalle JC, Renan-Druart CA, et al (1992) Séméiologie IRM des tumeurs du foie. Revue Imagerie Médicale 4: 17-29
20. Li KC, Glazer M, Quint LE, et al (1988) Distinction of hepatic cavernous hemangioma from hopatic metastases with MR imaging. Radiology 169: 409-415
21. Lombardo DM, Baker ME, Spritzer CE, et al (1990) Hepatic hemangiomas versus metastases: MR differentiation at 1.5 T. AJR 155: 55-59
22. Martin E (1990) Carcinome hépato-cellulaire fibrolamellaire. In: O Blétry (ed) Les 365 nouvelles maladies. Flammarion Médecine-Sciences, Paris, pp 47-48
23. Mathieu D, Grenier PH, Larde D, et al (1984) Portal vein involvement in hepatocellular carcinoma: dynamic CT features. Radiology 152: 127-132
24. Mathieu D, Larde D, Vasile N, et al (1983) Etude de l'angioscanner hépatique normal et au cours de tumeurs hépatiques: caractéristiques hémodynamiques et morphologiques. Gastroenterol Clin Biol 7: 961-968
25. Mitchell DG, Stark DD (1992) Liver. In: DD Stark, W Bradley (eds) Magnetic Resonance Imaging, 2nd edn. Mosby-Year Book, St Louis, pp 1652-1768
26. Osteaux M, Wilms G, Darras TH, et al (1981) Tomographie computée du foie: acquis récents. Radiologie J CEPUR 1: 79-89
27. Osteaux M, Blétry O, Benhamou JP (1991) Foie. In: D Buthiau (ed) TDM et IRM Cliniques. Frison-Roche, Paris, pp 611-631
28. Rummeny E, Weissleder R, Sironi S, et al (1989) Central scars in primary liver tumors: MR features specificity, and pathologic correlation. Radiology 171: 323-326
29. Scherrer A, Vincent P (1992) Recherche des métastases hépatiques. Revue Imagerie Médicale 4: 569-572
30. Soyer Ph, Van Beers B, Barge J, Kazerouni F, Lacheheb D, et al (1993). Tomodensitométrie des lymphomes hopatiques. Revue Imagerie Médicale 5: 325-331
31. Soyer Ph, Lacheheb D, Levesque M (1993) Le porto-scanner. Revue Imagerie Médicale 5: 633-638
32. Soyer Ph, Levesque M, Legmann P, Fajadet P (1992) Imagerie par résonance magnétique des tumeurs hépatiques malignes de l'adulte. J Radiol 73: 219-227
33. Soyer Ph, Roche A, Levesque M, Legmann P (1991) CT of fibrolamellar hepatocellular carcinoma. J Comput Assist Tomogr 15: 533-538
34. Soyer Ph, Levesque M, Sihassen C, Zeitoun G, Roche A, Mignon E (1992) Etude comparative du porto-scanner et de l'imagerie par résonance magnétique à haut champ dans la détection des tumeurs hépatiques. Revue Imagerie Médicale 4: 221-226
35. Vullierrne MP, Vilgrain V, Menu Y, Nahum H (1991) Communications porto-caves intrahépatiques au cours de l'HTP: aspects échographiques et tomodensitométriques. Revue Imagerie Médicale 3: 105-109
36. Van Beers B, Demeure R, Pringot J, et al (1990) Dynamic spin-echo imaging with Gd-DTPA: value in the differentiation of hepatic tumors. AJR 154: 515-519

CHAPTER 24

Tumors of the biliary system

Clinicians
D. Nizri, M. Gozy, F. Guinet,
R. Dendale, D. Khayat

Radiologists
D. Buthiau, F. Gelbert

Cancers of the bile ducts (BD) and gallbladder (GB) are rare: bile ducts cancers representing 2% and gallbladder cancers 3-6% of all cancers with a different incidence depending on the sex and age of the patient [4, 5, 7, 11, 12 ,15]:
- bile ducts cancers are more common in men with a sex ratio of 1 to 4;
- gallbladder cancers are more common in women with a sex ratio of 6.7;
- there is a clear predilection for elderly patients.

The tumors may be first detected in very different circumstances:
- during the investigation of non-specific symptomatology such as:
  - epigastric and hypochondrial pain (BD 50%; GB 79-90%);
  - variable degree of jaundice associated with pruritis (BD 97%; GB 34-40%);
  - syndrome of neoplastic disease with a palpable right hypochondrial mass of variable mobility on respiration (often corresponding to a markedly advanced unresectable cancer);
  - fever, ascites, nausea and vomiting (53%), alteration in the general state of the patient with loss of weight (42% of cases);
- as part of an examination performed for deranged liver function tests with a cholestatic picture present in 80% of cases;
- as an incidental finding during biliary surgery (0.5%); note that 88% of gallbladder cancers are associated with lithiasis;
- during the investigation for some other abdominal pathology;
- 0.01-0.4% of bile ducts tumors are detected at autopsy.

Ultrasound is usually requested initially and may suggest the diagnosis, particularly for gallbladder cancers. This is more difficult for cancers of the bile ducts if the tumor is fairly localized, although ultrasound will demonstrate dilatation of the intrahepatic bile ducts in the majority of cases.

It should be noted that the bile duct is often obscured by the first part of the duodenum and therefore poorly visualized on ultrasound.

Ultrasound may be used in the staging for the demonstration of lymphadenopathy and even invasion of the vessels at the porta hepatis.

In the majority of cases with bile ducts dilatation, transhepatic cholangiography (PTC) is indicated which has the advantages of being able to clearly visualize the biliary tree and to allow, in certain cases, decompression of the bile ducts. Endoscopic retrograde cholangiopancreatography (ERCP) may also be requested which has the disadvantage of only visualizing the portion of the bile duct distal to a complete obstruction.

It is possible to predict the resectability of lesion in the majority of cases by a combination of arteriography and PTC.

CT (rarely MRI) which unlike the preceding techniques is non-invasive may be useful to help localize an obstruction of the bile ducts, to determine its nature and assess the extent of the lesion.

Cancer of the gallbladder [7, 9]

Indications for CT and MRI

CT

First, it is complementary in making the diagnosis by demonstrating the lesion at the level of the middle hepatic fissure within the gallbladder bed. However, it is particularly useful for detecting local spread into the liver (30-40% of cases), pancreatic head, portal vein, bile duct and locoregional or distant lymph nodes. The presence of distant metastases is a sign of a markedly advanced tumor.

MRI

Although it is the fifth commonest cancer of the digestive tract, very little work has been done as yet on the role of MRI. Its role seems essentially to be limited by the absence of specificity (fig. 24.1), notably in the differentiation of an inflammatory lesion or even a interposed loop of bowel following cholecystectomy.

Signs

CT

CT may show an irregular, slightly enhancing mass, sometimes with a central necrotic zone [9]. Focal or extensive thickening of the gallbladder wall is frequently seen, as are associated with gallbladder calculi (more than 90% of cases). A cholecystitis may be encountered which is seen more commonly in the friable papillary adenomas due to obstruction of the cystic duct or the presence of a porcelain gallbladder (in 15-20% of gallbladder cancers).

CT will demonstrate any contraindication to surgical resection such as secondary hepatic involvement in segments IV and V, contiguous spread to the middle hepatic fissure and gallbladder bed, routinely resected in practice. Similarly, surgery is contraindicated if there is significant lymphadenopathy around the vascular pedicles or celiac axis, concomitant involvement of the bile ducts (the frequency of which may be greater than or equal to 80%) at the level of the superior biliary confluence, and tumor encasement of the right and left hepatic arteries or portal veins or

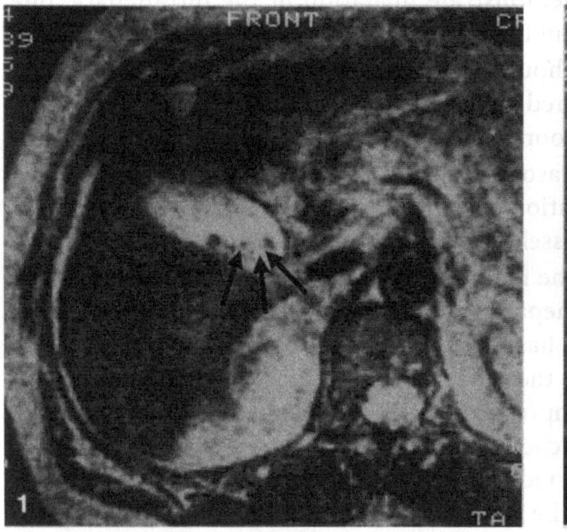

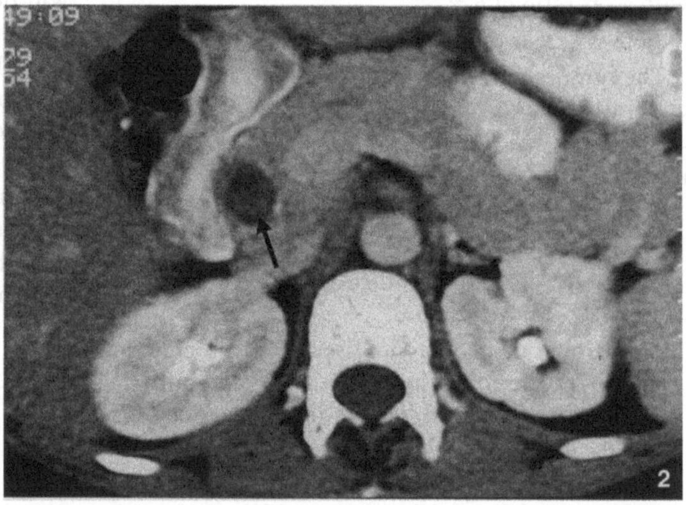

Fig. 24.1. Gallbladder cancer on axial T2-MRI: there is a non-specific, heterogeneous, endoluminal nodularity of the posterior wall of the gallbladder *(arrows)*, which cannot be differentiated especially from an inflammatory condition or even simple gallbladder calculi

Fig. 24.2. Cholangiocarcinoma on post-contrast CT: in this patient of 40 years old presenting with jaundice and a general deterioration in health, CT demonstrates dilatation of the retropancreatic portion of the common bile duct with an intracanalicular soft tissue lesion exhibiting intermediate enhancement *(arrow)* corresponding to a small cholangiocarcinoma of the distal extrahepatic bile duct spleno-mesenteric trunk. In all these different situations, the treatment is only palliative by percutaneous or endoscopic biliary drainage, possibly associated with radiotherapy.

MRI

The lesion appears hypointense on heavily T2-weighted images in the form of gallbladder wall thickening which is hypointense to the adjacent hepatic parenchyma. The differentiation from an inflammatory pathology remains nonetheless difficult. Moreover there are recognized pseudomasses which may simulate a gallbladder lesion, for example interposition of bowel at the level of the middle hepatic fissure following cholecystectomy.

Gallbladder metastases

The majority are associated with hepatic metastases and particularly arise from primary ovarian cancer or melanoma. Metastases localized to the gallbladder may cause hydrocholecystitis.

CT appearances are non-specific, and gallbladder may be demonstrated during the investigation of a known primary tumor or an ultrasonically abnormal gallbladder. The appearance of the lesion has no specificity, and the diagnosis will only be really easy in the presence of known primary cancer. Otherwise histological confirmation is always necessary.

There is no known indication for MRI in this particular context.

Cholangiocarcinoma of the extrahepatic bile duct [4, 9, 15]

The preferential site is the superior biliary confluence.

Indications for CT and MRI

CT assists in making the diagnosis and is indispensable in the assessment of the extent of the lesion.

Currently there is no indication for MRI since it has no particular advantage and may even be misleading due to partial volume effects.

Signs

On CT, the lesion is often small, frequently enhanced, and is better seen on thin sections centered on the common bile duct (fig. 24.2). Biliary dilatation stops at the same level as the tumor. The assessment of extension should look for involvement of the intrahepatic bile ducts, notably the confluence of the right biliary ducts and left hepatic duct. This search should also include an evaluation of locoregional or distant lymph nodes, hepatic spread particularly to the caudate lobe, vascular involvement of the hepatic artery, portal vein or inferior vena cava with or without associated atypical vascularization and perfusion abnormalities on angio-CT (fig. 24.3).

MRI may show an infiltrative mass in the porta hepatis extending along the portal vein, but partial volume effects with the portal vessels and biliary ducts are common. Increased signal due to biliary stasis and hepatic edema may be the cause of the hyperintensity

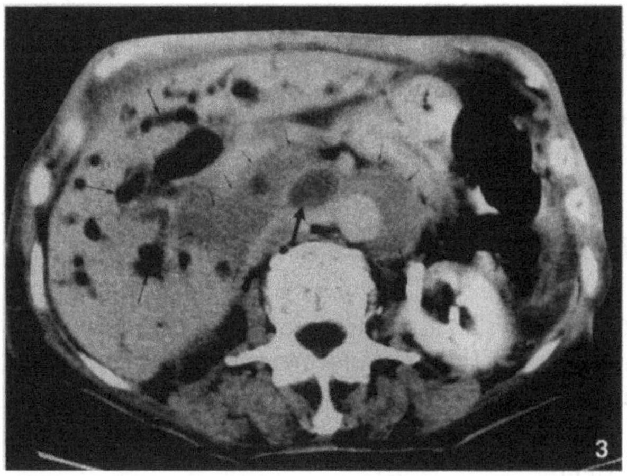

Fig. 24.3. Cholangiocarcinoma of the superior biliary confluence on post-contrast CT. The lesion itself is not directly visible, but there is marked locoregional lymphadenopathy *(small arrows)* and dilatation of the intrahepatic bile ducts *(medium arrows)* as a result of the tumor itself and obstruction at the porta hepatis by the lymphadenopathy. There is encasement of the inferior vena cava *(large arrow)* which is displaced away from the spine and contains an occlusive endoluminal thrombus

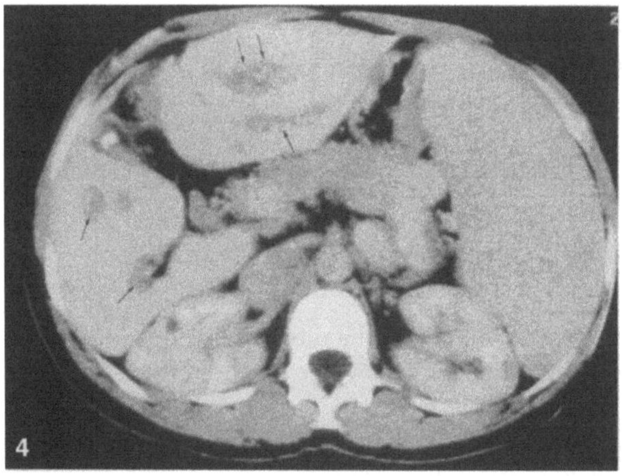

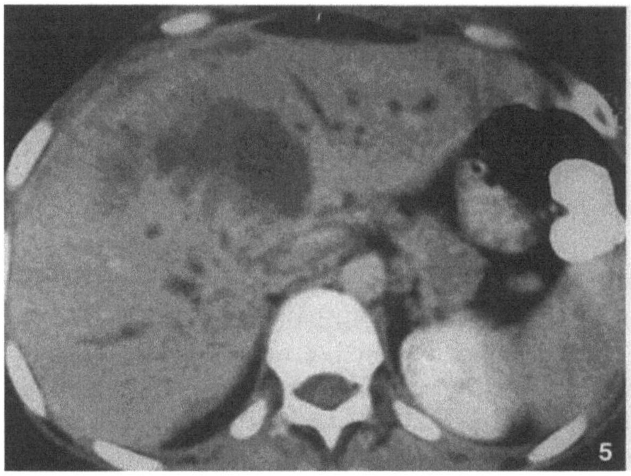

Fig. 24.4. Sclerosing cholangitis in a patient with abdominal involvement by AIDS: there is associated dilatation and narrowing of the intrahepatic bile ducts with obstruction of the peribiliary spaces by non-specific lymphomatous infiltrate

Fig. 24.5. Cholangiocellular carcinoma on post-contrast CT: combination of extensive but solitary, fairly well circumscribed hepatic metastasis with biliary dilatation occurring in a healthy liver

on T2-weighted imaging and is sometimes extensive with geographical or linear contours located usually either side of the portal vein. However, this appearance is non-specific with numerous possible differential diagnoses; lymphatic metastasis in the porta hepatis, hepatitis, cholangitis (fig. 24.4), recent biliary obstruction, surgery or rejection of a liver transplant, lymphatic obstruction, and periportal edema, the latter being associated with cholangiocarcinoma which sometimes causes an overestimation of the extent. As a general rule, MRI shows biliary dilatation less clearly.

Cholangiocellular carcinoma

This consists of lesions arising in small caliber intrahepatic bile ducts within a healthy liver. The appearance is one of a hepatic tumor without true biliary obstruction.

Indications for CT and MRI

CT provides an accurate diagnosis of the presence of intrahepatic tumor involvement, as well as the assessment of extent prior to the almost routine surgery.

MRI demonstrates well the intrahepatic tumor extent.

Signs

On CT, the tumor mimics hepatic involvement by metastasis (fig. 24.5) appearing circumscribed, nodular, often solitary. There is often weak and peripheral enhancement with central necrosis. CT can look for the presence of hematogenous spread to the lungs, or lymphatic spread, especially to the celiac axis nodes.

On MRI, the lesion is hypointense on T1-weighted imaging and hyperintense on T2-weighted imaging, usually heterogeneous with central necrosis. The borders of the tumor are often better defined by this technique, but the intrahepatic biliary dilatation is again less clearly shown than on CT.

Conclusion

CT, which is performed after ultrasound, has a central role in the evaluation of gallbladder and bile duct tumors and secondarily in the detection of the complications of biliary surgery. In addition, the performance of a single examination gives a complete assessment of the abdominal and thoracic spread. In addition, thoracic CT helps to determine the size of the radiotherapy field if post-operative treatment is being contemplated.

The indication for MRI is very limited mainly due to its lack of specificity, confusing appearances in gallbladder cancer, partial volume effects with the liver, periportal fatty tissue, and bile ducts for cholangiocarcinomas. However, it demonstrates more clearly the intrahepatic spread of cholangiocellular carcinomas.

References

1. Ament AE, Haaga JR, Viedenmann SD, et al (1983) Primary sclerosing cholangitis: CT findings. J Comput Assist Tomogr 7: 795-800
2. Berk RN, Armbuster TG, Saltzstein SL (1973) Carcinoma of the porcelain gallbladder. Radiology 106: 29-31
3. Cameroon JL, Sanfey H (1987) Surgical management of proximal cholangio carcinomas. In: Wanebo HJ (ed) Hepatic and biliary cancer. Marcel Dekker, New York, pp 395-415
4. Faintuck J, Levin B (1987) Diagnostic of bile duct cancer. In: Wanebo HJ (ed)Hepatic and biliary cancer. Marcel Dekker, New York, pp 299-338
5. Gibby DG, Hauks JB, Waneboth J, et al (1985) Bile duct carcinoma: diagnostic and treatment. Ann Surg 202:139
6. Greenberg M, Rubin JM, Greenberg BM (1983) Appearance of the gallbladder and biliary tree by CT cholangiography. J Comput Assist Tomogr 7: 788-794
7. Houry S, Lacaine M, Huguier M (1987) Cancer de la vésicule bilaire. In: Encyclopédie des cancers, cancers digestifs. Flamarion Médecine-Sciences, Paris, pp 284-301
8. Kane RA, Jacobs R, Katz J, et al (1984) Porcelain gallbladder: ultrasound and CT appearance. Radiology 152: 137-141
9. Menu Y, Erlinger S (1992) Voies biliaires. In: Buthiau D (ed) TDM et IRM cliniques - Pathologie abdomino-pelvienne. Frison-Roche, Paris, pp 105-113
10. Menu Y, Lorphelin JM, Scherrer A, et al (1985) Sonographic and computed tomographic evaluation of intrahepatic calculi. AJR 145: 579-583
11. Reding R, Duard JL, Lebeau G, Lauwes B (1988) Résultats de l'enquête AFC. In: Launois B, Cubertafond P (eds) Les cancers des voies biliaires extrahépatiques. Masson, Paris, p 58
12. Sako K, Seitzing GL, Garbide E (1957) Carcinoma of the extra hepatic bile duct. Review of the literature and report of six cases. Surgery 41: 416
13. Smathers RL, Lee JK, Heiken JP (1984) Differenciation of complicated cholecystitis from gallbladder carcinoma by computed tomography. AJR 143: 255-259
14. Sorensen K, Glazer G, Francis I (1982) Diagnosis of cystic extasia of intrahepatic bile ducts by computed tomography. J Comput Assist Tomogr 6: 486-489
15. Weibling HH, Dockerty MB, Waugh JM (1949) Carcinoma of the extrahepatic bile ducts. Surg Gynecol Obstet 86:429

CHAPTER 25

Cancer of the esophagus

Clinicians
E. Malaurie, B. Chiche, F. Hecht, M. Gozy, D. Nizri, D. Salandre, M. Bouaziz, P. Piedbois, J.-P. Le Bourgeois, J.-L. Misset

Radiologist
D. Buthiau

The main symptom of cancer of the esophagus is dysphagia leading to the performance of an endoscopic examination. This will visualize the lesion in the majority of cases and allow the biopsies to be taken for histological analysis.

In a few cases, endoscopy will need to be complemented by other investigations, and it is here that CT or MRI have a role to play.

Indications for CT and MRI

The positive diagnosis of the lesion is only rarely made by one or other of these examinations. The only noteworthy example is the presence of a submucosal lesion which may be missed endoscopically or when endoscopy is normal, and other investigations, namely x-ray upper GI under pressure, pH test, and esophageal manometry are negative. Rarely there may be the accidental detection of a lesion during an examination performed for another pathology, for example mediastinal, spinal, cardiopulmonary, hematological or infectious.

The value of these investigations resides primarily in the assessment of the local extent of an endoscopically insuperable lesion (wall involvement), and the presence of lymph node involvement and distant spread (thoracic and high subdiaphragmatic) which helps choose the appropriate treatment. In addition, these investigations can be used to determine the relationships of the tumor with certain critical organs (important prior to radiotherapy) and to monitor progress following treatment.

CT

CT has an important role in the treatment decision by its ability to appreciate the tumor volume (fig. 25.1), to look for a second localization already suggested or demonstrated by the endoscopy, to assess tracheobronchial (fig. 25.1), subdiaphragmatic and lymphatic (fig. 25.2) spread. CT can also:

- demonstrate any contraindications: involvement of the celiac (figs 25.2 & 25.3), supraclavicular nodes or massive mediastinal lymphadenopathy, tracheobronchial invasion, and invasion of unresectable structures;
- plan the surgical technique depending on the relationships of the tumor by evaluating spread preoperatively:
  - to the vital organs (pericardium, trachea, aorta),
  - to lymph nodes (mediastinal, supraclavicular and celiac) (figs 25.2 & 25.3),
  - to the upper esophagus which is often poorly assessed intra-operatively; however, the assessment of the middle and lower thirds of the esophagus is less contributory. According to the series in the literature, attempted curative surgery is possible in 20-45% of esophageal cancers;
- plan the position of treatment volumes and determine anatomical relationships of the critical organs (spinal cord, heart, and lungs; superior pole of the left

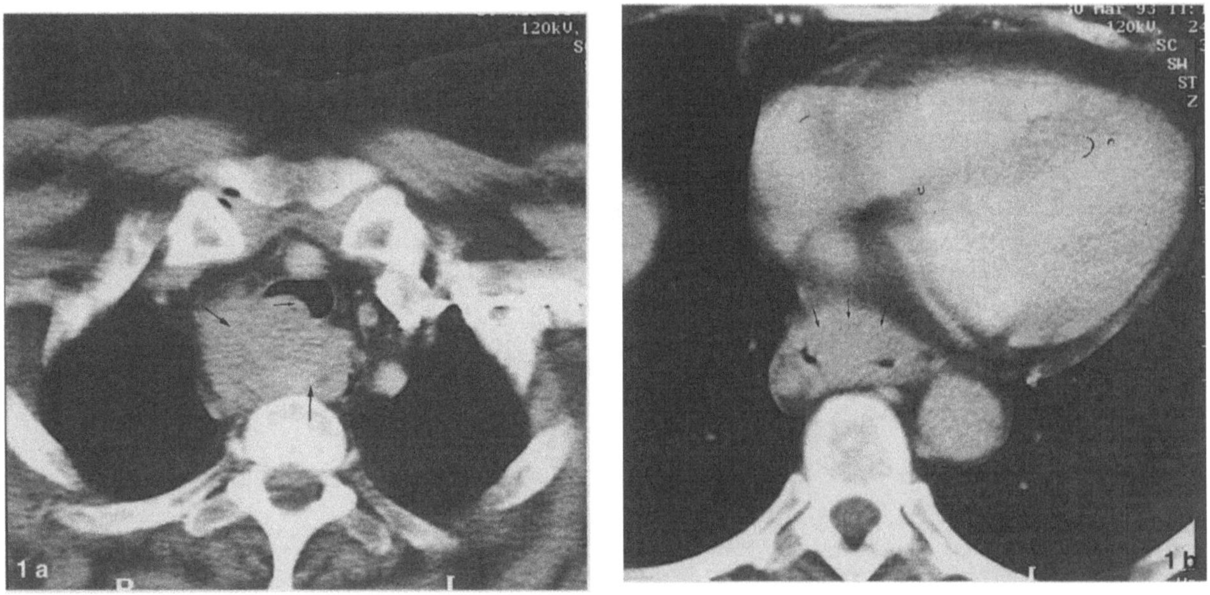

Fig. 25.1 a, b. Cancer of the esophagus on CT. **a** Cancer of the upper third of the esophagus on post-contrast CT: an extensive lesion *(large arrows)* associated with inseparable locoregional lymphadenopathy, an eccentric esophageal lumen and endoluminal spread into the right postero-lateral aspect of the trachea *(small arrow)*; **b** cancer of the esophagus on post-contrast CT: concentric thickening predominantly anteriorly *(small arrows)* with stenosis of the esophageal lumen without any sign of peri-esophageal spread

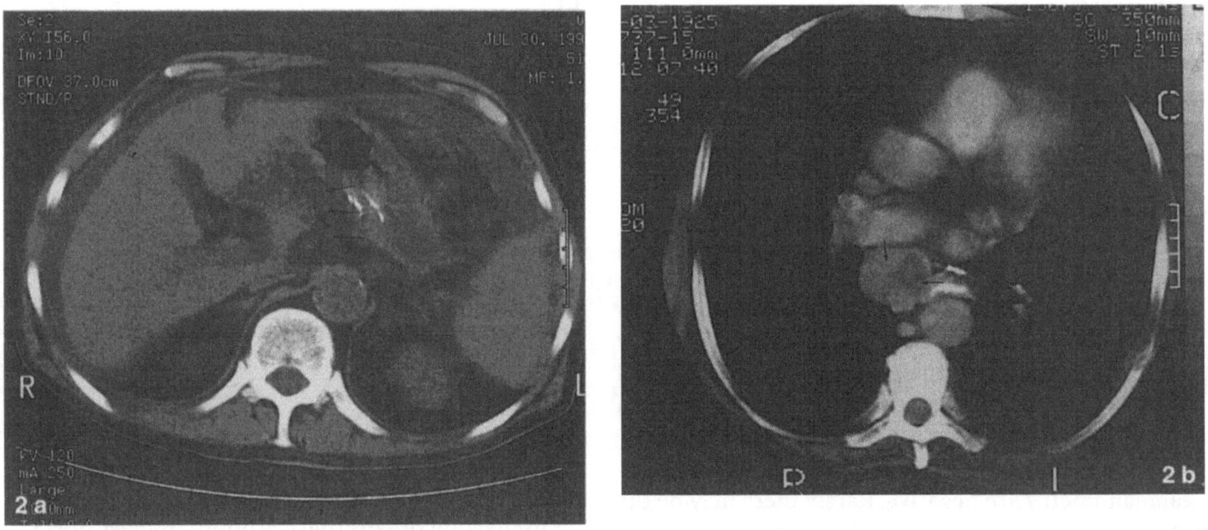

Fig. 25.2 a, b. Lymph node spread from esophageal cancer. **a** Celiac lymph node involvement affecting the nodes on the lesser curvature within the lesser omentum *(small arrows)*. In addition, there is infiltration into the peritoneum appearing as irregular thickening of the intraperitoneal fat with peri-hepato-splenic ascites; **b** subcarinal lymphadenopathy *(arrows)* from esophageal cancer arising in the upper third (not visible on this section)

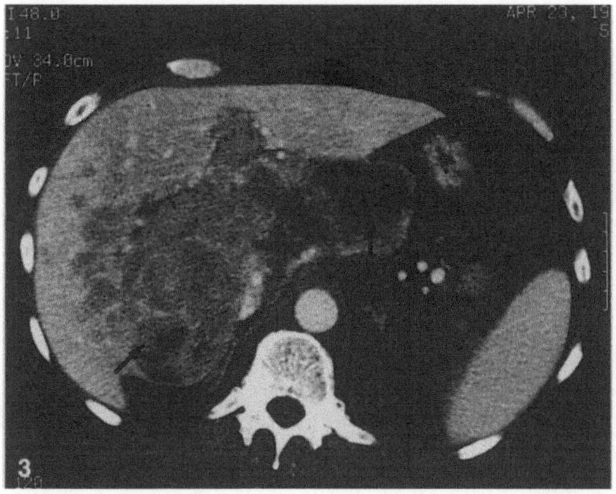
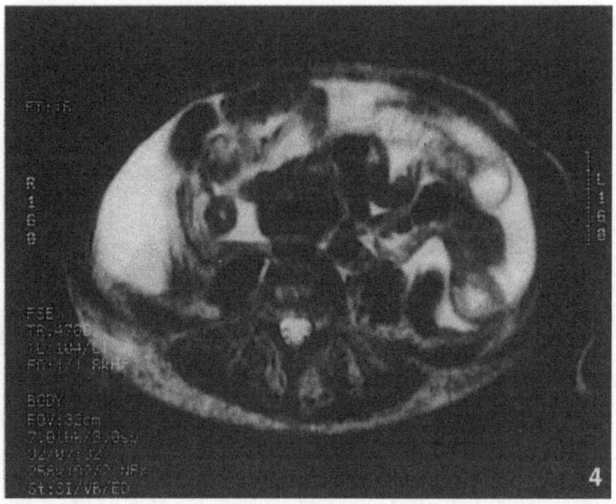

Fig. 25.3. Lymphadenopathy in the celiac and porta hepatis regions (*large arrows*)due to lymph node involvement by cancer of the cardia on post-contrast CT. There is an extensive right and left portal vein thrombosis *(small arrows)* due to obstruction at the porta hepatis and fissure for the ductus venosus

Fig. 25.4. Miliary peritoneal carcinomatosis visible only in the form of diffuse ascites surrounding the ileo-colic bowel loops on sagittal T2 MRI. Micronodular involvement of the peritoneum is not directly discernible using this technique

kidney for irradiation of the celiac axis), and also obtain an accurate dosimetry when radiotherapy is contemplated;
- assess the response to adjuvant treatment (radio- and/or chemotherapy), and determine any indication for a second operation;
- monitor the progress of the lesion, as well as the follow-up of esophagoplasties and detect any recurrence.

Endo-esophageal ultrasound also is important in the evaluation of locoregional spread.

MRI

This has a limited role (fig. 25.4) and is less reliable and of less diagnostic value compared to CT, apart when looking for endoluminal spread.

Signs

CT

There are no specific morphological or density changes to differentiate particularly a benign from a malignant lesion. CT can assess the tumor size, especially prior to radiotherapy, and look for a possible other localization, determine the distance between the superior border of the aortic arch and the upper limit of the tumor (supra- or subaortic lesion). CT can also evaluate all these features prior to any treatment and following any possible adjuvant chemotherapy. CT has no real value in determining the resectability of a lesion since the non-visualization of the peri-esophageal fatty tissue is not specific for tumor infiltration and is therefore not a reliable criterion for planning treatment.

Mediastinal spread:

- Tracheobronchial spread: the only reliable criteria are the demonstration of the endo-tracheo-bronchial nodule (fig. 25.1 a) to correlate with the endoscopic findings, which may or may not cause an endoluminal stenosis. The other significant sign is irregular thickening of the tracheobronchial wall. Simple contiguity between the esophagus and trachea, with or without extrinsic compression and displacement, and loss of the intervening fat plane represent in no way reliable criteria of pathological involvement.

- Spread into the mediastinal fat should be suspected in the presence of soft tissue replacement of the fat planes situated between the esophagus, carina, left main bronchus, trachea, aortic arch or descending aorta or at the level of the aortopulmonary window.

- Spread to the aorta is suspected when the lesion is in direct contact over more than 90° although this is not a specific sign.

Table 25.1. Normal CT and MRI anatomy of the esophagus [1]

Measurements (CT)		
Normal	Diameter: 1 cm (variable, depending on the degree of distension by air) Length: 26 cm Wall thickness: average 2 mm, always < 3 mm	
Pathological	Wall thickening Symmetrical - esophageal varices - inflammation: esophagitis, reflux - hiatus hernia - post-irradiation (mediastinal fibrosis) - infection (monoliasis) - hypertrophy	 Asymmetrical - primary or secondary malignant tumor - tumor, inflammation, initially extra-esophageal infection with direct contiguous spread into the esophagus

There are eight distinct anatomical levels described from superior to inferior:
- cervical esophagus, from the pharyngo-esophageal junction to the base of the neck (CT often limited to this level);
- level of the thoracic apex;
- superior mediastinal esophagus;
- level of the aortic arch;
- level of the carina or left main bronchus;
- subcarinal esophagus;
- retrocardiac esophagus (posterior to the left atrium);
- posterior inframediastinal esophagus (gastro-esophageal junction) which may appear on CT as a mass of the superior part of the lesser curvature of the stomach near to the fissure for the ductus veinosus

Table 25.2. Therapeutic approach depending on the CT findings (reproduced from B. Gayet et al [3])

In cases of mediastinal invasion on CT, the treatment will either call for chemotherapy alone or combined with radiotherapy, or for an initial thoracotomy, or for chemotherapy followed by thoracotomy after improvement in the CT appearances.

In cases of metastatic spread through a non-resectable structure on CT which has been confirmed histologically, the patient is incurable; nonetheless palliative by-pass surgery using a segment of intestine may be indicated. The aim of laser treatment is to improve patient comfort. It should be remembered that this situation may be dramatically changed by adjuvant chemotherapy or radiotherapy or a combination of the two.

In cases of two synchronous tumors, the treatment is:
- a thoracotomy immediately if the superior limit is poorly defined: however, it is often well shown by endoscopy and confirmed by CT;
- or surgery extended into the neck if the position of the tumor is supra-aortic.

– Spread into the pericardium, diaphragm, pleura or cardiac chambers should be suspected in the presence of irregularities or focal nodules, localized thickening or an effusion, contiguous with the lesion although these are not again specific features.

– Spread to the chest wall, often well shown on CT which commonly appears as bone lysis associated with a frequently biconvex, extrapleural chest wall mass.

– The diagnosis of lymph node spread to the middle anterior mediastinal (fig. 25.2 b), posterior, inframediastinal and celiac (fig. 25.2 a) groups depends on size criteria and not on the internal structure of the node (cf. Investigation of thoracic lymph nodes, chapter "Bronchopulmonary cancer"). The upper limit of normal is 6 mm for the celiac nodes.

– Metastastic disease is particularly well shown on CT which assesses the liver, adrenals, retroperitoneal lymph nodes and lungs in a single examination. CT has a significant role in the diagnosis of hepatic metastatic lesions which are more often central than subcapsular.

In the follow-up of patients, CT can detect complications such as pulmonary or subphrenic abscess, med-

Table 25.3. Spread of esophageal cancers on CT [1]

Wall	– asymmetrical non-specific thickening
Trachea, bronchi	– displacement by extrinsic compression: insufficient sign of pathological involvement – irregularities of the wall and endoluminal nodules (stenosis): reliable sign – involvement predominantly of the carina and by direct contiguous spread to the posterior walls
Peri-esophageal fat planes	– loss of the fat line – non-specific – inconstant – only of value if seen on two adjacent sections
Pericardium, left atrium, aorta	– suspected but not confirmed – angle of contact between tumor and aorta; if > 90°: certain invasion; if < 45°: rarely involved; between 45 and 90°: equivocal invasion (in 50% of cases)
Chest wall	- bone (vertebral) and muscle involvement
Diaphragm and pleura	– diagnosis suggested but not absolute – limited for the treatment
Lymphadenopathy	– size criteria – investigation of all the territories from the supraclavicular level to the infra-mediastinal and celiac levels

Table 25.4. CT classifications of cancers of the esophagus

a) Classification of Wutrz et al and TNM (1988) [7]

Primary tumor (T)	
T1	Tumor not visible or mass < 10 mm in diameter
T2	Mass between 10 and 20 mm in diameter
T3	Mass > 20 mm in diameter without any sign of mediastinal invasion
T4	As above + sign of spread to mediastinal structures
Lymph nodes (N)	
N0	No detectable lymphadenopathy
N1	Regional lymphadenopathy (mediastinal and/or perigastric)
Distant metastasis (M)	
M0	No distant metastasis
M1	Distant metastases present (including celiac and cervical lymphadenopathy)

(*) The staging classification is interchangeable with that of the UICC (1977); the diameter criteria for lymphadenopathy are unchanged.

b) Proposed new classification (G. Gayet et al) [3]

Stage I	a	tumor thickness < 1 cm, Na–
	b	tumor thickness < 1 cm, Na
Stage II	a	tumor thickness 1 cm
	b	Nb or Nc
Stage III	a	non-resectable tumor or lymphadenopathy
	b	metastasis or distant lymphadenopathy (paraaortic, supraclavicular, etc.)

Na: peri-esophageal node or node of the cardia; Nb: mediastinal node; Nc: coronary gastric lymph node chain

iastinitis, encysted pleural effusion with or without an empyema, or anastamotic leak. It can also be used to follow-up esophagoplasties and to look for recurrences which are often poorly demonstrated by upper GI x-ray since they are extramucosal.

MRI

Apart from the 3-dimensional studies which demonstrate possible endocavity spread (left atrium), MRI has no particular role in making the diagnosis; the esophageal lesion is better delineated on a T2-weighted sequence although there are significant unfortunate artefacts. Injection of the paramagnetic contrast agent gadolinium does help to define the pathology, but the increase in the signal intensity of the tumor may "hide" the lesion by rendering it isointense to the surrounding fatty tissue.

Conclusion (tables 25.1-25.4)

CT and particularly MRI have no diagnostic role in current practice in esophageal cancer.

However, CT is essential in the assessment of thoracic and abdominal spread allowing correlation of the CT criteria with those of endo-esophageal ultrasound and surgery (tables 25.3 & 25.4). CT accurately localizes the lesion prior to radiotherapy, distinguishes the intra- and extramural lesions, assesses spread to the mediastinum, pleura, viscera and lymph nodes (dependent on simple size criteria) and helps plan radiotherapy.

CT can be used in post-treatment follow-up, particularly after radiotherapy or adjuvant chemotherapy and in the search for recurrent disease.

MRI is rarely indicated in this disease and has no additional value apart from the detection of endoluminal or endocavity spread to adjacent organs when compared to CT.

References

1. Aboulker C, Buthiau D, et al (1991) Œsophage. In: Buthiau D (ed) TDM et IRM Cliniques. Frison Roche, Paris, pp 650-667
2. Becker CD, Barbier P, Porcellini B (1991) CT evaluation of patients undergoing transhiatal esophagectomy for cancer. J Comput Assist Tomogr 10: 607-611
3. Gayet B, Frija J, Cahuzac J, Fékété F (1988) Intérêt de la TDM dans le cancer de l'œsophage; étude prospective et "aveugle". Gastroenterol Clin Biol 12: 23-28
4. Halvorsen RA, et al (1986) Esophageal Cancer Staging by CT: long term follow-up study. Radiology 161: 147-151
5. Mauro MA, et al (1986) CT after uncomplicated esophageal sclerotherapy. AJR 147: 57-60
6. Recht MP, et al (1989) Recurrent esophageal carcinoma at thoracotomy incisions: diagnostic contributions of CT. J Comput Assist Tomogr 13: 58-60
7. Wurtz A, Castaner P (1988) Carcinomes malpighiens de l'œsophage thoracique: quelle classification tomodensitométrique ? Gastroenterol Clin Biol 12: 921- 925

CHAPTER 26

Tumors of the gastrointestinal tract (excluding esophagus): cancer of the stomach, duodenum, small bowel, colon, rectum and anus

Clinicians
B. Chiche, E. Malaurie, D. Nizri, F. Hecht, D. Salandre, P. Piedbois, E. Vuillemin, L. Zelek, J.-P. Le Bourgeois, D. Khayat

Radiologists
C. Aboulker, D. Buthiau, P. Schmit

Morphological assessment of the gastrointestinal tract (GIT) was, until not so long ago, "limited" to endoscopy and/or conventional radiology. Both these methods of examination provide a direct visualization of the mucosa but only an indirect assessment of the wall and extraluminal structures (extrinsic and intramural pathology).

This hole to a large extent is filled by the new imaging techniques such as conventional and endoscopic ultrasound, computed tomography (CT) and magnetic resonance imaging (MRI). These are able to visualize the wall of the gastrointestinal tract and surrounding tissues. In addition, they can give an overall assessment of the whole abdomino-pelvic cavity. However, these techniques cannot replace the classical examinations due to lack of visualization of he mucosa (apart from endoscopic ultrasound). These different examinations are of great value in oncology, not only for the initial assessment of locoregional and general spread but also for repeated follow-up examinations. This results in more accurate treatment planning and prognostic information.

This chapter concentrates on CT which nowadays is the most commonly performed examination due to the technical advances in image reconstruction and the amount of pathological information assimilated specifically from CT.

Ultrasound and MRI are indicated more specifically in certain pathologies.

Indications for CT and MRI

CT

CT is usually performed to assess the extent of a lesion following the prior detection of a mucosal tumor by endoscopy and/or conventional radiology.

More rarely it is performed as the first examination, demonstrating a tumor arising in the digestive tract. Such is the case in the investigation of the cause for:

- a symptomatic or asymptomatic abdominal mass detected incidentally;
- an acute abdomen with the demonstration of an obstruction;
- vague presenting symptoms (loss of energy, elevation of the ESR, unexplained fever, iron-deficiency anemia).

CT is able to localize the tumor with a view to percutaneous biopsy or prior to radiotherapy. It also has an important role in post-treatment follow-up for the detection of recurrences or iatrogenic complications.

MRI

The indications for MRI are infrequent and will be highlighted during the course of this chapter.

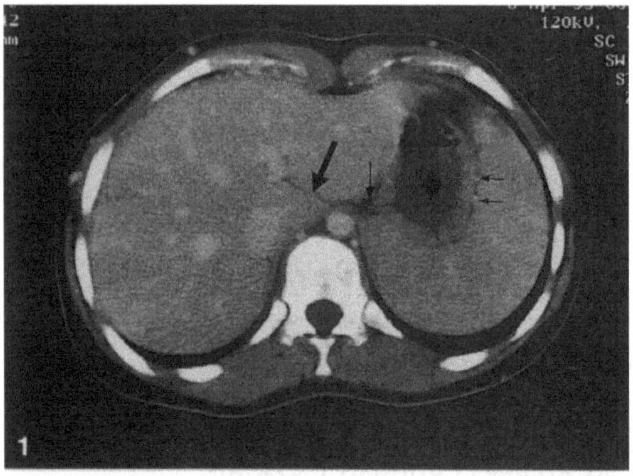

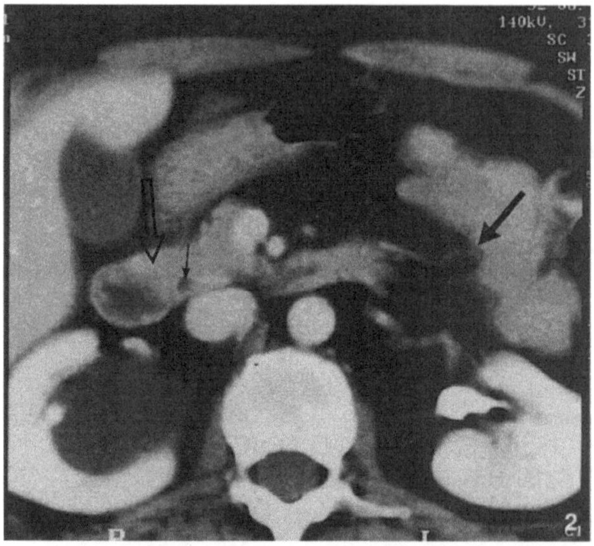

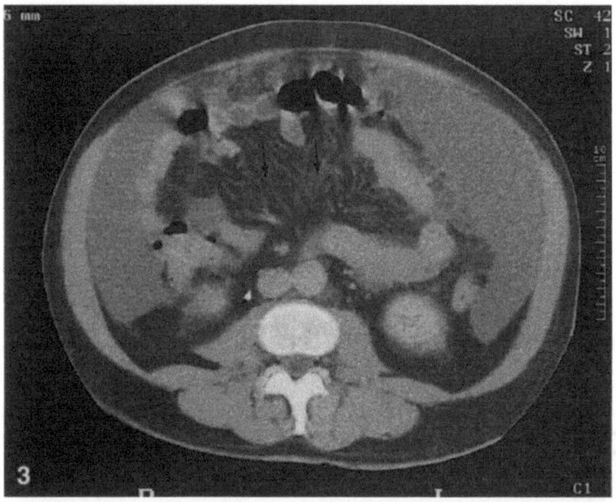

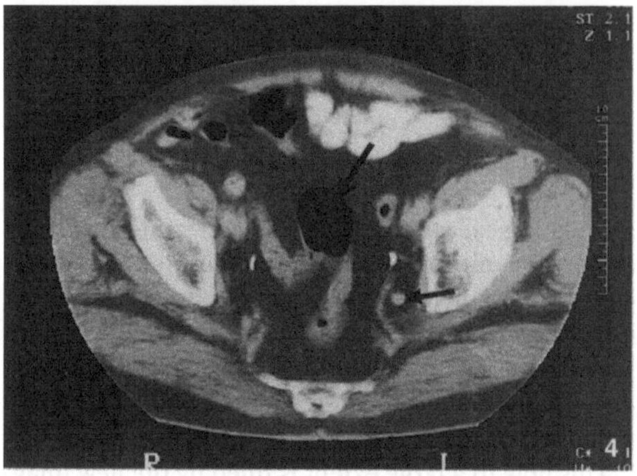

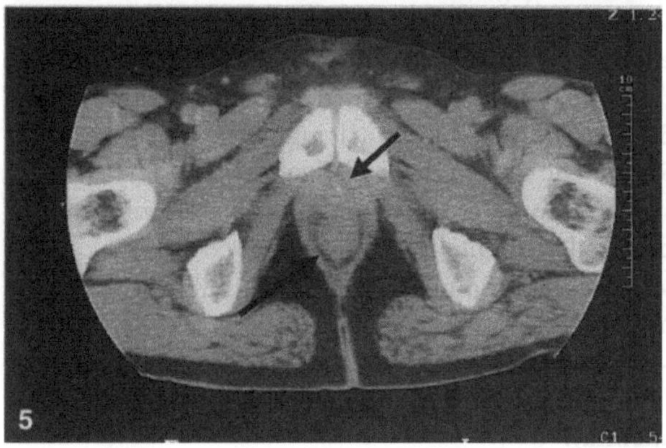

Fig. 26.1. CT: normal stomach. The cardia *(medium arrow)* is the landmark for the fissure of the ductus venosus (Arantius' canal) *(large arrow)*. The gastric fundus (*) is partially filled with residual fluid and air, and some air bubbles are caught in the gastric folds. Small external nodules correspond to the gastro-epiploic vessels *(small arrows)*

Fig. 26.2. Normal duodenum. Inferior portion of the second part merging with the pancreatic head *(hollow arrow)*, good visualization of the distal main biliary tract *(small arrow)*, empty small bowel loops simulating an abdominal mass, but the relationship with one of the segmental mesenteric vessels gives the diagnosis *(large arrow)*

Fig. 26.3. CT: normal mesentery *(small arrows)* in a patient with ascites. Fan-like distribution of the segmental mesenteric vessels which diverge towards the small bowel loops

Fig. 26.4. CT: sigmoid and rectosigmoid junction. Distension of a sigmoid loop by an air bubble *(large arrow)* and small subcentimeter sized left internal iliac lymph node *(small arrow)*

Fig. 26.5. CT: perineal rectum and anal canal *(large arrow)*; bulbar urethra, dorsal artery of the penis *(small arrow)*

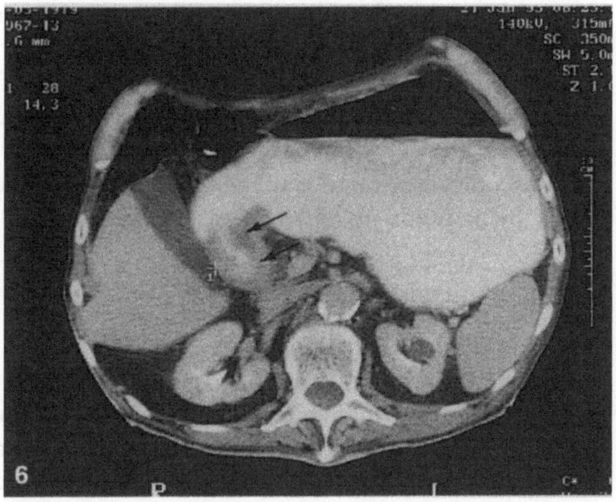

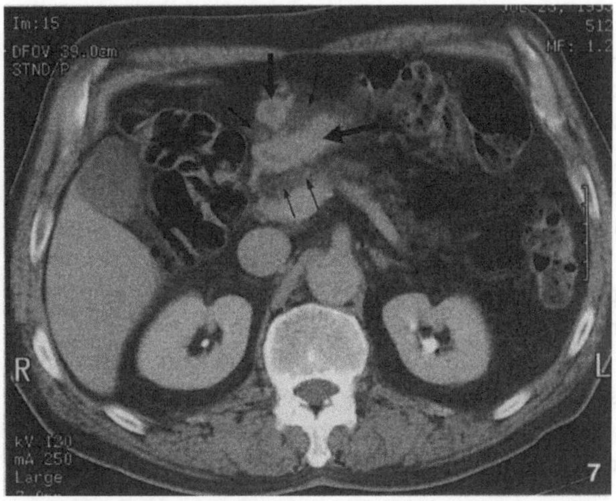

Fig. 26.6. CT: gastric cancer. Cuff of circumferential thickening of the antral wall *(arrows)* (14 mm) adjacent to the gallbladder *(cross and 1)* and inferior vena cava. Subtle changes in the peri-antral fat. At surgery, peritoneal carcinomatosis with multiple granulations which were not visible on the CT, and invasion of the gallbladder wall

Fig. 26.7. CT: gastric cancer. Perilesional peritoneal invasion from a cancer of the antrum *(large arrow)* appearing as increased density in the peri-antral fatty tissue *(small arrows)* and metastatic lymph nodes *(medium arrow)*

Other investigations

Of the other investigations, endoscopic ultrasound is a very useful technique in the initial assessment of the tumor extent, particularly in determining the depth of mural infiltration and involvement of adjacent lymph nodes. This helps to determine more accurately as to whether preoperative radiotherapy is indicated. In addition, it is possible to monitor anastamoses.

Anatomy of the digestive tract on CT

See figures 26.1-26.5.

Radiological signs according to the pathology

Adenocarcinomas of the GIT

These include primary tumors, metastases and tumor invasion by direct contiguous spread to the organs of the digestive tract.

Although not belonging to the same pathological entities, metastases and invasion by direct contiguous spread are suspected to be due to adenocarcinomas; wall thickening is not specific, the appearance often being identical; spread occurring via the mesocolon either in the bowel-regional viscera direction or in the reverse direction.

Imaging is involved in the initial assessment prior to any treatment to determine prognosis and, subsequently, in the follow-up of patients who have been treated or are undergoing treatment.

Stomach

Adenocarcinomas (figs 26.6 & 26.7)

Mural thickening is polymorphic

It may appear in the form of a vegetation manifesting as an intraluminal filling defect; alternatively there may be mural thickening of variable degree and extent, sometimes cicumferential but very rarely diffuse as in linitis plastica (1%). The advanced stages of this latter condition are associated with microgastria.

Transmural infiltration is suspected in the presence of mural thickening [22] of greater than 2 cm which is highly suggestive of serosal infiltration, or by changes in the fat plane (ill defined increased density of the fat, dense linear bands...).

Lymph node enlargement is very common (> 80%) and usually occurs in the celiac, coronary gastric and splenic lymph node chains, porta hepatis with possible biliary obstruction, retrocrural and median retroperitoneal spaces.

Possible spread to the regional organs includes:
- cancers of the gastric fundus invading the left lobe of the liver, diaphragm, cardia and lower esophagus, as well as the spleen via the intermediate gastrosplenic ligament;
- cancer of the antrum extending into the pancreas, transverse colon, left lobe of the liver and gallbladder.

Imaging is often disappointing for the diagnosis of peritoneal (parietal peritoneum, lesser omentum) metastases.

The detection of secondary deposits in the liver, spleen, adrenal and lung is common.

In addition, ovarian tumors (Kruckenberg tumors) may mimic primary ovarian tumors.

Results

In the initial staging of gastric cancer, CT is disappointing [12, 22, 23, 35, 39].

In the study by Sussmann [36], the staging was incorrect in 47% of patients, underestimated in 31% and overestimated in 16%.

Lymph node involvement is often underestimated with a sensitivity of 67%; the assessment is difficult along the greater curvature. In addition, confluent lymph node masses often coalesce in a tumor mass. One advantage of CT must be emphasized, namely the visualization of the retroperitoneal and retrocrural lymph nodes which are not routinely assessed surgically.

Spread to the pancreas is even more difficult to predict with a sensitivity of only 27% [39] to 60% [12].

Peritoneal carcinomatosis is not apparent in 30% of patients.

Despite well aware of these limitations, Scatarige [35] suggests a routine CT coupled with ultrasound for the following reasons:
- the presence of one or several lymph node or visceral metastases obviates the need for exploratory laparotomy in the knowledge that the tumor will be even more extensive. However, this does not rule out palliative by-pass surgery or wide excision;
- an exploratory laparotomy with excision may be contemplated in the presence of an isolated cancer. This will include an assessment of the abdominal extent, often underestimated on CT;
- CT has a particular value in the assessment of regions not included in the laparotomy (i.e. posterior inframediastinal space, retroperitoneal space, adrenals...).

In the post-therapeutic follow-up, CT is indicated for the detection of a peri-anastamotic recurrence in conjunction with endoscopy for a mucosal recurrence, and endoscopic ultrasound is better for mural recurrence. CT may also detect a lymph node recurrence, or hepatic metastasis.

MRI has no proven role apart from the theoretical advantage of its ability to perform sagittal and coronal sections for the detection of diaphragmatic spread.

Endoscopic ultrasound is valuable for cancers of the cardia, pylorus and juxtapyloric gastric antrum.

Gastric metastases

These are rarely isolated findings.

Bronchial carcinoma, breast cancer and malignant melanoma have a high metastatic potential by the hematogenous route. Tumor infiltration occurs from the submucosa towards the serosa, mesocolon and omentum.

Full thickness involvement of the wall results in a pseudolinitis appearance which is often extremely difficult to distinguish from the primary linitis plastica. Lymphadenopathy is, however, much more infrequent in the pseudolinitis, and the commonly associated infiltration of the omentum causes spicules along the gastric borders. The level of the tumor markers (CA 15-3) and the clinical context are also important factors.

Contiguous spread

This occurs via the ligaments: gastrocolic for the cancers of the transverse colon, gastrosplenic for cancers of the pancreatic tail.

Duodenum and small intestine

Adenocarcinomas [15, 26, 35]

These are infrequent, arising mainly in the duodenum and jejunum, and present with chronic bleeding or partial obstruction. The diagnosis is often made at the stenotic stage with associated proximal dilatation. They may be responsible for dilatation of the bile ducts due to direct compression, invasion of the common bile duct or compression by lymphadenopathy.

There is often a paucity or absence of intra-abdominal fat which prevents precise delineation of the mural thickening and spread to adjacent organs; attempts to determine resectability of the tumor are disappointing.

Lymph involvement is rare. The diagnosis is obtained by endoscopy.

Ultrasound and endoscopic ultrasound have a role in the preoperative assessment (locoregional and distant spread).

CT is useful for the differential diagnosis of duodenal extension from regional cancers: pancreatic head (difficult diagnosis due to the paucity or absence of the fatty interface), common bile duct, gallbladder, gastric antrum, ascending colon, right kidney and lymphadenopathies (lymph node metastases from bronchial, breast, or skin cancers or lymphoma).

Tumors of the ampulla of Vater are differentiated by the associated symptomatology (icterus, bleeding). Ultrasound and sometimes endoscopic ultrasound are sufficient for the pre-treatment assessment. CT has a role in large ampullary lesions in attempting to differentiate them from a pancreatic carcinoma: the ampullary tumor appears as a filling defect projecting into the duodenal lumen.

Metastases

Initial involvement is submucosal as with the stomach and cancer, the differentiation from a primary cancer is impossible.

Colon and rectum (figs 26.8-26.11)

The colo-rectal cancers are the commonest of the GIT cancers (25,000 new cases per year in France). 75% of the colorectal cancers occur in the rectosigmoid region. In view of its frequency and the rich anatomy within the pelvis, cancer of the rectum is described in this paragraph.

The principle treatment for rectal cancers is surgery and provides almost the only chance of "cure" for stages A and B1 for which the survival rate is 90-95%.

Adjuvant treatment is given the tumor with stage B2 or more.

The incidence of pelvic recurrence can be reduced by 50% with external radiotherapy (EORTC, NSABD). The addition of chemotherapy (5FU) further improves the results in terms of local control and survival rate. The treatment strategies must be understood by the radiologist who will influence the imaging examinations and the content of the report.

Surgical treatment:

- High rectum: rectosigmoid resection with end-to-end or side-to-end anastamosis;
- Mid and low rectum: the decision to perform sphincter conserving surgery depends on the cancer-free margin: a minimum of 2 cm between the inferior margin of the tumor and the levator ani muscles; above this, a colo-anal anastamosis is possible; below this, an abdominoperineal resection (APR) with a permanent left sided colostomy in necessary. Sphincter conservation may be possible after preoperative radiotherapy. The level of mural spread relative to the anal sphincter therefore represents a critical factor in the choice of surgery or preoperative protocol.

Preoperative radiotherapy in the case of an infiltrative tumor reduces the rate of pelvic recurrences. Recent studies have clearly shown that the addition of adjuvant chemotherapy increases the survival rate of these patients.

The initial assessment is undertaken by a digital rectal examination, proctoscopy and colonoscopy with biopsy, CT and endoscopic ultrasound when the tumor is accessible. Barium enema is requested by the majority of clinicians because it gives an overall view of the tumor and the rest of the colon and is the only objective element available to the surgeon preoperatively. The tumor can be classified using this approach (table 26.1).

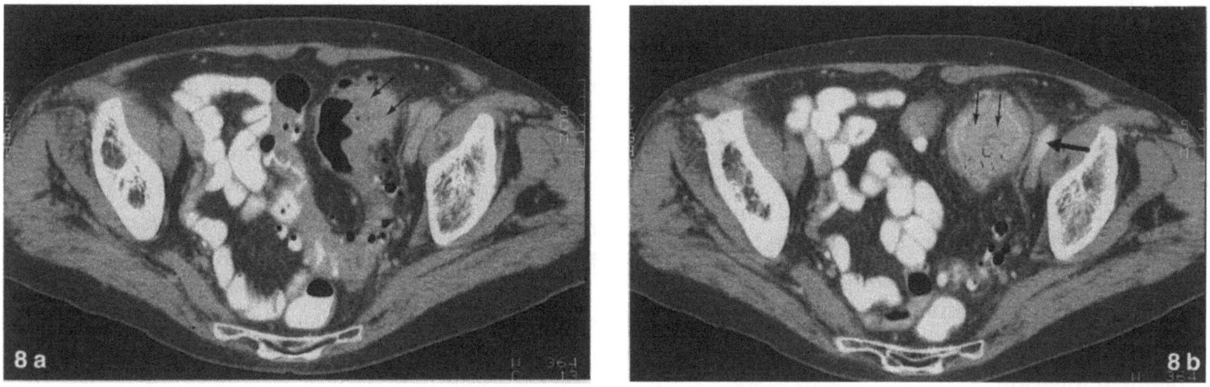

Fig. 26.8 a, b. CT: sigmoid cancer. Barium enema demonstrated a stenosis in a segment of sigmoid colon with diverticular disease in a febrile patient. The diagnosis of a sigmoid cancer with break of the serosa can be made on CT, and the bowel enhanced wall mass *(small arrows)* has spiculated borders and compresses the left internal iliac vein *(large arrow)*

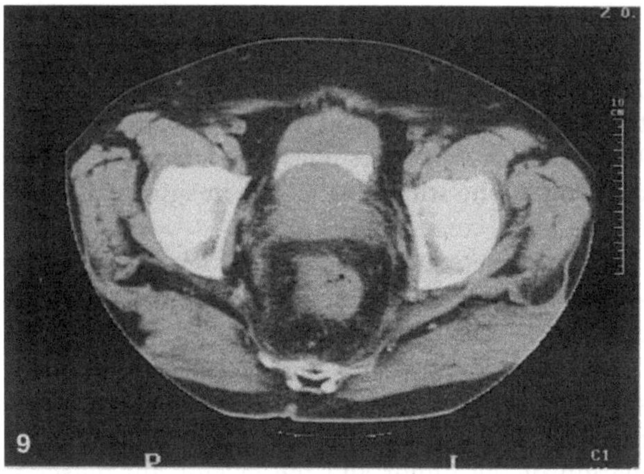

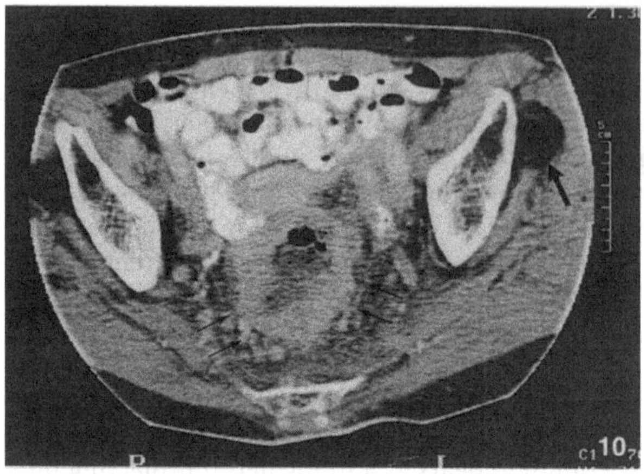

Fig. 26.9. CT: rectal cancer. Circumferential thickening of the rectal wall; indistinct rectal contour with small linear and punctiform opacities in the perirectal fat suggestive of a break of the serosa, confirmed at operation

Fig. 26.10. CT: large rectal cancer; the periphery of the tumor *(small arrows)* is indistinct and the perirectal fat is completely heterogeneous, speckled with numerous nodular and linear densities. Incidental lipoma of the left gluteus minimus *(large arrow)*

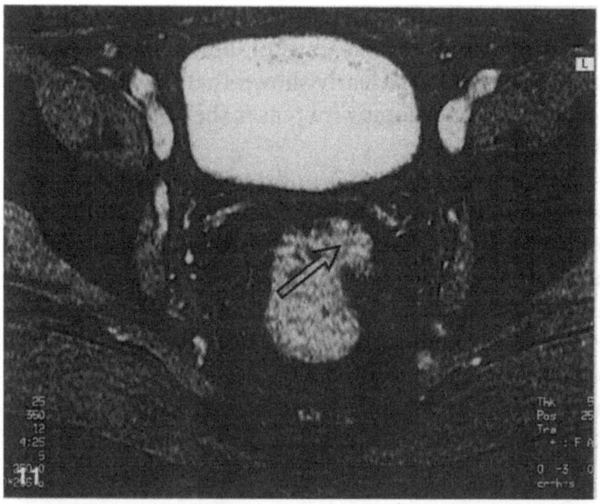

Fig. 26.11. MRI: rectal cancer. Axial post-gadolinium T1-weighted image. Almost circumferential bowel wall thickening with spiculated borders related to a subserosal break *(hollow arrow)*

Initial assessment

• *CT*

The tumor: it is polymorphic with endoluminal, often ulcerated nodules; ulcero-infiltrative appearance with mural thickening > 5 mm; endo- or exoluminal mass, often ulcerated on the mucosal aspect and containing several areas of necrosis, sometimes with calcifications (mucoid adenocarcinoma). However, it is usually not visualized.

Regional invasion

Apart from the changes in the fat already described, thickening of the perirectal fascia is a good indicator of invasion of the peripheral fat.

Extension may involve the internal genitalia (seminal vesicles or prostate, uterus or ovaries), urinary tract (bladder with a possible fistula in cases of intravesical air, adjacent ureteric dilatation), pelvic small bowel loops, pelvic musculature (obturator internus, piriformis, sacrococcygeus, gluteus maximus...), the parametrium, sacrum or coccyx...

Lymph node (perirectal, pedicular, mesenteric) spread is present in 33% of cases at the time of diagnosis.

Metastases

Hepatic metastases (present in 40% of cases), sometimes contain areas of calcification.

Table 26.1. Classification of rectal cancers

Duke's	Modified Duke's by Astler and Coller	CT classification according to Thoeni	TNM according to UICC	MRI classification according to Guinet
A: limited to the bowel wall	A: limited to the mucosa, negative nodes	I: endoluminal nodule without wall thickening	T1: mucosal and/or submucosal involvement	T1: limited to the bowel wall
B: extension beyond the bowel wall without lymph node involvement	B1: invasion of the muscle without break of the serosa and without lymph node involvement	II: wall thickening > 5 mm without invasion of the regional fat	T2: limited to the serosa or perirectal fat	T2: involvement of the serosa and perirectal fat
	B2: involvement of the serosa without perirectal invasion, without lymph node involvement			
C: with lymph node involvement	C1: lymph node involvement, tumor limited to the rectal wall	IIIA: bowel wall thickening of mass with locoregional spread	T3: spread to the perirectal organs	T3: limited to adjacent organs
	C2: lymph node involvement, tumor extending beyond the serosa	IIIB: IIIA + spread to the pelvic side wall muscles	T4: spread beyond adjacent organs	T4: spread beyond adjacent organs
		IV: distant metastases	N0: no lymphadenopathy	N1: pararectal lymph node involvement
	D: distant metastases		N1: pararectal and inferior mesenteric nodal involvement	N2: mesenteric nodal involvement
			N2: iliac and para-aortic nodal involvement	N3: iliac and para-aortic nodal involvement
			M: metastases	M: metastases

Ovarian metastases (between 5 and 8%) may appear identical to primary ovarian tumors (Kruckenberg tumor). For this reason, a primary GIT cancer must be excluded for any ovarian tumor. Conversely, the presence of ovarian metastases must be excluded in any GIT cancer. Bilateral oophorectomy is the treatment of choice in post-menopausal women.

Adrenal lesions and peritoneal spread are not uncommon.

Differential diagnosis

CT is usually performed as a second line investigation following endoscopy and biopsy, and therefore the differential diagnosis is rarely a problem.

However, it is not possible on CT to diagnose the benign or malignant nature of an endoluminal nodule detected on a routine scan. Any bowel wall thickening due to inflammatory procto-colitis or inflammatory spread from pancreatitis can simulate a GIT tumor, but the clinical context gives a clue to the diagnosis.

Perforation of the tumor, with or without an abscess collection, is often difficult to distinguish from sigmoiditis due to the marked regional inflammatory changes; the presence of mural thickening, focal or diffuse, should always raise the suspicion of cancer and may alter the treatment strategy.

Colonic metastases, rarely isolated, cannot be differentiated from colon cancer by their CT appearances alone; similarly colonic or rectal endometriosis may also be difficult to distinguish.

In the presence of a frozen pelvis, it is difficult to determine the original organ of the primary cancer. The clinical history from the patient is important and may provide clues (hematuria, rectal bleeding, vaginal bleeding).

What is the role of CT in the staging of rectal cancers [2, 3, 19, 21, 29, 31, 40-43]?

Numerous authors have reported the results of CT in the assessment of rectal cancers. The results are disappointing and difficult to compare due to the extremely variable methods of assessment, some relatively old studies and series which include patients in very different stages of the disease. In addition, some studies do not include a lymph node assessment or group together the perirectal and pedicular nodes (apart from in the most recent study by Guinet [21]).

The initial examination was only performed correctly in 60% of cases in Thompson's series [42], 71% in Guinet's [21], 81% in Van Waes' [43]; 92% in Thoeni's [40], but this latter series included a large number of advanced cancers.

Infiltration of the perirectal fat appears "fork-shaped" in 60-79% of cases [2, 19].

The underestimation of tumor extent is due to the fact that CT cannot differentiate the different layers of the bowel wall, and its inability to visualize micro-breaks of the serosa and micro-invasion of the regional fat.

The lower limit of the tumor is less well defined than by rectal examination or colonoscopy.

The sensitivity for lymph node detection is poor, 22% in a study by Thompson [42]. Guinet [21] distinguishes the perirectal from the pedicular lymph nodes (sensitivity 63%). The specificity is mediocre; the size of the node is the only criterion to indicate tumor involvement, an enlarged node may simply be inflammatory, and a small node may be infiltrated by tumor.

CT therefore is of little value in the initial assessment of early stage tumors. It is more useful however, for more advanced stages of the disease as shown in the study by Thoeni [40] by demonstrating spread to viscera and regional muscles.

It is likely, however, that the routine performance of fine sections (2 mm) will improve the accuracy rates.

Endoscopic ultrasound brings a new dimension by its ability to distinguish the different layers of the bowel wall allowing assessment of intramural and perirectal tumor spread with an accuracy rate varying from 83-92% [14].

The sensitivity of lymph node assessment increases to 82%, but the specificity remains poor (59%) for the same reasons as CT.

It is less accurate than CT in the determination of the distance between the inferior margin of the tumor and the levator ani muscles, but this can be improved by the use of a linear probe.

• *MRI [18, 20, 21, 29]*

Axial sections from the level of the anal margin to the common iliac vessels are complemented by sagittal or coronal section.

The tumor appears hypointense on T1-weighted imaging, well silhouetted by the signal void of the insufflated air and by the high signal intensity of the peripheral fat.

The peripheral fat is assessed on T1-weighted imaging, appearing hyperintense. Extraserosal spread appears as a heterogeneity in the fat; a viscus involved by tumor appears enlarged with a signal identical to that of the tumor on T2-weighted imaging.

Lymph node assessment: the perirectal lymph nodes are hypointense on T1-weighted imaging within the hyperintense fat.

MRI can estimate the distance between the lower limit of the tumor and the insertion of the levator muscles with the anus in planes that CT cannot perform (sagittal sections: anterior or posterior tumor, coronal sections: laterally situated tumor).

Guinet [21] found similar results for preoperative assessment in a comparative study using MRI and CT in 21 patients. The assessment of spread was accurate in 76% of cases on MRI alone and 71% on CT. In addition, MRI was no better than CT in the assessment of the upper and lower limits of the tumor, and both remain inferior to the rectal examination. The sagittal sections do not improve the accuracy of tumor localization .

At the moment, MRI does not give any additional information in the local staging even though some authors consider it that it is better for the assessment of tumor spread into the perirectal fat. The future of MRI is undoubtedly related to the detection of small hepatic metastases for which it would appear to be more accurate than CT.

In practice, there is no unanimously accepted protocol, and the examination technique varies with personal experience and depends mainly on the local availability. We have tried to define an examination protocol which can be modified depending on the findings of the initial clinical examination.

For the assessment of the wall and perirectal fat, the clinical and rectal examinations guide the choice of investigation:

- in the presence of an extensive tumor, the rectal examination revealing a fixed mass and perirectal lymph nodes, CT is performed straight-away and will give a relatively accurate anatomical assessment;
- in the presence of a localized tumor, endoscopic ultrasound alone is sufficient. For tumors which do

not extend beyond the muscle, surgical treatment alone is indicated. If endoscopic ultrasound demonstrates an infiltrative tumor or associated satellite lymphadenopathy, surgery is complemented by radiotherapy and, in many cases, chemotherapy.

In the presence of rectal stenosis, endoscopic ultrasound is replaced by CT. However, the current popularity for preoperative radiotherapy makes it necessary to perform a pelvic CT even though this is not strictly necessary for staging purposes. A combination of ultrasound and CT is sufficiently reliable for assessment of the liver and the rest of the abdomen.

• *Classification of tumors of the rectum*

There are numerous classifications which are set out in table 26.1. Most surgeons use the Duke's classification. Endoscopic ultrasound, by its ability to analyze the bowel wall, combined with CT more closely approaches the TNM classification proposed by the International Union Against Cancer (UICC).

Follow-up (figs 26.12-26.14)

Pelvic recurrences result from tumor micro-aggregates persisting from the time of surgical excision which was judged to be macroscopically clear. Metastases occur from systemic micro-emboli arising from the tumor, and the incidence is sometimes increased by surgery.

Locoregional radiotherapy for rectal cancers reduces the risk of recurrence (cf treatment of rectal cancer). However, this does not treat the distant micrometastases.

The frequency of local recurrence is variable and depends on the stage and treatment, and the majority occur within the first two years.

The recurrence rate is primarily dependent *on the degree of intramural tumor extension:* the frequency is virtually nil for cancers confined to the muscle wall and increases to 25% for those involving the serosa and/or perirectal fat [10].

The presence of lymphadenopathy increases the rate recurrence which is 4% in the absence of nodal involvement rising to 50% with lymph node spread [10].

Recurrences are often associated with involvement of the lymph nodes of the regional small bowel, pelvic carcinomatosis and distant metastasis.

The patients at high risk can be identified by the pre- and peroperative assessment in order to plan subsequent follow-up.

Wide surgical excision is the only curative treatment which is always difficult in performing an anterior resection or an abdomino-perineal resection. It is for this reason that the diagnosis should be made as early as possible by regular follow-up examinations; quick repeat surgery would theoretically improve the prognosis. This can be greatly facilitated by previous radiotherapy.

The incidence of distant metastases increases with the degree of bowel invasion and the presence of lymph node involvement.

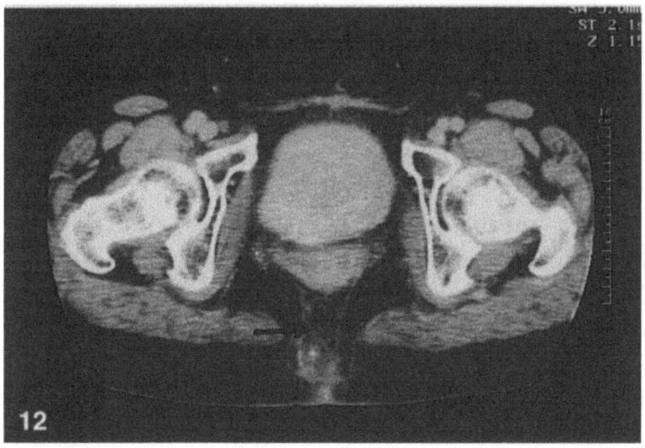

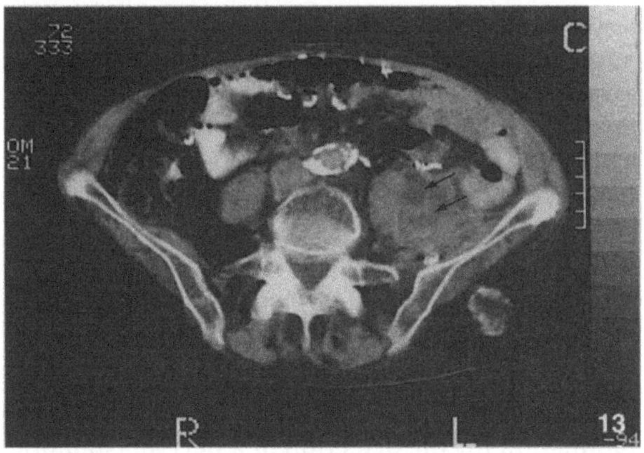

Fig. 26.12. CT: CT appearances at an early stage following radiotherapy and abdomino-perineal resection for anal cancer. The rectal bed is filled by posterior displacement of the vesico-genital structures. Post-treatment linear densities in the posterior fat *(arrow)*. Any changes in this appearance are suspicious

Fig. 26.13. CT: recurrence of cancer of the left colon following anterior resection and anastamosis. Heterogeneous mass between the spine and left iliac wing involving the iliacus and psoas muscles *(arrows)*

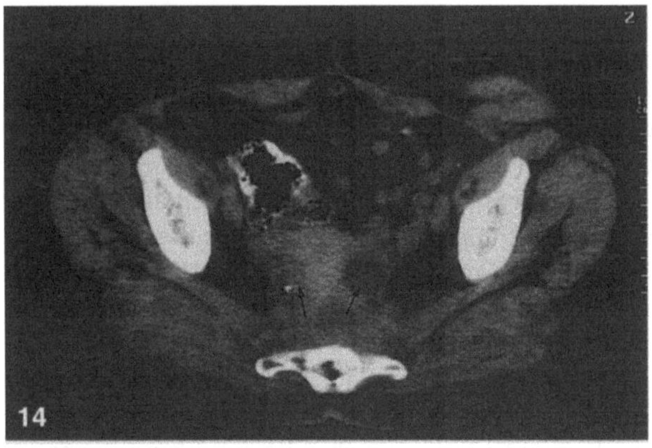

Fig. 26.14. CT: recurrence of rectal cancer after abdomino-perineal resection. Large presacral heterogeneous mass with indistinct borders containing necrotic areas *(arrows)*

The detection of pelvic recurrences [6, 10, 14, 17, 29, 37, 42] is made by:

- clinical examination, particularly rectal and vaginal examination that are extremely important, followed by a battery of appropriate investigations in cases of a suspected abnormality. In male patients after an abdomino-perineal resection, the perineum is inaccessible; in females, a vaginal examination allows a good clinical assessment;
- tumor markers, ACE and CA 19-9: their levels improve the predictive value. However, there is a large number of false positives (CA 19-9).

A persistent elevation of their levels on successive blood tests is highly suspicious of tumor progression (recurrence or metastasis).

– Following anterior resection of the rectum, the recurrence may be mucosal, submucosal or peri-anastamotic:

- endoscopy is the best examination for a mucosal recurrence and should be performed every six months for three years; it is also able to examine the rest of the colon in the search for new lesions, polyps or cancers. Barium enema, as the second line investigation following failed endoscopy, is sometimes useful in the detection of mucosal or submucosal lesions;
- theoretically, endoscopic ultrasound has an important role in the detection of a submucosal or peri-anastamotic recurrence; however, anastamotic scarring or a stenosis at the suture line may cause problems.

In this instance, CT is indicated as the second line examination for the detection of a peri-anastamotic recurrence. It is therefore important to have a reference baseline scan performed at least 2-3 months after surgery.

– Following an abdomino-perineal resection, a vaginal examination is only possible for clinical follow-up and becomes extremely important.

There is complete agreement among different authors that CT has a vital role in this situation.

Abdomino-perineal resection results in a "rearrangement" of the pelvic structures with a polymorphic appearance; it is for this reason that a baseline examination is necessary one or two months following the treatment to allow time for the post-operative or post-radiotherapy changes to settle. Any alteration from this initial post-operative scan should be considered to be suspicious.

The rectal bed is replaced by altered fatty tissue and becomes heterogeneous due to the numerous dense bands of scar tissue.

CT may demonstrate an homogeneous, essentially midline and symmetrical mass with boundaries which may or may not be well defined, a concave outline and a diameter often less than 3 cm; this structure may reduce in size over several months or remain unchanged. This stability is reassuring and suggestive of a fibrotic process.

CT should be performed every six months for the first three years; any change in the imaging appearances is always suspicious with a mass or an increase in the size of a nodule which was initially classified as benign.

Recurrent disease is globular, greater than 5 cm in size, causing compression on the adjacent viscera; there is often associated regional lymphadenopathy, pelvic carcinomatosis, metastasis... The lesion is enhanced in a heterogeneous fashion with areas of necrosis.

The diagnosis of a recurrence is more difficult in the presence of a poorly defined infiltration, particularly following radiotherapy. Serial measurements of tumor markers can be of great value in this situation. The differential diagnosis is hematoma or abscess in the first few months following surgery. It is relatively easy to differentiate a hematoma by its natural evolution and solitary nature; an abscess may be associated with inflammatory lymph node enlargement, changes in the adjacent fat, mural thickening at the anastamosis and sometimes mimics recurrent disease.

If there is any doubt, a CT guided biopsy is indicated using a large needle (16 or 18 gauge).

MRI [4, 18, 20] has a role in the differentiation between tumor (hypointense on T1-weighted imaging and hyperintense on T2-weighted imaging) and fibrosis (hypointense on both T1- and T2-weighted imaging).

However, false positives have been described in the presence of fibrosis mixed with inflammatory and hemorrhagic processes which are more likely after pre- or post-operative radiotherapy. Similarly, false negatives may occur in certain tumors which evoke an intense desmoplastic reaction giving a low signal intensity on T2-weighted imaging. If doubt remains in the presence of a heterogeneous mass of intermediate signal intensity, only biopsy can provide a definitive answer.

Anus [32, 36, 37]

Most cancers (90%) of the anal canal are due to the Malpighian epithelioma (subpectinal zone) and cloacal epithelioma (transitional zone). Sarcomas and malignant melanomas are much more infrequent, and the cancers of the anal margin of the cutaneous type are not dealt with here. The treatment has been revolutionized by adjuvant chemotherapy and radiotherapy which conserve the sphincter function. The small tumors of less than 5 cm without lymphadenopathy can be treated by external radiotherapy and curietherapy (radium treatment). The larger tumors or those with associated lymphadenopathy cannot have curietherapy and are treated by a combination of external radiotherapy and chemotherapy. Surgical intervention by abdomino-perineal resection is reserved for failures of combined radio-chemotherapy in cases of non-sterilization of lesions, local or lymph node recurrence, or finally in the presence of a large destructive process which does not allow conservation of the anal sphincter.

Initial assessment

This is achieved by a combination of rectal examination which assesses tumor infiltration and detects perirectal lymph nodes, vaginal examination, proctoscopy and biopsy, a search for inguinal lymphadenopathy, pelvic CT and the more recently introduced endoscopic ultrasound.

The pathological CT appearances of cancers of the anus are excellently described by Scherrer [36] in a series of 26 patients using contrast enhanced fine sections.

The tumor

The tumor may be invisible with a normal CT appearance (6 out of 26 cases). It is sometimes directly visible as a small hypodense area within the anorectal musculature (5 out of 26 cases). Alternatively it may be apparent by only indirect signs when it is isodense (11 out of 26 cases): symmetrical bulging of the anal sphincter; asymmetry and irregularity of the levator ani, asymmetry of the perianal fat; linear opacities in the ischio-rectal or ischio-anal fossae suggesting tumor permeation.

Lymph nodes

The perirectal lymph nodes drain into the inferior mesenteric group; the accessory hypogastric node is rarely involved.

The incidence of pelvic lymph node involvement correlates with the size of the tumor, its localization on the superior anal canal and an undifferentiated histology.

Rectal examination under general anesthesia is performed to detect perirectal lymph nodes; CT has a fairly good sensitivity because the involved lymph nodes are often larger than those in rectal cancers. The role of endoscopic ultrasound in this study is described in the section on rectal cancers.

Distant lymph node spread involves the superficial inguinal group, particularly the supero-medial group (separated from the infero-medial group by the crossing of the long saphenous vein) which drain to the external, common iliac and para-aortic nodes. They drain mainly the cancers of the inferior canal and can be assessed by clinical examination and CT.

The prognosis deteriorates with increasing size of the tumor, superior localization and initial involvement of the inguinal and/or pelvic lymph nodes.

Follow-up

There is a fine margin between insufficient radiotherapy required for sterilizing the lesion and excessive radiation which is responsible for radionecrosis, occurring in 11.7% of cases [32].

Pelvic (iliac and inferior mesenteric) lymph node recurrences often occur within 18 months of radiotherapy, and the prognosis is bleak.

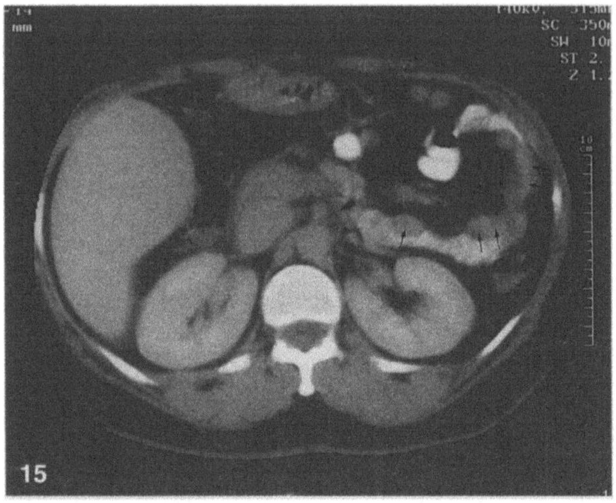

Fig. 26.15. CT: jejunal lymphoma. Nodular submucosal thickening of the bowel wall indenting the jejunal lumen *(arrows)*

The presence of inguinal recurrences has a slightly better prognosis. Metastases most commonly occur in the liver and lungs.

CT detects possible iatrogenic complications, assesses the tumor growth (when visible), the lymph node size, and detects distant metastases. It has a vital role following an abdomino-perineal resection (cf Rectum).

Bowel wall tumors

These are extramucosal lesions which are predominantly due to the lymphomas.

Lymphomas [8, 27, 28, 44, 45] (fig. 26.15)

Primary non-Hodgkin's lymphomas (NHL) rarely arise in the digestive tract (5% of all NHL, increasing incidence associated with HIV).

On the other hand, involvement of the digestive tract is common in the nodal form of NHL: 43% [27], justifying routine investigation of the digestive system in the initial assessment (endoscopy, CT and ultrasound).

In adults, the stomach is involved in about 50% of cases, small bowel in around a third of cases, the colon (cecum), rectum and duodenum being much more rarely involved. The ileocecal junction is the commonest site in children.

Initial assessment

CT demonstrates a non-specific mural thickening, often greater than 3 cm; the mural thickening is homogeneous, rarely heterogeneous with several necrotic areas; the external contours are often lobulated, and the internal borders are irregular and associated with hypertrophy of the folds and ulceration; one or several segments of the bowel may be involved (suggestive diagnostic feature); the regional fat is unaltered.

Disease outside the digestive tract in NHL is investigated by ultrasound and CT, and by lymphography in Hodgkin's disease (HD) and NHL.

Lymph node involvement

This is frequently considerable; the nodes are often globular, separate or matted together in a mass around the mesenteric vessels. There should be a complete assessment of the lymph nodes which includes accurate measurements to compare with subsequent examinations.

The abdominal lymph nodes are theoretically well assessed by ultrasound unless there are technical difficulties (gas, obesity...).

Lymphography "forgets" the hypogastric and celiomesenteric nodes but can detect pathological lymph nodes which are of normal size and has a role in the monitoring of disease progression.

CT has well recognized limitations; it only assesses size, misses involvement of normal sized nodes and cannot diagnose the entirely inflammatory nature of some enlarged nodes. It has a role in guiding biopsy of a solitary mass. The mediastinal lymph node chains are analyzed by CT which demonstrates lymphadenopathy in a third of cases, not previously apparent on standard radiographs [44].

MRI has results comparable to CT in the investigation of lymphomas, with the same limitations [8]; it provides a better study of the splenic and mesenteric lymph node chains and is sometimes indicated if CT appearances are atypical or there is a contraindication to CT due to allergy to iodinated contrast.

Assessment of the viscera

This should be routine (liver, spleen, kidneys, CNS, bone marrow....).

The clinical forms are numerous:
- the lymphoma may involve a whole segment of the digestive tract giving a pseudolinitis appearance or manifest as an isolated submucosal nodule which is difficult to diagnose;
- the lumen is often dilated (pseudo-aneurysmal form) due to the destruction of the submucosal nerve plexus; there are also stenosing forms which are initially difficult to diagnose when isolated;
- there may be minimal or even absent lymph node infiltration;
- high grade non-Hodgkin's lymphomas have been described in the context of AIDS which are sometimes the presenting feature. Involvement is more often multifocal and atypical by its predilection for the ano-rectal region. CT appearances are essentially identical: any rapidly enlarging lymph node mass should raise the suspicion of a lymphoma and requires histological confirmation by ultrasound or CT guided biopsy;
- in the cases of NHL arising in patients on immunosuppressant treatment, the clinical picture is similar to that of AIDS.

Follow-up

This consists of monitoring the evolution of the initial tumor size by imaging method:
- the plain abdominal x-ray, lymphography, ultrasound;
- CT is the examination of choice because it is able to obtain accurate and comparable measurements on sections at identical levels from one examination to the next. In particular, it is the best examination for the follow-up of bowel wall thickening. It can detect any residual mass for the biopsy;
- MRI has a role in the differentiation between a sterile residual mass and an active lesion; the presence of hyperintense zones on T2-weighted imaging is very suggestive of persistent disease activity or a recurrence [46] with an accuracy rate of approximately 85% [28].

Involvement of the GIT in other malignant hematological conditions [5, 9]

The malignant hematological conditions are generalized systemic diseases which may affect the whole body. In such cases, submucosal infiltration of the digestive tract is almost inevitable, usually asymptomatic, and does not alter the treatment.

It may be radiologically undetectable or appear as several, sometimes ulcerated, submucosal nodules or rarely as a focal mass which may or may not be responsible for specific GIT symptoms (the infrequent "pseudo-appicillary" forms of acute leukemia in children).

The radiological diagnosis is often made accidentally, CT having been performed in the overall staging of the disease extent in the abdomen, thorax, and brain, and MRI in the assessment of bone and brain (when CT is negative in a symptomatic patient).

In the case of chronic lymphoid leukemia (CLL) and Waldenstrom's disease, bowel wall thickening is often multifocal, multinodular and associated with locoregional lymphadenopathy. The presence of a tumor of the digestive tract during the evolution of a CLL should always suggest the development of a high grade non-Hodgkin's lymphoma (Richter's syndrome).

In multiple myeloma [9], secondary bowel involvement is exceptional, occurring at a late stage, and involving particularly the stomach. The presence of bowel involvement does not influence the chemotherapy treatment strategy. It must be differentiated from a solitary plasmocytoma which is an infrequent tumor of the stomach, small bowel or colon, and is included in the NHL group of diseases.

GIT involvement is extremely uncommon in the acute leukemia and the chronic myeloid leukemia.

Kaposi's sarcoma

This is very common in AIDS patients, sometimes associated with a lymphoma; there are multiple moderately enlarged lymph nodes; the associated lesions are generalized (skin, thorax, liver, spleen...).

Involvement of the GIT is common, often in the rectum.

Mural thickening manifests as multiple submucosal nodules, sometimes confluent and circumferential.

Connective tissue tumors [25, 30, 34]

CT together with ultrasound are performed following the detection of a symptomatic or asymptomatic abdominal mass or for an extrinsic mass detected by endoscopy or conventional radiological techniques.

Apart from assessing the tumor size and spread, CT can also help in the differentiation of masses arising from adjacent organs in the region, but this diagnosis

is not always easy; the following features are all taken into consideration;
- the adjacent viscera are intact;
- the tumor is well outlined by the fat, is in contact with the bowel and separate from the viscera, sometimes associated with mucosal involvement resulting in thickened folds, ulceration or an endoluminal nodule;
- the bowel lumen is stretched by an intrinsic mural mass but compressed by an extrinsic mass;
- the acute angle of contact with the bowel wall is suggestive of a bowel wall tumor.

Ultrasound or CT guided biopsy will give the diagnosis in difficult cases, but the diagnosis is usually established at exploratory laparotomy.

Leiomyosarcoma [34]

This is a very infrequent tumor (1-3% of malignant tumors of the stomach), often presenting with hemorrhage; lesions arising in the stomach can be demonstrated by endoscopy and appear as mucosal erosions of minimal significance and gastric wall compression. The demonstration of compression, stretching and separation of opacified loops of bowel are suggestive features of a tumor on the small bowel meal.

CT demonstrates an exoluminal, spherical or oval tumor which is often large [25] (more than 12-15 cm); it appears heterogeneous, containing many areas of necrosis, but calcifications are rare.

There are alterations in the mucosa, often hypertrophied and ulcerated. Lymph node metastases are uncommon. Metastastic disease tends to occur by direct contiguous spread to the viscera and by hematogenous dissemination to the liver, bones and lungs.

The differential diagnosis is essentially with a leiomyoma when the tumor is small:
- the benign leiomyoma is typically homogeneous but often heterogeneous when its size is greater than 5 cm;
- calcifications are rare but more common than in a leiomyosarcoma;

Some tumors are almost completely necrotic resulting in a pseudocystic appearance which may suggest the diagnosis of a cystic lymphangioma or a pancreatic cyst.

Leiomyoblastoma

This is considered to be a tumor of intermediate grade malignancy; lymph node and hepatic metastases have been described. The tumor appearance is polymorphic: the mass is of variable size, heterogeneous, often of fluid density and multiloculated.

Other malignant connective tissue tumors

These are much more infrequent (schwannosarcoma, fibrosarcoma, liposarcoma...).

CT is performed as the initial examination, but there are no specific diagnostic features apart from the fatty content of lipomatous tumors.

MRI has a role after treatment in the detection of tumor recurrences which appear hyperintense on T2-weighted imaging whereas scar tissue is hypointense.

Carcinoid tumors [11]

These tumors rarely present with a syndrome of flushing but more often with symptoms related to the gastrointestinal tract. The serotonin and HIAA levels confirm the diagnosis.

The commonest site is the appendix in which it is almost always benign and discovered histologically. The ileum is the second commonest site (30% of carcinoids) and the most likely source of carcinoid metastasis.

Morphological assessment is obtained using CT and small bowel meal. In the early stages of a submucosal nodule, only the small bowel meal is likely to be positive whereas the CT is negative; the progression of the tumor is slow and insidious with trans-serosal spread towards the mesentery and lymph nodes.

The value of CT is predominant in the assessment of the mesentery by demonstrating a stellate soft tissue mass associated with retraction of small bowel loops on their mesenteric border. This mesenteric reaction is sometimes the cause of extrinsic stenosis of the small bowel with proximal dilatation.

The liver is the commonest site for metastases.

Mucocele of the appendix [13, 33]

The appendix is the commonest site for a mucocele; the cystadenocarcinoma is much more infrequent than the benign cystadenoma (80%).

The lesion is detected by ultrasound or CT, either accidentally or during the investigation of a pelvic mass.

CT appearances are the same in the early stage of development: a small rounded mass of fluid density, sometimes with thin peripheral calcifications. The diagnosis is easy for a retrocecal tumor but more difficult in the pelvis where other causes of pelvic cystic masses need to be considered (sometimes with thin peripheral calcifications). Rupture of a cystadenocarcinoma results in peritoneal spillage and a pseudomyxoma peritonei due to gelatinous material throughout the peritoneum for which the prognosis is bleak. CT may also visualize either multiple small fluid levels scattered throughout the peritoneal cavity or free ascites. This ascites is different due to its gelatinous nature, leaves an imprint on the liver or spleen and displaces the bowel loops laterally (whereas they are centrally placed in classical ascites).

Treatment is surgical comprising of removal of the initial tumor and multiple gelatinous foci. Complete resection is rarely achieved, and recurrences are frequent. Intraperitoneal chemotherapy may be useful.

CT is the best investigation for follow-up and detection of small persistent or recurrent gelatinous foci.

The second commonest cause of a pseudomyxoma peritonei is a cystadenocarcinoma of the ovary; much more rarely, causes are cancers of the stomach, bile duct or pancreas.

Iatrogenic complications [16, 38]

These are predominantly due to post-radiation damage to bowel loops within the irradiation field and have become very uncommon since the development of very high energy equipment and the use of multiple beams. Acute lesions appear as hypodense and circumferential wall thickening due to submucosal edema.

The lesions in the chronic stage appear as a mural thickening in fixed, rectilinear, adherent bowel loops due to mesenteric fibrosis. There is sometimes associated segmental dilatation proximal to a fibrotic stenosis.

In these patients, the differentiation from a recurrence is often difficult; the absence of peritoneal thickening, ascites, lymphadenopathy or a mass are features in favor of a post-radiation lesion. In cases of doubt, percutaneous biopsy is indicated, particularly if serial tumor markers are suggestive of a recurrence.

Other complications are not specific to the cancer (abscess, hematoma...). The local complications of intra-arterial chemotherapy are very rarely seen, and the imaging findings have not been described.

Conclusion

Significant progress has been made in cancers of the GIT due to the development of radio- and chemotherapy treatments. Imaging of the digestive tract previously was restricted to contrast examinations. Nowadays the new imaging techniques can provide a direct assessment of the bowel wall and surrounding tissue. Endoscopic ultrasound is even able to differentiate the different layers of the wall. The combination of these techniques has led to an improved initial staging accuracy. Currently, imaging of the GIT using CT seems to be the most accurate due to the advances in image reconstruction and the performance of an examination specifically adapted for the digestive tract.

CT is the examination of choice in all pathologies apart from certain circumstances for which endoscopic ultrasound and MRI appear to be superior.

For adenocarcinomas, CT assessment of peritumoral spread is mediocre and should be confirmed by endoscopic ultrasound. CT has a role in extensive tumors for the evaluation of the liver when endoscopic ultrasound cannot be performed.

For the post-treatment follow-up, particularly after abdomino-perineal resection, CT has a central role.

In other pathologies, CT is the main investigation for detecting spread and recurrences. Guided biopsy must be performed if there is any doubt.

MRI has a role both in the examination of the brain and bone prior to the treatment of hematological disorders, and in the follow-up of patients by helping to differentiate active from sterile residual masses.

References

1. Aboulker C, Buthiau D, Cady J, et al (1991) Exploration du tube digestif en TDM et IRM: estomac, intestin grêle, côlon, rectum, anus. In: Buthiau D (ed) TDM et IRM cliniques. Frison-Roche, Paris
2. Adalsteinsson B, Glimelius B, Graffman S, et al (1985) CT in staging rectal carcinoma. Acta Radiol (Diagn) (Stockh) 26: 46-50
3. Balthazar EJ, Megibow AJ, Hulnick D, et al (1988) Carcinoma of the colon: detection and prooperative staging by CT. AJR 150: 301-306
4. Benhaim M, et al (1989) Intérêt de l'IRM dans le dépistage et le bilan d'extension locorégionale des récidives post-opératoires des cancers du rectum. Med Chir Dig 18, 3
5. Brunet R, Hoerni B (1983) Localisations digestives des hémopathies malignes. Encycl Med Chir Paris, Estomac- Intestin, 9088 A10, 11
6. Bruneton JN, Normand F, Lagrange JL, et al (1988) Apport de la scanographie dans la surveillance des cancers colorectaux traités par chirurgie radicale. J Radiol 69: 501-507
7. Buthiau D (1991) Réalisation des examens TDM et IRM: notions générales. In: Buthiau D (ed) TDM et IRM cliniques. Frison-Roche, Paris

8. Buthiau D, Jasmin C, Gabarre J, et al (1991) Indications de la TDM et de l'IRM en hématologie. In: Buthiau d (ed) TDM et IRM cliniques. Frison-Roche, Paris
9. Bersani D, Etcharry F, Tauzin C,et al (1990) Maladie de Kahler à localisation gastrique. A propos d'une observation. J Radiol 71: 667-672
10. Cady J, Godefroy J, Sibaud O (1988) Les récidives locorégionales après résection anastomose colo-rectale pour cancer. La Letttre Chirurgicale 62
11. Cockey BM, Fishman EK, Jones B, et al (1985) Computed tomography of abdominal carcinoid tumor. J Comput Assist Tomogr9: 38-42
12. Cook AO, Levine BA, Siriner KR, et al (1986) Evaluation of gastric adenocarcinoma: abdominal computed tomography does not replace cœliotomy. Arch Surg121: 603606
13. Cordolliani YS, Simon P, Wannin G, et al (1988) Tumeurs muco-secrétantes rétrocæcales de l'appendice (Mucocèle). A propos de trois cas diagnostiqués radiologiquement. J Radiol 63: 741-750
14. Detry R, Gigot JF, Gérard R (1988) Performance de l'échographie endorectale en pathologie tumorale du rectum. Gastroenterol Clin Biol 12: 810-813
15. Farah MC, Jafry SZHj Schwab RE, et al (1987) Duodenal neoplasms. Role of CT. Radiology 162: 839-843
16. Fischman EK, Zinreich ES, Jones B (1984) Computed tomography: diagnosis of radiation ileitis. Gastrointest Radiol 9: 149-152
17. Guenelli N, Briccoli A (1985) La récidive pelvi-périnéale après amputation du rectum pour cancer. Ann Gastroenterol Hepatol 21: 343-346
18. Goldberg HI, Thoeni RF (1989) MRI of the gastrointestinal tract. Radiol Clin North Am 27: 4
19. Grabe E, Lierse W, Winckler R (1383) The perirectal fascia: morphology and use in staging of rectal carcinoma. Radiology 149: 241-246
20. Guinet C, Buy JN (1988) IRM des cancers du rectum. Ann Gastroenterol Hepatol 24: 159-164
21. Guinet C, Ghossain M, Buy JN et coll (1990) Etude comparative de l'IRM et de la TDM dans le bilan préopératoire des cancers du rectum. J Radiol 71: 357- 363
22. Hada M, Hihara T, Kakishita M (1984) Computed tomography in gastric carcinoma: thickness of gastric wall and infiltration to serosa. Radiat Med 2: 27-30
23. Kleinhaus U, Militiani D (1988) Computed tomography in the preoperated evaluation of gastric carcinoma. Gastrointest Radiol 13: 97- 101
24. Malafosse M, Fourtanier G (1987) Le traitement des cancers du rectum. Monographie de l'Association Française de Chirurgie. Masson, Paris
25. Megibow AJ, Balthazar EJ, Hulnick H, et al (1985) CT evaluation of gastrointestinal leiomyomas and leiomyosarcomas. AJR 144: 727-731
26. Merine D, Fishman EK, Jones B (1989) CT of the small bowel and mesentery. Radiol Clin North Am 27: 743-752
27. Miaux Y, Frija J, Laval-Jeantet M (1991) Imagerie des lymphomes. Journées Francophones de Radiologie. Société Française de Radiologie Médicale, Cours de perfectionnement post-universitaire 5-7-8 novembre 1991
28. Piedbois P, Levy E, Rotman N, et al (1993) Evaluation of a follow-up procedure in patients recciving adjuvant chemotherapy for resectable colorectal cancer. Proc Am Soc Clin Oncol 12: 544
29. Portalez D, Carcy JB, Teisseire R, et al (1988). Imagerie du rectum normal, pathologique et opéré. Encycl Med Chir Paris, Radiognostic IV, 33480 A05, 11
30. Pradel J, Bruel JM, Guiry M, et al (1988) Tumeurs gastrointestinales à développement exoluminal. intérêt de l'examen TDM. Feuillets de Radiologie 28: 309-316
31. Pradel J, Taourel P, Bruel JM (1992) Tomodensitométrie en pathologie gastrointestinale: piège, luxe ou nécessité? Journées Francophones de Radiologie. Société Française de Radiologie Médicale. Cours de perfectionnement post-universitaire 5-7 novembre 1992 et 8 novembre 1992
32. Richelme H, Ceccanti JP, Alfonsi JP, et al (1983) Tumeurs malignes de l'anus. Encycl Med Chir Paris, Estomac Intestin, 9084, D 10: 11
33. Rieux D, Laufenburger A, Soulier A, et al (1985) Aspects tomodensitométriques de la maladie gélatineuse du péritoine. A propos de 5 cas. J Radiol 66: 297-302
34. Scatarige JC, Fishman EK, Jones B, et al (1985) Gastric leiomyosarcoma: CT observation. J Comput Assist Tomogr 9: 320-327
35. Scatarije JC, Disantis DJ (1989) CT of the stomach and duodenum. Radiol Clin North Am 27: 687-706
36. Scherrer A, Reboul F, Martin D, et al (1990) CT of malignant anal canal tumours. Radiographics 10: 433-453
37. Stines J, Regend D, Becker S, et al (1986). Le diagnostic radiologique des récidives locales des cancers du rectosigmoïde et du canal anal. Feuillets de Radiologie 26: 115-123
38. Stines J, Regend D, Barlier C, et al (1986) L'imagerie dans le grêle radique. Feuillets de Radiologie 28: 441-458
39. Sussmann STK, Halvorsen RA, Illescas FF, et al (1988) Gastric adenocarcinoma: CT versus surgical staging. Radiology 167: 335-340
40. Thoeni RS (1981) Detection and staging of rectal and rectosigmoid cancer by computed tomography. Radiology 141: 135-138 .
41. Thoeni RS (1989) CT evaluation of carcinoma of the colon and rectum. Radiol Clin North Am 27: 731-741
42. Thompson WM, Halvorsen RA, Foster WL, et al (1986) Preoperative and postoperative CT staging of rectosigmoid carcinoma. AJR 146: 703-710
43. Van Waes PFGM, Koehler PR, Feldberg MAM (1983) Management of rectal carcinoma: impact of computed tomography. AJR 140: 1137-1142
44. Yana C, Frija J, Rain JD (1989) Imagerie fonctionnelle en hématologie. Encycl Med Chir Paris, Sang, 13000, N40,3
45. Zerhouni EA (1988) Rôle de la résonance magnétique dans le bilan des lymphomes. In: Vasile N (ed) IRM corps entier. Vigot, Paris
46. Zerhouni EA, Fishman EK, Jones B (1988) Principles and technics. In: Fishman EK, Jones B (ed) Computed tomography of the gastrointestinal tract. Churchill Livingstone, New York, pp 1-16

CHAPTER 27

Primary retroperitoneal tumors

Clinicians
J.-C. Piette, B. Wechsler, B. Chiche, D. Nizri

Radiologists
D. Buthiau, J.-M. Faintuch

The primary retroperitoneal tumors arise from the connective tissue, nervous and vestigial structures which are situated in the retroperitoneal space. They are separate from the retroperitoneal organs and major vessels. Usually it is necessary to exclude lymphomatous lymph node disease.

These lesions are large at the time of diagnosis; in fact, the presenting symptoms are essentially due to compression of organs and neighboring structures.

However, the exact diagnosis of some lesions may be difficult due to the uncertainty in recognizing the site of origin and anatomical limits, the histological nature, or the histological criteria of a benign or malignant lesion.

These difficulties have led to the creation of a histological grading system [5] which gives some indication of the metastatic potential of the tumor. This represents one of the principal parameters for deciding on adjuvant treatment after surgery.

Indications and signs for CT and MRI

CT

CT is the fundamental investigation which has the ability to:
- visualize the tumor;
- confirm its retroperitoneal location and exclude an intraperitoneal tumor or a lesion originating from an abdominal organ;
- assess its volume, extent and relationship to adjacent viscera;
- detect lymph node spread and possible metastases;
- help in the diagnosis of its precise nature by appreciating its soft tissue composition and guiding cytological or histological biopsies;
- monitor its evolution during and after treatment [2].

Positive diagnosis

This is of variable difficulty and is aimed at appreciating the retroperitoneal location and extraparenchymal nature of the lesions. It is much harder if the tumor is large, and there is significant spread to adjacent organs. A number of signs have been described to infer the retroperitoneal nature of a mass:
- anterior displacement of the kidney and/or adrenal gland relative to the mass arising posterior to these organs in the posterior pararenal space;
- anterior displacement of adherent colon, duodenum, pancreas and splenic vein;
- anterior displacement of the inferior vena cava, a non-specific sign which is sometimes seen in hepatic tumors of the posterior sector.

The accuracy of CT in determining the retroperitoneal nature of a mass varies 86-90% depending on the series. The greatest difficulties are encountered with very large and extensive masses arising from the anterior pararenal space.

The second stage in the diagnostic process consists of excluding both retroperitoneal masses originating in lymph nodes or the retroperitoneal organs, and the non-neoplastic masses (retroperitoneal fibrosis). The size and extent of the mass are the principal features which predispose to errors. Confusion with adrenal tumors or large lymph node masses in midline perivascular distribution is common. Hemorrhagic or infected tumors are rarely confused with simple abscesses or hematomas.

Diagnosis of spread

On CT, there are limited definite criteria of spread to adjacent organs. Only tumor proliferation within the adjacent parenchyma or encasement of a vessel with or without associated stenosis is unequivocal sign of extension.

The preservation of a fat plane may indicate a possible plane of cleavage, but microinvasion of the fat cannot be excluded.

Three-dimensional reconstruction on the latest generation spiral CT scanners demonstrates more accurately the relationships of the tumor to the adjacent organs.

Diagnosis of the nature of the tumor

The accuracy rate quoted for CT is variable depending on the authors and criteria used for the assessment of spread. Although lymph node spread is rare in this type of tumor, the presence of hepatic, pulmonary or bony metastases confirms the malignant nature of the tumor; their density may be very different from that of the primary tumor.

CT is able to appreciate certain components of the lesion: calcification, fat, cystic components and septa. CT angiography can assess the degree of vascularization. However, density measurements can only give an approximate diagnosis of the histological nature. Like ultrasound, CT can be used to guide percutaneous biopsy for cytological and/or histological examination. The failure rate (10-20%) is related to the difficulty in penetrating the tumor tissue and the slenderness of the biopsy fragments compared to the very heterogeneous composition of the tumor and to the presence of inflammatory or necrotic areas. Biopsy is only of value if positive.

Mesenchymal tumors (fig. 27.1)

Malignant tumors of fatty origin

Liposarcomas (fig. 27.1 a) are the commonest retroperitoneal mesenchymal tumors; they represent 7-25% of retroperitoneal sarcomas, and 10% of liposarcomas arise in the retroperitoneum. These tumors develop from the constituents of fat with a variable degree of differentiation. Four types have been described: the lipogenic (highly differentiated), pleomorphic, myxoid and round cell forms. CT appearances depend on the histological type (fig. 27.1 a).

The well differentiated tumors are dominated by the areas of fat density with linear or radial septa.

The other histological forms contain areas of fatty and soft tissue, fluid and more rarely calcification density.

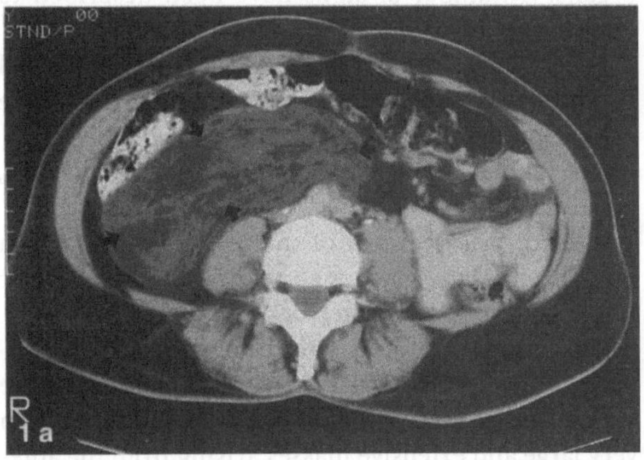

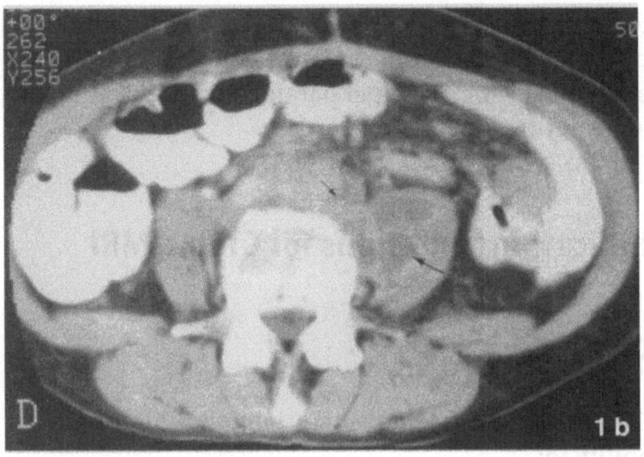

Fig. 27.1 a, b. Mesenchymal tumor on CT. **a** Retroperitoneal mesenchymal tumor (liposarcoma) on post-contrast CT: the lesion *(arrows)* contains multiple areas of fatty density with linear and radial septa and areas of pleomorphic soft tissue density; **b** retroperitoneal cystic lymphoma on post-contrast CT demonstrates cystic areas within the left psoas *(medium arrow)* in contiguity with the left latero-aortic retroperitoneal lymphadenopathy *(small arrow)*

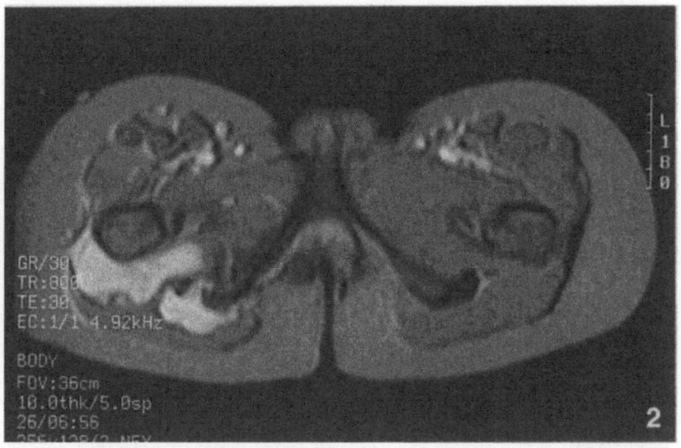

Fig. 27.2. Angiosarcoma on MRI demonstrates spread to the right buttock region from a retroperitoneal lesion appearing clearly hyperintense

The assessment of spread by CT is essential before surgical treatment; peritoneal spread (via the mesentery) is possible and should be suspected in the presence of ascites.

The rates of local recurrence vary between 53 and 85%, depending on the degree of differentiation of the tumor; hepatic, pulmonary or bone metastases may occur.

The differential diagnosis is with a retroperitoneal accumulation of fat (lipomatosis) which does not exert any mass effect on the adjacent organs.

Tumors of vascular origin

These are more often benign and dominated, particularly in children, by the cystic lymphoma (fig. 27.1b). The common malignant tumor is the angiosarcoma (MRI appearance: fig. 27.2).

Tumors of histiocytic origin

These are recently described tumors; their phylogenetic and histological nature are controversial. The architectural variability of these tumors explains the large number of synonyms: histiocytosarcoma, histiocytofibrosarcoma (fig. 27.3), fibrohistiosarcoma, fibroxanthosarcoma.

On CT, they appear heterogeneous with central hypodense zones due to necrosis and enhanced following contrast injection. They have a predilection for the peri- or pararenal regions of the retroperitoneum. Infiltration of adjacent organs is characteristic of these tumors; recurrences and metastases are common.

Other mesenchymal tumors

Arising from smooth or striated muscle, the malignant forms are much commoner than the benign forms.

Tumors of neuro-ectodermal origin

These occur more frequently in children in whom the commonest is neuroblastoma:
- the malignant forms of the ganglioneuroma have a very variable evolution, sometimes they are encapsulated and associated only with locoregional spread;
- the malignant forms of the neuroglial tumors are dominated by malignant schwannomas and malignant degeneration of neurofibromas (15-20% of neurofibromas);
- the malignant forms of paragangliomas arising from the paraganglionic system are responsible for lymph node and bone metastases.

Tumors of vestigial origin

Teratomas are rarely retroperitoneal, and 25% of these are malignant. Two anatomical forms, "cystic or solid", are possible made up of mature or immature tissues; the diagnosis is suggested by the presence of a lesion containing areas of fatty and soft tissue density as well as large calcifications. Choriocarcinoma rarely develops in the retroperitoneum. It has the same histological features of malignancy as in the other localizations, particularly in the gonads.

MRI [4] (figs 27.2 & 27.3)

The 3-dimensional capability of MRI is helpful in the pre-surgical assessment of extension (figs 27.2 & 27.3). However, its failure to improve the specificity compared to CT and the non-visualization of calcification have prevented this technique from making any significant contribution.

Only the lipomatous liposarcoma appears hyperintense on T1-weighted imaging and this suggests its fatty nature.

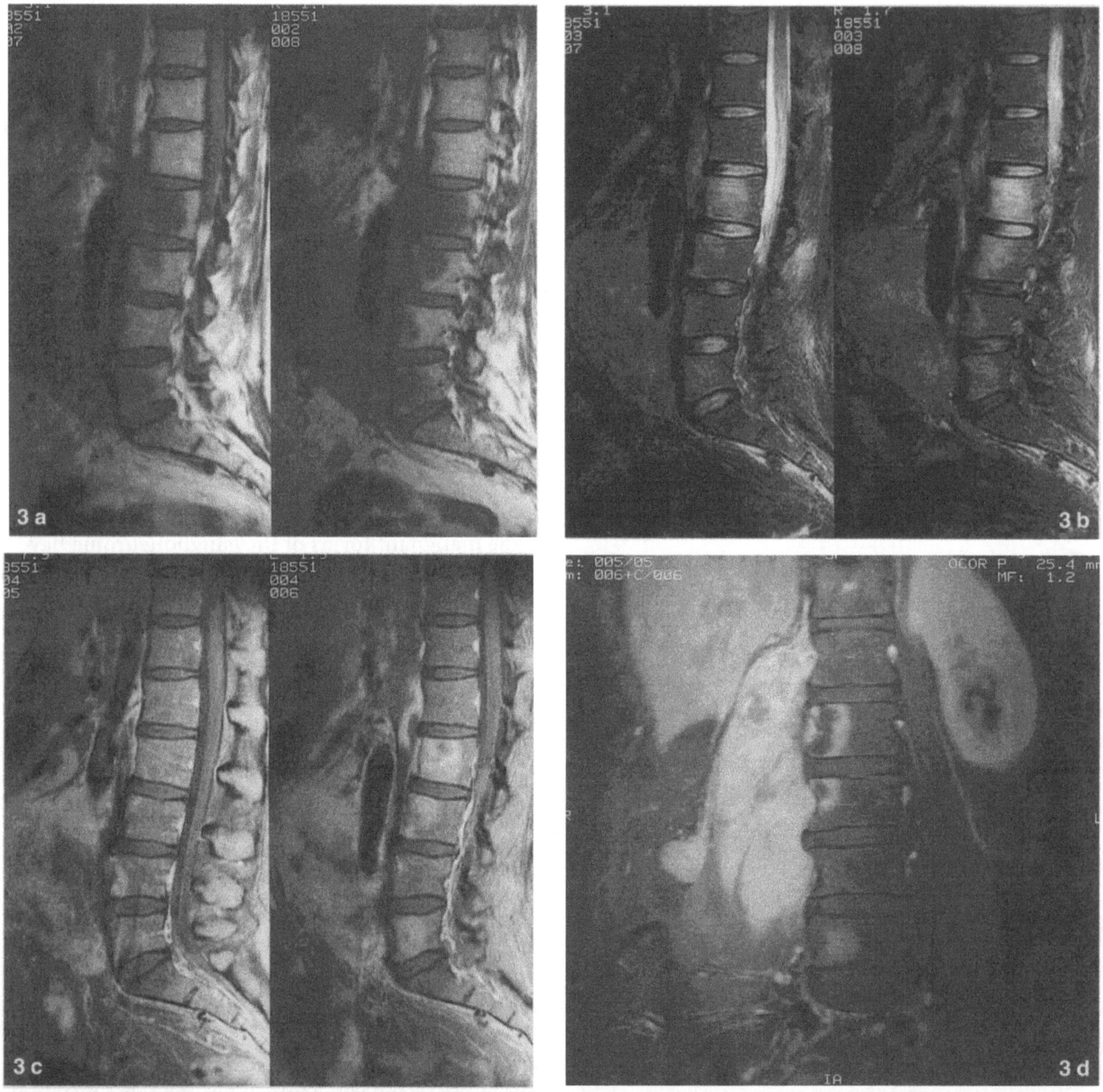

Fig. 27.3 a-d. Histiocytofibrosarcoma on MRI. **a** Sagittal T1 section; **b** sagittal T2 section; **c** post-gadolinium sagittal T1 section; **d** post-gadolinium coronal T1 section; the examination provides a 3-dimensional assessment of tumor spread demonstrating pre-and peri-aorto-caval retroperitoneal invasion, infiltration of the whole right psoas, right crus of the diaphragm and right latero-lumbar muscle masses. There is infiltration of the right L1-L5 neuroforamina and direct invasion of the vertebral bodies, particularly L2 and L3. The injection of contrast agent (**c, d**) gives better delineation of the lesion and demonstrates enhancement in the epidural space which does not correspond to true epidural infiltration but to hypervascularization due to epidural venous collateral resulting from obstruction of the inferior vena cava

Conclusion

Primary retroperitoneal tumors have for a long time been considered as infrequent and large tumors which are difficult to diagnose and present late.

Ultrasound and particularly CT have totally replaced the classical radiological techniques in the diagnosis and preoperative evaluation. Despite its limitations in the assessment of spread and the nature of the tumors, CT is still the most accurate initial radiological technique. It is also of value in the follow-up of these lesions. MRI does not give any significant further information as to the nature of the lesion. However, it does appear to be sensitive in the detection of areas of fat. Its major advantage is related to its multiplanar capability in the pre-surgical work-up (figs 27.2 & 27.3).

References

1. Buthiau D, Piette JC (1991) Rétropéritoine. In: Buthiau D (ed) TDM et IRM cliniques. Frison-Roche, Paris, pp 693-698
2. Guivarch M (1986) Tumeurs rétropéritonéales primitives. Encycl Med Chir Paris, Reins organes génito-urinaires 18102 A 10, 7
3. Laurent F, Drouillard J, Dorcier F, et al (1988) Scanographie des tumeurs rétropéritonéales primitives. Feuillet de Radiologie 28: 349-358
4. Lee JKT (1989) Retroperitoneum in Computed Body Tomography and MRI correlation. Raven Press, New York, pp 743-753
5. Suit H, Russel W, Martin R (1985) Sarcoma of soft tissue: clinical and histopathological parameters and response to treatment. Cancer 35: 1478-1483
6. Waligore MP, et al (1981) Lipomatous tumors of the abdominal cavity: CT appearence and pathologic conditions. AJR 137: 539-545

CHAPTER 28

Malignant retroperitoneal fibrosis

Clinicians
B. Wechsler, J.-C. Piette, D. Nizri,
C. Chapelon-Abric

Radiologists
D. Buthiau, J.-M. Faintuch

Malignant disease is the cause of 75% cases [3] of retroperitoneal fibrosis. Many primary malignancies have been implicated: breast, lung, thyroid, gastrointestinal tract, genito-urinary system, lymphomas and sarcomas; 50% of fibroses of neoplastic origin are due to the recurrence of a known cancer or the spread from a clinically apparent cancer.

Any insult may induce a post-radiotherapy or post-surgery fibrosis.

Before the advent of the new imaging techniques (CT and MRI), intravenous urography (IVU) was the examination of choice for diagnosing retroperitoneal fibrosis by demonstrating the typical appearances of bilateral ureteric stenosis with displacement and associated pelvicalyceal dilatation of variable severity depending on the degree of obstruction. Contrast studies of the retroperitoneal vessels (cavography, arteriography) also showed involvement of these structures by the fibrotic process.

CT and MRI not only demonstrate the same signs as the "old" investigations but also directly visualize the fibrosis itself.

Indications for CT and MRI

CT (fig. 28.1)

CT demonstrates the fibrosis and defines its relationships to structures adjacent to the aorta (inferior vena cava, ureters+++).

- CT can search for the underlying etiology or another localization, and guide biopsy which is only of value if positive;
- it is reproducible and can monitor progress on treatment;
- however, it is of limited value for patients in renal failure in whom the injection of a contrast agent is effectively contraindicated.

MRI

The role of MRI is yet to be defined; its 3-dimensional capability, particularly the coronal and sagittal planes, and the non-requirement of a contrast agent would seem to be obvious advantages.

It is able to demonstrate the relationships of the fibrosis to the retroperitoneal vessels, as well as extension into the pelvis and obstructive hydronephrosis.

However, it cannot determine reliably the nature of the fibrotic process.

Signs

CT

The appearances of the fibrotic plaque in retroperitoneal fibrosis are very variable: midline (fig. 28.1) or asymmetrical, well or poorly defined, localized or extensive. It is of soft tissue density, similar to that of

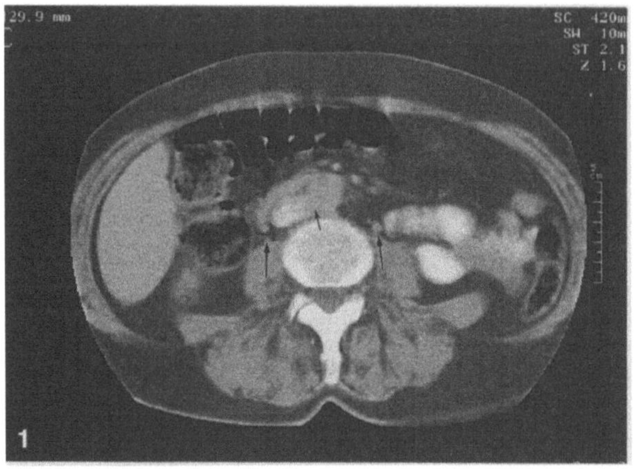

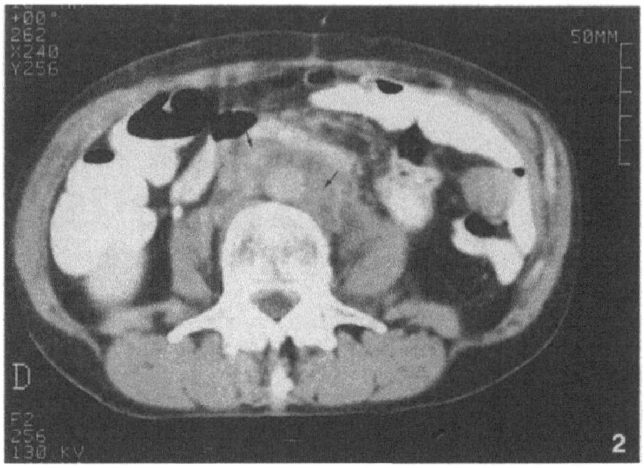

Fig. 28.1. Retroperitoneal fibrosis on post-contrast CT: early stage of malignant fibrosis secondary to a breast tumor at a stage prior to ureteric encasement: the fibrosis *(small arrow)*, confirmed histologically at the time of hepatectomy for secondary hepatic lesions, appears as an inter-aortico-caval small soft tissue density which is neither encasing, breaking or obstructing the ureters *(medium arrows)*

Fig. 28.2. Retroperitoneal lymphadenopathy causing vascular encasement by soft tissue on post-contrast CT with lobulated anterior borders. The lymphadenopathy was due to a cancer of the cervix. Note that the enlarged nodes *(arrows)* are responsible for extrinsic compression of the third part of the duodenum and encasement with detachment of the inferior vena cava from the spine posteriorly

adjacent muscle. Following contrast injection, the degree of enhancement varies depending on the inflammatory nature of the plaque [4].

The commonest localization is below the aortic bifurcation at the level of the sacral promontory with subsequent cranial extension towards the renal hila anterior to the lumbar vertebral bodies; encasement of the ureters is responsible for uni- or bilateral hydronephrosis. In cases of vascular invasion, the inferior vena cava (IVC) has a laminated appearance without evidence of thrombosis and the aorta-iliac bifurcation appears to be cemented into the fibrosis with loss of the clear fat plane of cleavage with the fibrosis.

The differential diagnosis between idiopathic and malignant retroperitoneal fibrosis is difficult. Bilateral ureteric obstruction at the L4-L5 level with medial displacement, and a slow progression are more suggestive of a benign process.

On the other hand, in a patient with a previous history of cancer, a stenosis inferior to the L5 level, an extensive fibrosis reaching the muscles of the side wall, a heterogeneous appearance with necrotic hypodense zones following contrast injection, and displacement of the aorta away from the vertebrae posteriorly [2] are all features more indicative of malignant retroperitoneal fibrosis. Although these features are suggestive, none of them are truly specific, and they are not always present.

The presence of retroperitoneal lymphadenopathy is not necessarily a feature in favor of malignant retroperitoneal fibrosis but is included in the differential diagnosis; some criteria for differentiating between these two entities have been described:

- vascular encasement with anterior borders which are lobulated (lymphadenopathy) (fig. 28.2) or flat or regularly curvilinear (fibrosis);
- fibrosis is centered on the aorta or often on the IVC.

MRI (fig. 28.3)

MRI would immediately appear to be useful due to its 3-dimensional capability, particularly the coronal and sagittal planes (fig. 28.3), and the non-requirement for contrast injection; the relative contraindications for administering iodinated contrast in patients in renal failure should be remembered and this renders the interpretation of CT very difficult.

MRI can define the relationships of the fibrosis to the major vessels (fig. 28.3), as well as spread to the pelvis and obstructive hydronephrosis. The vascular structures appear relatively hypointense on T1-weighted imaging since the vessels remain patent and can be clearly distinguished from the intermediate signal intensity of the fibrosis.

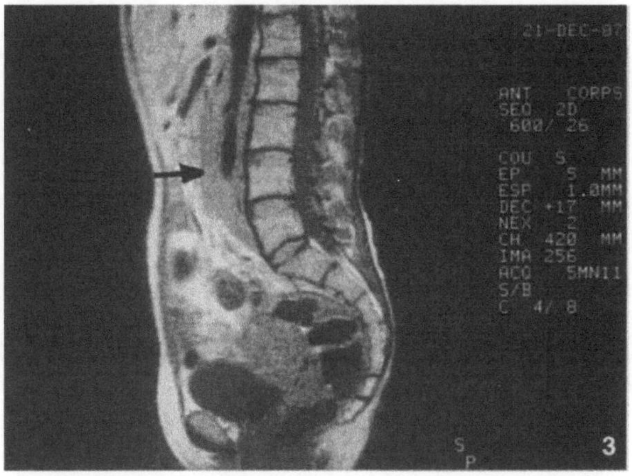

Fig. 28.3. Retroperitoneal and, to some extent, pelvic fibrosis on sagittal T1 MRI. The lesion *(arrow)* is arising anterior to the lumbar spine, encasing the aorta and extending into the upper part of the pelvis; there is significant extension of this lesion with ureteric encasement, displacement of the aorta from the vertebrae posteriorly suggestive of malignant retroperitoneal fibrosis (courtesy of Dr C. Chapelon-Abric et al. In: D. Buthiau (ed) Clinical imaging in gynecology. Vigot, Paris)

The signal of the retroperitoneal fibrosis is usually weak on T1-weighted imaging irrespective of the etiology. If the signal remains hypointense on T2-weighted imaging, a benign etiology is likely; however, high signal intensity on T2-weighted imaging is compatible either with a malignant cause or a benign lesion containing inflammatory changes [1].

Finally, although the extent of the lesion is well demonstrated, the small lesions limited to the retroperitoneum are less well assessed than on CT.

Conclusion

The diagnosis of retroperitoneal fibrosis may be suspected and detected on intravenous urography and/or ultrasound: these examinations are extremely sensitive for the demonstration of ureteric obstruction by the fibrosis. For subsequent investigation, CT remains the examination of choice for the diagnosis (fig. 28.1) and assessment of the extent of these lesions.

MRI is of value due to its 3-dimensional capability which accurately determines the extent of the lesion. MRI is performed instead of CT if iodinated contrast agent is contraindicated.

The current limitation of imaging is the absence of any specific feature in favor of a malignant etiology in the presence of retroperitoneal fibrosis.

References

1. Arrivé L, Hricak H, Tavares NJ, Miller Th (]989) Malignant versus non malignant retroperitoneal fibrosis: differentiation with MR imaging. Radiology 172: 139-143
2. Buthiau D, et al (1988) TDM et IRM en Gynécologie Obstétrique. Diffusion Sanofi-Labaz: 62
3. Chapelon-Abric C, Piette JC, Wechsler B, Buthiau D, Ziza JM, Godeau P (1993) Fibroses pelviennes. In: Buthiau D, Dargent D, et al (eds) Imagerie Clinique en Gynécologie. Vigot, Paris, pp 369-372
4. Chishom RA, Coltart RS, Cooper P, Diton AK (1986) Circonferential para-aortic masses: computed tomographic observations. Clin Radiol 37: 531-535
5. Godeau P, Chapelon-Abric C, Piette JC (1991) Fibroses systémiques idiopathiques. In: MF Khan, A Peltier, O Meyer, JC Piette (eds) Les maladies systémiques. Flammarion Médecine-Sciences, Paris, pp 1115-1136
6. Koep L, Zuidema GD (1977) The clinical significance of retroperitoneal fibrosis. Surgery 81: 250-257
7. Stephen E, Amis Jr (1991) Retroperitoneal fibrosis. AJR 157: 321-329

CHAPTER 29

Cancer of the pancreas

Clinicians
B. Chiche, B. Wechsler, J.-C. Piette, E. Malaurie, D. Nizri, D. Salandre, E. Vuillemin, G. Cohen-Aloro, D. Khayat

Radiologists
D. Buthiau, J.-M. Faintuch

Over the last few years, the diagnosis and staging of pancreatic tumors have been revolutionized by the advent of ultrasound, computed tomography (CT), magnetic resonance imaging (MRI) (whose role is yet to be defined), and more recently endoscopic ultrasound. Although CT and MRI have not, until now, altered the survival times of patients, they have replaced the other more invasive techniques (ERCP, PTC, arteriography) and can select out the operable lesions [1].

Indications and signs of CT and MRI

Tumors of the pancreas arise from the three groups of pancreatic cell-types: the acinar cell, the ductal cell, the endocrine cell.

Ductal or canalicular adenocarcinoma

The aim of imaging is to confirm the presence of a pathological mass, to differentiate a malignant from benign condition, and to assess the chances of successful surgery when there is a cancer.

Ductal adenocarcinoma is the commonest of the pancreatic tumors (90%) and usually occurs in the head of the pancreas.

CT (figs 29.1 & 29.2)

It appears as a mass which at the time of diagnosis usually causes an alteration in the size, contours and shape of the organ. It is rarely calcified and hypodense before contrast injection; following the injection of contrast, it appears as a localized or diffuse, clearly enhancing heterogeneity of the gland associated with hypodense or frankly fluid density areas.

Sometimes there is a localized loss of symmetry of the pancreatic contours with or without alterations in the intra- or peripancreatic density at this site. On the other hand, it may appear as a suspicious homogeneous area within a heterogeneous pancreas (physiological cases of fatty involution).

Thus, the signs may be subtle such as simple convexity of the pancreatic outline or hypodensity of the abnormal pancreatic parenchyma relative to the healthy parenchyma.

The detection of pancreatic carcinomas is easier in the fatty pancreas because the very hypodense structure of the pancreas is absent within the tumor which is clearly visible on the unenhanced images.

The other CT signs for the diagnosis of a pancreatic carcinoma are related to the phenomena of ductal obstruction and secondary parenchymal atrophy induced by the tumor:
- dilatation of the extra- and sometimes intrahepatic bile ducts;
- dilatation of the duct of Wirsung (fig. 29.2 a)
- atrophy of the pancreatic parenchyma proximal to the obstruction (fig. 29.2 a);
- pseudocysts proximal to the obstruction.

The role of CT is therefore to stage the tumor, particularly to determine its resectability. The following radiological signs are considered to indicate non-resectability [5];

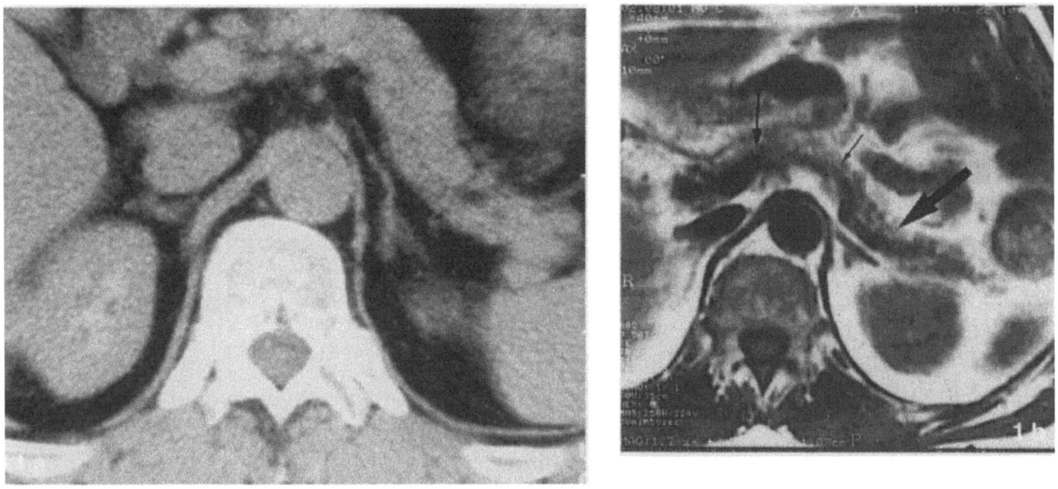

Fig. 29.1 a, b. Normal anatomy of the pancreas on CT (**a**) and MRI (**b**). The pancreas has a smooth or multilobulated contour with fatty involution in obese individuals. It is orientated obliquely from left to right, and supero-inferiorly extending from the splenic hilum on the left to the duodenal loop on the right. In both these examples, it is possible to see the regions of the proximal head, isthmus (neck), body and tail, and the junction of the head and isthmus *(medium arrow)*, isthmus and body *(small arrow)*, and body and tail *(large arrow)*. The symmetrical contours and intraglandular homogeneity are more important than the actual dimensions of the pancreas. The usual measurements found are as follows: 20 mm at the level of the head, 10-20 mm in the region of junction of the body and tail, 5-10 mm in the region of the premesenteric isthmus, and 4-7 cm in the cranio-caudal direction. Wirsung's duct is visible in 70% of cases, and should measure no greater than 2-3 mm in diameter. The pancreas belongs to the anterior pararenal space in the retroperitoneum. It is separated from the stomach by the lesser sac which is limited inferiorly by the transverse mesocolon. The lesser sac is formed by the fusion anteriorly of the prepancreatic peritoneal folds. These relationships explain certain routes of tumor spread

- invasion of organs or regions adjacent to the pancreas, especially the perivascular space around the superior mesenteric artery;
- obstruction or invasion of the inferior vena cava, celiac trunk, hepatic artery, superior mesenteric artery or vein;
- total or partial obstruction of the portal vein (fig. 29.2 c); sometimes with thrombosis of the splenic vein resulting in splenic infarction;
- lymph node spread is often difficult to separate from the tumor itself (fig. 29.2 b). This justifies the necessity to perform thin sections with contrast; the lymph node chains involved are the peripancreatic, lumbo-aortic, as well as the periportal and perivascular renal nodes.

Although CT can detect distant metastatic spread which affects, in decreasing order of frequency, the peritoneum, liver and lungs, it is inaccurate in micro- and sometimes even macronodular peritoneal involvement.

The commonest causes of an erroneous diagnosis of a malignant primary pancreatic adenocarcinoma on CT are: chronic pancreatitis (fig. 29.3 a), malignant lymphoma, pancreatic metastases (fig. 20.3 b), tumor of the ampulla of Vater (fig. 29.3 c).

Chronic pancreatitis is the difficult but critical diagnosis to make because the treatment is different; the diagnosis of pancreatitis is sometimes (60% of cases) highly probable in the presence of significant coexistent calcifications in the gland, false cysts, dilatation of Wirsung's duct and the absence of lymph node lesions. However, small sized calcifications can be seen in both conditions, and the differential diagnosis may become extremely difficult, even at open operation.

A tumor may be associated (see above) with areas of pancreatitis proximally or peritumoral inflammatory changes.

Lymph node involvement can occur in pancreatitis and tends to be limited and non-confluent with only of a moderate degree.

The sensitivity of CT [9] is dependent on the size of the tumor and is poor for lesions whose diameter is less than 2 cm. However, pancreatic cancers are generally detected at a late stage and the overall sensitivity is therefore 70-80%. When the tumor arises in the pancreatic head, the diagnostic accuracy rates of ultrasound and CT are similar. On the other hand, CT is clearly superior for lesions in the body and tail, particularly in the assessment of resectability. The sensitivity for vascular extension is 60-85% [8], and this is

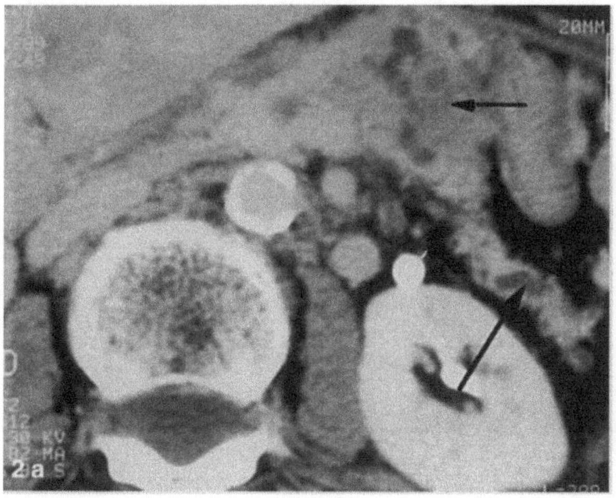

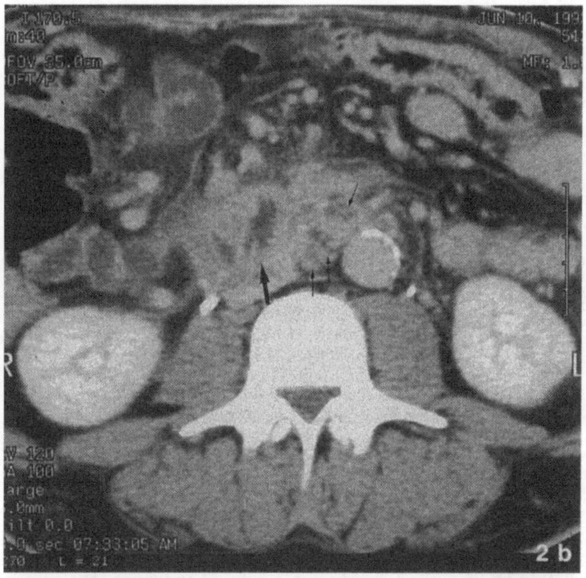

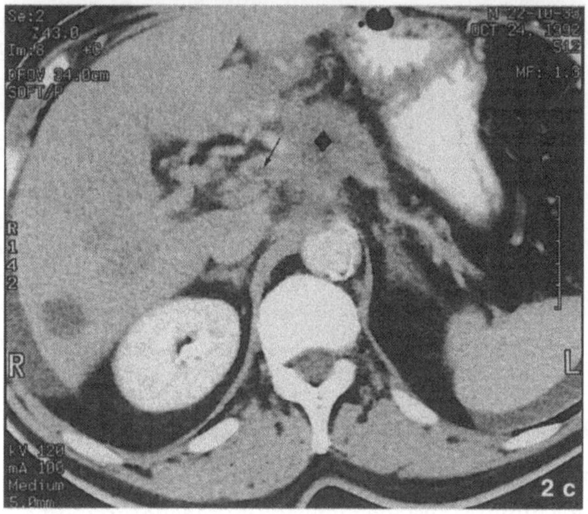

Fig. 29.2 a-c. Ductal or canalicular adenocarcinoma on post-contrast CT. **a** Cancer in the region of the isthmus and junction of the pancreatic body and neck *(small arrow)*. There is a significant heterogeneity and also soft tissue mass containing micro-pseudocysts and necrotic hypodense zones. Note the atrophy of the body and tail proximal to the pancreatic parenchymal obstruction and the dilatation of Wirsung's duct *(large arrow)*. **b** Cancer arising in the uncinate process *(large arrow)*. This partially necrotic lesion is compressing the inferior vena cava and is associated with lymph node spread to the inter-aorto-caval and pre-aorto-caval nodes *(small arrows)* situated at the medial border of the tumor; **c** cancer of the pancreatic isthmus *(diamond)* associated with mesenterico-portal spread in the form of a neoplastic thrombus *(arrow)*. Note the hypodense hepatic metastases and perihepatic ascites

further improved by the advent of continuous rotation scanners. However, the sensitivity is poor for the detection of metastatic lymph nodes (20%).

MRI (fig. 29.1)

MRI does not give any additional information concerning the staging or resectability of a pancreatic tumor, nor does it help in the differential diagnosis with other pancreatic and ampullary tumors, nor in the distinction between inflammatory and neoplastic disease. It does, however, appear to be more sensitive than CT for the detection of small size tumors using the FLASH and FSSE sequences. On these sequences, the tumor is usually of low signal intensity relative to the adjacent parenchyma [15].

On the traditional sequences, (T1- and T2-weighted), the pathological appearances are variable depending on the soft tissue, fluid and/or hemorrhagic content of the lesion:

- variable tumor signal intensity; hypo-, iso-, or hyperintense with heterogeneity of the peripancreatic fat;
- high signal on T1-weighted imaging indicating a hemorrhagic content;
- hypointense on T1-weighted imaging and hyperintense on T2-weighted imaging indicative of pseudocystic fluid content;
- variable signal intensity on T1- and T2-weighted imaging for the mucinous and necrotic lesions, often of low signal on T1- and slightly increased signal on T2-weighted imaging.

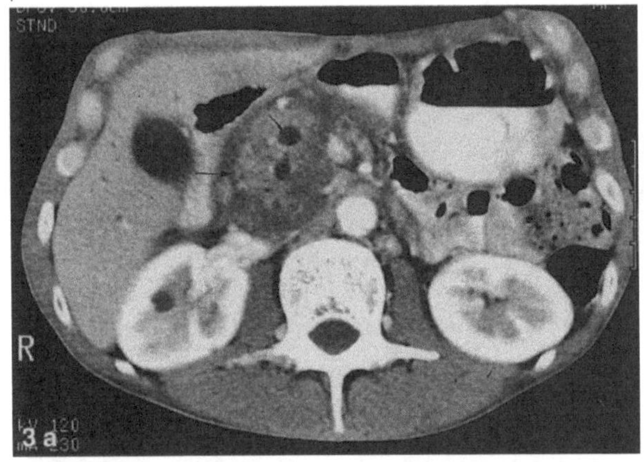

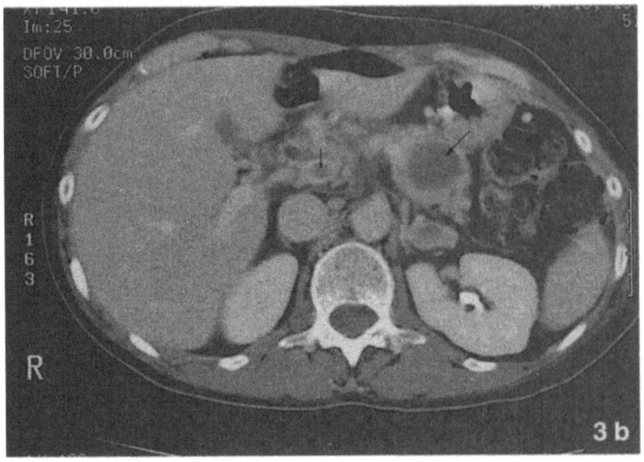

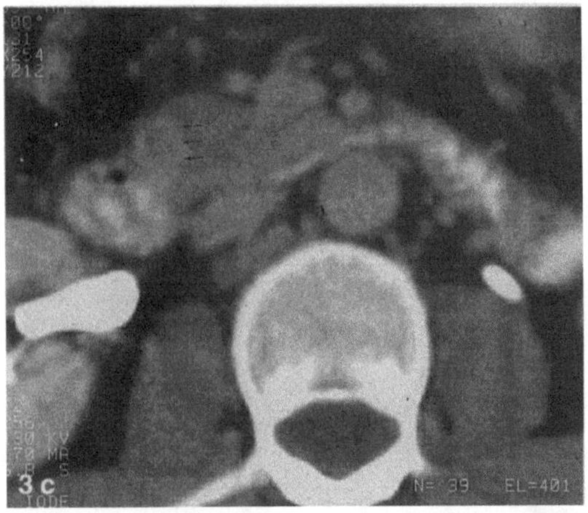

Fig. 29.3 a-c. Differential diagnosis of pancreatic cancers on CT. **a** Hypertrophic chronic pancreatitis involving the head and, to a lesser degree, the isthmus with marked hypertrophy of the pancreas *(large arrow)* and a pseudocystic heterogeneity *(small arrow)*. **b** Pancreatic metastasis *(large arrow)* from a bronchial carcinoma. Note the extensive superior mesenteric thrombus *(small arrow)*; **c** lesion of the ampulla of Vater on post-contrast CT *(arrows)*. Even though the tumor is seen projecting slightly into the distended duodenal lumen, and the differential diagnosis with a pancreatic lesion remains difficult, endoscopic ultrasound certainly being of value in this case

Cystic tumors (fig. 29.4)

These comprise of the serous cystadenoma and mucinous tumors (cystadenoma and cystadenocarcinoma) with a malignant potential.

For all these lesions, MRI [10] (fig. 29.4 b) is superior to CT in the detection of cystic lesions but is less sensitive for calcification and the visualization of the intracystic walls.

The serous cystadenoma or benign microcystic adenoma is a small benign lesion (3-4 cm) comprising of a multilocular fluid-filled cystic cavity with thin septa, calcifications being infrequent.

The mucinous cystic tumors [5] are large macrocysts measuring on average 9-10 cm in diameter containing nodules and thick, sometimes calcified septa. They almost exclusively occur in the body and tail of the pancreas. The lesions are made up of multiple cysts (fig. 29.4a), each of several centimeters in diameter, separated by septa which sometimes calcify, rarely giving a fine multicystic appearance. Their mucinous content is of higher density than that of a serous cystadenoma; the large multicompartmentalized lesions often have nodular borders.

Differential diagnosis:

These cystic lesions are often difficult to distinguish, apart from the clinical and biochemical context, from the following conditions:

- necrotic adenocarcinoma,
- subacute or focal chronic pancreatitis with calcifications and pseudocyst formation,
- necrotic lymph nodes (lymphoma, tuberculosis) but have an extrapancreatic location,
- pancreatic lymphangioma or cysts occurring in von Hippel-Lindau disease.

Endocrine tumors

These can be classified into two groups: quiescent non-functioning tumors and hormonally active tumors.

The inactive tumors are often large, up to 20 cm in diameter, clearly enhanced on CT relative to the normal pancreatic tissue and may cause hepatic metasta-

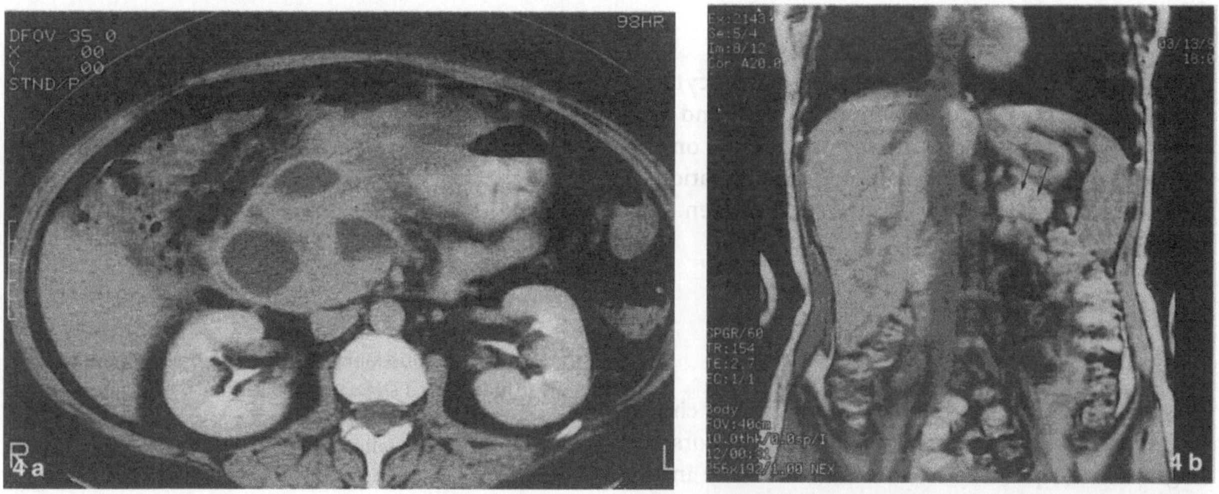

Fig. 29.4 a, b. Cystic tumor of the pancreas on CT and MRI. a Multi-macrocystic cystadenocarcinoma of the pancreatic head on post-contrast CT; b cystic tumor of the body and tail *(arrows)* of high signal on a coronal T1-weighted MRI image indicating hemorrhagic changes

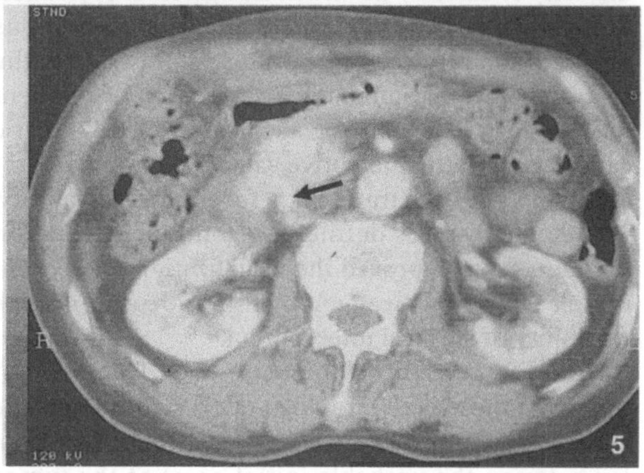

Fig. 29.5. Active pancreatic endocrine tumor on post-contrast CT (continuous rotation scanner); there is a small zone of 6 mm in diameter *(arrow)* involving the posterior portion of the pancreatic head region (well defined at this early stage following the injection of contrast agent) at which time the pancreatic enhancement is more intense, confirmed histologically

ses. Calcifications are more common than in adenocarcinomas whereas necrotic or pseudocystic appearances are much more uncommon and vascular involvement less frequent. MRI demonstrates a homogeneous, large soft tissue mass which usually respects the fat planes and vascular pedicles.

The hormonally active tumors may be solitary or multiple, and are often small (fig. 29.5) (insulinoma, gastrinoma), less than 2 cm, and therefore their detection requires the performance of fine sections; the lesions are often isodense, more rarely hyperdense (fig. 29.5) or hypodense relative to the adjacent parenchyma. Calcifications are uncommon and more frequently occur in the malignant forms. The sensitivity of CT is 40% (insulinoma and gastrinoma) and the specificity is 80%. MRI has not proven to be superior to CT. There are no macroscopic features favoring malignancy apart from calcification and the presence of metastases.

For this type of tumor, arteriography and phlebography of the pancreatic and peripancreatic veins with sampling for hormonal levels still have a role [4]; endoscopic ultrasound seems promising, particularly for insulinomas (sensitivity 82%, specificity 95%) [12].

Other rare tumors

Lymphoma

Isolated pancreatic involvement is exceptionally rare: spread into the pancreas from adjacent disease is characteristic. It is usually associated with lumbo-aortic, retroperitoneal, mesenteric or peripancreatic lymphadenopathy.

Solid papillary epithelial tumor [6]

This is a solid and cystic (hemorrhagic necrosis), often large tumor affecting young women. MRI is beneficial in this lesion due to the high signal intensity on T1-weighted imaging.

Others

Intrapancreatic metastases (fig. 29.3b), plasmocytoma and pleomorphic carcinoma are infrequent and lack any distinctive signs. The diagnosis depends on the clinical context and/or histopathologic examination of a guided pancreatic biopsy or surgical specimen.

Conclusion

CT seems, therefore, to be the examination of choice for the diagnosis and staging of pancreatic tumors; the diagnosis of a pancreatic mass can be made in the majority of cases by CT which also gives an evaluation of local spread and accurately guides percutaneous needle biopsy. According to most authors, it is the essential examination in the investigation of a patient in whom there is a strong suspicion of a pancreatic cancer. On CT, the predictive value of possible resectability is less accurate than for non-resectability. Technical advances on the new continuous rotation scanners have improved the visualization of adjacent vessels whose involvement by tumor determines the feasibility of surgical intervention.

However, the developments in CT have not improved the overall prognosis of exocrine pancreatic adenocarcinomas. There is, in fact, a consistent time lag between the probable initial onset of the tumor and the first clinical presenting signs of the disease. Tumors are, therefore, are often detected at a stage well beyond any possibility of cure.

The challenge today is to try and detect tumors of less than 15 mm in diameter before any minor symptoms are apparent:

- new MRI sequences seem to have a higher sensitivity for the detection of these small lesions;
- endoscopic ultrasound particularly appears to be the technique of choice for the detection of "mini-tumors". In addition, on the one hand, it can stage the lesion according to the TNM classification with an accuracy of 92% [7] in a series of 43 patients and, on the other hand, can differentiate pancreatic from ampullary lesions. The sensitivity for the detection of lymph node spread is less (74%) due to the poor penetration of the ultrasound beam into the deep tissues.

The role of "invasive imaging" (vascular studies, percutaneous transhepatic cholangiography, ERCP) is nowadays virtually non-existent in the diagnosis of pancreatic tumors. However, interventional radiology (see chapter 42) has preeminent role in the management of patients in whom the tumor is often advanced;

- alcohol ablation of the perisplanchnic nerves for pain relief;
- chemo-embolization of hepatic metastases;
- the placement of endoprostheses via the endoscopic or percutaneous route for the frequent situation of invasion of the common bile duct is a particularly important technique.

References

1. Buthiau D, Bousquet O, Chigot JP (1992) Pancréas. In: D Buthiau (ed) TDM et IRM Cliniques, Abdomen-Pelvis. Frison Roche, Paris, PP 171-190
2. Dupuy DE, Costello P, Ecker CP (1992) Spiral CT of the Pancreas. Radiology 183: 815-818
3. Freeny PC, Marks WM, Rgava JA, Traverso LW (1988) Pancreatic ductal adenocarcinoma diagnosis and staging with dynamic CT. Radiology 166: 125-133
4. Galiber AK, Reading CC, Charboneau JW, et al (1988) Localization of pancreatic insulinoma: comparaison of pre and intraoperalive US with CT and angiography. Radiology 166: 405-408
5. Itoch S, Shiguchi T, Ishigacki T, et al (1992) Mucin producing pancreatic tumors: CT finding and histopathologic correlation. Radiology 183: 81-86
6. Kuni O, Shigeru F, Masataka O, et al (1992) Solid and papillary epithelial neoplasm of the pancreas: MR Imaging and pathologic correlation. Radiology 184: 567-570
7. Lok Tio T, Tygat GNJ, Cikot RJ(1990) Ampullopancreatic carcinoma: preoperative TNM Classification with Endosonography. Radiology 175: 455-461
8. Mask E, Baher (1991). Pancreatic adenocarcinoma: are there pathognomonic changes in the fat surrounding the superiormesenteric artery. Radiology 180: 613-614
9. Megibow AJ (1992) Pancreatic adenocarcinoma: design the examination to evaluate the clinical questions. Radiology 183: 297-303
10. Minami M, Itai Y, Ohtomo K, et al (1989) Cystic neoplasm of the pancreas: comparaison of MR Imaging with CT. Radiology 171: 53-56
11. Mitchell D, Shapiro M, Schuricht A, Barhot D, Rosato F (1992) Pancreatic disease: findings on state of the Art MR images. AJR 159: 533-538
12. Rosch T, Lightdale CS, Bolet JT, et al (1992) Localization of pancreatic tumors by endoscopic ultrasonography. N Engl J Med 326: 1721-1726
13. Semelka RC, Krocher MA, et al (1991) Pancreatic disease: prospective comparison of CT, ERCP, and 1.5 MRImaging with dynamic Gadolinium Enhancement and Fat Suppression. Radiology 181: 785-791
14. Steiner E, Stark DD, Hahn PF, etal (1989) Imaging of pancreatic neoplasm: comparison of MR and CT. AJR 152: 487-491
15. Vellet AD, Romano W, Bach DB, et al (1992) Adenocarcinoma of the pancreatic ducts: comparative evaluation with CT and MR Imaging at 1.5 T. Radiology 183: 87-95

CHAPTER 30

Cancer of the kidney

Clinicians
A. Foulet, D. Paraiso, B. Gosselin, J. Biserte, E. Mazeman

Radiologists
L. Lemaître, P. Martinat, Y. Robert

Adenocarcinoma of the kidney is the commonest form of primary renal tumor in the adult. Early diagnosis is possible for this tumor due to its characteristic mode of spread and generally slow growth rate. In a third of cases, the diagnosis is made incidentally when the patient is still asymptomatic. In the metastatic phase, the presenting signs are variable depending on which organs are involved, and will guide the choice of investigations.

The appearance of successive techniques such as ultrasound, computed tomography (CT) and more recently magnetic resonance imaging (MRI), has improved diagnostic sensitivity and also provided a more accurate staging of these tumors.

Cancer of the kidney represents 3% of all adult cancers. 86% of these tumors are adenocarcinomas with an average incidence in Western Europe of 7/100 000 people. There is a clear male predominance with a sex ratio of 2:1. The peak age incidence is between the sixth and seventh decades. However, lesions occurring in young adults are not rare [40].

Several predisposing factors have been incriminated:
- smoking; this increases the incidence of renal adenocarcinoma by a factor of 5;
- von Hippel-Lindau disease: a renal neoplasm occurs in 1/3 cases;
- chronic hemodialysis significantly increases the incidence, and the figure quoted varies in the literature but is around 3%.

Review of anatomopathology and prognostic factors

See figs 30.1-30.9 and tables 30.1 & 30.2. In brief, it should be remembered that, in the absence of an effective treatment, the prognosis depends on the anatamo-clinical criteria such as:
size of the tumor, involvement of the vessels and lymph node chains, presence of metastases, histological type. In fact, the five year survival rate drops from nearly 100% for tumors strictly localized to the kidney to 50% if there is involvement of the renal vein, to 33% in cases of perinephric invasion and less than 10% in the presence of metastases.

Malignant tumors

Renal adenocarcinoma or renal cell carcinoma

Initially described by Grawitz in 1183, it is also known under the name of Grawitz's tumor or hypernephroma, terms which today have been abandoned.

Macroscopic appearance

Renal adenocarcinoma may have different macroscopic appearances [15, 28]. It usually develops in the renal cortex without any preference for either pole, more rarely in the medulla (tubulopapillary form). The tumor is often large, measuring 5-10 cm [15]. It is multifocal in 4.5% of cases and bilateral in 0.5-1.5%.

The tumor is typically made up of pale yellow or orange-yellow tissue of firm or resistant consistency. It can appear as a solitary nodule (fig. 30.1) which is well defined by a fibrous pseudocapsule. Alternatively, it appears as a lobulated lesion formed by several coalescent nodules (fig. 30.2), or as a less well defined mass (fig. 30.3) extending into the collecting system, displacing and invading the capsule and perirenal fat, often containing hemorrhagic or necrotic areas. Sometimes it appears cystic, either as a result of tumor necrosis (fig. 30.4) or de novo (fig. 30.5) [23, 58]. In this

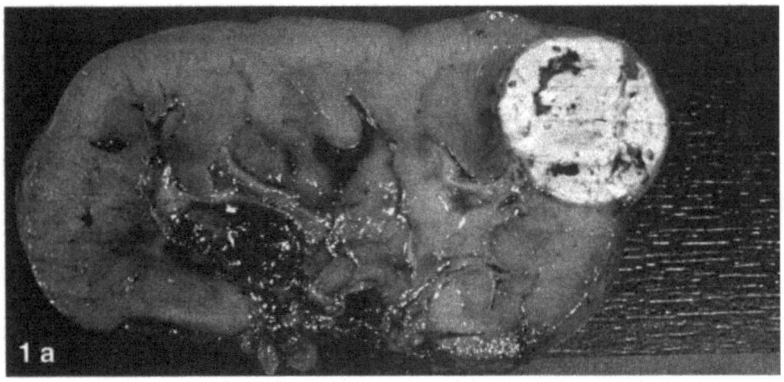

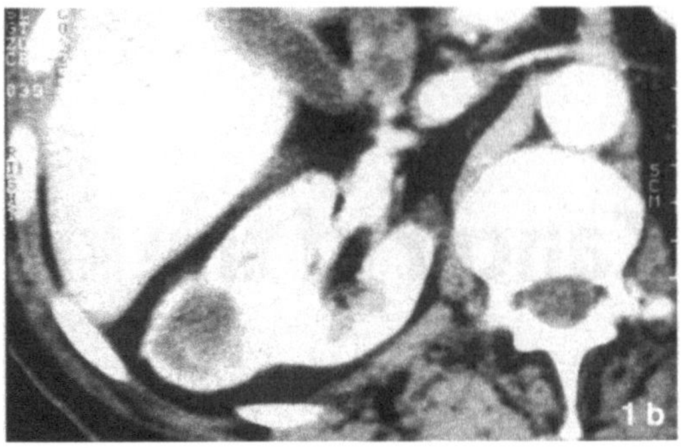

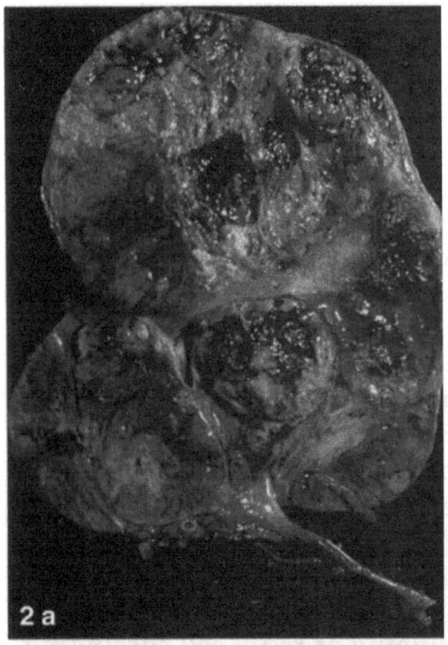

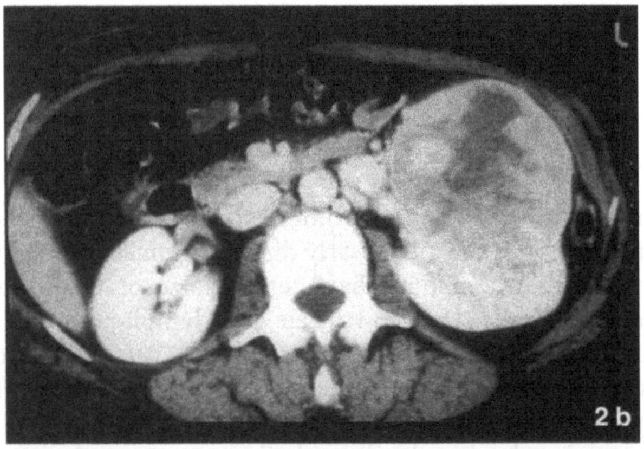

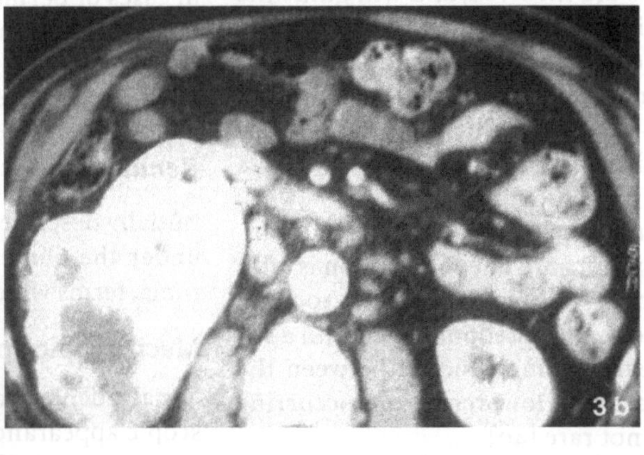

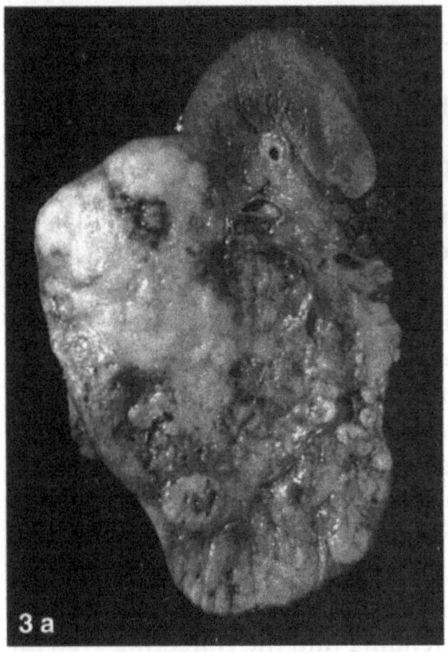

Figs 30.1-30.5. Macroscopic appearances of renal adenocarcinomas

Fig. 30.1 a, b. Nodular form. **a** Macroscopic appearance: well defined tumor, typically pale yellow, relatively homogeneous with several of areas of necrosis; **b** post-contrast CT images in the cortical stage: hypervascular, relatively homogeneous mass

Fig. 30.2 a, b. Multinodular form. **a** Macroscopic appearance: lobulated tumor formed by several coalescent nodules with more numerous areas of necrotico-hemorrhagic change; **b** post-contrast CT section performed in the tubular stage: well defined mass formed from several nodules with large hypodense zones corresponding to necrotico-hemorrhagic changes

Fig. 30.3 a, b. Massive form. **a** Macroscopic appearance: massive form with well defined borders, marked invasion of the renal parenchyma with preservation of the upper pole; **b** CT sections performed in the cortical phase: large hypervascular mass with significant necrotico-hemorrhagic changes only preserving a small cap of renal parenchyma antero-superiorly

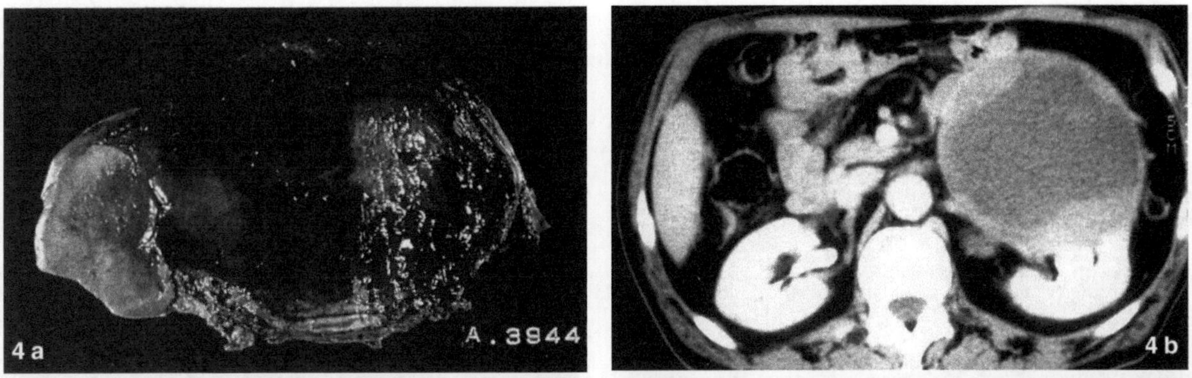

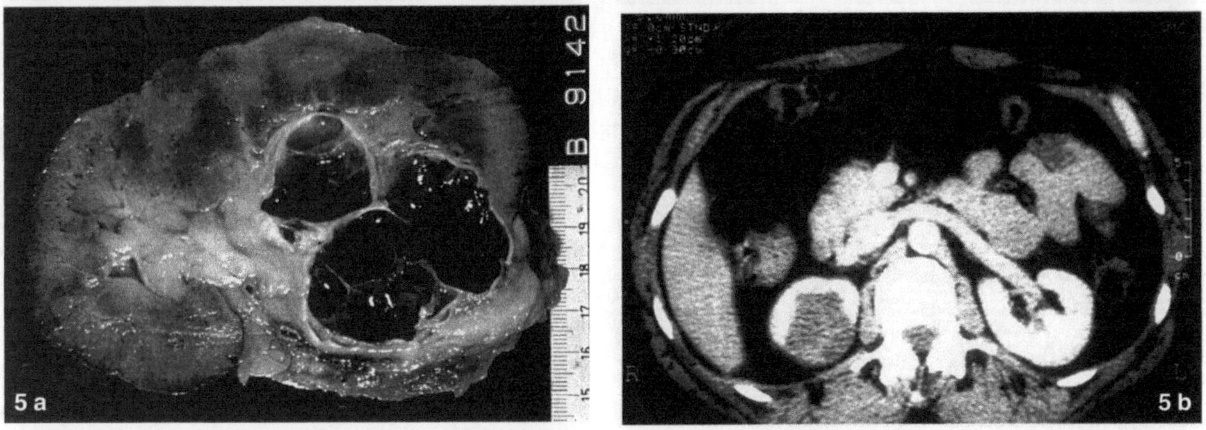

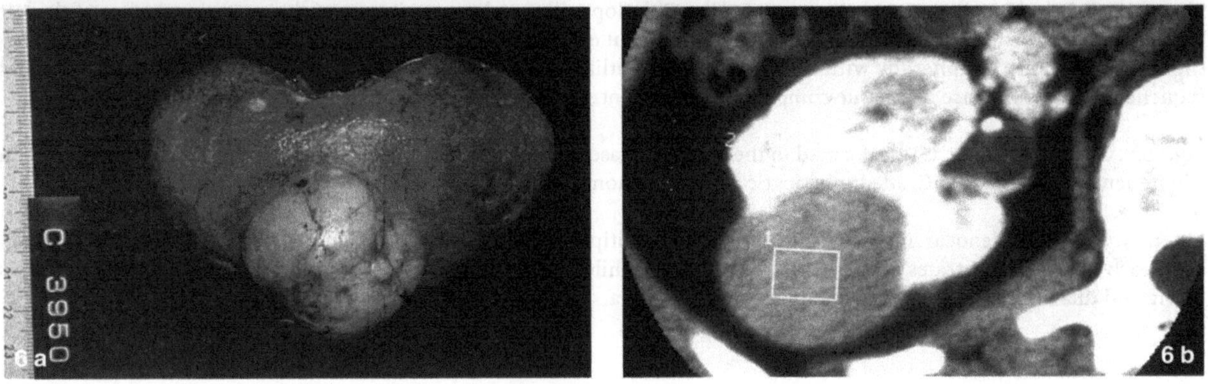

Fig. 30.4 a, b. Pseudocystic form. **a** Macroscopic appearance: pseudocystic form due to tumor necrosis; **b** CT section in the late calyceal phase: large tumor mass arising in the anterior portion of the kidney largely of fluid consistency due to hemorrhagic necrosis highlighted by the dense nodular tissue in the periphery

Fig. 30.5 a, b. Cystic form. **a** Macroscopic appearance: cystic form composed of several cavities filled with a lemon yellow, even hemorrhagic fluid, separated from each other by fibrous septa of variable thickness; **b** post-contrast CT: a mass without perfectly rounded contours formed from several fluid filled structures separated by thin and dense walls: microscopic examination demonstrated cystic carcinoma of the kidney with neoplastic cells lining the cavities or massed together within the fibrous walls

Figs 30.6-30.9. Specific features of primary tumors of the renal parenchyma

Fig. 30.6 a, b. Tubulopapillary carcinoma (grade I). **a** Macroscopic appearance: well defined tumor corresponding histologically to a tubulopapillary carcinoma; **b** post-contrast CT in the cortical phase: weakly enhancing, hypovascular, and well defined tumor

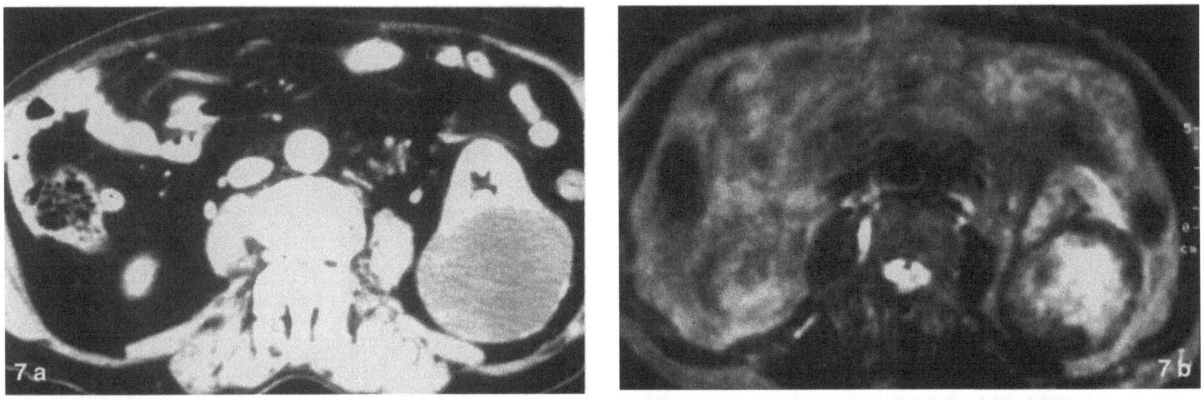

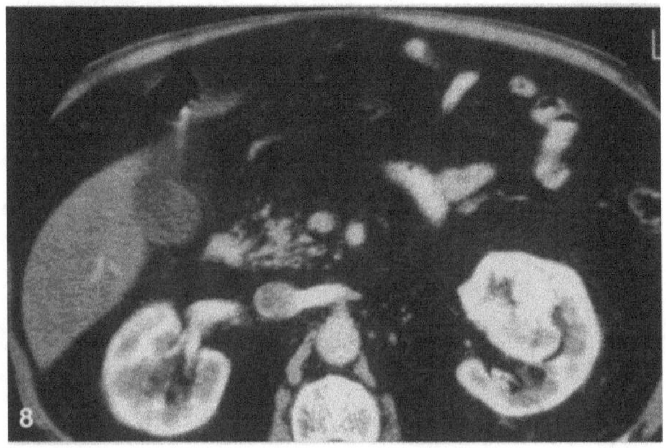

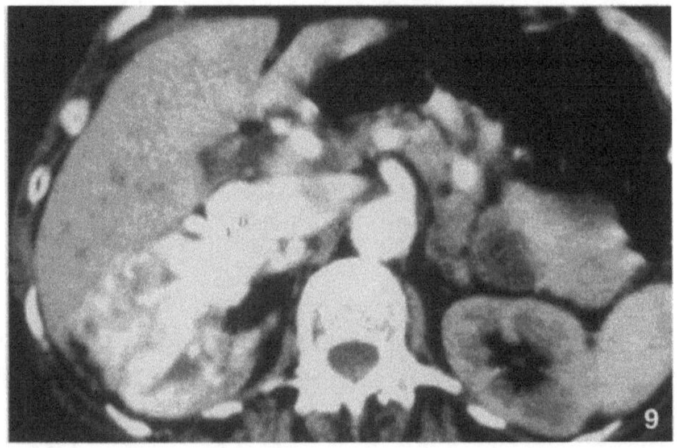

Fig. 30.7 a, b. Tubulopapillary carcinoma (grade II). **a** Tubulopapillary adenocarcinoma of the posterior surface of the left kidney. Post-contrast CT in the tubular phase: mass of about 6 cm in diameter, completely hypodense, comprising of very slight heterogeneity peripherally with fine calcification outlining the external contour of the lesion. **b** MRI T2-weighted sequence. The hypointense soft tissue component is well contrasted with the hyperintense necrotic component

Fig. 30.8. Oncocytic tumor. CT performed in the cortical phase: mass on the anterior lip of the kidney, highly vascular with a hypodense stellate center. Grade II oncocytic adenocarcinoma at histology

Fig. 30.9. Clear cell adenocarcinoma of the kidney with multiple arteriovenous tumor shunts. Post-contrast CT performed at an early stage demonstrates multiple vessels at the renal hilum and within the tumor itself associated with early venous filling and dilatation of the renal vein and inferior vena cava

case, the tumor is more often formed by several cavities filled with a yellow lemon-colored or even hemorrhagic fluid, separated from each other by fibrous walls of variable thickness. It may be mistaken for a benign multilocular cyst. The presence of pale yellow areas in the cyst wall or within the septa is suggestive of renal carcinoma.

Evolution

The natural growth rate of a renal carcinoma is estimated to be, on average, 0.5 cm/year. Arising within the renal parenchyma (proximal convoluted tubules or distal collecting system) [15, 37], the tumor progressively invades the capsule, perirenal fat and the adjacent organs. Spread to the renal collecting system is responsible for the presence of hematuria, urographic abnormalities and tumor dissemination along the excretory system which is still rare.

Metastastic spread occurs by two routes:

- lymphatic: metastatic spread to lymph nodes is seen in 60% of cases in autopsy series. Initially the intrarenal lymphatic network is involved, in close relationship to the venous network, followed subsequently by the latero-aortic and aorto-caval lymph node chains. The most frequently involved lymph nodes, however, are in the lumbo-aortic and mediastinal regions;
- hematogenous, with tumor thrombus in the renal veins and subsequently the IVC. This often occurs at

Table 30.1. Robson's classification

Stage	Extent	5 year survival rate (13)
Stage I	Tumor confined within the capsule	73%
Stage II	Tumor extending beyond the capsule but not beyond the renal bed	68%
Stage III		
Stage IIIA	Extension into the renal vein or IVC	51%
Stage IIIB	Metastatic lymphadenopathy in the renal pedicle or lumbo-aortic lymph node chains	60%
Stage IIIC	Venous or lymph node spread	43%
Stage IV		
Stage IVA	Extension beyond the renal bed	
Stage IVB	Distant metastasis	20%

Table 30.2. TNM Classification

Classification of the tumor	Description	5 year survival (Tumor T × N0)
Stage T1	Intraparenchymal tumor < 5 cm in size	> 80%
Stage T2	Intraparenchymal tumor > 5 cm in size	50%
Stage T3	Renal lesion which does not extend beyond the renal bed	N0 rare
T3a	Extension into the perirenal fat	
T3b	Extension into the renal vein	
T3c	Extension into the IVC	
T3d	Extension into the supradiaphragmatic IVC	
Stage T4	Regional spread to adjacent organs	N0 exceptional
Lymph node invasion	**Description**	
Stage N0	No lymph node involvement	
Stage N1	Presence of solitary unilateral adenopathy	10%
Stage N2	Presence of multiple nodal involvement	
Stage N3	Presence of multiple and fixed lymphadenopathy	
Metastases	**Description**	
Stage M0	No metastasis	
Stage M1	Metastasis present	< 6%

an early stage and is caused by richly vascularized neoplastic tissue whose histopathological and radiological characteristics are identical to those of the primary tumor. In conjunction with other criteria, this determines the prognosis as well as the surgical approach.

Complete obstruction of the renal vein induces the development of a collateral venous network from the gonadal and perispinal veins which explains the presence of metastases in both these locations.

Distant metastases are present in 25% of cases at the time of diagnosis [28]. They are dominated by pulmonary metastases (76% in autopsy series) and lymph node metastases (66% of cases). Other sites include bone (42%), adrenals (17%), pancreas (14%), brain (6%) and skin [28,44].

Tumor staging is defined in terms of the clinical, radiological and histopathological findings. There are two classification systems principally used [24]:

- Robson's classification (table 30.1), established in 1969, is the first. Although simple, it has the disadvantage of grouping together in the same stage (stage III) some features which have a very different prognostic significance (venous and lymph node invasion);
- the TNM classification of the OMS from 1988 (table 30.2) is preferable. This classification system is more precise although the differentiation between certain stages may seem artificial. The 5 year survival rates for stages T3a and T3c are very different whereas those for T1, T2 and T3a or T3b are comparable.

The slow natural growth rate of renal adenocarcinomas should render possible an early diagnosis, while the tumor is still localized. This raises the question of the impossibility of even considering a mass screening program due to the absence of a clearly proven risk factor and the difficulty of characterizing small lesions (even using all imaging modalities). The frequency of multifocal lesions must be underlined with the resultant implications on conservative treatments. This occurs with an incidence of between 7 and 17% depending on the series.

Histopathology and prognostic factors

The **histological forms** of the carcinomas are very variable. They are distinguished by:
- the architecture:
  - the compact or highly vascular acinar forms;
  - the tubular forms;
  - the tubulopapillary forms in which the papillae contain a vascular-connective tissue axis usually punctuated with calcospherites (minute intracellular spherical deposits of calcoglobulin) and infiltrated with foamy macrophages (fig. 30.6);
  - the cystic or pseudocystic forms due to tumor necrosis (fig. 30.4); the truly cystic forms (fig. 30.5) in which neoplastic cells lodge in one or several sites adjacent to the cavity or in a mass within the fibrous septa;
- the cell type [28, 70]:
  - clear cell carcinoma, more than 75% of which consists of polygonal cells with a visibly empty cytoplasm, rich in glycogen and lipids;
  - oxophil cell carcinoma, more than 75% of which consists of polygonal eosinophilic cells, rich in multiple micro-organites on electron microscopy;
  - mixed cell carcinoma containing equal proportions of clear and oxyphilic cells;
  - basophil cell carcinomas (of a tubulopapillary structure);
  - the recently identified chromophobe cell carcinomas, made up of cells with clear or eosinophilic cytoplasm with discrete vacuole, unique by their micropolysaccharide content and the presence of carbonic anhydrase [37, 76];
  - sarcomatoid cell carcinomas with independent fusiform tumor calls and multiple cytonuclear atypias. They are usually associated with typical zones of renal cell carcinoma. However, immunohistochemistry (cells positive for antikeratin antibodies, EMA) may be necessary to exclude a true sarcoma.

Prognostic factors: the most commonly used histological grading system for prognosis is that of Susan Führman which combines simplicity with a precision of definition and reproducibility [28, 54, 70].

Grade I: presence of small regular nuclei (< 10 μm) without nucleoli.

Grade II: presence of slightly irregular nuclei (around 15 μm) with nucleoli visible at high magnification.

Grade III: presence of very or slightly irregular nuclei (around 20 μm) with nucleoli visible at low magnification.

Grade IV: appearances similar to grade III but with nuclear atypia (multilobulated nuclei).

This grading system seems to correlate well with the survival rate independent of the stage. In stage I disease, grades I and II are associated with a ten year survival rate without recurrence of 100%. This falls to less than 50% for grades III and IV.

Other prognostic histological features are more contentious [14, 28, 54, 63, 70]. The homogeneous, sarcomatoid forms tend to have a poor outlook. On the other hand, the chromophobe cell and the tubulopapillary cell carcinomas (when composed predominantly of basophil cells) are associated with a favorable prognosis [57, 70, 76].

Ploidy and cytogenetics: the ploidy of the tumor population is one of the most recently studied prognostic criteria. Aneuploidy seems to correlate with the nuclear grading and more advanced stage. The percentage of cells in phase S has no particular significance. However, the results to date are still too limited for the use of ploidy as an independent prognostic indicator [1, 5, 16, 18, 39, 52].

Cytogenetic studies of renal tumors have demonstrated non-hazardous chromosomal alterations which vary depending on the type of tumor (anomaly of the short arm of the chromosome 3 in clear or eosinophilic cell carcinomas, trisomy 17 in tubulopapillary carcinomas, trisomy 7 in both types of tumor) [32, 38, 49].

In the basophil cell tubulopapillary tumors, the presence of multiple chromosomal abnormalities seems to correlate with a more aggressive tumor with a greater metastatic potential [38].

Other malignant tumors

Sarcomas represent 1% of all malignant renal neoplasms [28]. Leiomyosarcomas are the commonest (40-60%) and have an intraparenchymal or pericapsular localization [28]. The other histological types are even more infrequent: fibrosarcoma, malignant histiocytofibroma, liposarcoma [15], rhabdomyosarcoma, vascular sarcomas…

Their histological appearance does not differ from that of sarcomas elsewhere. The histoprognosis

Table 30.3. Modes of presentation of renal cancer

1) Symptomatic forms a) Urological symptoms – Frank hematuria, insidious, intermittent, painless and recurrent – Lumbar pain or renal colic – Palpable mass in the flank or lumbar region b) Medical symptoms – General • Fever • Deterioration in general health • Chronic inflammatory syndrome • Metastasis – Hematological • Anemia • Polycytemia – Cardiovascular • Resistant hypertension • Thrombo-embolism – Paraneoplastic syndromes: • Stauffer's syndrome (non-metastatic hepatomegaly) • Polyneuropathy • Hypercalcemia...
2) Forms detected incidentally: (more than 50% of cases for the tumors < 5 cm) Detected during a paraclinical examination: ultrasound or CT

defines 2-4 grades depending on the classification and depends on several different criteria; differentiation, cellularity, anisokaryotosis and anisocytosis, number of mitoses, the presence of tumor necrosis [27].

The nephroblastoma in the adult is extremely rare [15].

Rare cases of primary small cell renal carcinomas have been described [75].

Benign tumors

The differential diagnoses are comprised primarily of the adenoma, oncocytoma, angiomyolipoma, Bolande's tumor, benign mesenchymal tumor and tumor of the juxtaglomerular apparatus.

Clinical features

Hematuria is the chief presenting sign of a renal cancer. However, these tumors may present with a number of other, sometimes misleading, symptoms (table 30.3).

The availability of examinations such as ultrasound and CT has resulted in an increase in the number of renal masses detected incidentally [2, 8, 60], a better prognosis being associated with those lesions which are suitable for a conservative treatment. This mode of detection seems to be the commonest in our experience, the symptomatic forms corresponding to the more advanced cancers.

Imaging

As a result of the early detection of renal masses [73] and the advent of conservative operative techniques, the clinician requires an accurate staging of the tumor as well as a prediction of the operative difficulty. The radiologist is helped in achieving this by the use of the different examination techniques, each with their own indications, contraindications and limitations.

Indications for CT, MRI and other imaging techniques

Intravenous urography (IVU)

This is an essential first line examination performed in cases of hematuria or alternatively at the time of a

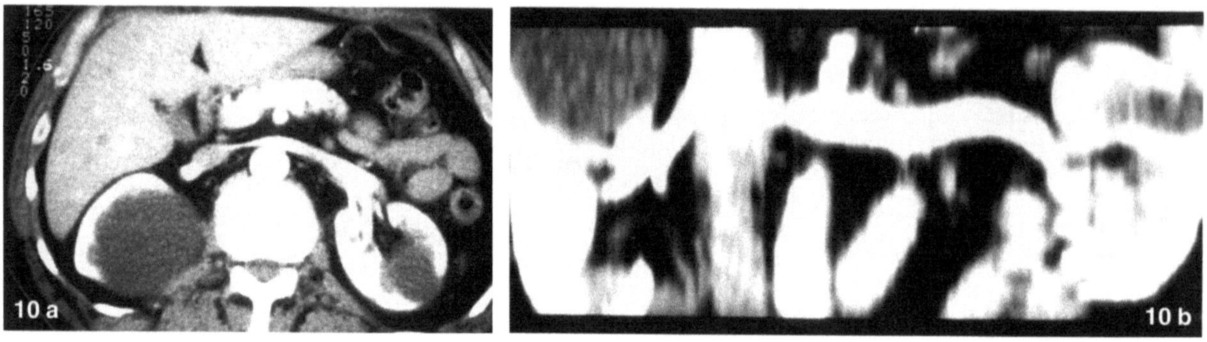

Fig. 30.10-30.14. Assessment of spread of renal carcinomas

Fig. 30.10 a, b. Anatomy of the renal veins. **a** Axial post-contrast CT in the cortical phase: good opacification of the left renal vein which lies in the axial plane of section and right renal vein located in an oblique plane running from infero-superiorly and latero-medially and appearing on this section as a dense opacity adjacent to the inferior vena cava. **b** Multiplanar reconstructions from a spiral acquisition obtained in a 24 second breath hold, sections performed every 5 mm and reconstructed every 3 mm. On this oblique reconstruction, the orientation of the right renal vein is highlighted, as well as the position of the left renal vein. Note the multiple cysts in the renal parenchyma bilaterally

CT examination (scano-urography), particularly for tumors detected incidentally or incidentally. IVU is especially targeted to assess the collecting system in order to detect invasion of the pelvicalyceal system and to give some idea of the function and morphology of the contralateral kidney.

This examination is unable to characterize the tissue or determine the intralesional vascularity. It is also poor for the detection of small intraparenchymal masses: although the sensitivity is good for masses greater than 3 cm (85%), there is a sharp fall below this size and is no greater than 10% if the tumor measures less than 1 cm in diameter [78]. This latter point is particularly important for lesions located on the anterior and posterior surfaces or for masses which do not deform the renal contour. However, urography provides a more satisfactory study of the renal poles than ultrasound, particularly the upper pole of the left kidney which is more difficult to assess ultrasonically.

Abdominal ultrasound

Due to its simplicity of use and safety, ultrasound has rapidly become an indispensable complementary examination in any patient presenting with abdominal symptoms. It enables early detection of asymptomatic renal masses explaining the high frequency nowadays of the incidental discovery of these lesions. Ultrasound gives a detailed assessment of the renal parenchyma and accurately defines the solid or cystic nature of the mass. The sensitivity of this technique is definitely superior to urography for tumors smaller than 3 cm although the latter seems to be better for the larger tumors [69,78]. The examination is completed by a color doppler ultrasound study which improves the definition of the vascular character of the mass and its spread into the renal vein and inferior vena cava.

There are no known contraindications to ultrasound. However, it may be technically difficult to perform due to the patient's habitus, interposition of bowel loops (flexures of the colon) or general immobility of the patient. In addition, certain tumors are difficult to assess, either due to their localization (particularly in the upper pole of the left kidney which is difficult to access ultrasonically), or the small size of the tumor or its echopattern relative to the normal parenchyma. The presence of calcification within the center or periphery of the tumor may also result in suboptimal visualization [69]. Ultrasound is of no value in the study of the excretory tracts except in the presence of significant ureteric dilatation.

Although ultrasound, particularly color doppler ultrasound, tends not to be reproducible and is operator dependent, the value of this technique should not be underestimated and it may in some cases provide invaluable information to the clinician.

CT

Like ultrasound, CT has become an essential examination in the assessment of a renal tumor. It is able in a very simple and reproducible fashion to diagnose, characterize and stage the tumor. In the majority of cases, single ultrasound examination is sufficient to confirm the diagnosis and assess tumor extent. For the purpose of clarity, we have separated the diagnostic stage from the staging process.

The constant improvements in equipment (microelectronics and computers) have led to a significant reduction in the acquisition time for each section making the performance of angiographic CT possible [55]. More recently, the arrival of a new generation of continuous rotation scanners employing a "spiral" mode technique enable the whole of the renal areas to be studied in a single pass. This latter technique has become the examination of choice for renal tumors due to its ability to study the tumor in the nephrographic phase as well as having the potential to perform higher quality multiplanar reconstructions, all achieved with a reduced examination time (fig. 30.10).

MRI

Using strong magnetic fields, this technique has raised hopes since its appearance concerning the tissue characterization of tumors. Unfortunately these have all proven to be false hopes, and it is currently not possible to differentiate a benign from a malignant tumor [64].

This technique has several advantages over CT and is complementary to it. Firstly, it has the advantage of a multiplanar capability for the assessment of the renal poles and the inferior vena cava. Second, it uses a gadolinium based contrast agent [66], which is minimally allergenic and does not affect renal function [34, 65]. Finally, the T2-weighted sequences analyze the water content of tissues providing an improved differentiation between tumor necrosis and viable tumor.

The MRI examination routinely consists of T1- and dual echo T2-weighted sequences (with early and late echoes) to define the different tissue constituents within the tumor.

As a subsequent examination, a dynamic breath hold study [71] using a specially adapted sequence after the injection of a paramagnetic contrast agent is able to follow the kinetics of tumor enhancement. If renal vein or caval spread is suspected, a flow sensitive sequence can be performed.

The great improvements in MRI with advent of rapid sequences, breath hold sequences, better spatial resolution with the use of a 512 × 512 matrix, and the reduction in artefacts have resulted in improved sensitivity compared to older generation scanners, and one can only surmise the possibilities and role of this technique in the future.

Angiography

Selective renal arteriography, previously widely used in the investigation of renal tumors, no longer has a role in the routine preoperative assessment since the development of CT, ultrasound and MRI. It is reserved for large hypervascular tumors and for those associated with large intratumoral arteriovenous shunts. Arteriography is often requested with the aim of devascularizing the tumor preoperatively in order to facilitate the surgical resection. The other indications for this technique include the presence of a tumor in a solitary kidney for which the production of a map of the vascular anatomy is useful to the surgeon if a partial nephrectomy is being considered [6, 12, 53].

The same applies to inferior vena cavography, the indication for which is an ambiguous appearance on the other previous investigations [6, 41, 42]. The value of routine urographic exposures centered on the kidneys should be remembered following an intravenous iodinated contrast injection administered during any diagnostic investigation not specifically targeted at the kidney. This is particularly relevant following arteriography where the image may sometimes detect a urographic abnormality leading to a complementary examination.

Bone scintigraphy

The aim of this radioisotope examination using technetium-99m methylene diphosphonate (MDP) is the detection of bony secondary deposits which usually appear as areas of increased uptake at the site of the metastasis. This test should be requested in the presence of clinical or biochemical evidence suggestive of a bony metastasis; the interpretation of the images is sometimes difficult due to the absence of specificity of an area of increased uptake which can equally well be seen in degenerative or infective disorders.

Signs

Following the diagnosis of a solid renal tumor, the radiologist must provide the clinician with as accurate as possible assessment of the locoregional and systemic extent of the disease in order to determine the prognosis, treatment and surgical intervention. Ultrasound and particularly CT and MRI give valuable information and enable the clinician to tailor the treatment decisions more and more to the clinical picture presented by the patient.

Characterization of renal tumors (renal adenocarcinoma)

See figs 30.1-30.9 and table 30.4.

CT

CT has become the reference examination in the morphological assessment of renal tumors and provides the clinician with a great deal of information.

On the unenhanced images, a third of renal adenocarcinomas contain calcifications which are distributed either centrally (67% of cases) or peripherally [79].

The presence of punctate calcification within a renal mass is infrequent but very suggestive of a renal tumor. Although typically hypodense (32% of cases) or isodense (32%) relative to the cortex before the injection of contrast, intrinsically hyperdense forms are not rare (32%) [79]; the malignant tumors in adults do not contain islands of fatty density.

There are three possible appearances on the post-contrast CT:

- the classical form of a well vascularized tumor exhibiting a typically intense and transient enhancement in the arterial phase (figs 30.1-30.3): on the later images, the measured tumor density is greater than that on the pre-contrast scan despite appearing relatively more hypodense compared to the normal cortex [79]. Due to the vascular changes, the contrast enhancement is more marked peripherally than centrally where necrotico-hemorrhagic phenomena are common;
- more rarely, the hypovascular tumors exhibit little or no enhancement, necessitating the performance of delayed images for the detection of even minimal enhancement. Comparison with the ultrasound study is essential in these cases [51] (fig. 30.6);
- the cystic renal masses are more difficult to analyze and require a meticulous assessment of the whole lesion, particularly its wall to look for any nodularity (figs 30.4, 30.5, 30.7) which is suggestive of a neoplastic process. Comparison of the ultrasound, CT and even MRI examinations is important in the diagnosis of these cystic renal masses. Bosniak and colleagues have proposed a classification, staging in four grades with the atypical features encountered in a cystic mass [3, 12, 13]. This has led to a treatment strategy which is dependent on the degree of these atypias and the suspicion of cancer.

Table 30.4. Staging accuracy of renal tumors by CT

Authors	Year of the study	Number of patients	Staging included accuracy (%)
Love et al	1979	17	89
Probst et al	1981	40	85
Karp et al	1981	24	70
Cronan et al	1982	23	91
Plainfossé et al	1983	12	75
Elder et al	1984	31	62
Rinsho et al	1987	34	82
Fein et al	1987	27	67
Kishi et al	1987	18	61
Johnson et al	1987	100	91
Mc Kintryand, Mc Ilrath	1987	21	78
London, Messios, et al	1988	28	72
Zeman, et al	1988	121	90
Miles, et al	1990	70	72
Dinney, et al	1992	314	68
Hatcher, et al 1992	653	64	
	Mean		76

MRI

MRI has initially been disappointing due to the lack of inherent contrast between the tumor and the normal adjacent renal cortex [19, 64]. More recently, the introduction of new sequences (fat suppression, rapid sequences) [71] coupled with the injection of gadolinium has definitely changed this state of affairs. As a result of these improvements, MRI has become more sensitive and could in future compete with CT in the diagnosis of these tumors.

The signal intensity of the tumor is very variable and non-specific on T1-weighted and T2-weighted imaging. Due to the histological diversity of renal tumors, it is not possible to make the diagnosis with certainty. Generally, the tumor appears as a heterogeneous mass distorting the renal outline, of intermediate signal intensity between that of the renal medulla and cortex on T1-weighted imaging [29, 46].

The combination of the T1- and T2-weighted sequences can distinguish the necrotic and hemorrhagic areas from the soft tissue zones. The hemorrhagic areas appear hyperintense on T1 whereas the necrotic areas have a less intense signal. On T2-weighted imaging, the signal intensity of necrotic and hemorrhagic tissues is variable depending on their composition and the degree of T2-weighting. Generally they are clearly hyperintense.

The injection of gadolinium associated with the use of fast sequences provides a dynamic study of the enhancement pattern [71]. The tumor tissues appear hypervascular and heterogeneous with peripheral enhancement in the majority of cases [26].

In the case of hypovascular tumors, the T2-weighted sequences may demonstrate hypointense soft tissue areas which are easy to differentiate from the hyperintense necrosis (fig. 30.7).

As with both the previous techniques, in the presence of a mass composed almost exclusively of fluid, it is necessary to analyze both the wall of the mass and its contents [19, 26, 34]. Following the injection of gadolinium, the presence of enhancement of the wall or a soft tissue portion of the mass should be looked for. However, the accuracy of MRI is limited by the poor spatial resolution of the current machines.

Tumor spread (figs 30.10-30.14)

The investigation of a renal mass should routinely include an analysis of various anatomical structures which may be involved by the lesion: CT has major role in this (table 30.6).

Extension by contiguous spread

Assessment of invasion of the capsule and perirenal region remains the area for which the different imag-

Table 30.5. Classification of atypical cysts

Type	Description
Category 1: Benign cyst	Rounded appearance, thin walls without septa. Homogeneous density (< 20 HU), no enhancement following contrast
Category 2: Complicated cyst	Presence of: – thin septa – fine and regular calcification – hyperdense contents *Follow-up is usually indicated*
Category 3: Indeterminate lesion	Presence of: – ill-defined borders – thick and irregular septa – thick and irregular calcification – multilocular appearance *Partial nephrectomy is indicated*
Category 4: Malignant tumor	Presence of: – thick walls (> 3 mm)/ nodularity – enhancement following contrast injection *Extended nephrectomy is necessary*

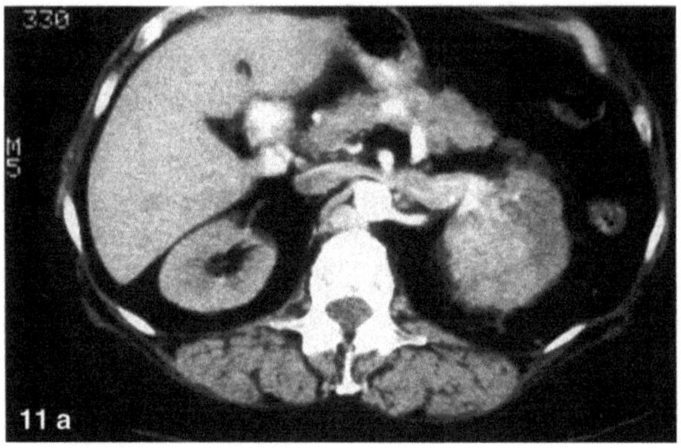

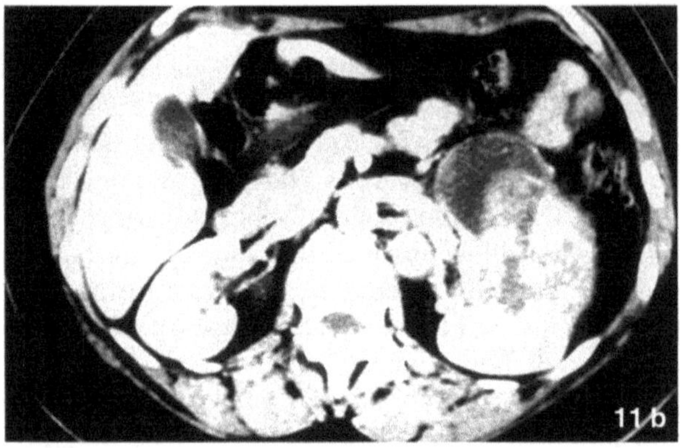

Fig. 30.11 a, b. Staging of a renal adenocarcinoma. **a** CT performed in an early phase: tumor located in the superior pole of the left kidney; enlargement of the renal vein proximal to the aorto-mesenteric space due to dense solid vascularized tissue. **b** CT in the early cortical phase, tumor with dual composition, vascularized soft tissue and necrotic hypodense tissue anteriorly. The left renal vein is clear, and 2 cm diameter adenopathy is visible posterior to the left renal artery and vein

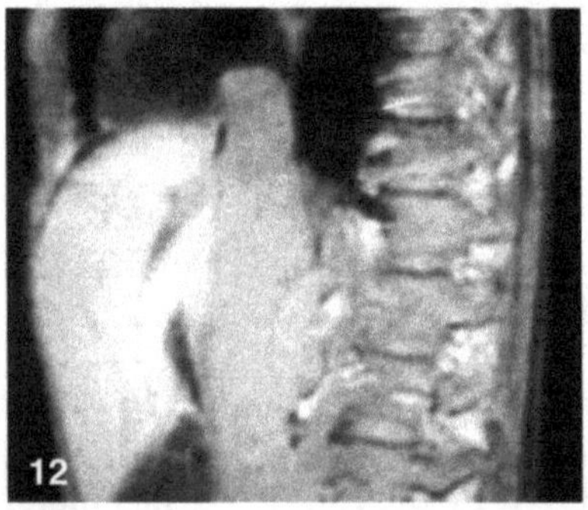

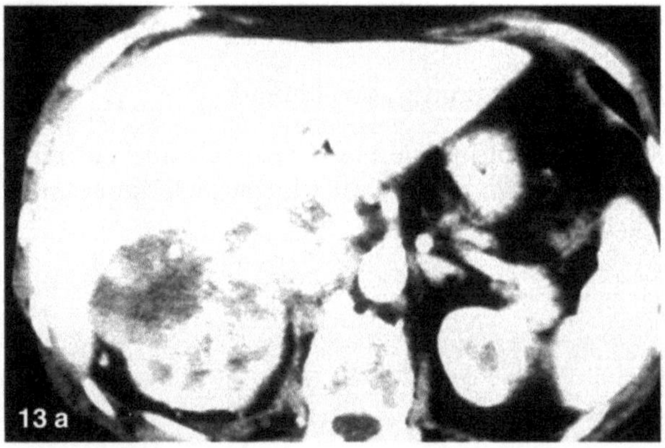

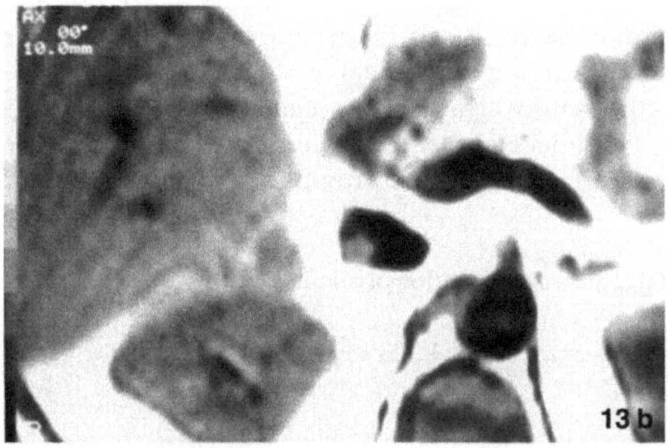

Fig. 30.12. Thrombosis of the inferior vena cava from a right renal adenocarcinoma. Sagittal MRI through the IVC: large thrombus involving the whole of the IVC and extending into the right atrium

Fig. 30.13 a, b. Clear cell adenocarcinoma with spread into the IVC. **a** CT at an early cortical phase. Hypervascularization of the wall of the IVC associated with a central filling defect within which are visible intratumoral bands: neoplastic thrombus of the IVC secondary to a adenocarcinoma of the anterior portion of the right kidney. **b** Axial T1-weighted MRI section. Filling defect in the right postero-lateral aspect of the IVC silhouetted by the low signal of the patent lumen: thrombus limited to the IVC secondary to a right renal adenocarcinoma

ing techniques have the poorest sensitivity. It is in fact currently impossible to demonstrate microscopic invasion. On the other hand, an area of fascial thickening can simply be due to inflammatory change [33].

The conventional imaging techniques (IVU, arteriography...) are of no value in the detection of this invasion. Ultrasound does not visualize the renal capsule and therefore cannot make this diagnosis. Only

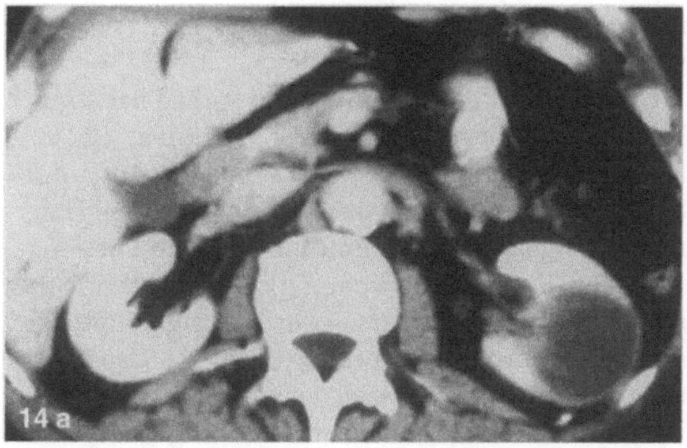

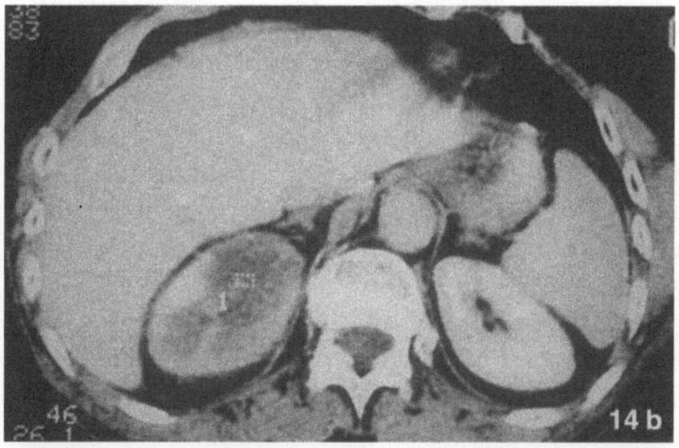

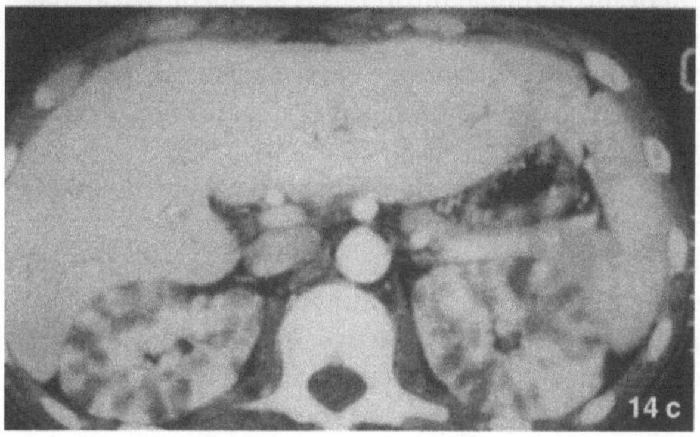

Fig. 30.14 a-c. a Squamous bronchial carcinoma. Left renal mass. Post-contrast CT: rounded hypodense lesion which barely deforms the renal outline, "globular" appearance: metastasis from a squamous cancer proven by percutaneous CT guided biopsy. **b** Infiltrative urothelial tumor. Tumor invading the renal tract, infiltrating the anterior part of the superior pole of the right kidney; nephrographic filling defect with irregular contours but without deformity of the renal outline. Small intratumoral vessels visible in the early phase following contrast injection. **c** Bilateral lymphomatous lesions involving the kidneys. Post-contrast CT: multiple hypodense nodules filling the renal parenchyma bilaterally

invasion of adjacent organs can be suggested ultrasonically by the presence of an area within the implicated organ which is in direct contact with the tumor and has an identical echopattern.

On CT, this invasion is suspected by the presence of a solid mass measuring more than 1 cm in diameter within the perirenal space [47]. This must be differentiated from the nodular-appearing structures secondary to the principally venous collateral circulation occurring in cases of renal vein thrombosis or the large hypervascular tumors. Comparison of the pre- and post-contrast images, as well as assessing the images immediately above and below, will avoid this pitfall [80].

The presence of fascial thickening adjacent to the tumor of variable regularity does not necessarily indicate invasion, inflammatory changes around the mass being frequent. A striated or spiculated appearance in the perirenal fat, although suspicious, is entirely nonspecific. Due to the axial plane of section, an evaluation of the adjacent organs can be difficult and may be helped by image reconstruction in the most appropriate plane. Invasion is also suspected in the presence of a heterogeneous area within the organ in continuity with the tumor [47].

On MRI, the assessment of capsular and perirenal invasion is improved by using fast breath hold sequences which give improved visualization of the fascia and reduce movement artefacts. The pathological appearances of perirenal invasion are similar to those described for CT with technical advantage of multiplanar sections. The pitfall of capsular varices is more easily avoided due to the signal characteristics of blood flow within them.

Finally, the invasion of adjacent organs is more easily detected on MRI by the demonstration of loss of the normal signal of the involved organ in contact with the tumor. The normal signal is replaced by a high signal intensity on T2-weighted imaging with irregular borders in the case of hepatic or muscle invasion and by high signal intensity on T1-weighted imaging in cases of splenic involvement [46]. The use of sagittal or coronal sections may useful in these cases.

Venous spread

Venous involvement represents one of the major elements in the staging process [43]. It must, therefore, be detected as accurately as possible because, to a large degree, this influences the surgical approach and technique. The use of often complementary techniques can appreciate invasion of the trunk of the renal vein with a satisfactory sensitivity. However, using current techniques it is very difficult to demonstrate the small thrombi within the intrahilar portion of the renal vein and its branches. The study of the renal vein is usually restricted to the portion beyond the hilum of the kidney.

On B-mode ultrasound, the diagnosis is suggested by the presence of a dilated renal vein containing echogenic material which may extend distally into the inferior vena cava and right atrium. The demonstration of intraluminal thrombus is an unequivocal diagnostic sign although it is not possible to determine as to whether it is tumor or simple thrombus. However, there are possible sources of error, and these should not be forgotten.

The presence of a dilated vein without thrombus may correspond to increased flow due to the hypervascular tumor or be related to the presence of intratumoral arteriovenous shunts. This ambiguity can easily be overcome by the use of color doppler ultrasound which clearly demonstrates the normal patency of the vein in these cases. In addition, certain anatomical variants (double renal veins) may be the source of false negatives. Finally, the investigation and assessment of the renal vein may sometimes be difficult in the presence of a large tumor.

The finding of color doppler ultrasound is similar to that of B-mode ultrasound, the technique giving a clearer demonstration of the venous pedicle and its collateral branches.

On CT, venous invasion appears as enlargement of the involved vein containing a hypodense filling defect following contrast injection which may or may not obstruct the vein (fig. 30.11) [42, 47, 59, 68]. This sign is sometimes associated with arteriolo-capillary opacification of the thrombus in the arterial phase, thus indicating its neoplastic nature (15% of cases) [33]. On the other hand, the presence of a venous collateral network is of little significance and may be due to a hypervascular mass or a venous thrombus.

Invasion of the inferior vena cava (fig. 30.13 a) follows the same finding; however, although CT can demonstrate well the inferior limit of the thrombus, it is difficult to localize the upper limit due to the axial plane of section and flow phenomena [33, 42, 68]. Unlike thrombus, flow phenomena have irregular outlines which occur at the site of a venous ostium and are not central.

Mural invasion of the vein appears as an interruption of the vessel wall. This sign is difficult to appreciate due to the poor contrast and the predominantly intrahepatic localization of the suprarenal inferior vena cava [56].

On MRI, the detection of venous spread has a much higher sensitivity for the inferior vena cava (figs 30.12 & 30.13b) [33, 45, 48, 67, 68]. The signal intensity of the tumor thrombus follows that of the tumor itself (intermediate signal on T1-weighted imaging and heterogeneous on T2-weighted imaging). On the other hand, simple thrombus appears of variable signal intensity depending on the age of the clot [59, 68]. Usually the tumor thrombus is associated with enlargement of the involved vein and enhanced following gadolinium injection [26, 68]. Invasion of the wall of the vein appears as an interruption or irregular thinning of the hypointensity of the wall on T2-weighted imaging [59, 68].

Due to the use of multiple planes, the superior limit of the thrombus can be accurately assessed, as well as determining as to whether the thrombus is neoplastic or simple.

On cavography, the thrombus appears as an intraluminal filling defect arising from one of the renal veins. Previously it was the reference examination for detecting venous spread. However, cavography can miss a thrombus within the renal vein or a posteriorly situated thrombus which explains its inferior sensitivity compared to MRI.

Lymph node spread

Although lymph node invasion is one of the major prognostic criteria, it is often impossible to demonstrate a microscopic involvement.

The conventional imaging techniques (IVU, arteriography...) have no role in the assessment of lymph node involvement.

Ultrasound may demonstrate the presence of peri-aortico-caval lymphadenopathy, but there are no specific ultrasound criteria which can indicate definite involvement. CT is a more reliable investigation for the detection of lymph node involvement (sensitivity of 68% and specificity of 50%). Any lymph node whose transverse diameter exceeds 1 cm and/or enhanced following contrast injection is considered to be involved (fig. 30.11b) [47, 48]. However, this arbitrary criterion of size is susceptible to the risk of both false positives (reactive inflammatory lymphadenopathy) and false negatives (microscopic invasion) [33, 41].

On MRI, lymph node spread is equally well visualized, although the signal intensity is non-specific. Generally lymphadenopathies appear isointense on T1-weighted imaging and hyperintense on T2-weighted imaging [34, 46].

Distant spread

Due to the mode of spread via the venous system, pulmonary metastases are the most frequently encountered secondary lesions. Pulmonary metastases are usually evident on a plain chest x-ray and have no distinctive features.

Hepatic involvement is often detected by ultrasound or CT. On MRI, hepatic metastases appear hypointense on T1-weighted imaging and hyperintense on T2-weighted imaging relative to the normal hepatic parenchyma [46].

Bone metastases, often detected by bone scintigraphy and standard radiographs, may also be picked up on MRI in the form of a mass appearing hypointense on T1-weighted imaging and hyperintense on T2-weighted imaging relative to the bone marrow [46].

Other metastatic sites of this cancer should be looked for if there is a clinical indication.

There should be a routine and careful assessment of the contralateral kidney to exclude multiple tumors. There are several possibilities to account for multiple lesions: these include either a metastasis, a contralateral cancer, or polyadenomatosis. The presence of multiple cystic and solid lesions raises the suspicion of von Hippel-Lindau disease.

Follow-up

In our experience, abdominal CT both with and without contrast agent is currently the examination of choice for the follow-up of renal cancer and has a satisfactory sensitivity for the detection of possible recurrences. Apart from local recurrence, the contralateral kidney should be carefully assessed to detect a contralateral cancer which occurs in about 10% of cases. The examination should be performed about 6 months after surgery and subsequently on an annual basis.

Ultrasound cannot adequately assess the nephrectomy bed because of interference by bowel loops. It may, however, detect secondary lesions which were imperceptible on the initial study and can evaluate the contralateral kidney. In cases of doubt over the possibility of a recurrence, a repeat MRI should be performed.

The follow-up of patients treated by immunotherapy (interleukin-2 and interferon) is also achieved by CT and ultrasound, the frequency of which depends on the protocol adopted. This treatment is still under evaluation but gives a response rate of about 15-20% with prolongation of the average survival rate and in several cases has affected a complete remission.

Other primary tumors of the kidney

The sarcoma is a rare tumor occurring with a frequency of 1.3% (the Mayo Clinic) over a period of ten years. This figure may be an overestimate as a result of diagnostic errors, essentially histological confusion with sarcomatoid carcinomas, clear cell sarcomas or even angiomyolipomas.

Among the various types of sarcoma, the liposarcoma would appear itself to be quite rare, but it shares with the osteosarcoma with the unusual characteristic of having a specific recognizable imaging feature. The principal problem is determining the site of original tumor:

- in the majority of cases, the liposarcoma arises from the extrarenal retroperitoneal tissues causing some degree of displacement of the kidney, only invading it at a late stage;
- true tumors of renal origin are very infrequent: the tumor arises from the capsule, intrarenal vessels or the tissues of the renal sinus. The differential diagnosis with a retroperitoneal sarcoma is not possible with these often large lesions, and the best criteria remain histopathological (subcapsular invasion of the renal parenchyma).

Renal metastases and lymphoma of the kidneys are essentially suggested by the presence of multiple solid tumors of the renal parenchyma. These lesions are often missed ultrasonically as their echogenicity is close to that of the normal parenchyma. They are characterized on CT by their hypovascularity and intrarenal localization but cause little or no deformity of the renal outline. In the cases of a solitary lesion, the clinical context, the CT criteria and particularly percutaneous biopsy (usually under CT guidance) which provides the histology are used to confirm the metastatic or lymphomatous nature of the lesion (fig. 30.14 a, b).

Tumors of the excretory system only really pose a problem in the forms which infiltrate the renal parenchyma. These tumors usually arise in the calyces, and this localization results in early parenchymal involvement; hematuria is the principal symptom of these urothelial tumors. Certain characteristic CT features should be underlined. The external morphology of the kidney is normal, and its overall dimensions are only moderately increased. The boundaries between the tumor and parenchyma are indistinct and irregular. As a rule, the tumor is hypovascular and appears as an area of density lower than that of the renal parenchyma, even on the early images, without significant enhancement following the injection of contrast. The images in the urographic phase confirm the presence

Table 30.6. Sensitivity of the different imaging techniques

	Tumor	Capsule	Perirenal	Adjacent organs	Renal vein	Inferior vena cava	Lymph nodes	Excretory tract	Liver	Bone
ASP	+/-	-	-	-	-	-	-	-	-	+
IVU	+	-	-	-	-	-	-	++++	-	+
US	++++	-	+/-	+	++	++	+	-	+++	-
CT	++++	++	++	+	++	+++	+++	-	++	+
MRI	+++	+	++	+++	++	++++	+++	-	+++	+++
Arterio	++	-	-	-	+/-	+/-	-	-	-	-
Cavo	-	-	-	-	++	+++	-	-	-	-

of enhancement or amputation of a calyx or in the territory of a calyx (fig. 30.14 b).

Conclusion

Renal cancer is more and more commonly detected incidentally as a result of the routine performance of ultrasound and CT. These tumors are often slowly growing over many years. However, tumors of less than a centimeter in size are still difficult to demonstrate, and the absence of an easily recognizable area does not allow an assessment of the mass.

Within a few years, CT has become the essential examination for tumor characterization and staging (table 30.6). The advent of new techniques, such as spiral CT, has further improved the sensitivity of this modality.

Although MRI currently has a rather marginal role in the assessment of renal tumors, the constant improvements in the machines and imaging sequences will enable it in the future to equal or even surpass the diagnostic accuracy of CT.

The improvements in the diagnosis, localization and staging of these lesions have opened the way to conservative treatments, either by necessity for multiple lesions or a solitary functioning kidney, or as the primary treatment of small intrarenal tumors confined to one pole or periphery of the kidney.

References

1. Al Abadhi H, Nagel R (1988) Prognostic relevance of ploidy and proliferative activity of renal cell carcinoma. Eur Urol 15: 271-276
2. Amendola MA, Bree RL, Pollack HM, Francis IR, Glazer GM, Jafri SZH, Tomaszewski JE (1988) Small renal cell carcinomas: resolving a diagnostic dilemma. Radiology 166: 637-642
3. Aronson S, Frazier HA, Baluch JD, et al (1991) Cystic renal masses: usefulness of the Bosniak classification. Urol Radiol 13: 83-90
4. Baltarowich o, Kurtz AB (1987) Sonographics evaluation of renal masses. Urol Radiol 9: 79-87
5. Banner BF, Ernstott MS, Bahnson RR, Titus-Erbstoff L, Taylor SR (1991) Quantitative DNA analysis of small renal cortical neoplasms. Hum Pathol 22: 247-253
6. Benson MA, Haaga JR, Resnick MI (1989) Staging renal cell carcinoma: what is sufficient? (abst) Radiology 172: 586
7. Birnbaum B, Bosniak MA, Megibow AJ, Lubat E, Gordon RB (1990) Observation on the growth of renal neoplasms. Radiology 176: 695-701
8. Black WC, Dwyer AJ (1990) Renal cell carcinoma: earlier discovery and increased detection. Radiology 174: 280-281
9. Boccon-Gibod L, Ben Lagba N (1992) Néphrome mésoblastique congénital atypique (tumeur de Bolande atypique). Arch Anat Cytol Pathol 40: 333-336
10. Bosniak MA (1991) Management of the small (1.5 cm) renal parenchymal tumor. Radiology 181: 288
11. Bosniak MA (1991) Differentiating between benign and malignant cystic lesions of the kidney (abst). Radiology 181:293
12. Bosniak MA (1991) Small (3 cm) renal parenchymal tumors: detection, diagnosis, and controversies. Radiology 179: 307-317
13. Bosniak MA (1986) The current radiological approach to renal cysts. Radiology 158: 1-10
14. Brucher Ph, Brunier G, Ferriere JM, Leguilloum (199]) Etude critique du pronostic de l'adénocarcinome rénal et essai de classification, à propos d'une série de 322 dossiers. Sem Hop Paris 67: 336-375
15. Cabanne F, Pages A, Billerey CL, Oppermann A, Carbillet JP (1993) Pathologie génitale masculine. Uropathologie: reins - tumeurs. Masson, Paris, pp 239-270
16. Chassevent A (1992) Analyse d'ADN par cytométrie en flux des carcinomes à cellules rénales. Arch Anat Cytol Pathol 40: 307-311
17. Cochand-Priollet B, Molinie V, Vieillefond A (1992) Les tumeurs oncocytaires du rein. Analyse des connais-

sances actuelles et création d'un groupe d'étude. Arch Anat Cytol Pathol 40: 244-249
18. Currin SM, Lee SE, Walther PJ (1990) Flow cytometric assessment of deosyribonucleic acid content in renal adenocarcinoma: does ploidy status entrance prognostic stratification over stage alone? J Urol 143: 458-463
19. Choyke PL (1988) MR imaging in renal cell carcinoma. Radiology 169: 572-573
20. Davidson AJ, Davis CJ Jr, et al (1988) Infiltrative renal lesions: CT-sonographic-pathologic correlation. AJR 150: 1061-1064
21. Denys A, Hélénon O, Souissi M, Attlan E, Chrétien Y, Dufour B, Moreau JF (1991) Doppler pulsé et couleur des masses rénales: corrélation angiographique et anatomopathologique. J Radiol 72: 599-608
22. Deslignères S, Flam T, Vachert-Lavenu MC, Debré B (1992) Tumeur rénale exceptionnelle chez une jeune femme: le néphrome mésoblastique cellulaire ou atypique à forme partiellement kystique. Arch Anat Cytol Pathol 40: 297-300
23. Deslignères S (1992) Tumeurs kystiques à cellules claires du rein. Arch Anat Cytol Pathol 40: 255-260
24. Dinney CPN, Awad SA, Gajewski JB, Belitsky P, Lannon SG, Mack FG, Millard OH (1992) Analysis of imaging modalities, staging systems, and prognosis indicators for renal cell carcinoma. Urology 39: 122-129
25. Dunnick NR (1992) Renal lesions: great strides in imaging. Radiology 182: 305-306
26. Eilenberg SS, Lee JKT, Brown JJ, Mirowitz Tartar VM (1990) Renal masses: evaluation with gradient-echo GdDTPA-enhanced dynamic MR imaging. Radiology 176: 333-338
27. Enzinger FM, Weiss SW (1988) General consideration in soft tissue tumors, 2nd Edn. Mosby, St Louis, pp 1-18
28. Farrow GM (1989) Diseases of the kidney: neoplasms of adult. In: Murphy WN (ed) Urological pathology. WB Saunders, Philadelphia, pp 423-482
29. Fein AB, Lee JKT, Balfe DM, et al (1987) Diagnosis and staging of renal cell carcinoma: comparison of MR imaging and CT. AJR 148: 749-753
30. Felson B, Wiot JF (1987) Renal neoplasms. Sem Roentgol 22: 227-315
31. Ferry JA, Malt RA, Young RH (1991) Renal angiomyolipoma with sarcomatous transformation and pulmonary metastases. Am J Surg Pathol 15: 1083- 1088
32. Fleming S (1993) The impact of genetics on the classificaton of renal carcinoma. Histopathology 22: 89-92
33. Fritzsche PJ, Millar C (1992) Multimodality approach to staging renal cell carcinoma. Urol Radiol 14: 3-7
34. Fritzsche PJ (1989) Current state of MRI in renal mass diagnosis and staging of RCC. Urol Radiol 11: 210-214
35. Foster WL Jr, Roberts L Jr, Halvorsen RA Jr (1988) Sonography of small masses with indeterminant density characteristics on computed tomography. Urol Radiol 10: 59-67
36. Gelb AB, Robert RB, Weiss LM. Medeiros L (1993) Stage I renal cell carcinoma. A clinicopathologic study of 82 cases. Am J Surg Pathol 17: 275-286
37. Gerharz CD, Molle E, Storkel S, Ramp U, Thoenes W, Gabbert EE (1993) Ultrastructural appearance and cytoskeletal architecture of the clear, chromophilic and chromophobe types of human renal cell carcinoma in vitro. Am J Pathol 142: 851-859
38. Gogusev J, Fournet JC, Couturier J, Beroud C, Patey N, Augusti M, Chretien Y, Paraf F, Adafer E, Droz D (1993) Carcinome à cellules rénales: aspects récents. Actualités Néphrologiques. Flammarion Médecine-Sciences, pp 65-83
39. Grignon DJ, Ayala AG, El Naggar A, Wishnow KI, Ro JY, Swanson DA, Mc Lemore D, Giacco GG, Guinee VF (1989) Renal cell carcinoma. A clinicopathological and DNA flow cytometric analysis of 103 cases. Cancer 64: 2133-2140
40. Haillot O, Lanson Y (1992) Epidémiologie et dépistage du cancer du rein de l'adulte. Rev Prat 10: 1211 -1215
41. Hatcher PA, Paulson DF, Anderson EE (1992) Accuracy in staging of renal cell carcinoma involving vena cava. Urology 39: 27-30
42. Hélénon O, Denys A, Rotkopf L, Souissi M, Cornud F, Moreau JF (1992) Imagerie du cancer du rein de l'adulte. Rev Prat 10: 1217-1229
43. Hietala SO, Ekelund L, Ljungberg B (1988) Venous invasion in renal cell carcinoma: a correlative clinical and radiologic study. Urol Radiol 9: 210-216
44. Hiroshi S (1981) Distant metastasis of renal adenocarcinoma. Cancer 48: 1487-1491
45. Horan JJ, Robertson CN, Choyke PL, et al (1990) Detection of renal cell carcinoma extension into the renal vein and inferior vena cava: a prospective comparison of venacavagraphy and magnetic resonnance imaging (abst) Radiology 175 :589
46. Hricak H, Theoni RF, Carroll PR, Demas BE, Marotti M, Tanagho EA (1988) Detection and staging of renal neoplasms: a reassessment of MR imaging. Radiology 166: 643-649
47. Johnson CD, Dunnick NR, Cohan RH, Illescas FF (1987) Renal adenocarcinoma: CT staging of 100 tumors. AJR 148: 59-63
48. Kabala JE, Gillatt DA, Persad RA, et al (1991) Magnetic resonance imaging in the staging of renal cell carcinoma. Br J Radiol 64: 683-689
49. Kovacs G, Szùcs S, Eichner W, Maschek HJ, Wahnschaffe U, De Riese W (1987) Renal oncocytoma. A cytogenetic and morphologic study. Cancer 59: 2071-2077
50. Kuijpers D, Jaspers R (1989) Renal masses: differential diagnosis with pulsed doppler US. Radiology 170: 59-60
51. Levine E, Hunttrakoon M, Wetzel LH (1989) Small renal neoplasms: clinical, pathologic, and imaging features. AJR 153: 69-73
52. Ljungberg B, Larsson P, Stenling R, Roos G (1991) Flow cytometric deoxyribonucleic acid analysis in stage I renal cell carcinoma. J Urol 146: 697-699
53. London NJM, Messios RB, Kinder RB, Smart JG, Osborn DE, Watkin EM, Flynn JT (1989) A prospective study of the value of conventional CT, dynamic CT, ultrasonog-

raphy and arteriography for staging renal carcinoma. Br J Urol 64: 209-217
54. Medeiros LJ, Gelb AB, Weiss LM (1988) Renal cell carcinoma. Prognostic significance of morphologic parameters in 121 cases. Cancer 61: 1639-1651
55. Miles KA, London NJM, Lavelle JM, et al (1991) CT staging of renal carcinoma: a prospective comparison of three dynamic computed tomography techniques. Eur J Radiol 13: 37-42
56. Mindell HJ (1989) Pitfalls in sonography of renal masses. Urol Radiol 11: 215-216
57. Molinie V, Dauge-Geffroy MC, Cochand-Priollet B, Vieillefond A (1992) Tumeurs tubulo-papillaires du rein. Une entité à part de pronostic discuté. Arch Anat Cytol Pathol 40: 261-265
58. Murad T, Komaiko W, Oyasu R, Bauer K (1991) Multilocular cystic renal cell carcinoma. Am J Clin Pathol 95: 633-637
59. Myneni L, Hricak H, Carroll PR (1991) Magnetic resonance imaging of renal carcinoma with extension into the vena cava: staging accuracy and recent advances. Br J Urol 68: 571-578
60. Ninomiya N (1992) Small renal cell carcinoma: pathologic and radiologic correlation. Radiology 184: 493-497
61. Patel SK, Stack CM, Turner DA (1987) Magnetic resonance imaging in staging of renal cell carcinoma. Radiographics 7: 703
62. Porena, Vespesiani, Rosi P, et al (1992) Incidentally detectod renal cell carcinoma: role of ultrasonography. JCU 20: 395
63. Reis M, Faria V (1988) Renal carcinoma. Reevaluation of prognostic factors. Cancer 61: 1192- 1199
64. Quint LE, Glazer GM, Chenevert TL, Fechner KP, Gikas PW, Shireman PK, Grossman HB, Li KC (1988) In vivo and in vitro MR imaging of renal tumors: histopathologic correlation and pulse sequence optimization. Radiology 169: 359-362
65. Rofsky NM, Weinreb JC, Bosniak MA. Libes RB, Birnbaum BA (1991) Renal lesion characterization with gadolinium-enhanced MR imaging: efficacity and safety in patients with renal insuficiency. Radiology 180: 85-89
66. Rominder MB, Kenney PJ, Morgan DE, Bernreuter WK, Listinsky JJ (1992) Gadolinium-enhanced MR imaging of renal masses. Radiographics 12: 1097-1116
67. Roubidoux MA, Dunnick NR, Sostman HD, Leder RA (1992) Renal carcinoma: detection of venous extension with gradient-echo MR imaging. Radiology 182 : 269-272
68. Roy C, Splitter G, Saussine C, Kastler B, Jacqmin D, Bourjat P (1992) Envahissement tumoral de la veine cave inférieure: évaluation de l'échographie, de la tomodensitométrie et de l'IRM. Revue Imagerie Médicale 4: 485-492
69. Roy C, Tuchmann C (1993) Petits cancers rénaux: apport de l'échographie et des autres techniques d'imagerie au diagnostic. J.E.M.U, 14: 23-30
70. Saint André JP, Vieillefond A, Sault MC, De Fromont M, Croue A (1992) Pourquoi et comment grader les carcinomes rénaux. Arch Anat Cytol Pathol 40: 238-243
71. Semelka RC, Shoenut JP, Krocker MA, Mac Mahon RG, Grcenberg HM (1992) Renal lesions: controlled comparison between CT and 1.5-T MR Imaging with nonenhanced and gadolinium-enhanced fat-suppressed spin-echo and breath-hold FLASH techniques. Radiology 182: 425-430
72. Skolnick ML (1928) Renal lesion characterisation. Radiology 182: 285
73. Smith SJ, Bosniak MA, Medibow AJ, Hulnick D, Horii SC, Raghvendra BN (1989) Renal cell carcinoma: earlier discovery and increased detection. Radiology 170: 699-703
74. Studer UE, Scherz S, Scheidegger Jr, et al (1991) Enlargement of regional lymph nodes in renal cell carcinoma is often not due to metastases (abst). Radiology 178: 589
75. Tetu B, Ro JY, Ayala AG, Ordonez NG, Johnson DE (1987) Small cell carcinoma of the kidney. A clinicopathologic, immunohistochemical and ultrastructural study. Cancer 30: 1809-1814
76. Vieillefond A, Paradis V, Gros Ph, Bouvier R, Croue A, Saint André JP (1992) Est-il utile d'isoler parmi les carcinomes du rein, une variante à cellules chromophobes? Arch Anat Cytol Pathol 40: 250-254
77. Vieillefond A, Quillard J, Boulais S, Martin E, Soubielle C, Benoit G, Jardin A (1988) Oncocytomes du rein et adénocarcinomes à oncocytes. Ann Pathol 8: 33-43
78. Warshauer DM, Mc Carthy SM, Strect L, Bookbinder MJ, Glickman MG, Richter J, Hammers L, Taylor C, Rosenfield AT (1988) Detection of renal masses: sensitivities and specificities of excretory urography/linear tomography, US and CT. Radiology 169: 363-365
79. Zagoria RJ, Wolfman NT, Karstacdt N, Hinn GC, Dyer RB (1990) CT features of renal cell carcinoma with emphasis on relation to tumor size. Invest Radiol 25: 261- 266
80. Zeman RK, Cronan JJ, Rosenfield AT, Lynch JH. Jaffe MH, Clark LR (1988) Renal cell carcinoma: dynamic thin-section CT assessment of vascular invasion and tumor vascularity. Radiology 167: 393-396

CHAPTER 31

Malignant tumors of the adrenal glands

Clinicians
J.-C. Piette, M. Schlumberger, D. Nizri, E. Vuillemin, D. Khayat

Radiologist
D. Buthiau

The contribution of CT and MRI is particularly important for adrenal tumors, notably CT (fig. 31.1) in the assessment of cancer spread, and MRI which is able to avoid more invasive techniques such as percutaneous biopsy and phlebography. Since the advent of these techniques, a new entity has arisen, namely the incidental detection of apparently non-secreting adrenal masses which require clinical and endocrinological investigation to help determine the histological diagnosis and treatment approach.

Hypersecreting lesions [14]

The diagnosis is clinical, biochemical and hormonal. Imaging may suggest the etiology, assess spread and enable follow-up of the lesion.

Bilateral adrenal hypertrophy of extrapituitary origin

This is essentially the paraneoplastic Cushing's syndrome resulting from ectopic secretion of ACTH by a neuro-endocrine tumor: medullary carcinoma of the thyroid, cancer of the endocrine pancreas, thymic and bronchial carcinoid, pheochromocytoma...

CT can demonstrate alterations in the morphology of both adrenals (fig. 31.2); the shape and density of the adrenals are preserved with an increase in the volume, sometimes globular and asymmetrical, the appearance of the adrenal outlines may be convex, rectilinear or sometimes nodular. There is no particular indication for MRI as it gives identical information without any alteration in the associated signal intensity.

Given the absence of signal change, the distinction between the hyperplastic and micronodular adrenal is relatively difficult to define. In the nodular forms, there may be very variable alterations in the signal. Usually the appearance of the adrenals is identical to that seen in the typical pituitary Cushing's disease.

Malignant cortical adrenalomas

In about 20% of cases, these lesions are not associated with hormonal hypersecretion. However, when present this may be a hypercortisolism, associated with signs of hypermineralocorticosteroidism, and hyperandrogenism or feminization. These are infrequent lesions.

Indications for CT and MRI

Both techniques have an important role in the identification of the adrenal mass, the diagnosis and assessment of spread. MRI does not demonstrate the calcification, but its 3-dimensional capability helps to diagnose the point of origin of a large tumor mass as well as locoregional spread (for example diaphragmatic).

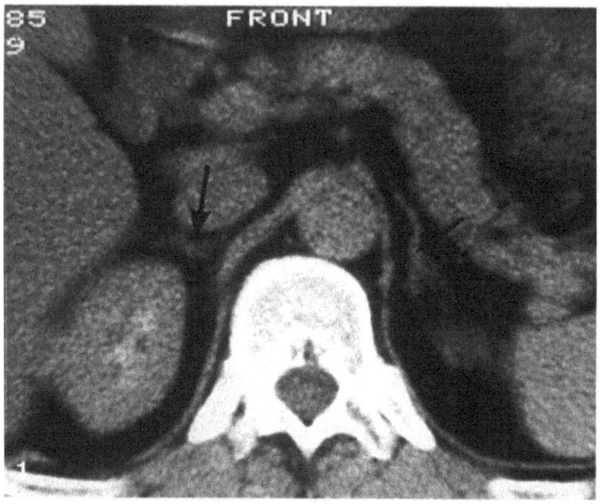

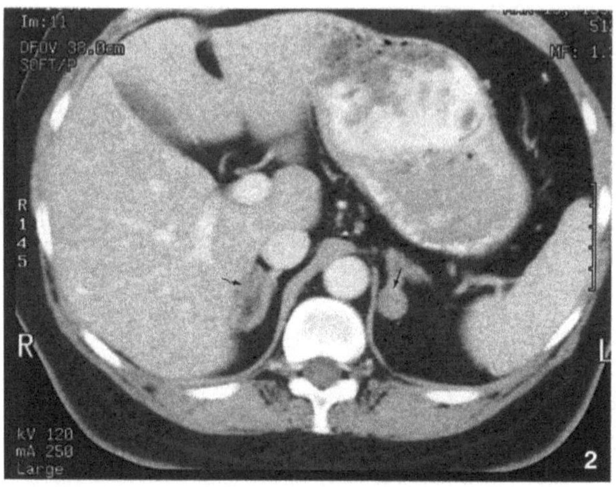

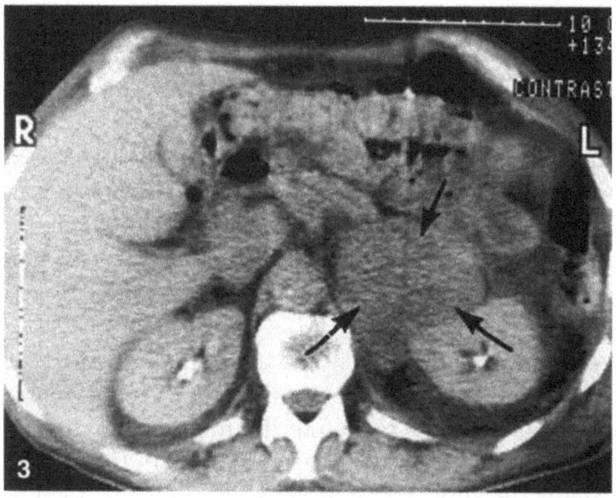

Fig. 31.1. Normal appearances of the adrenals on post contrast CT: the adrenals *(arrows)* are well demonstrated on CT. The right adrenal is situated at the level of T12, posterior to the inferior vena cava and coming into close contact with the right hemidiaphragm medially *(arcuate ligament)*. The lower and more anterior left adrenal is in close relationship to the pancreatic body anteriorly, the kidney posteriorly and the left hemidiaphragm medially. The thickness of the limbs of either adrenal glands should not normally exceed 5 mm. Its borders are normally rectilinear or slightly concave. The cortex and medulla cannot be differentiated

Fig. 31.2. Bilateral hypertrophy of the adrenals of extrahypophyseal origin in a case of paraneoplastic Cushing's syndrome; the appearance on post-contrast CT is that of an asymmetrical increase in the volume of the adrenals bilaterally with rectilinear outlines on the right and convex and nodular configuration on the left

Fig. 31.3. Malignant cortico-adrenaloma on post contrast CT: soft tissue homogeneous lesion of 55 mm in diameter *(arrows)* lying anterior to the left kidney causing locoregional compression of the kidney and bowel without any sign of direct extension

Signs

On CT, there is a rounded or lobulated mass of very variable size, a diameter of > 5 cm being highly suggestive of malignancy (fig. 31.3). It is difficult to appreciate the adrenal origin of a mass in the presence of a large lesion, but the following features are helpful: on the right side, a lesion of hepatic origin displaces the inferior vena cava (IVC) postero-medially whereas an adrenal tumor displaces it anteriorly: any pancreatic mass is anterior to the splenic vessels, the opposite applies to adrenal lesions. The differentiation from a tumor of the upper pole of the left kidney requires the performance of thin sections through the angles of contact and the demonstration of a normal adrenal.

Intratumoral calcifications are quite common, as are areas of necrosis, the source of the heterogeneity of these tumors.

In a single examination, CT is able to detect spread to the IVC, spleen, liver, lymph nodes, peritoneum, pericardium, or lung.

MRI demonstrates a mass of low signal intensity on T1-weighted imaging and high signal intensity on T2-weighted imaging, often containing areas of necrosis and hemorrhage, the calcifications showing as signal voids (fig. 31.4). The 3-dimensional study, and particularly the sagittal images on T1-, T2-weighted imaging and the STIR sequence, accurately define the craniocaudal extent and spread to the IVC, liver, spleen, intestine and pancreas. Extension into other adjacent

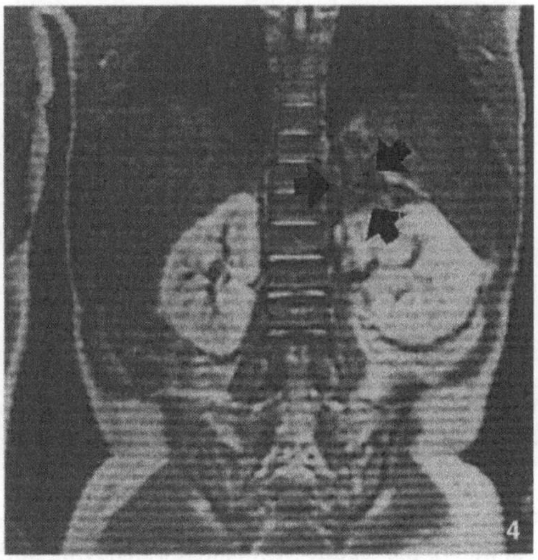

Fig. 31.4. Malignant cortico-adrenaloma on coronal T2-weighted MRI section. There is a soft tissue mass of slightly increased signal containing areas which appear a little more intense due to necrosis, and multiple calcifications visible as signal voids resulting in an overall reduction in the signal intensity of the lesion

organs is more difficult to appreciate on MRI. Caval spread is particularly well demonstrated following gadolinium injection, reducing the indications for cavography. The coronal and sagittal images help to differentiate the adrenal lesion from a mass of renal origin, and these planes of section also demonstrate diaphragmatic involvement.

Malignant pheochromocytomas

These represent 10% of pheochromocytomas which themselves are rare tumors (3/1,000) and arise in the adrenal medulla. In practice, it is important as far as the clinician is concerned to make the diagnosis of a pheochromocytoma, confirm it biochemically, localize the lesion and attempt to determine its benign or malignant nature preoperatively based on the criteria of size, content, spread, and associated secondary lesions using CT and MRI. Malignancy is proven by the presence of neoplastic tissue in which there are no sympathetic structures.

There should be a routine search for the malignant forms in patients resistant to treatment and also in associated disorders such as multiple endocrine neoplasia IIA (MEN IIA), also called Sipple's syndrome (pheochromocytoma, medullary cancer of the thyroid, parathyroid hyperplasia), or in the context of MEN IIB (pheochromocytoma, medullary cancer of the thyroid and multiple neurinomas). The pheochromocytomas in the MEN syndromes are particularly malignant. Other associations have been described; the familial paragangliomatoses, neurofibromatosis 1 and the von Hippel-Lindau type of neurodermatoses. Ectopic lesions are commoner in these forms. As a result, CT which is an excellent examination for the assessment of the adrenals and retroperitoneum, should be complemented by an MRI as soon as there is the suspicion of an ectopic form or when the lesion is small. In practice, investigation commences with MIBG scintigraphy which determines whether or not the pheochromocytoma takes up the isotope, localizes the tumor and looks for metastases. This ultimately determines whether complete surgical excision is feasible.

Indications for CT and MRI

CT (fig. 31.5a) localizes the lesion or lesions, detects possible metastases and demonstrates the relationships with the adjacent viscera and vessels prior to surgery. In cases of extra-adrenal pheochromocytomas, CT helps in the search for ectopic lesions along the major vessels, the axis of the vena cava, the bladder wall (fig. 31.5b), and the organ of Zuckerkandl (thoracic, abdominal and pelvic CT). However, this search for ectopic lesions by CT, as well as the demonstration of a recurrence or metastasis is difficult. This explains the multiplicity of complementary investigations, particularly scintigraphy [3].

MRI has made a significant contribution in the investigation of malignant pheochromocytoma as much within the adrenal as in the ectopic forms. According to some authors, MRI should be the initial examination of choice. In fact, about 90% of the ectopic lesions are situated close to the major vessels and the performance of coronal T1- and axial T2 sections greatly facilitates their detection.

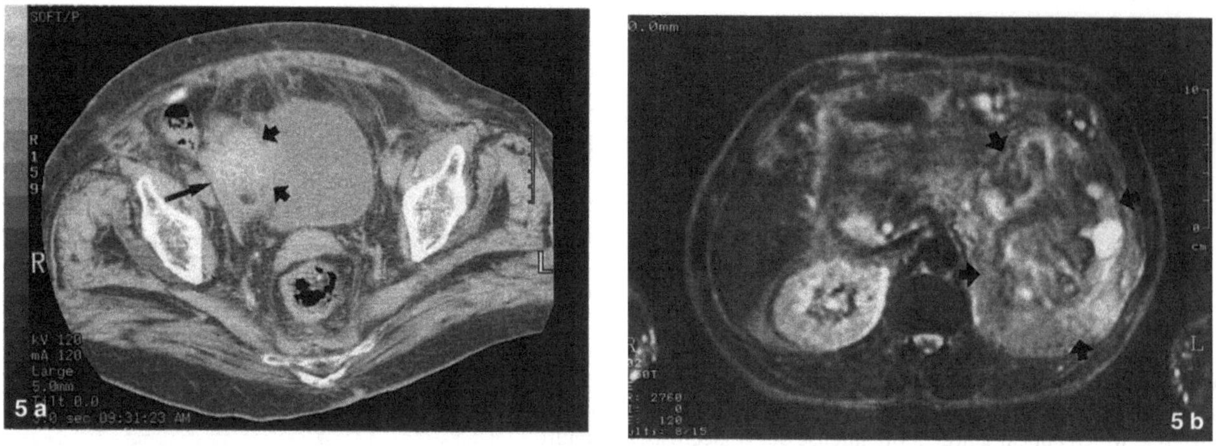

Fig. 31.5. a Ectopic malignant pheochromocytoma on post contrast CT: presence of a soft tissue mass visible in the right lateral wall of the bladder *(small arrows)*, having both an endo- and extravesical component, extending to the right umbilico-prevesical fascia *(large arrow)* and internal iliac fascia. On CT, this lesion of soft tissue density is not specific, and the diagnosis of its nature depends on the histology. **b** Malignant pheochromocytoma on an axial T2-weighted MRI section: presence on the left of a heterogeneous necrotic and hemorrhagic mass *(arrows)* with more or less multilobulation compressing the bowel, occupying the major part of the left hypochondrium and displacing the kidney inferiorly and the spleen superiorly (these organs are not visible on this section)

Table 31.1. Diagnostic algorithm for an incidentaloma (reproduced from M. Marichez et al) [14]

First case scenario

Adrenal tumor detected accidentally (CT). Radiological investigations normal; size 3 cm

↓

MRI

← Homogeneous signal reducing on T2
↓
Benign lesion
↓
Follow-up: clinical, biochemical, CT

→ Heterogeneous signal increasing on T2
↓
Percutaneous biopsy
- dangerous
- diagnostic yield very poor, even on the operative specimen, the main differential diagnosis is between a benign adenoma [23] and a malignant cortico-adrenaloma CT and can be extremely difficult

↓
Surgery preferable

Second case scenario

Adrenal tumor
Detected accidentally (CT or ultrasound)
Normal biochemical investigations
Mass > 3 cm or calcified, or heterogeneous, or bilateral

↓

MRI + MIBG

Whatever the signal characteristic (to exclude a non-secreting pheochromocytoma preoperatively)

↓

Surgery

Signs

On CT, the tumor is often very well defined, slightly calcified and appears heterogeneous following contrast injection. In extreme cases, the lesions may be encapsulated. For the ectopic forms (fig. 31.5a), the axial plane of section is a limiting factor as the area which needs to be covered is large (thorax, abdomen and pelvis). As a result, there are many false positives and negatives (vascular structures, bowel, lymph nodes...).

On MRI, however, the lesions located in the adrenals are of intermediate signal intensity on T1-weighted imaging, frequently heterogeneous on T2-weighted imaging (cystic or hemorrhagic necrosis), and often multilobulated (fig. 31.5b). MRI can also detect possible lymph node involvement (although this is better demonstrated on CT), secondary hepatic involvement or bone metastases on the sagittal or coronal T1-weighted images. The relationship of the mass to the spleen, pancreas, kidney, liver or diaphragm as well as the vessels and drainage pedicle are better demonstrated on the 3-dimensional study.

According to some authors, the conventional T2-weighted sequences are more sensitive than MIBG scintigraphy in the ectopic forms [4]. The STIR and more recently the fat suppression sequences are more accurate for the detection of ectopic lesions. MRI provides a concomitant assessment of other associated pathologies (e.g. neurinoma, von Hippel-Lindau disease).

Non-secreting lesions [14]

These lesions may be picked up incidentally and present the problem of an adrenal or extra-adrenal incidentaloma (table 31.1). The benign or malignant nature and non-secreting character of the lesion must therefore be established.

The tumors are sometimes detected in the assessment of the adrenals as part of the staging process of a tumor or during the investigation of any abdominal or lumbar tumor.

Adrenal metastases and the diagnostic problem of differentiation from a benign non-secreting adenoma [14] (fig. 31.6)

It is generally considered that any lesion less than 3 cm on CT presents a real problem in the differential diagnosis. The presence of an adrenal metastasis should be suggested by the following features: a mass greater than 3 cm, with a variable degree of irregularity (fig. 31.6a), frequently heterogeneous and bilateral, arising asymmetrically and sometimes calcified.

MRI can give additional information for masses less than 3 cm because, although the signal intensity is weak or intermediate on T1, there is an increase in the signal intensity on T2-weighted imaging in metastases which is not seen in benign adenomas irrespective of whether or not they are secreting lesions.

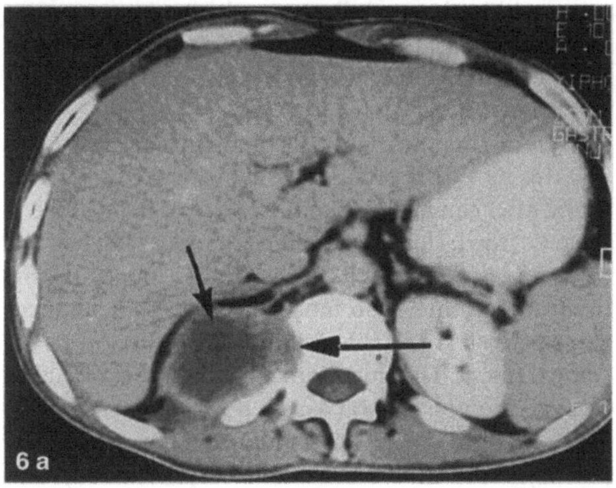

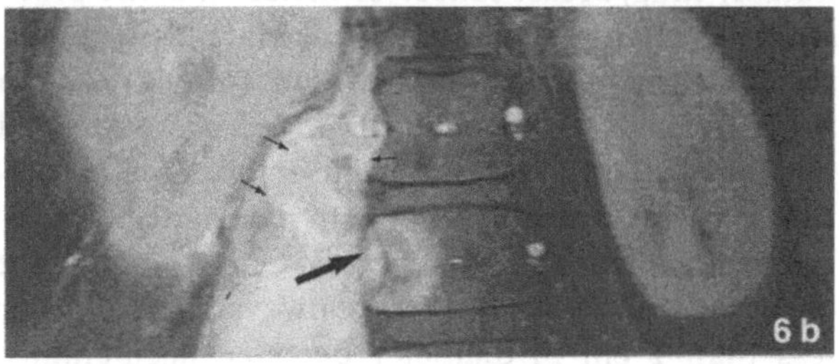

Fig. 31.6. a Right adrenal metastasis on post-contrast CT; extensive necrotic lesion of 4 cm diameter *(small arrow)* situated posterior to the inferior vena cava and arising in the medial limb of the right adrenal with spread to the spine, costotransverse and costovertebral areas *(large arrow)*. **b** Post-contrast MRI demonstrates well the superior spread of the lesion *(small arrow)* and its spinal involvement by contiguous extension *(large arrow)* with abnormal signal of the adjacent bony medulla

The differentiation remains nonetheless difficult, and the following features are taken into account:
- the incidental detection of a non-secreting adenoma occurs in 2-9% of patients depending on the series. Conversely, secondary deposits in the adrenal are common, the fourth commonest site after lung, liver and bone. In total, more than 50% of the adrenal lesions detected in cancer patients correspond to benign adenomas. The size criterion is only moderately contributory since the diameter of benign adenomas can reach 4 cm [4]. As a rule, lesions greater than 5 cm are presumed to be malignant (primary or secondary), and bilateral involvement is considered to be metastatic. However, these criteria are not specific;
- MRI has a sensitivity between 70 and 95% for the detection of metastases, but while the sensitivity increases, the specificity decreases. It is known that some metastases have a pseudo-adenomatous appearance and the signal intensity may be altered by cystic, necrotic or hemorrhagic changes. Moreover, the signal intensity of an adenoma can be changed physiologically during periods of stress; the blood products or hemosiderin may reduce the signal intensity of a metastasis and mimic an adenoma. The numerous studies which have assessed the signal intensity of the adrenal lesion relative to the adjacent organs (particularly the liver) or relative to the fat have not taken into account the inherent signal changes of these structures (ferric content...). The calculation of the T2 values at low or mid-field does not appear to have any significant value. This is less true for the high field system, but the risk of error remains.

In those patients presenting with a known cancer, notably lung, breast cancer or melanoma, the probability that a non-functioning adrenal mass is metastatic clearly increases (more than 40% of cases in some series). 17% of small cell cancers are associated with adrenal metastases. Despite an increased sensitivity, MRI is probably unable to distinguish a non-secreting adenoma, a metastasis or a malignant cortico-adrenaloma. It is true, however, that a tumor less than 2 cm in diameter detected accidentally, whose signal decreases between the first and second echo on the T2-weighted sequence is suggestive of a non-secreting benign adenoma and simply requires follow-up without biopsy, initially at three monthly intervals.

The role of gadolinium injection using rapid gradient echo sequences appears promising. Non-secreting adenomas seem to be little altered by the injection unlike the malignant lesions (fig. 31.6 b) and also pheochromocytomas [4]. These findings still require confirmation.

Adrenal lymphoma

CT is very sensitive but non-specific although its accuracy is superior to ultrasound. MRI is only of value as the last resort in cases of discordance or doubt.

Adrenal involvement appears on CT as an enhancing tumor mass, sometimes necrotic, inflammatory or hyperdense due to blood. The appearances are entirely non-specific.

On MRI, the mass appears hyperintense on T1-weighted imaging in the presence of chronic blood breakdown products and on T2-weighted imaging in the presence of necrosis; sometimes a simple infiltration does not cause any change in the signal but only a loss of the normal anatomy.

Non-secreting pheochromocytoma

True non-secreting pheochromocytomas have been reported. In these cases, MRI has a definite role for raising the possibility of the diagnosis preoperatively so that all the necessary anesthetic and surgical precautions can be taken. In addition, the significant risk of percutaneous fine needle aspiration should not be forgotten.

Neuroblastoma

This lesion particularly involves children under 2 years of age; it is infrequent in the adult. It can occur at any location within the sympathetic nervous system; 40% of cases occur in the adrenals where it arises within the medulla. It may be benign or malignant with a variable degree of malignancy, metastases being essentially to bone and lymph nodes, and is rapidly progressive.

CT confirms the diagnosis of an adrenal mass and assesses its extent preoperatively with MIBG scintigraphy. MRI can also define the extent of the disease.

On CT, the lesions are calcified in more than half the cases and are usually large, heterogeneous with soft tissue, cystic and even fatty densities. The enhancement pattern is variable depending on the soft tissue compartment. The injection of contrast is essential to localize the vessels and assess possible encasement. MRI, with the help of gadolinium, evaluates the patency of the vessels and can detect possible adjacent venous thrombosis, as well as hepatic or bony spread. The study in three planes defines the extension, and demonstrates the heterogeneity of the lesion. Calcification is visible as a signal void.

Conclusion

CT and MRI have a particularly important role in the investigation and complete assessment of the spread of malignant adrenal tumors, as much by their sensitivity as by their non-invasive nature. The main problem is the differentiation between a non-secreting adenoma and a primary or secondary tumor, and this is still difficult. MRI is insufficient and should be complemented by a CT guided percutaneous biopsy since the demonstration of adrenal metastases determines the treatment. The diagnostic strategy should follow a logical chronological sequence starting first with the clinical features, then the biochemical levels and finally, if required, the imaging findings.

References

1. Bernardino ME (1988) Management of the asymptomatic patient with an unilateral mass. Radiology 166: 121-123
2. Chang A, Glaser HS, Lee JKT, et al (1987) Adrenal gland: MR imaging. Radiology 163: 123-128
3. Chatal F, Charbonnel B (1985) Comparison of iodobenzylguanidine imaging with CT locating pheochromocytoma. J Clin Endocrinol Metab 61: 769-772
4. Choyke PL, Doppman JL (1992) Adrenal glands. In: DD Stark, WG Bradley Jr (eds) MRI, 2nd edn. Mosby-Year Book, St Louis, pp 1880-1902
5. Falke THM, Te Strake L, Sandler MP, et al (1987) Magnetic resonance imaging of the adrenal glands. Radiographics 7: 343-370
6. Falke THM, Te Strake L, Shaff MI, et al (1986) Magnetic resonance imaging of the adrenals: correlation with computed tomography. J Comput Assist Tomogr 10: 242-253
7. Glazer HS, Weyman PJ, Sagel SS, et al (1982) Non functioning adrenal masses: incidental discovery on computed tomography. AJR 139: 81-85
8. Glazer JM, Woolsey EJ, Borello J, et al (1986) Adrenal tissue characterization using MR imaging. Radiology 158: 73-79
9. Krestin MD (1989) Adrenal masses: evaluation with fast gradient-echo MR imaging and Gd-DTPA-enhanced dynamic studies. Radiology 171: 675-680
10. Leroy-Willig A, Roucayrol JC, Luton JP, et al (1987) In vitro adrenal cortex characterization by NMR spectroscopy. Magn Reson Imaging 5: 339-344
11. Leroy-Willig A, Luton JP (1989) L'imagerie par résonance magnétique des glandes surrénales. J Urol 95: 305-308
12. Luton JP, et al (1990) Clinical features of adrenocortical carcinoma, prognostic factors and the effect of mitotane therapy. N Engl J Med 322: 1195-1201
13. Marichez M, Desprez E, Taieb A (1988) Les surrénales, apport de l'imagerie spectroscopique. In: IRM corps entier. Springer-Verlag, Paris, pp 199-210
14. Marichez M, et al (1992) Surrénales. In: Buthiau D (ed) TDM et IRM cliniques, Abdomen-pelvis. Frison-Roche, Paris, pp 209-223
15. Miyake H, Maeda H, Tashiro M, et al (1989) CT of adrenal tumors: frequency and clinical significance of low attenuation lesions. AJR 152: 1005-1007
16. Reinig JW, et al (1986) MRI of undeterminated masses. AJR 149: 493-496
17. Shah HR, Love L, Williamson MR, et al (1989) Hemorrhagic adrenal metastases: CT findings. J Comput Assist Tomogr 13: 77-81
18. Velchik MG, Alavi A, Kressel HY, et al (1989) Localization of pheochromocytoma: MIBG, CT and MRI Correlation. J Nucl Med 30: 328-336
19. Welch TJ, Sheedy HPF, Johnson CD, et al (1989) CT-guided biopsy: prospective analysis of 1000 procedures. Radiology 171: 493-496

CHAPTER 32

Cancer of the bladder

Clinician
M. Housset

Radiologists
D. Buthiau, D. Vadrot

Of all bladder pathologies, tumor involvement is the most important. Cancers of the bladder are common; they effect four men for one woman, the average age being 65 years. In the majority of cases, it is a primary urothelial (transitional cell carcinoma). The other histological types are rare, adenocarcinoma, sarcoma, lymphoma, epidermoid. The main problems posed by cancer of the bladder concern the detection, tumor characterization and staging.

Tumor detection and characterization currently depend on cystoscopic examination which demonstrates the tumor and allows biopsies to be taken which confirm the diagnosis and define the histological grade.

The prognosis and treatment strategies of bladder cancer depend on the position, histology, and particularly the tumor extent. It is essential to distinguish the superficial tumors which are confined to the mucosa from the infiltrative tumors (diagram 32.1). The tumors which only infiltrate the superficial muscles can, in certain cases, be treated by partial cystectomy depending on their location and size. Otherwise, as with the tumors involving the deep muscle layers, they require total cystectomy. Radiotherapy is usually reserved for patients with contraindications to surgery or who refuse total cystectomy.

Only peroperative surgical examination can provide an exact staging assessment for classifying the tumor according to the TNM classification (table 32.1). However, the aim is to obtain an accurate tumor staging prior to surgery. Clinical examination even under general anesthesia, cystoscopy and intravenous urography are inadequate and frequently underestimate the degree of bladder wall invasion [13].

CT and magnetic resonance imaging (MRI) can help in the pre-surgical assessment of spread with a good predictive value for the likely difficulty that will be encountered during surgery. CT and MRI are also used for the assessment of bladder involvement by other pelvic tumors. These techniques also complement cystoscopy, particularly if the vesical involvement is limited to the deep planes without mucosal involvement.

The detection of post-operative complications and follow-up after treatment also represent important roles of imaging as local and/or distant metastatic recurrences are common in the evolution of bladder cancers. In fact, it is essential to attempt to detect early recurrences using these imaging methods and to help distinguish post-radiation or post-surgical fibrosis from zones of active recurrent tumor.

Diagnosis and staging of bladder cancers [5]

Indications for CT and MRI

The detection and characterization of lesions depend not on CT or MRI but on cystoscopy. However, these two imaging techniques form part of the investigations for detecting lymphatic and locoregional spread, once the biopsy has demonstrated involvement of the lamina propria. Even if there is an unfavorable picture,

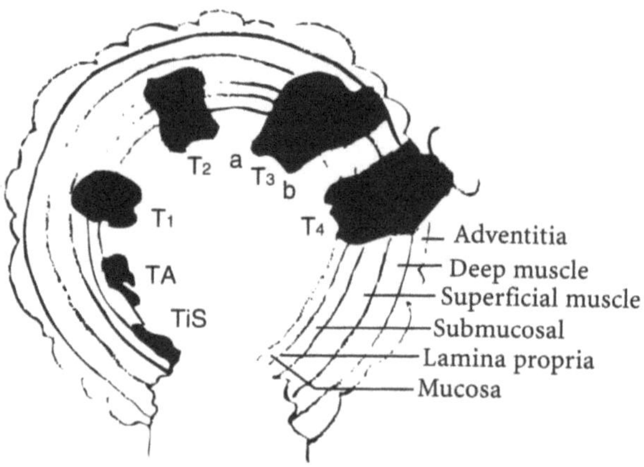

Diagram 32.1. Staging of bladder cancers

Fig. 32.1. Infiltrative cancer of the bladder on post contrast CT. There is thickening with an irregular inner border of the posterior and postero-lateral wall of the bladder bilaterally, predominantly on the right *(small arrows)*; the distinction of submucosal, mucosal and muscle involvement is not possible

Fig. 32.2. Infiltrative cancer of the bladder involving the posterior and left postero-lateral wall on post contrast CT; the infiltrative lesion *(small arrows)* is associated with dilatation of the left ureter, not necessarily due to tumor invasion. The presence of ureteric obstruction is very characteristic of infiltrative tumors

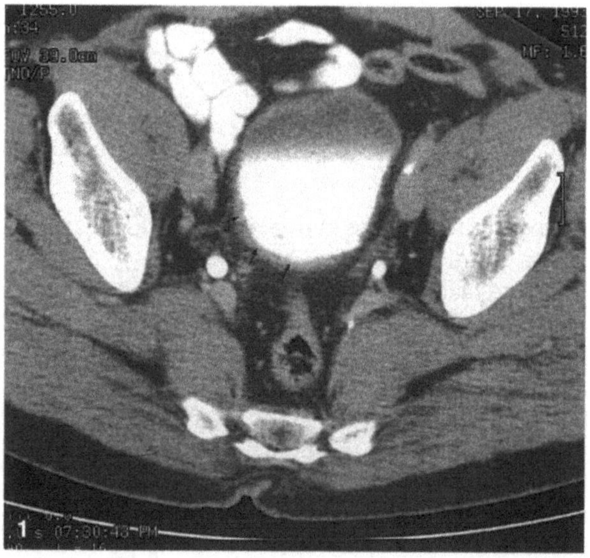

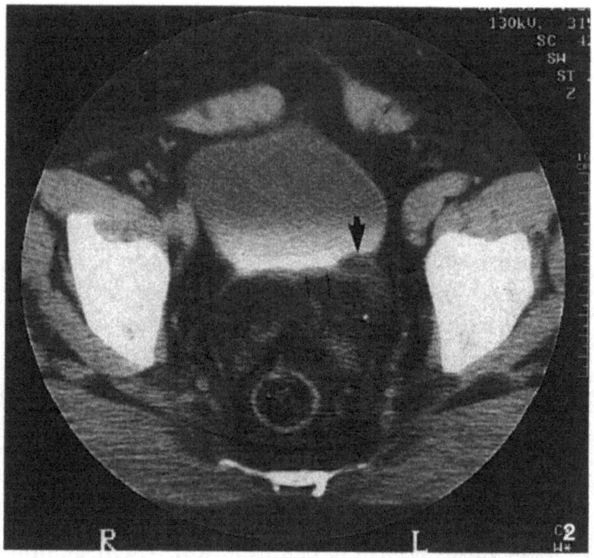

Table 32.1. TNN classification of bladder cancers (see diagram 32.1)

Tis	Cancer *in situ*
Ta	Tumor restricted to the mucosa
T1	Involvement of the lamina
T2	Involvement of the superficial muscle
T3A	Involvement of the deep muscle
T3B	Extension to the perivesical fat
T4A	Extension to adjacent organs
T4B	Extension to the pelvic side wall
N0	No lymph node involvement
N1	Single lymph node in the homolateral external or internal iliac chain
N2	Contralateral, bilateral or multiple lymph nodes in the internal or external iliac chain
N3	Fixed internal iliac node
N4	Common iliac, inguinal or para-aortic lymph node involvement
M0	No metastasis
M1	Metastasis present

these techniques are indispensable in certain cases if radiotherapy is contemplated. In fact, CT and MRI should be considered as a routine part of the assessment of local spread when there is evidence of infiltration of the muscle at resection. If there is only an infiltration of the lamina propria, the indications for imaging depend on the macroscopic nature of the tumor and its degree of differentiation.

Signs

CT (figs 32.1-32.5)

CT can clearly define the size of the lesion once it has reached a size of at least 8-10 mm. The localization of the tumor and its nodular, endoluminal infiltrative nature are equally well demonstrated (figs 32.1-32.4). When the lesion causes a localized thickening of the

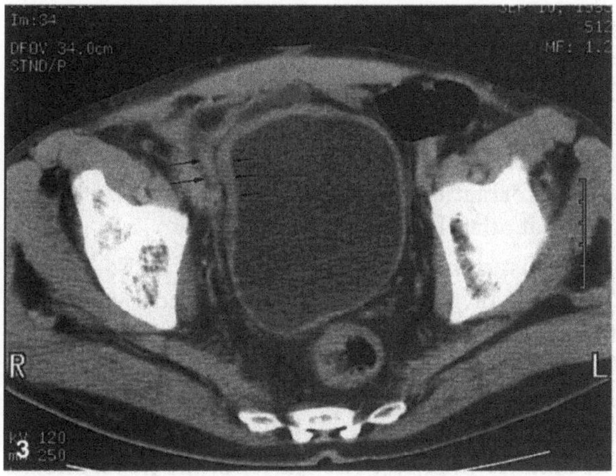

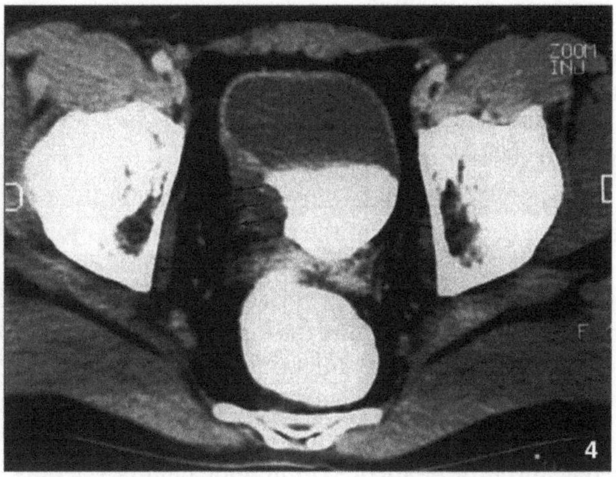

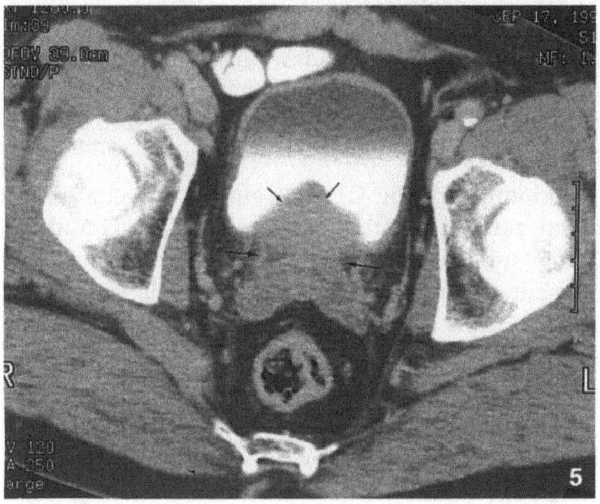

Fig. 32.3. Infiltrative tumor of the lateral and right antero-lateral wall of the bladder on CT. In this full bladder, the thickening of the bladder wall is clearly greater than 3 mm *(small arrows)*. There is inhomogeneity of the fatty tissue adjacent to the lesion. Note particularly a thickening of the prevesico-umbilical fascia on the right *(large arrows)* related to invasion of the perivesical fat in a stage 3B tumor

Fig. 32.4. Post-contrast CT of stage T3B bladder tumor: the right postero-lateral tumor of the bladder extends onto perivesical fat appearing as an irregular soft tissue lesion *(large arrows)* (courtesy of Dr L. Arrivé et al. In: D. Buthiau (ed) "Clinical CT and MRI" Frison-Roche, Paris)

Fig. 32.5. Cancer of the bladder on post-contrast CT with spread to the seminal vesicles. Filling-in of the right and left vesico-seminal angles *(large arrows)*, but no significant morphological change or asymmetry of the vesicles. Spread to the prostate is suggested by the regular impression on the bladder base *(small arrows)*, and this was confirmed surgically

bladder wall, the physiological upper limit of normal of the wall thickness in a full bladder is taken to be 3 mm (fig. 32.3). The depth of bladder wall involvement cannot be determined (the distinction of submucosal, mucosal and muscle involvement, in other words stages T1, T2 and T3A, is not possible). In cases of infiltration of the perivesical fat, CT shows an inhomogeneity of the fatty tissue adjacent to the lesion with indistinct borders (fig. 32.4). It should be remembered, however, that an irregular appearance to the bladder wall-fatty tissue interface may be seen in stage T3A in which there is involvement of the bladder wall without invasion into the adjacent fat. In stage T3B, when there is invasion of the perivesical fat, CT demonstrates inhomogeneous changes in the paravesical fat density. There may even be areas of abnormal soft tissue with an infiltrative appearance or nodules with round or oval masses. Cases of subtle involvement may give the appearance of "grass fire" in the form of fine strands adjacent to the bladder wall. At this stage there is no involvement of the pelvic side wall or adjacent organs (preservation of the fat planes between the different structures). In all these forms, CT is able to appreciate any possible obstruction of the upper urinary tract. This can be confirmed, if necessary, by performing a urologic CT.

In stage T4A, involvement of an adjacent organ by direct spread manifests as a persistent mass between the bladder and organ with invasion of the adjacent fat plane. This extension is well demonstrated in the seminal vesicles (fig. 32.5), with a filling of the vesico-seminal angle, asymmetry or disorganization of the seminal vesicle [7]. Spread to the prostate is only suggested (fig. 32.5) by the propagation of the tumor at the bladder base into a deformed and enlarged prostate gland. Extension to the rectum is quite difficult to confirm and is demonstrated as thickening of the pelvic tissue planes, the prerectal aponeurosis , and the anterior or antero-lateral rectal wall.

In stage 4B, the pelvic side wall involvement manifests by a propagation of the soft tissue process to the pelvic side. The diagnosis is even more likely if this process is extensive. If the contiguity extends over less than or equal to 3 or 4 mm, the diagnosis of extension is equivocal [4, 14]. The injection of a contrast agent does not improve the diagnostic accuracy.

Lymph node involvement may occur in any of the pelvic and lumbo-aortic lymph node chains. CT only demonstrates an increase in volume, the physiological upper limit of normal being a short axis diameter of 1.5 cm for the external iliac, ilio-femoral, common iliac and obturator nodes, and 1 cm for the hypogastric and lumbo-aortic nodes. Only lymph node sampling is able to confirm lymphatic involvement by tumor, even if this is to some extent linked to the size of the node.

Abdomino-pelvic CT is useful in the search for metastases. Apart from assessing the pelvis and the lymph nodes, it can also look for hepatic lesions, complemented by ultrasound. The routine application of a bony window is necessary for the detection of bone metastases in the spine and pelvis.

MRI (figs 32.6-32.8)

The sagittal and coronal sections are particularly well adapted for the analysis of tumors of the dome and the base of the bladder [4, 15]. The axial sections provide information on the presence and size of the tumor at other locations.

The distinction between stages T1 and T2, namely tumors involving the lamina propria and invading the superficial muscle layer is not possible on MRI. However, these stages are characterized by the preservation of a continuous hypointense line outlining the bladder which indicates a normal deep muscle layer of the bladder wall [17]. The clarity of the hyperintense zone when there is a chemical shift phenomenon has the same significance. The perivesical fatty tissue is normal.

The invasion of the deep muscle layers in stage T3A disease appears as a focal interruption of the black line of the normal bladder wall with normal adjacent perivesical fat. In cases of only moderate involvement of the muscle, there may still be preservation of the hypointense peripheral line.

In stage T3B, MRI demonstrates loss of the hypointense muscle layer of the bladder with associated changes in the perivesical fat. This may either be in the form of a reduction in the signal intensity of the fat or a local infiltration of soft tissue intensity which may

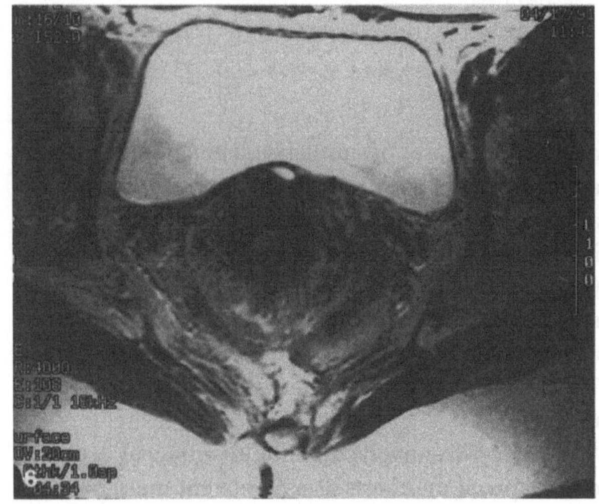

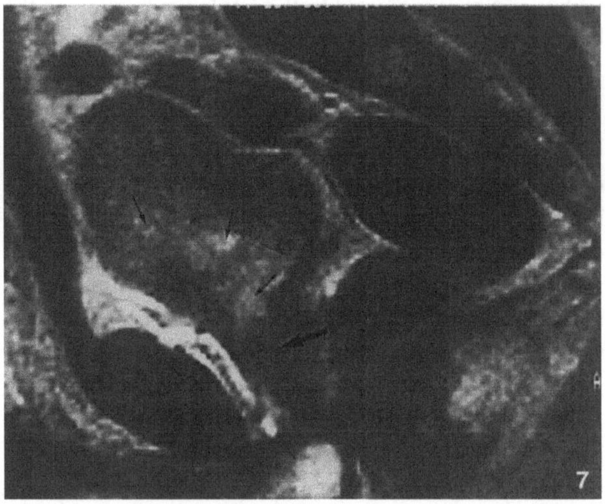

Fig. 32.6. Normal appearance of the bladder on axial T2 MRI; full bladder, the bladder wall is regular and hypointense on T2-weighted imaging

Fig. 32.7. Cancer of the bladder on sagittal T2 MRI: the nodular lesion *(small arrows)* is clearly hyperintense on T2-weighted imaging whereas the prostate *(large arrow)* remains of low signal. This difference in signal intensity between the lesion and prostate suggests sparing of the latter structure by the tumor be nodular but without involvement of the pelvic side wall or pelvic organs [12] (fig. 32.8).

In stages T4A and B, the spread to the pelvic organs is associated with contiguity of the mass with the involved organ and invasion of the fat plane between these two structures. The signal intensity of the visceral spread is identical to that of the tumor on all imaging sequences [6, 8]. In addition, there is always invasion of the surrounding fat, apart from the cases of prostatic spread. Prostatic involvement occurs directly by contiguous spread of bladder base tumors through the bladder wall. The differential diagnosis with a benign lesion is always difficult. Signs which help in the diagnosis of prostatic area spread are: the absence of contrast between the suspicious prostatic area and the tumor whatever the sequence used (fig. 32.7), interruption of the line between the lesion and the prostate, and loss of a clear inter-prostato-vesical cleavage plane. Apart from filling-in of the vesico-seminal space, involvement of a seminal vesicle may manifest as deformity, abnormal orientation or even a simple focal abnormality of signal intensity: hypointense area relative to the controlateral seminal vesicle within a normally hyperintense seminal vesicle on T2-weighted imaging (signal intensity greater than that of fat). This sign is of significance even if there is no associated morphological abnormality. Spread to the ureter or urethra is difficult to diagnose. Ureteric dilatation is not synonymous with invasion. Ureteric obstruction is very rarely seen in non-infiltrative tumors.

The use of a gadolinium contrast agent does not improve the definition of spread to the deep muscle layers of the bladder [16] but does provide better definition of necrotic and soft tissue areas.

Lymphatic extension depends on the demonstration of hypertrophied lymph nodes that cannot be differentiated from hyperplastic or inflammatory lymph nodes. The volumetric criteria are identical to those for CT.

Apart from the demonstration of bone metastases in the pelvis which appear hypointense on T1-weighted imaging, hyperintense on T2-weighted imaging and enhanced with gadolinium, MRI does not guarantee an assessment of distant metastases.

Both CT and MRI are useful methods for the staging of bladder tumors but are nonetheless unable to detect early microscopic invasion or to differentiate neoplastic lesions from simple inflammatory changes. The value of CT and MRI is roughly the same [7, 14], MRI being slightly superior for the appreciation of the spread onto the seminal vesicles and prostate [1].

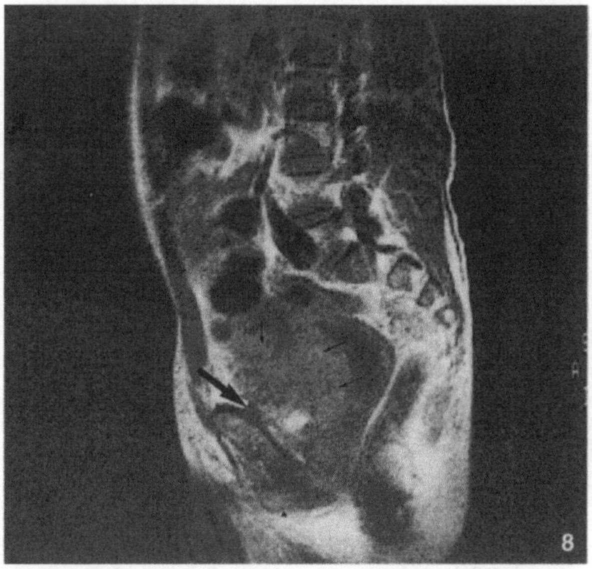

Fig. 32.8. Tumor of the bladder wall following percutaneous biopsy. Sagittal MRI demonstrates a nodular lesion *(small arrows)* seemingly associated with anterior spread into the prevesical fat in Retzius' space *(large arrows)*, and this is a pitfall that may be encountered following biopsy or transurethral resection (TUR)

Bladder involvement by other pelvic tumors [5]

Bladder wall involvement is routinely looked for in the preoperative work-up of cancers of the uterus and rectum. In fact, surgical resection is sometimes possible at the price of an extensive operation requiring total exenteration. CT and MRI are of particular value and are complementary to cystoscopy which may be negative if the bladder wall involvement is limited to the outer muscle layers.

CT demonstrates the contiguity between the tumor mass and the bladder wall with loss of the adjacent fat, associated with focal or nodular thickening of the bladder wall (fig. 32.9].

The 3-dimensional capability of MRI, particularly in the sagittal plane, is particularly suited to detect a vesical involvement by uterine cancers. Loss of the fat tissue along the posterior surface of the bladder and located between the bladder and the uterus, continuity between the bladder wall and the uterine tumor, and loss of the hypointense line of the bladder wall on T2-weighted imaging represent important presumptive features, and bladder invasions which are even

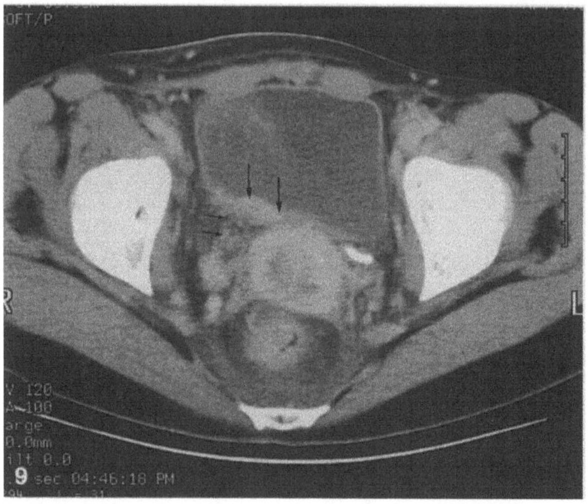

Fig. 32.9. Bladder extension from other pelvic tumors: post contrast CT demonstrates contiguity between the tumor of the uterine cervix and the bladder wall with progressive loss of the adjacent fat *(small arrows)* and nodular thickening of the bladder wall *(large arrows)*

more suggestive when there is endoluminal nodular involvement of the bladder.

As a general role CT, particularly in cancers of the uterus, forms an almost routine part of the initial staging process. The exceptions are the extremely limited tumors with normal lymphography which are treated by surgery straight-away.

Post-treatment follow-up [5]

Indications

For early post-operative complications, CT is indicated initially for the detection of a pelvic collection, such as a lymphocele, urinoma, hematoma or abscess. At a later stage, CT will help in the detection of recurrent disease. If the patient has been treated by radiotherapy alone without surgery or following anterior resection, there are interpretive difficulties posed by changes linked to the radiotherapy or surgery resulting in rigidity and thickening of the bladder wall.

As yet there is no definite proof as to the benefit of performing routine follow-up with CT or MRI in these previously treated patients. These investigations should be performed in the presence of any clinical signs such as fever, edema of the lower limbs, pelvic pains or urinary problems.

Signs

CT

In the early post-operative period, the usual problem is that of a pelvic collection. This may be due to a hematoma which has an intrinsically high density, an abscess appearing as a heterogeneous thick walled lesion, a thin walled urinoma of fluid density, or a lymphocele, also thin walled and fluid density located at the level of a lymphatic vessel. Bone infection and particularly osteitis pubis should routinely be looked for.

In the longer term, the post-radiation bladder manifests as a reduction in the bladder capacity, increased density of the perivesical fat (from the second or third month following radiotherapy), and thickening of the bladder wall. The exact nature of a soft tissue mass detected 4-6 months following treatment is difficult to determine on CT. A multinodular mass is more commonly active residual disease, whereas an infiltrative area of soft tissue density without any extrinsic compression or discrete mass is more likely to be synonymous with post-treatment fibrosis. However, an unequivocal diagnosis is impossible, even after contrast injection, since inflammation and active tumor both are enhanced.

MRI

MRI is more accurate than CT for the demonstration of recurrent disease in the later stages but would appear to be less useful for the assessment of the early complications.

During the first three months following radiotherapy, vesical inflammation appears as a significant increase in the signal intensity and thickening of the wall, particularly at the trigone. The signal intensity of the bladder wall and perivesical fat reduces from the third month onwards [21]. Circumferential thickening of the bladder wall is visible from the 4th to 6th month. There is also an associated reduction in the signal intensity and size of the pelvic organs, particularly the uterus [3].

MRI morphological criteria for the distinction of post-therapeutic fibrosis from recurrent tumor are identical to CT. The evolution of the signal intensity on T2-weighted imaging are additional complementary features of MRI: recurrences have an increased signal on T2-weighted imaging whereas fibrosis appears of low signal from 6 months (or better, one year) following treatment. A compressive mass of high signal on T2-weighted imaging situated away from the treatment area is suggestive of recurrence. On the other hand, a poorly defined, of low signal on T2-weighted imaging soft tissue area which may or not be infiltrative, and without extrinsic compression is relatively characteristic of fibrosis. There must always be a delay of at least 6 to 12 months before this differentiation is of any value, the distinction being unreliable before this time due to the persistence of inflammatory changes. The injection of gadolinium has no demonstrable advantages, its role being close to that of the use iodinated contrast in CT.

Conclusion [5]

CT and MRI are essential for staging and should be routinely used preoperatively for invasive tumors. They are too cumbersome, costly and inaccurate for the detection of the tumor itself. The diagnosis is first confirmed by a cystoscopy at which the biopsy can be performed for histological analysis. It is useful to combine the clinical findings (pelvic examination) with the imaging findings for T3B and T4 tumors.

These techniques can perform "lymph node staging", particularly CT, and can forewarn the surgeon of possible operative difficulties. Their limitations are essentially: the non-detection of microscopic disease, the inability to distinguish tumor and inflammatory changes or to discriminate the different layers of the bladder wall.

For follow-up, the problems depend on the type of lesion. Superficial lesions can be followed-up by cystoscopy alone. For infiltrative tumors, there is a particular risk of lymph node recurrence and/or a metastasis following a total cystectomy (less than 10% failure rate following cystectomy). In these cases, ultrasound is less useful. MRI is seemingly superior to CT in the differentiation between fibrosis and recurrence in the presence of a soft tissue lesion detected outside the treatment area (particularly after one year).

References

1. Amendola MA, Glazer GM, Grossman HB, Aisen AM, Francis IP (1986) Staging of bladder carcinoma: MRICT-surgical correlation. AJR 146: 1179-1183
2. American Joint Committee for Cancer Staging and EndResults Reporting (1978) Manual for staging of cancer. Whiting, Chicago
3. Arrivé L, Chang YCF, Hricak H, Brescia RJ, Auffermann W, Quivey JM (1989) Radiation-induced uterine changes: MR imaging. Radiology 170: 55-58
4. Arrivé L, Guinet C, Buy JN, Malbec L, Vadrot D, LavalJeantet M (1985) Imagerie par résonance magnétique de la région pelvienne. Résultats préliminaires. J Radiol 6: 771-777
5. Arrivé L, Richard F, Vadrot D (1992) Vessie. In: Buthiau D (ed) TDM et IRM Cliniques, Abdomen-Pelvis. Frison-Roche, Paris, pp 253-263
6. Barentsz JO, Lemmens JAM, Ruijs SK, et al (1988) Carcinoma of the urinary bladder: MR imaging with a double surface coil. AJR 151: 107- 112
7. Bryan PJ, Butler HE, Lipuma JP, Resnick MI, Kureh ED (1987) CT and MR imaging in staging bladder neoplasms. J Comput Assist Tomogr 11: 96-101
8. Buy JN, Moss AA, Guinet C, Ghossain MA, Malbec L, Arrivé L, Vadrot D (1988) MR staging bladder carcinoma: correlation with pathologic findings. Radiology 169: 695-700
9. Chang YCF, Arrivé L, Hricak H (1989) Gynecologic tumor imaging. Semin Ultrasound CT MR 10: 29-42
10. Dershaw DD, Scher HI (1988) Serial transabdominal sonography of bladder cancer. AJR 150: 1055-1059
11. Fisher MR, Hricak H, Crooks LE (1985) Urinary bladder MR imaging. Part I: Normal and benign conditions. Radiology 157: 467-470
12. Fisher MR, Hricak H, Tanagho EA (1985) Urinary bladder MR imaging. Part II: Neoplasm. Radiology 157: 471-477
13. Golding RP, Van Zanten TEG, Tierie AH, et al (1987) Intravenous urography as a prognostic indicator in vesical carcinoma. Cancer 60: 883-886
14. Husband JES, Olliff JFC, Williams MP, Heron CW, Cherryman GF (1989) Bladder cancer staging with CTand MR imaging. Radiology 173: 435-440
15. Koelbel G, Schmiedl U, Griebel J, Hess CF, Kueper K (1988) MR imaging of urinary bladder neoplasms. J Comput Assist Tomogr 12: 98-103
16. Neuerburg JM, Bohndorf K, Sohn M, Toufl F, Guenther RW, Daus HJ (1989) Urinary bladder neoplasms: evaluation with contrast-enhanced MR imaging. Radiology 172: 739-743
17. Rholl KS, Lee JKT, Heikon JP, Ling D, Glazer HS (1987) Primary bladder carcinoma: evaluation with MR imaging. Radiology 163: 117-121
18. Richard F, Arrivé L, Vadrot D, Camey M (1985) Imagerie par résonance magnétique des tumeurs de vessie. Communication personnelle à la SFU, Paris
19. Richard F, Sotto H, Plougastel ML, Camey M (1986) Chimiothérapie néo-adjuvante associée à la cystoprostatectomie radicale dans les tumeurs urothéliales de vessie. In: Neo-adjuvant Chemotherapy. Colloque INSERM. John Libbey Eurotext 137: 705-709
20. Sandler CM, Hall JT, Rodriguez MB, Corriere JM (1986) Bladder injury in blunt pelvic trauma. Radiology 158: 633-638
21. Tavares NJ, Arrivé L, Demas BE, Quivey J, Hricak H (1988) Bladder morphology following radiation therapy: assessment with MR imaging. Radiology 169: 169-175
22. Vallancien G, Veillon B, Caharten M, et al (1986) Can transabdominal ultrasonography of the bladder replace cystoscopy in the follow-up of superficial blader tumors? J Urol 136: 32-34

CHAPTER 33

Cancer of the uterine cervix

Clinicians
Y. Darbois, D. Dargent, D. Nizri, J.-V. Chantelard, G. Lefebvre, H. Charreyre, A. Wacrenier, E. Vuillemin, D. Khayat

Radiologists
D. Buthiau, J.-D. Picard

The diagnosis of cancer of the cervix is clinical and histological. Imaging has no role to play in the diagnosis but has an important role in staging and determining the treatment strategy. Imaging has also a considerable role in the post-treatment follow-up for the detection of recurrence [5].

For staging purposes, we use the International Federation of Gynecology and Obstetrics (FIGO) classification system which depends on the clinical findings. It is possible to further simplify this classification by considering separately the locally limited cancers (centro-pelvic) which are the stage IB and the proximal stages IIA and IIB lesions, and the clinically more extensive cancers represented by the distal stage IIB and stages III and IV (table 33.1) [5].

Table 33.1. The FIGO classification

Stage	0	TIS N0 M0: cancer *in situ*
Stage	I	T1 N0 M0: cancer limited to the cervix
	IA1	T1 A1 N0 M0: early stromal invasion
	IA2	T1 A2 N0 M0: depth of 5 mm or less; extent of 7 mm or less
	IB	T1 B N0 M0: larger lesion than T1A2
Stage	II	T2 N0 M0: tumor beyond the uterine cervix but within the limits of the pelvic region (pelvic side wall, inferior third of the vagina)
	IIA	T2 A N0 M0: no parametrial infiltration
	IIB	T2B N0 M0: parametrial infiltration
Stage	III	
	IIIA	T3 N0 M0: tumor involving the boundaries of the pelvic region (pelvic side wall, inferior third of the vagina)
	IIIB	T1 - 3 N1 M0: tumor associated with metastatic lymphadenopathy
Stage	IV	
	IV A	T4 N0 or 1 M0: tumor invading the bladder or rectum or extending beyond the pelvic region with or without lymphadenopathy
	IV B	T1 - N0 or 1 M1: cancer with distant metastases

The limited cancers

The therapeutic approaches are variable for these types of tumors. Some authors advocate the use radiotherapy whereas others prefer surgery. In France, a combination of radiotherapy and surgery is often proposed although the chronological order of these treatments is variable.

Some authors propose surgery alone in the most favorable cases. Imaging has a vital role in supplementing the clinical findings in order to obtain an accurate staging of the disease [5].

Lymph node involvement is seen in 5-15% of stages IB and IIA and approximately 20% of stage IIB tumors. There is a resultant fall in the 5 year survival rate from 80-90% down to 45-60% for those limited forms which are associated with lymph node involvement. It should be remembered that the primary lymph node drainage sites are the interiliac, obturator, hypogastric and sacral lymph nodes.

The presence of lymph node involvement is closely related with the size of the primary lesion, the depth of invasion and the histological grade. These are also all parameters which determine the risk of local recurrence in those tumors without lymph node involvement.

Adenocarcinomas, which represent 10-15% of cervical cancers and up to 35% in a recent series in the literature, and adenosquamous carcinomas (2-5% of cases) seem to have a higher recurrence rate, despite the absence of a more marked affinity for lymphatic spread.

Involvement of adjacent structures, either infiltration of the vesico-vaginal septum or posterior rectum, has prognostic implications and generally precludes surgery, or necessitates very extensive surgery initially for isolated anterior or posterior involvement.

In conclusion, imaging has an important role for [5]:

- assessing tumor volume;
- determining the degree of invasion;
- demonstrating possible lymphadenopathy;
- detecting parametrial invasion;
- demonstrating invasion of the vesico-vaginal septum or rectal wall posteriorly.

The search for distant metastases is less important in the limited forms of the disease: 5% of stage IB and 9% of stage IIA present with a disseminated disease. However, more than 15% of stage IIB (and almost 25% of stage IV) have metastatic disease at presentation

• Assessment of tumor volume. Two distinct types must be considered. The first is the nodular exocervical lesion, the measurement of which is essentially clinical. On the other hand, infiltrative tumors of the cervix, as well as the exophytic tumors associated with an infiltrative component, cannot be reliably evaluated clinically. In these cases, imaging can play a useful complementary role (measurement of volume and spread towards the uterine body).

• Appreciation of parametrial invasion. Imaging has an important role here. In effect, pelvic examination, although reliable, has a significant margin of error due to difficulties in differentiating of tumor infiltration, obstetric sclerosis and local inflammation.

• Infiltration of the vesico-vaginal septum and rectal wall posteriorly. Here, also radiology has an important role. There are significant errors associated with internal pelvic examination, palpation, cystoscopy and proctoscopy, and even palpation under cystoscopic control.

Table 33.2. Investigation of lymph node spread (From D. Buthiau, D. Dargent. Imagerie clinique en gynécologie. Paris, 1993 [5])

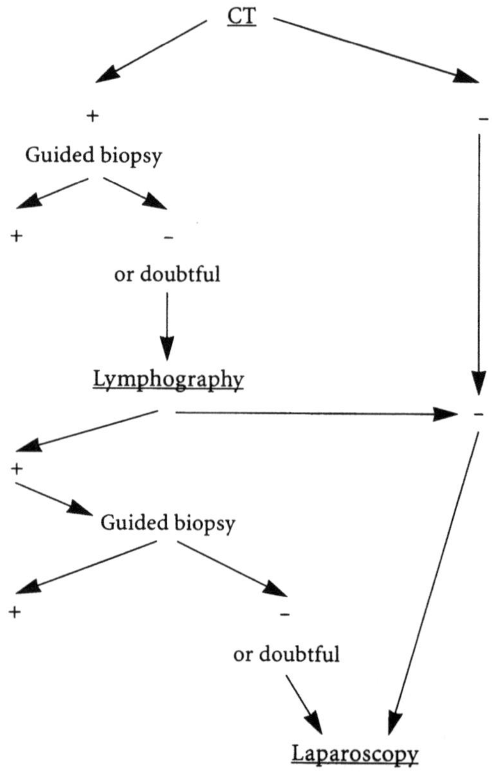

• Lymph node invasion (table 33.2). Classically, lymphography used to be the only method of making this diagnosis. Nowadays, laparoscopy has no considerable role but is being used more and more commonly. However, it can be avoided if imaging, particularly CT, makes the diagnosis and enables a guided biopsy to be performed (under CT or ultrasound guidance). In addition, preoperative imaging will help to determine whether immediate surgery, diagnostic laparoscopy or ultrasound guided biopsy is indicated depending on the probability of lymph node involvement.

Extensive cancers

For these lesions, it is generally agreed that radiotherapy is the most appropriate treatment. There is still a place for chemotherapy and salvage surgery as second line treatments. Imaging provides the initial staging and subsequent follow-up both during and following treatment.

Pre-invasive stage of cancer of the cervix [5]

There is no indication for any of the imaging techniques in this early stage of the disease. The tumor detection depends on cytology and colposcopy, and the diagnosis on histology. Cervical cancers are usually diagnosed at this stage.

Invasive cancer of the cervix [5]

The diagnosis is easy in the presence of provoked or sometimes spontaneous metrorrhagia; occasionally there is only purulent leucorrhea. Clinical examination using a speculum and eventually colposcopy demonstrate a cervical lesion. Biopsy gives the histological type.

Staging is often more difficult and is achieved by vaginal or rectal examination or a combination of the two. The accuracy rate is better if they are performed under anesthesia by an experienced clinician. They provide an assessment of tumor volume, the parametria, as well as the vesico-vaginal and recto-vaginal septa, and the utero-sacral ligaments.

Role of CT and MRI [3, 5]

In cancer of the cervix, imaging only has a role in staging.

Conventional radiography

This is of secondary interest. A chest radiograph should not be omitted to look for pleuro-parenchymal secondary deposits. Intravenous urography is performed to detect compression or invasion of the urinary tract. Finally, in some very advanced cancers, a barium enema is performed if there is uncertainty about the presence of invasion of the rectosigmoid colon.

Lymphography

The indications for this technique have markedly reduced due to the reliability of CT. The internal iliac, paracervical and parametrial lymph nodes are not opacified by intrapedal injection.

Ultrasound

This can be of value, particularly if the examination is performed endovaginally or endorectally, and combined with color doppler. It may give some indication as to the degree of spread superiorly towards the isthmus, but assessment of spread inferiorly into the vaginal wall is more difficult. Ultrasound can measure the tumor volume. Finally, using transvaginal or better still axial transrectal sections, it can give information as to the presence of parametrial invasion. It has not negligible role in the assessment of the vesico-vaginal septum or rectal wall. However, CT and MRI are the essential radiological imaging techniques for the staging of cancers of the uterine cervix.

CT

This has a dual role:
- firstly, for all stages of the disease, it can assess the lymph nodes and look for possible metastases;
- secondly, it may be used to assess the local extent of the lesion itself for stages IIB and above, with a variable accuracy depending on the histological type.

MRI

MRI has a sensitivity between 75-83% and a specificity greater than 90% [5]. The sensitivity improves in the more advanced stage.

MRI (see figs 33.4 & 33.5) is superior to CT for the assessment of tumor volume (see fig 33.6). It is also more accurate than clinical examination in the case of an endocervical lesion or subepithelial spread.

Signs

CT

The primary cervical lesion

This is characterized on CT by an increase of the volume of the cervix. The appearance is usually non-specific, sometimes associated with enhancement following contrast injection (fig. 33.1) or a necrotic hypodensity (fig. 33.2).

More suggestive is the presence of a focal deformity with asymmetry (fig. 33.2).

Parametrial spread

This initially is seen as an irregular appearance to the lateral surfaces of the cervix. Subsequently, it appears

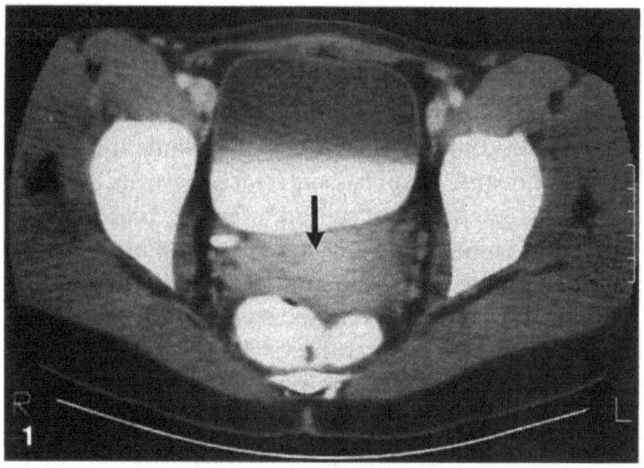

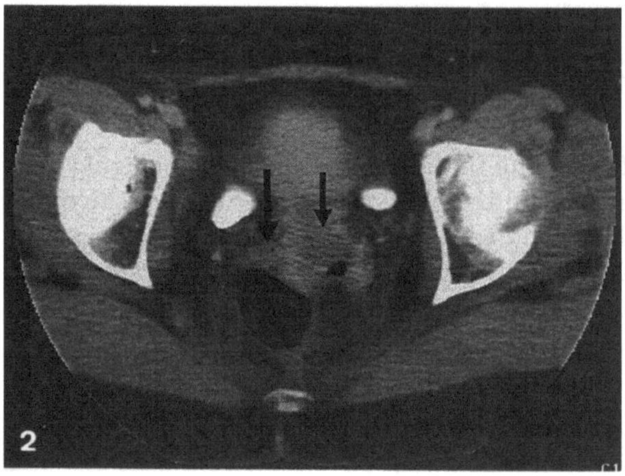

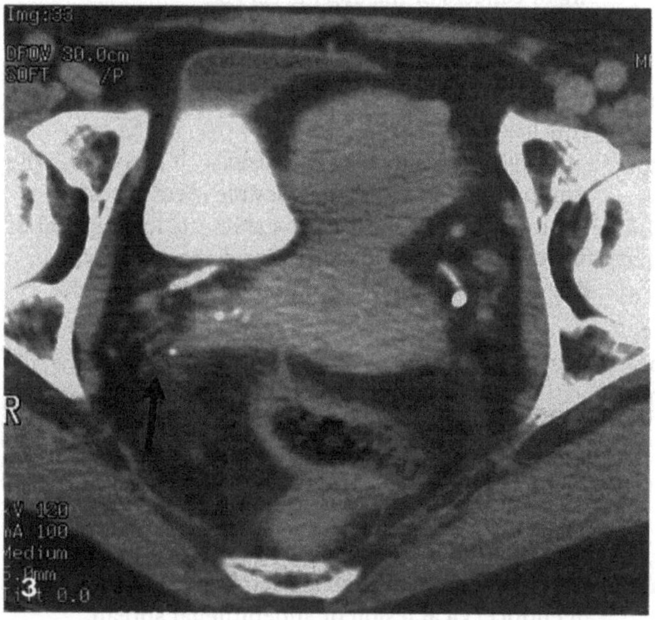

Fig. 33.1. Stage IB cancer of the cervix on post-contrast CT: non-specific enlargement of the volume of the cervix with apparent enhancement *(arrow)* which may equally be encountered in the physiological state at the centro-cervical level

Fig. 33.2. Stage IIB cancer of the cervix on post contrast CT: the lesion is necrotic *(small arrow)* and is associated with early filling-in of the fatty tissue between the cervix and the ureter and right internal iliac vessel *(large arrow)*, confirmed at surgery

Fig. 33.3. Stage IIB cancer of the cervix on post-contrast CT: the scan demonstrates non-specific enlargement of the cervix and almost complete filling-in of the fatty tissue between the cervix and internal iliac pedicle and right ureter. Note the involvement of the fat around the vessels and right internal iliac fascia *(arrows)* highly suggestive of a stage IIB, confirmed surgically

as a parametrial soft tissue mass, generally of a triangular or lobulated shape, which is contiguous with the cervix.

A supplementary feature is the presence of a soft tissue mass obliterating the lateral peri-ureteric fat planes. There may also be loss of the physiological fatty tissue in the pericervical and peri-ureteric regions. Invasion of the fatty tissue around the internal iliac vessels may also be noted (figs 33.2 & 33.3).

However, it must be underlined that these very suggestive appearances are not specific. In fact, inflammatory changes involving the parametria can give identical changes, particularly if there is superadded infection of the cervix. Moreover, if these changes are related to cancer spread then the cancer is always very extensive.

Spread to the pelvic side wall

This is seen as an irregular, linear soft tissue density of variable homogeneity extending in a continuous fashion to the pelvic walls.

The lesion is theoretically classified as IIIB when the parametrial mass infiltrates to within 3 mm of the pelvic wall, even if a small thin fat plane persists. The same applies when there is hydronephrosis or hydroureter indicating invasion of the lower ureter with dilatation of the whole length of the ureter and the pelvicalyceal system (also well seen on ultrasound).

Spread to the bladder or rectum

This is suggested by a focal loss of the perivesical or perirectal fat. This sign is classically associated with

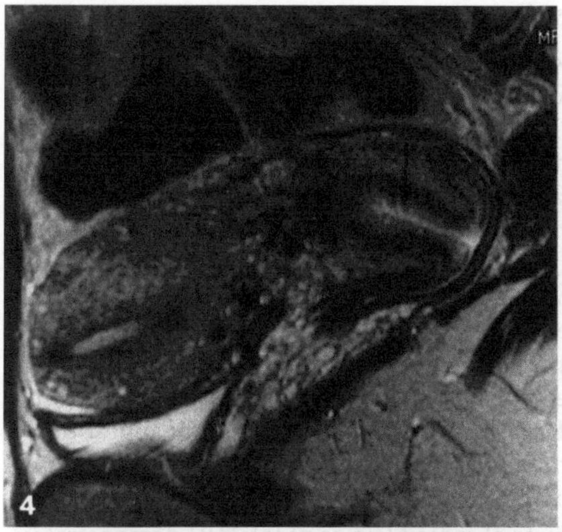

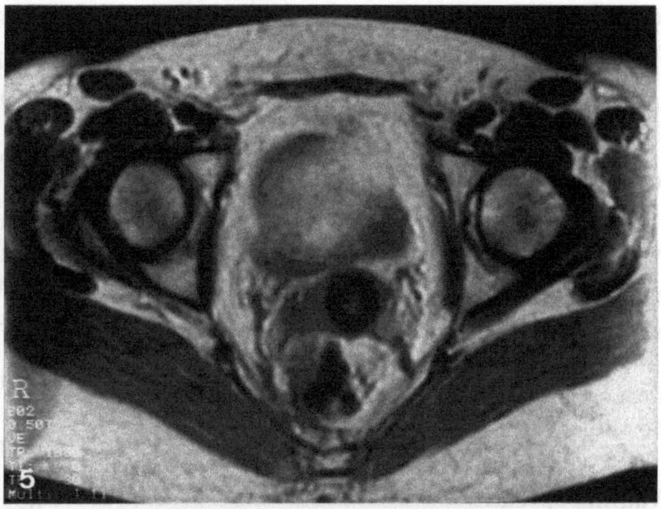

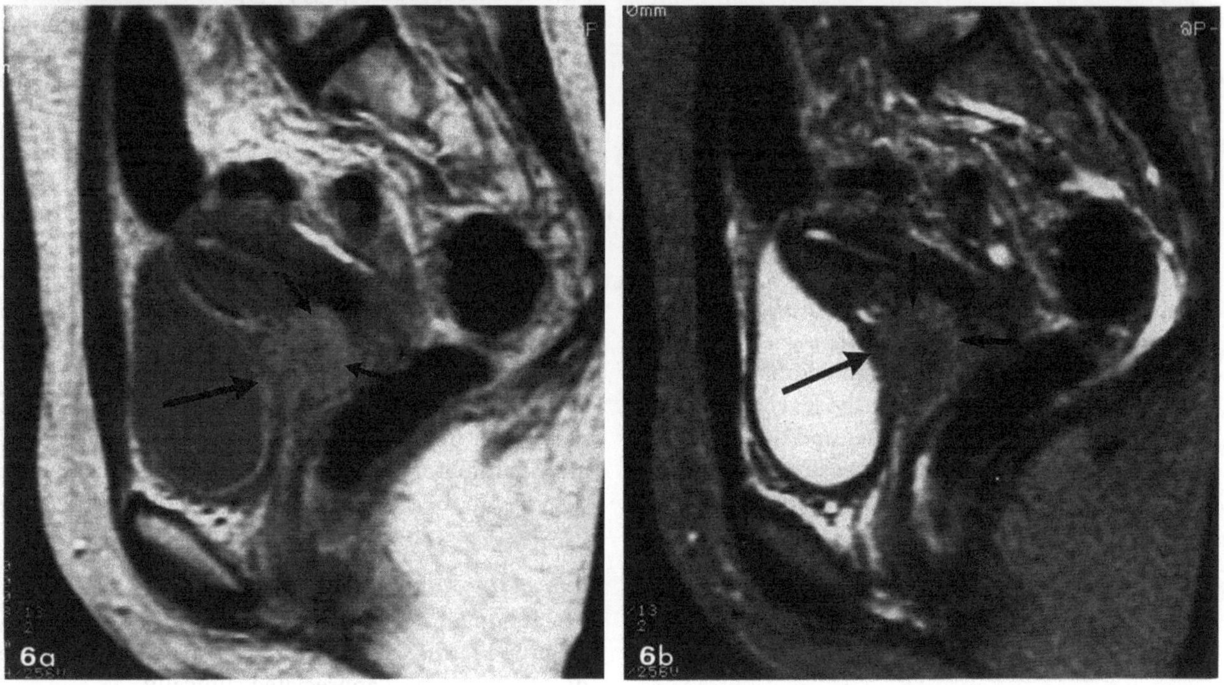

Fig. 33.4. MRI appearance of the normal cervix on a heavily T2-weighted sagittal section: the uterine cervix is of low signal due to the presence of fibro-elastic connective tissue. Note the endocervix and the plicae palmatae cervicis *(arrow)*

Fig. 33.5. Normal appearance of the cervix and parametria on axial T1-weighted MRI section: the cervix is formed by a hypointense cylinder peripherally and a hyperintense central area corresponding to the endocervix; the parametria are of intermediate to high signal intensity due to the presence of numerous vascular structures with slow flow

Fig. 33.6 a, b. Adenocarcinoma of the cervix on sagittal MRI, proton density (**a**) and T2-weighted (**b**). The lesion *(small arrows)* is hyperintense on the proton density sequence, well differentiated from the physiological hypointense cervix (visible superior to this lesion). It involves the anterior lip of the cervix, extends to the vagina (superior third) and is associated with loss of the inter-vesico-vaginal septum. Nonetheless, there is no change in the chemical shift artefact nor any sign of bladder wall involvement *(large arrow)*. Comparison with the surgical findings in this patient showed an agreement with infiltration of the septum but no involvement of the wall itself. Note that recognition of the difference in signal between the lesion and cervix makes it possible to assess tumor volume by MRI (the volume being sometimes slightly overestimated due to inseparable perilesional edema) asymmetrical thickening of the adjacent wall but is not specific.

There may be a nodular or irregular appearance of the bladder or rectal wall.

A further feature may be noted with the presence of an endoluminal filling defect due to tumor.

Vesico- or recto-vaginal fistula

This is a difficult pathology to demonstrate and is usually not visible. It should be remembered that the presence of intravaginal air has no pathological significance.The diagnostic accuracy of CT varies between 60 and 80%.

Vaginal spread

The appreciation of vaginal spread (stage IIA) is essentially clinical (sometimes aided by endovaginal ultrasound).

MRI

(figs 33.4-33.6)

Cervical lesion

MRI demonstrates an increase in the volume of the cervix on all sequences.

More particularly, on T2-weighted imaging there is a frankly hyperintense area at the level of the lesion itself. The signal is clearly higher and therefore differentiable from the low signal intensity of the adjacent cervical stroma, as well as of the myometrium and vagina.

The signal intensity of the tumor remains less than that of the endometrium, cervical canal or parametria. Adenocarcinomas, due to their higher water content, are more hyperintense (fig. 33.6) than squamous (epidermoid) cancers. The T1-weighted sequence gives good contrast between the tumor and paracervical fatty tissue which appears hyperintense, as well as the cylindrical mucosa of the cervical canal. The injection of a contrast agent further improves the differentiation between the tumor and the healthy peritumoral tissues.

Staging

• *Stage* 0:

MRI provides no useful information.

• *Stage I:*

MRI can accurately delineate the outline of the tumor.

• *Stage II:*

MRI can delineate the region of the tumor, particularly its superior limit:

- There may be endocervical tumor stenosis with proximal hemotometria or pyometria.

- Vaginal spread may be demonstrated in the form of tumor tissue infiltrating the vaginal walls in continuity with the cervical lesions. The administration of contrast agent can improve the sensitivity of the technique.

- Spread to the myometrium is suggested by the loss of the normal low signal intensity between the tumor and the myometrium. It may sometimes appear on T2-weighted imaging as a hyperintensity of the myometrium.

Parametrial spread (fig. 33.7) [5]. MRI demonstrates:

- an extension of the high signal intensity of the tumor into the parametrial region of one or both sides;
- an irregular contours of the lateral cervical wall with enlargement of the cervix;
- a loss of the parametrial fat plane situated between the lateral walls of the cervix and internal iliac vessels.

This appearance is of great importance because it can determine the proximal or distal nature of the involvement which allows distinction between the early or advanced stage IIB lesions. It must be noted that the association of several pathological criteria provides greater diagnostic certainty. In fact, there is the possibility of a diagnostic error in 10-15% of cases. This may either be a false positive diagnosis in the case of an inflammatory reaction or local infection, or false negative in the case of lymphatic micro-emboli (rapidly invasive cancers of young women).

• *Stage III*:

The lesion locally is usually very large.

Spread to the inferior third of the vagina is visible on MRI but is best appreciated clinically.

Spread to the lateral side wall of the pelvis is suggested by the loss of the physiological fat situated along the lateral pelvic muscle plane, particularly the piriformis and obturator muscles.

Loss of the physiological fatty tissue around the internal iliac pedicle or within 3 mm of the pelvic side wall indicates stage IIIB.

In extreme cases, there is alteration in the signal intensity of the muscles with enlargement and infiltration of the raphes. MRI is an excellent technique for demonstrating this spread.

• *Stage IV:*

The major sign of visceral invasion is the loss of the vesico-uterine or utero-rectal fat plane (figs 33.6 & 33.8).

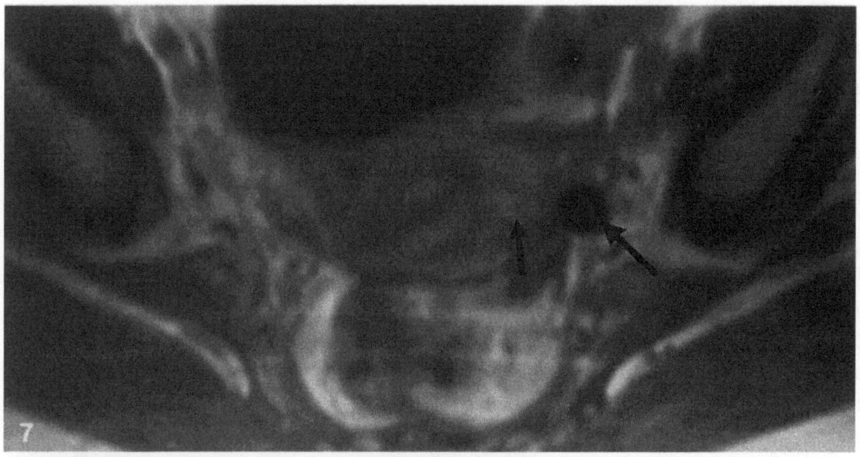

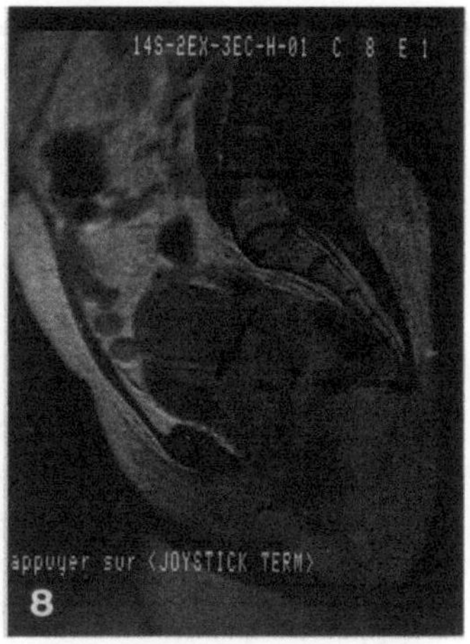

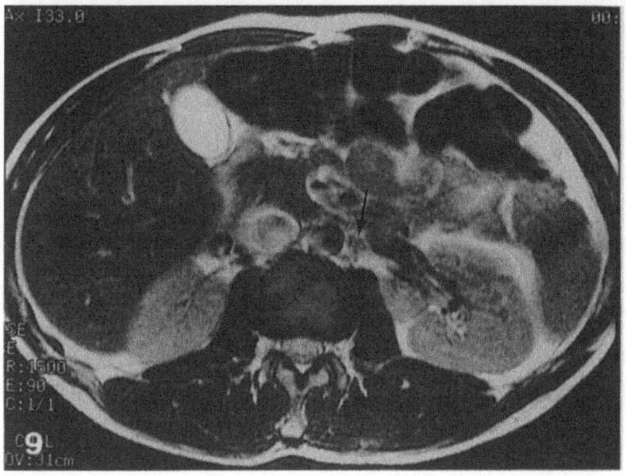

Fig. 33.7. Cancer of the cervix on an axial T1-weighted MRI sequence: the examination demonstrates spread of the hyperintensity on T1-weighted imaging *(small arrow)* into the left parametrial region with irregular contours and enlargement of the paracervical region, as well as loss of the tissue planes between the lateral wall of the cervix and left internal iliac vessels *(large arrow)*

Fig. 33.8. Cancer of the cervix with bladder involvement on a sagittal proton density MRI: MRI demonstrates the cervical lesion extending directly into the vesico-vaginal septum and posterior vaginal wall which is thickened with infiltration of the dome of the bladder *(arrow)*

Fig. 33.9. Lymph node in the retroperitoneum, left latero-aortic *(arrow)*, on axial T2 MRI. As with CT, MRI can only assess the volume and not the content of the node and therefore provides no additional information compared to CT

The reliability of this sign is considerably increased if there is alteration in the normal signal intensity of the bladder wall associated with local thickening indicating infiltration (fig. 33.8). Alteration in the chemical shift artifact also constitutes a good sign of invasion.

Whenever there is a doubt on the MRI images, proctoscopy and cystoscopy are indispensable for visceral extension and rarely provide information on spread to the walls.

Clinical forms

Cancer of the uterine cervix occurring in pregnancy: staging by MRI is very accurate. The technique does not use ionizing radiation, and the multiplanar capability of MRI is ideally suited to the changes in the cervico-isthmic region of the uterus which occur during pregnancy.

Clinical investigations

Cystoscopy

This remains the most reliable method for detecting involvement of the bladder mucosa. It is also possible to detect muscle involvement in the form of a flattened area revealed by "colposcopy"; this method consists of cystoscopic visualization of the trigone while mobilizing the tumor by digital pelvic examination.

Proctoscopy

This detects spread to the rectal mucosa.

Diagnostic surgical investigations

Laparotomy

This consists of immediate histological evaluation successively of the lumbo-aortic, subaortic and pelvic lymph nodes, and an assessment of possible parametrial involvement.

The therapeutic decision depends on this examination: surgery for non-disseminated cancers and radiotherapy for the more advanced lesions.

Lymph node sampling by laparascopic surgery

- Either by retroperitoneal pelviscopy (D Dargent) [5],
- or by classical intraperitoneal laparoscopy.

These more recent techniques allow a more accurate assessment of the pelvic lymph nodes. They have the advantage of requiring hospitalization of the patient for only two days but necessitate specific equipment and training.

Positive diagnosis and staging [3, 5]

A positive diagnosis is obtained from biopsy. Staging is achieved by a combination of operative techniques under locoregional anesthesia or preferably general anesthesia (particularly in elderly patients). The assessment includes vaginal and rectal examinations, cystoscopy and possibly proctoscopy. It is possible to have several clinicians performing this assessment in order to compare their opinions.

One can deduce the volume of the tumor, spread into the parametrium and bladder anteriorly resulting in a staging of the lesion according to the FIGO classification system.

The role of imaging [5]

Advanced forms

Imaging has an important role for these lesions.

CT provides assessment of lymph node involvement and follow-up under radiotherapy.

Ultrasound and in particular MRI can determine the tumor volume prior to radiotherapy and monitor progress.

Limited forms

The treatment for these lesions is disputed. Some authors prefer radiotherapy, and others advocate surgery. Some propose a combination of the two treatments.

Surgery alone, however, seems adequate for the less extensive forms.

Assessment of tumor volume

MRI is the most accurate and reproducible technique, superior or equivalent to ultrasound. This latter technique may be more sensitive using color doppler. This method has yet to be evaluated in a large series.

Lymph node involvement

CT has a dominant role in the assessment of lymph node involvement. MRI provides little additional information (fig. 33.9) and has the double problem of cost and limited geographical accessibility to machines. Ultrasound also has no significant contribution in this area. CT is, therefore, suggested as the initial examination of choice. If positive, CT guided fine needle aspiration for cytology or lymphography should be performed.

If CT is negative or the FNA is inconclusive, one can resort to lymphography which should lead on to a laparoscopy if itself is also negative or inconclusive (see table 33.2).

Parametrial and cervico-vaginal spread

Ultrasound may have a role in as much as some authors propose ultrasound guided parametrial biopsy. MRI, however, is less operative dependent and is generally preferred due to its superior or equal sensitivity to CT and superior specificity. MRI seems to be promising in the assessment of the vesico-vaginal septum, but this is still under evaluation.

Patient management in practice [5]

In the case of primary surgery

Operability is determined by the clinical and cystoscopic findings and the assessment of locoregional spread from the operative techniques. However, imaging can be useful in the preoperative assessment of lymphatic and parametrial spread. This may result in the choice of other treatment options when positive and avoid unnecessary surgical intervention, even celioscopy.

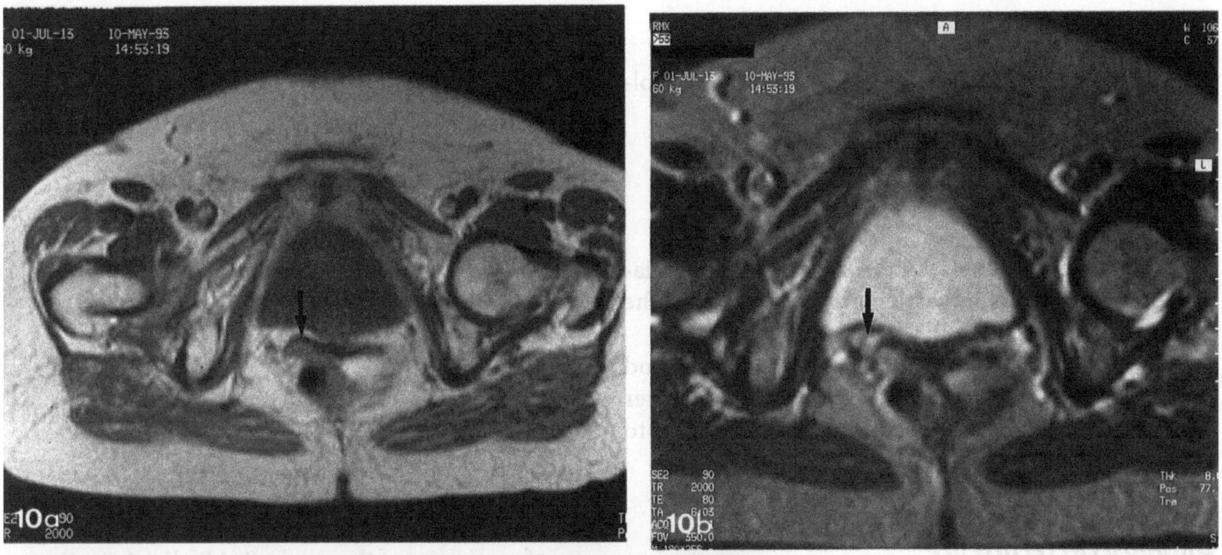

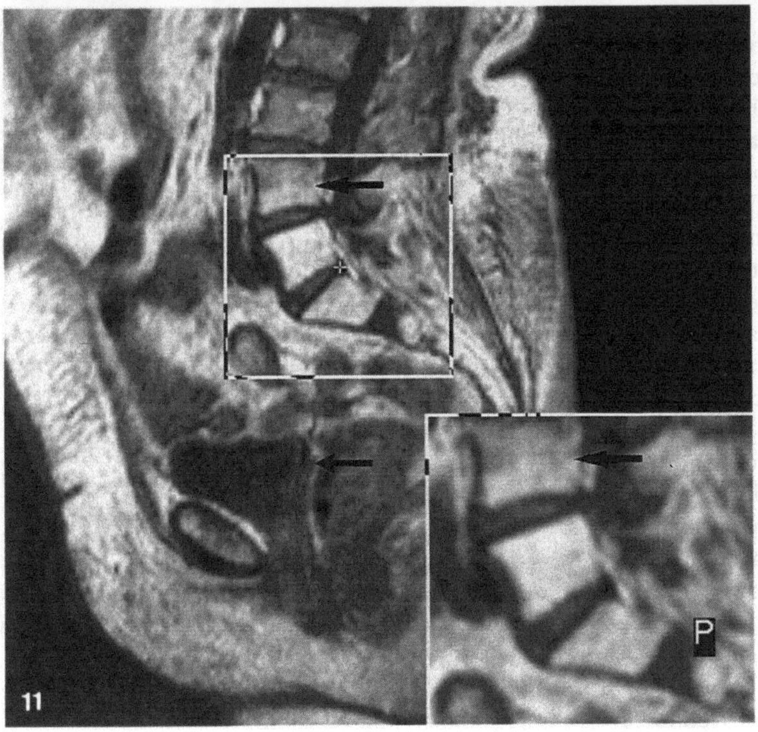

Fig. 33.10 a, b. Local recurrence of a uterine cancer on axial MRI proton density (**a**) and T2-weighted imaging (**b**). There is focal enlargement (in the order of 4 to 5 mm) of intermediate but already increased signal intensity on proton density (**a** *arrow*) and high signal intensity on T2-weighted imaging (**b** *arrow*). Note that on a, this area of recurrence with a slightly increased signal is well differentiated from the thin hypointense operative cuff which appears as a band of low signal intensity displaced by the lesion. Clinically there was a suspicious palpable asymmetry

Fig. 33.11. Baseline control following treatment: the operative cuff is of intermediate intensity on T1 *(small arrow)*. Note that the lumbosacral spine is of altered signal intensity (increased) with clear borders within the irradiation field *(large arrows)*

In the case of external beam radiotherapy, MRI can appreciate the anatomical relationships and volume of the tumor.

CT assesses pelvic and lumbo-aortic lymph node involvement. It will also determine the dosimetry depending on the extent of the tumor.

MRI and CT can also monitor the response of the tumor to radiotherapy treatment.

The combination of primary radiotherapy and surgery

Before radiotherapy, CT and MRI can determine the volume of the tumor and its relationships in order to establish the irradiation modalities.

The pelvic and lumbo-aortic lymph nodes are assessed at the surgical stage.

In the case of radiotherapy alone

CT and MRI are part of the initial assessment and follow-up.

Cancer of the cervix and pregnancy

The assessment of tumor volume and anatomical relationships of the tumor, particularly at the level of the isthmus, is more difficult.

MRI, with its ability to scan in the coronal, axial and particularly sagittal planes, demonstrates better spread superiorly into the isthmus or inferiorly into the vagina.

Diagnosis of recurrence

This presents in two forms. The vaginal recurrence is the easiest form as it is accessible to clinical examination. More difficult is that of centro- and latero-pelvic recurrence for which the endovaginal ultrasound findings seem promising. CT and MRI should be performed as complementary techniques if there is the least doubt (figs 33.10 & 33.11). It is important to remember the potentially helpful contribution of these two imaging techniques when a recurrence is not accessible to clinical examination, ultrasonically or x-ray guided biopsy. In these cases (central pelvic or presacro-coccygeal lesions or lateral sciatic notch, obturator region, isthio-coccygeal raphe...), CT is the initial imaging modality of choice on the condition that the examination technique is meticulous, and the initial reference baseline scan is routinely performed 6 months after the completion of all treatment. MRI has an acknowledged central role nowadays to evaluate "the activity" of a residual area or recurrence by its ability to differentiate fibrosis, hypointense on T2-weighted imaging, from a recurrence, hyperintense on T2. The injection of gadolinium has not proven to be of any additional value. Pre-treatment selective angiography determines the indication for chemoembolization or intra-arterial chemotherapy.

Conclusion

CT and MRI are not operator dependent but easily reproducible and provide a better assessment of visceral and lymph node spread (CT). MRI seems to be more accurate for parametrial invasion.

References

1. Bartoli JM, Moulin G, Di Stefano-Louineau D, Gaubert, JY, Delannoy L, Delpero JR, Blanc B, Kasbarian M (1990) Uterine cervix cancers: staging by magnetic resonance imaging. Ann Radiol (Paris) 33: 241-247
2. Bruneton JN, Merran D, Balu-Maestro C, Geoffray A, Rogopoulos A, Giordano P, Chauvel P, Monticelli J (1990) Echography and computed tomography in the evaluation and follow up of uterine cancers. Bull Cancer (Paris) 77: 689-694
3. Buthiau D, et al (1992) TDM et IRM en gynocologie pelvienne. In: Buthiau D, Piette JC, Khayat D, Nizri D (eds) TDM et IRM cliniques: Abdomen-pelvis. Frison-Roche, Paris, pp 266-291
4. Cobby M, Browning J, Jones A, Whipp E, Goddard P (1990) Magnetic resonance imaging, computed tomography and endosonography in the local staging of carcinoma of the cervix. Br J Radiol 63 (753): 673-679
5. Dargent D , et al (1993) Cancer du col utérin. In: Buthiau D, Dargent D (eds) Imagerie clinique en gynécologie. Vigot, Paris, pp 202-218
6. Dargent D (1990) Diagnostic, classification et pronostic des cancers du col utérin. Rev Prat "Cancers de l'utérus", 1
7. Egashira K,Nakamura K, Terashima H,Nakata H, Kashimura M (1992) MR imaging in uterine cervical cancer after radiotherapy. Radiat Med 10: 117-122
8. Flueckiger F, Ebner F, Poschauko H, Tamussino K Einspieler R, Ranner G (1992) Cervical cancer: serial MR imaging before and after primary radiation therapy -a 2-year follow-up study. Radiology 184: 89-93
9. Hawnaur JM, Johnson RJ, Hunter RD, Jenkins JP, Isherwood I (1992) The value of magnetic resonance imaging in assessment of carcinoma of the cervix and its response to radiotherapy. Clin Oncol (R Coll Radiol) 4: 11-17
10. Hirano Y, Kubo K, Hirai Y, Okada S, Yamada K, Sawano S, Yamashita T, Hiramatsu Y (1992) Preliminary experience with gadolinium-enhanced dynamic MR imaging for uterine neoplasms. Radiographics 12: 243-256
11. Houvenaeghel G, Rosello R, Delpero JR, Resbeut M, Jacquemier J, Guerinel G (1991) Locoregional extension of advanced cancer of the uterine cervix: prospective evaluation of results of clinical examination, endocavitary ultrasonography, TDM, MRI and histology. Bull Cancer (Paris) 78: 969-978
12. Janus CL, Mendelson DS, Moore S, Gendal ES, Dottino P, Brodman M (1989) Staging of cervical carcinoma: accuracy of magnetic resonance imaging and computod tomography. Clin Imaging 13: 114-116
13. Kim SH, Choi BJ, Kang SB, Choi YM, Han MC, Kim CW (1990) Uterine cervical carcinoma: comparison of CT and MR findings. Radiology 175: 45-51
14. Koster O (1990) Possibilities and limitations of radiology, CT and MRI in cases of tumors of the uterus and ovary. Rontgenblatter 43: 413-419

15. Lien HH, Blomlie V, Kjorstad K, Abeler V, Kaalhus O (1991) Clinical stage I carcinoma of the cervix: value of MR imaging in determining degrce of invasiveness. AJR 156: 1191-1194
16. Maranzano E, Latini P, Checcaglini F, Beneventi S, Panizza BM, Perrucci E, Baffa S, Rossi L, Caprino G (1990) Role of lymphangiography and abdomino-pelvic CT in uterine tumors. Radiol Med (Torino) 79: 599-602
17. Matsukuma K, Tsukamoto N, Matsuyama T, Ono M, Nakano H (1989) Preoperative CT study of lymph nodes in cervical cancer - its correlation with histological findings. Gynecol Oncol 33: 168-171
18. Milestone BN, Schnall MD, Lenkinski RE, Kressel HY (1991) Cervical carcinoma: MR imaging with an endorectal surface coil. Radiology 180: 91-95
19. Mizoe J (1990) Analysis of the dose-volume histogram in uterine cervical cancer by diagnostic CT. Strahienther Onkol 166: 279-284
20. Moore DH, Dotters DJ, Fowler WC Jr (1992) Computed tomography: does it really improve the treatment of cervical carcinoma? Am J Obstet Gynecol 167: 768-721
21. Parker LA, Mc Phail AH, Yankaskas BC, Mauro MA (1990) Computed tomography in the evaluation of clinical stage IB carcinoma of the cervix. Gynecol Oncol 37: 332-334
22. Raber G,Potzschke B (1989) The status of computerized tomography in the diagnosis of primary cervix cancer. Geburshilfe Frauenheilkd 49: 17-23
23. Russel AH, Walter JP, Anderson MW, Zukowski CL (1992) Sagittal magnetic resonance imaging in the design of lateral radiation treatment portals for patients with locally advanced squamous cancer of the cervix. Int J Radiat Oncol Biol Phys 23: 449-455
24. Santoni R, Bucciolini M, Chiostrini C, Cionini L, Renzi R (1991) Quantitative magnetic resonance imaging in cervical carcinoma: a report on 30 cases. Br J Radiol 64: 498-504
25. Schœppel SL, Ellis JH, La Vigne ML, Schea RA, Roberts JA (1992) Magnetic resonance imaging during intracavitary gynecologic brachytherapy. Int J Radiat Oncol Biol Phys 23: 169-174
26. Sironi S, Reloni C, Taccagni G, Del Maschio A (1991) Invasive cervical carcinoma: MR imaging after preoperative chimiotherapy. Radiol 180: 719-722
27. Sironi S, Reloni C, Taccagni G, Del Maschio A (1991) Carcinoma of the cervix: value of MR imaging in detecting parametrial involvement. AJR 156: 753-756
28. Sironi S, Zanello A, Rodighiero MG, Vanzulli A, Taccagni GL, Belloni C, Del Maschio A (1991) Invasive carcinoma of the cervix uteri (Stage IB-IIB) Comparaison of CT an MR for the assessment of the parametrium. Radiol Med (Torino) 81: 671-677
29. Sœters RP, Beningfield SJ, Dehaeck K, Levin W, Bloch B (1991) The value of magnetic resonance imaging in patients with carcinoma of the cervix (a pilot study). Eur J Surg Oncol 17: 119-124
30. Soyer P, Rigaud C, Masselot J, Michel G (1991) Evaluation of the role of MRI at 1.5 T in the staging of the initial extension of cancer of the uterine cervix. J Belge Radiol 74: 85-90.
31. Smith FW, Cherryman GR, Bayliss AP, Fullerton WT, Law AN, Robertson EM, Weir J, Donald RT, Mallard JR (1989) A comparative study of the accuracy of ultrasound, X-ray CT and low field MRI in the demonstration of cervical and tlterine malignancy. Magn Reson Imaging 7: 677-679
32. Yamada E (1991) Role of X-ray computed tomography in the evaluation of prognosis of cervical carcinoma. Nippon Sanka Fujinka Gakkai Zasshi 43: 205-212
33. Yamashita Y, Takahashi M, Sanada T, Miyazaki K, Okamura H (1992) Carcinoma of the cervix: dynamic MR imaging. Radiology 182: 643-648
34. Yokoyama T, Hiura M, Myoga H, Yorishima M, Tanaka M, Chiba T, Inatsuki S (1990) Computed tomography for the assessment of pelvic lymph node metastasis in cases of uterine cervical carcinoma. Gan No Rinsho 36: 495-498
35. Youosem DM, Magid D, Scott WW Jr, Fishman E K (1989) Treated invasive cervical carcinoma. Utility of computed tomography in distinguishing between skeletal metastases and radiation necrosis. Clin Imaging 13: 147-153
36. Zweizig S, Schlaerth JB, Boswell WD Jr (1991) Computed tomography of lymphogranuloma venereum mimicking cervical cancer. Comput Med Imaging Graph 15: 97-100

CHAPTER 34

Cancer of the endometrium

Clinicians
D. Dargent, Y. Darbois, D. Nizri, G. Lefebvre, J.-V. Chantelard, A. Wacrenier, H. Charreyre, E. Vuillemin, D. Khayat

Radiologists
D. Buthiau, N. Perrot

Radiological imaging represents a precious aid to the clinicians in the assessment of endometrial cancer. The positive diagnosis is clinical and histological. However, imaging could play an important role in the early detection or even screening in the future. On the other hand, it is currently only in the position to stage the cancer prior to commencing treatment.

Positive diagnosis; The importance of early detection [4, 6]

Adenocarcinoma of the endometrium is a cancer with a low mortality rate (it is only responsible for 13% of cancer deaths in this region whereas it represents nearly a half of the tumors). Many tumors are detected at autopsy. However, the prognosis depends on the stage of the disease. The tumor is frequently diagnosed at stage I (76%).

Over many years, the only methods of detection have been cytology and hysterography. The first is neither sensitive nor specific. The second offers a good sensitivity but has a clearly inadequate specificity.

Hysteroscopy nowadays has replaced these two methods. It can detect lesions at an early stage with a high reliability and guide biopsy sampling. However, it is difficult to propose it as a mass screening technique; it cannot be considered as a diagnostic method either for asymptomatic women or for women at risk (previous family history, obesity, diabetes). Endovaginal ultrasound on the other hand could be proposed. Its sensitivity is excellent, but its specificity has yet to be determined, particularly for the differentiation between hyperplasia and carcinoma. It is probable that this technique will progress further due to the improvements in ultrasound machines and probes resulting in a greater diagnostic accuracy. Nowadays, the ultrasound examination is completed by color doppler ultrasound which could provide complementary information to conventional transvaginal ultrasound in postmenopausal patients.

Diagnosis of spread [4, 6]

Tumor spread occurs in two stages:
- initially, there is infiltration of the myometrium, isthmus and uterine cervix inferiorly;
- subsequently, in a fashion similar to cervical cancer, invasion extends into the soft tissues of the pelvis with involvement of the parametrium, bladder and then rectum.

The treatment of endometrial cancer still limited to the uterus is essentially surgical. A hysterectomy with adnexectomy is performed during which the degree of spread is assessed with, if required, lymph node sampling. Medical imaging does have a role preoperatively to judge the involvement of the myometrium and uterus which determines the therapeutic approach (and assess uterine volume if a transvaginal surgical approach is being considered). It also contributes to the assessment of the pelvic and lumbo-aortic lymph nodes which are involved in 35% of the high grade stage I lesions.

When surgery is impossible, radiotherapy treatment is indicated. In this case, imaging will be necessary to plan the treatment and to monitor its efficacy.

Myometrial invasion

Myometrial involvement is sometimes difficult to evaluate on the operative specimen. In fact, adenocarcinoma infiltrates the myometrium in a variable fashion. It is judged, therefore, by locating the area where the healthy myometrium is thinnest. It should be known that the greater the depth of myometrial invasion, the greater the risk of distance metastases, particularly if there is involvement of the superficial third due to the presence of a large venous network at this level.

Endovaginal ultrasound and MRI are very accurate for assessing depth of infiltration, and the size of the uterine cavity which would seem to correlate with the risk of pelvic lymph node spread.

Spread to the uterine cervix

It is extremely important to demonstrate the involvement of the internal os of the cervix. In fact, this alters the staging of the tumor from T1 to T2. Hysteroscopy is the method of choice for making this diagnosis although it is sometimes difficult due to the presence of blood and a theoretical risk of tumor migration. The use of a flexible hysteroscope overcomes the difficulty resulting from deformity of the uterine cavity (e.g. submucosal myoma). However, it will only demonstrate mucosal infiltrations which are not the most significant in terms of prognosis. The most serious infiltrations are submucosal, and these can only be demonstrated by ultrasound and MRI.

The symptoms of cancers of the endometrium are very variable. In the premenopausal patient, menorrhagia and metrorrhagia are the usual symptoms. Following the menopause, the cancer classically results in abnormal discharges, usually metrorrhagia. Rarely it results in hydrorrhoea or sero-hemorrhagic discharges. Clinical examination demonstrates little. It will confirm the intra-uterine origin of the discharge if it is performed in the context of metrorrhagia. Internal pelvic examination often demonstrates a uterus of abnormal size for the age of the patient. A myomatous uterus can give this appearance, particularly prior to the menopause.

At the initial consultation, samples are taken at the level of the cervix and intra-uterine cavity, either for cytological examination (endocyte, cytobrush) or histological examination (microbiopsy using Cornier's instrument). However, this technique is not completely reliable, and in the case of a negative result a transvaginal ultrasound is required at the time of which hysteroscopy with biopsy is performed. CT and MRI are only indicated as third line investigations for staging and determination of the prognosis.

Applications of CT and MRI [4, 6]

Conventional radiography

This is primarily hysterography which is requested less and less commonly. Typically it demonstrates irregularities of the outline of the uterine cavity with the presence of notches, lacunae, tufts or cloud-like filling defects, and heterogeneous filling of the uterine cavity indicating surface irregularities due to a lesion situated on one of the surfaces. It is also possible to combine the technique with an intravascular injection.

In the vegetative forms, there is the appearance of a lacuna with irregular ragged outlines of boggy consistency.

In the infiltrative forms, the diagnosis is more difficult. An irregular serrated spiculated appearance of one of the surfaces of the uterine cavity may be seen.

Ultrasound

Only transvaginal ultrasound can provide images of adequate quality. This demonstrates hypertrophy of the endometrium. It should be remembered that in many cases there is no ultrasonic difference between simple hyperplasia and a cancer. Thickening of the endometrium, particularly in a postmenopausal patient, can be considered as highly suspicious and requires further investigations (hysteroscopy). In some cases the diagnosis may be more obvious with an irregular hyperplasia, loss of the junctional zone between the endometrium and myometrium with an indistinct and irregular outline of the endometrium suggestive of myometrial invasion. This can be measured and related to the overall thickness of the uterus. This technique needs to become more specific although it has an excellent sensitivity. In effect, if a

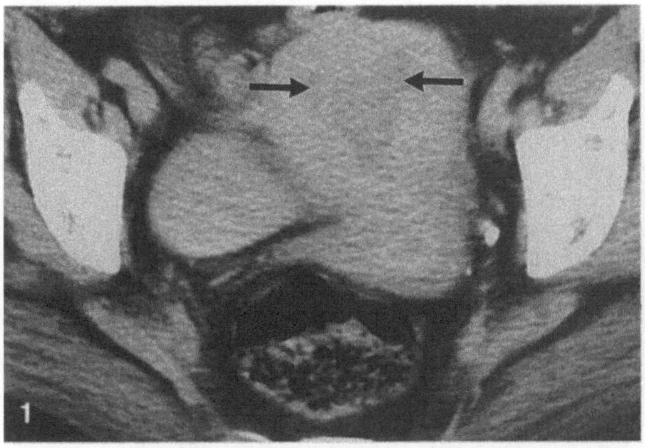

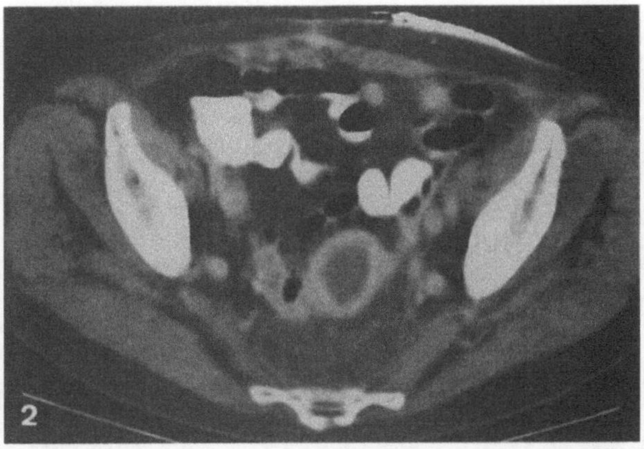

Fig. 34.1. Cancer of the endometrium on an axial post-contrast CT section: there is a hypodense area within the uterine cavity (partially anteflexed and anteverted uterus). The thickness of the endometrium on this section reaches 23 mm *(arrows)*. There is a reduction in the myometrial thickness, particularly clear at the level of the uterine fundus, which is an indirect sign of myometrial spread, but no evidence of deformity of the uterine outline, asymmetry, or abnormal enhancement is noted. No evidence of any suspicious cervical hypodensity

Fig. 34.2. Cancer of the body of the uterus on axial post-contrast CT: there is marked intra-uterine hypodensity with clear thinning of the myometrium due to diffuse myometrial spread, confirmed surgically

thin atrophic non-measurable mucosa is demonstrated on endovaginal ultrasound in a post menopausal patient, the risk of missing an endometrial cancer is virtually nil.

CT

CT has no value in making the diagnosis and is non-specific. However, it is still indicated for the assessment of the abdomino-pelvic lymph node chains, and the liver. It is also indicated following treatment, to monitor progress following radiotherapy and to detect recurrent disease provided that the initial base line examination is performed at least 4 to 6 months after the completion of all treatment.

MRI

The specificity of MRI is clearly superior to CT; it is able to accurately measure the endometrial thickness. However, MRI is rarely requested for this purpose in practice for two main reasons: firstly ultrasound, and particularly transvaginal ultrasound, is more accurate for this purpose; secondly there is limited access to the examination.

It should also be noted that MRI, like ultrasound, cannot differentiate hyperplasia of the endometrium from cancer.

However, MRI seems to be the best technique for assessing the depth of spread into the myometrium and cervix, as well as monitoring progress on treatment, particularly for those cases in whom surgery has not been performed. Finally, MRI with ultrasound should be performed to detect recurrence.

Signs [6]

CT

The lesion

This appears as a hypodense area situated within the uterine cavity (figs 34.1 & 34.2) and is strongly enhanced following contrast injection. There may be dilatation of the uterus with or without intracavity fluid retention in cases of endocervical obstruction. This appearance is difficult to differentiate from a small hemorrhagic effusion which is common in post-menopausal women not on hormone replacement treatment.

Myometrial spread

This appears as abnormal enhancement corresponding to intramyometrial spread of the endometrial cancer.

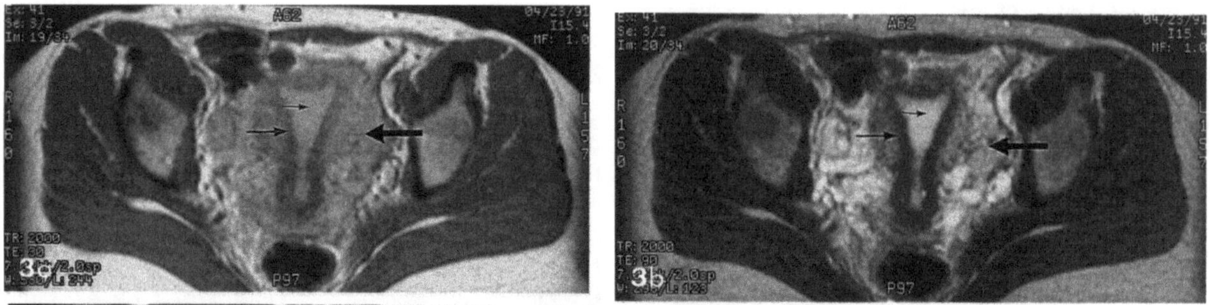

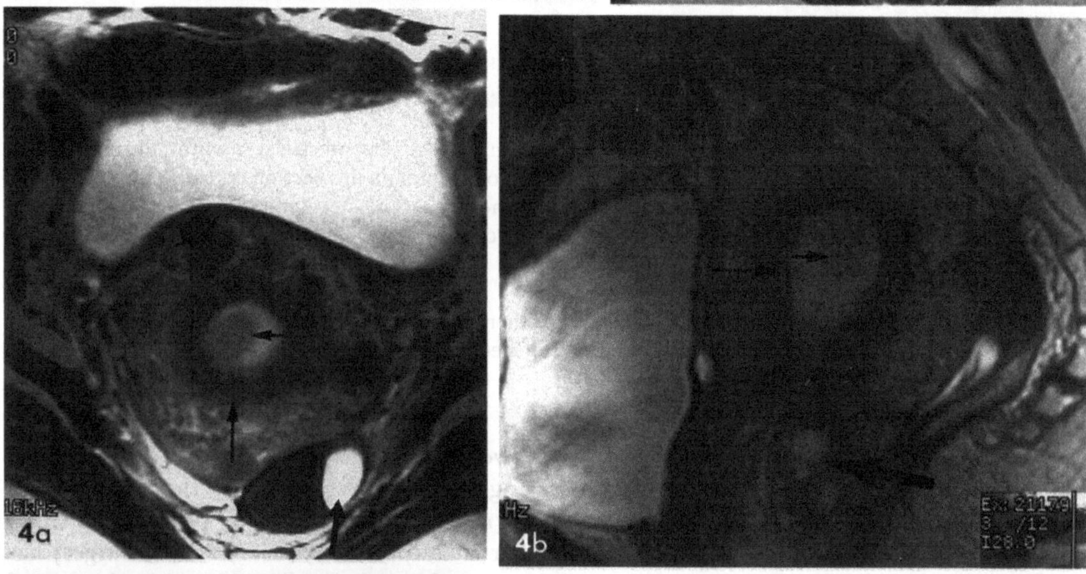

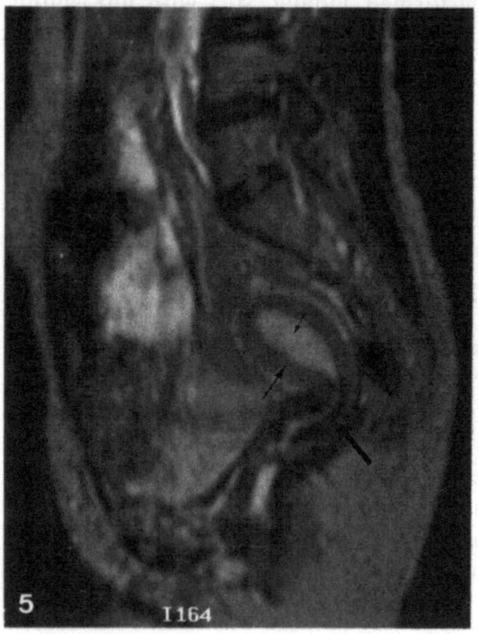

Fig. 34.3 a, b. Cancer of the endometrium on axial MRI proton density (**a**) and T2 (**b**). There is thickening of the endometrium (15 mm) within the uterine cavity without heterogeneity which may indicate the presence of retained debris or intracavity blood. The signal intensity is close to that of the normal endometrium. There is preservation of the physiological junctional zone located on the deep surface of the myometrium; *small arrow*: cancer of the endometrium; *medium arrow*: junctional zone; *large arrow*: myometrium. Note that the cervix is of physiological low signal intensity without the break of this hypointensity or any sign of infiltration. Note the enlargement of the uterine volume

Fig. 34.4 a, b. Cancer of the endometrium on MRI heavily T2-weighted axial (**a**) and sagittal images (**b**): there is definite thickening of the endometrium with a heterogeneous area of low signal intensity within the uterine cavity corresponding to the tumor itself *(small arrow)*. Preservation of the junctional zone *(medium arrow)*. The myometrium contains hypointensites corresponding to small calcified myomas (**a** *arrowhead*). Note the presence of Nabothian cysts within the cervix (**b** *large arrow*), and a small dermoid cyst of the left ovary in a retro-uterine position predominantly of lipid composition (**a** *large arrow*) (courtesy of General Electric)

Fig. 34.5. Carcinoma of the endometrium on sagittal T2-weighted image: note the enlargement of the endometrial cavity of identical signal intensity to the myometrium, this appearance being undifferentiable from simple hyperplasia or a submucosal polyp. The lesion *(small arrow)* is not associated with any disruption of the junctional zone *(medium arrow)*, and therefore there is no myometrial spread (confirmed surgically). Note the preservation of the physiological hypointensity of the cervix and the absence of any sign of cervical spread *(large arrow)*

There may be deformity of the uterine outline resulting in asymmetry. A reduction in the thickness of the myometrium, either localized or diffuse, may also be seen (fig. 34.2).

Cervical spread

Cervical spread is seen as an increase in the volume of the cervix with hypodensity of the stroma.

Ovarian spread

This is rare. The appearances are variable with both solid and liquid elements, generally heterogeneous, located in the adnexa. This appearance is very suggestive in a postmenopausal patient.

MRI

The lesion

The tumor appears hyperintense on T2-weighted imaging and its signal intensity is close to that of the normal endometrium (figs 34.3 & 34.5).

There is often a reduction in signal intensity on T2-weighted imaging relative to the normal endometrium (fig. 34.4).

The central endo-uterine zone can be measured and is considered to be suspicious if the thickness is more than 9 mm in a premenopausal woman and 5 mm in a postmenopausal woman not on hormone replacement therapy (figs 34.3-34.5).

The injection of a contrast agent may improve the demonstration of tumor infiltration and better differentiate the tumor from the intracavity debris, particularly from hemorrhagic material.

Myometrial spread (figs 34.3-34.7)

The most suggestive sign of myometrial invasion is disruption of the junctional zone (figs 34.3-34.7) (hypointense band on T1- and T2-weighted imaging located in the deep part of the myometrium). When present, this sign has a high diagnostic value. However, the junctional zone is not always visualized in postmenopausal women.

Sironi [18] gives a sensitivity and specificity of 74% for MRI in the appreciation of myometrial spread, and

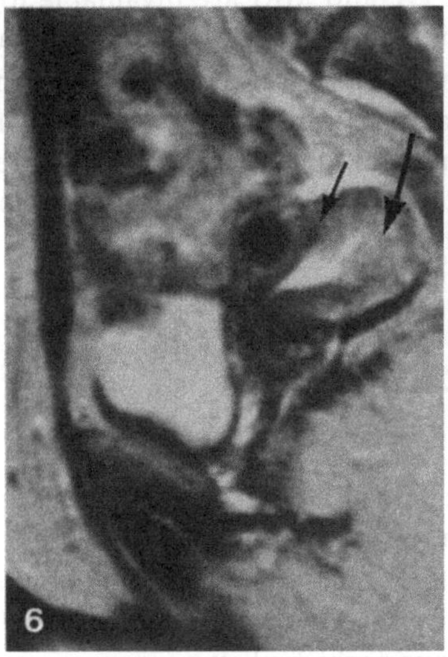

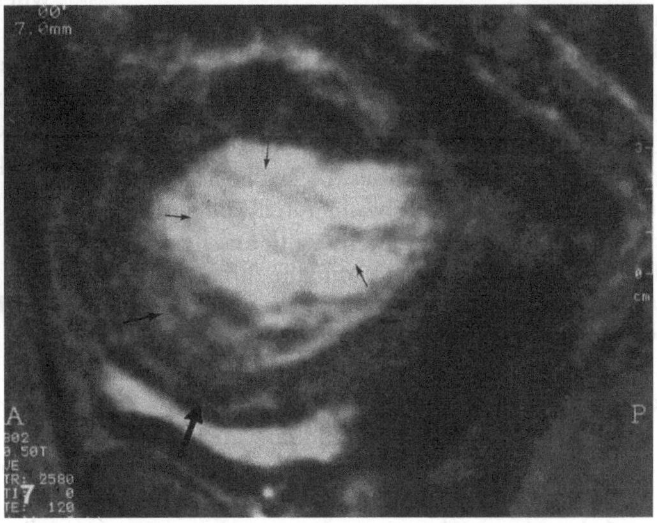

Fig. 34.6. Carcinoma of the endometrium with myometrial invasion on sagittal T2 MRI: note a disruption of the junctional zone in the region of the uterine fundus (retroverted uterus), this interruption *(small arrow)* occurring adjacent to the heterogeneous hyperintensity of the tumor in the uterine fundus *(medium arrow)*. Note also the presence of a rounded hypointensity in the anterior part, corresponding to a calcified myoma (image courtesy of Dr. Buthiau D (1993) Imagerie clinique en gynécologie. Vigot)

Fig. 34.7. Large endometrial carcinoma on sagittal T2 MRI: the lesion is heterogeneous made up of a polymorphic hyperintense region *(small arrow)* and an area isointense to the myometrium, itself heterogeneous *(medium arrow)* and a maximum thickness of 5 cm. This lesion is causing enlargement of the uterine volume. It is associated with definite narrowing of the myometrium inferiorly *(large arrow)* as well as the hypointense junctional zone which is irregularly and intermittently disrupted in the same area. Note the marked mass effect on the dome of the bladder a sensitivity of 88% with a specificity of 85% for the appreciation of deep myometrial spread (fig. 34.7). The diagnostic errors of MRI are due, in the majority of cases, to an overestimation of the depth of spread.

The injection of a contrast agent can improve the diagnostic accuracy.

The performance of the so-called dynamic sequences with sequential acquisitions following the injection of contrast further improves the visualization of the endometrial lesion.

Invasion of the endocervix (figs 34.3 & 34.5)

This manifests as an enlargement of the cervix with a heterogeneous appearance of the endocervical mucosa. Loss of the physiological low signal appearance of the cervix may be demonstrated, its signal intensity becoming similar to that of the tumor.

Patient management in practice [6]

Role of imaging in the diagnosis

In the postmenopausal patient, the presence of leucorrhoea, an abnormal hormonal status, metrorrhagia or a paradoxically enlarged uterus for the age and particularly if there are any risk factors (hypertension, diabetes, obesity), hysteroscopy is the complementary investigation which provides the diagnosis. However, endovaginal ultrasound should initially be performed in order to screen out patients with an endometrial thickness of less than the 5 mm, the threshold below which the risk of uterine cancer is almost nil, thus avoiding hysteroscopy.

For the thickness above 5 mm hysteroscopy should routinely be performed with directed biopsy.

Hysterosalpingography should nowadays be abandoned and replaced by a combination of endovaginal ultrasound and hysteroscopy. It should be remembered that the results of cytology are improved by using the aspiration technique which is very reliable if the cavity is regular and of average size.

Role of imaging in treatment management

The role of imaging is limited for the stage I cancers which represent 8 out of 10 cases in France. In fact, the treatment is abdominal hysterectomy or, in certain cases, laparoscopic or transvaginal hysterectomy. At the time of surgery, an indication for further complementary surgery may be found depending on the presence of parametrial or lymph node invasion. Histological assessment of the operative specimen gives the degree of myometrial and cervical invasion.

Medical imaging can detect extra-uterine spread, particularly hepatic or pulmonary.

However, not all patients presenting with a stage I endometrial carcinoma are operative candidates. In fact, obesity, the age of the patient or associated cardiac or respiratory problems can make surgery more dangerous or impossible. In these cases, vaginal hysterectomy is indicated if the volume and mobility of the uterus allow it. This method has the disadvantage of not being able to assess spread, particularly peritoneal, adnexal, nodal or hepatic metastases (not relevant for stage I disease).

The demonstration of extra-uterine spread, particularly on CT for the lymph nodes (see Chapter 33: Cancer of the cervix, section: Lymph node invasion), and on MRI for infiltration of the myometrium and cervix, is extremely valuable and will contraindicate vaginal hysterectomy in these patients in whom radiotherapy treatment would be more appropriate.

The same applies for stages II, III and IV cancers where CT and MRI are invaluable for radiotherapy planning and intracavity radium therapy.

Finally CT and MRI, probably preceded by an endovaginal ultrasound, are essential for the follow-up of patients and the detection of pelvic recurrences (see Chapter 33: Cancer of the cervix, section; Diagnosis of recurrence) (fig 34.8).

Conclusion [6]

Medical imaging for cancer of the endometrium has a role in the early detection and staging of disease.

Hysterosalpingography should be abandoned in this clinical context. It should be replaced by transvaginal ultrasound which plays an increasing role in the early diagnosis. It may perhaps be useful as a screening procedure in the future.

Ultrasound can be valuable in the staging, particularly for assessing the depth of myometrial invasion. It should be remembered that this examination is both operator and machine dependent.

Hysteroscopy is the key examination for making the positive diagnosis, particularly for the small lesions missed by ultrasound. During the procedure, directed biopsies can be performed.

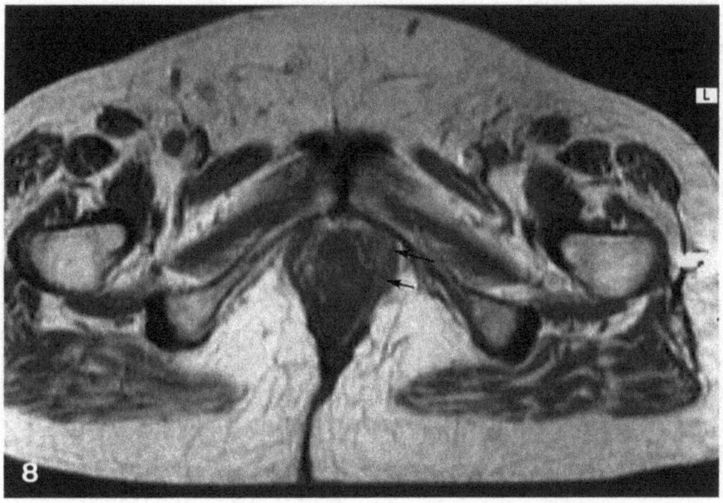

Fig. 34.8. Focal recurrence of carcinoma of the endometrium, 18 months following treatment: there is asymmetry of the levator ani muscle on the left *(arrows)* close to the urogenital diaphragm in the lower pelvis corresponding to an infiltrative recurrence with subtle involvement of the most anterior and medial part of the left inferior ischiorectal space

For staging, hysteroscopy is unable to appreciate infiltration into the myometrium. However, it can assess involvement of the isthmus and cervix, but only in a mucosal infiltration.

The CT examination demonstrates lymph node involvement and distant metastatic spread. It helps to plan the radiotherapy treatment and monitor the progress of the patient.

Nowadays, MRI is the best examination for assessing tumor volume and depth of spread into the myometrium. In cases treated by radiotherapy or adjuvant therapy it is able to monitor the treatment along with CT. It is also suggested, in combination with CT, in the follow-up after surgery for the detection of recurrences. According to D. Dargent [7], "Transvaginal ultrasound and MRI nowadays define with great accuracy the extent of endometrial cancers and particularly the degree of myometrial infiltration. However, as cancer of the endometrium is really a "surgical cancer", is it really necessary to spend money requesting examinations preoperatively when the operation itself provides much more information ? The answer is yes, and the reason for this is as follows: one no longer performs the same operation today for stage IA IB tumors (no infiltration or limited infiltration of the myometrium), stage IC tumors (less than 50% thickness of the myometrium) or stage II and III tumors" (table 34.1).

Table 34.1. Staging of endometrial cancers (D Dargent [7])

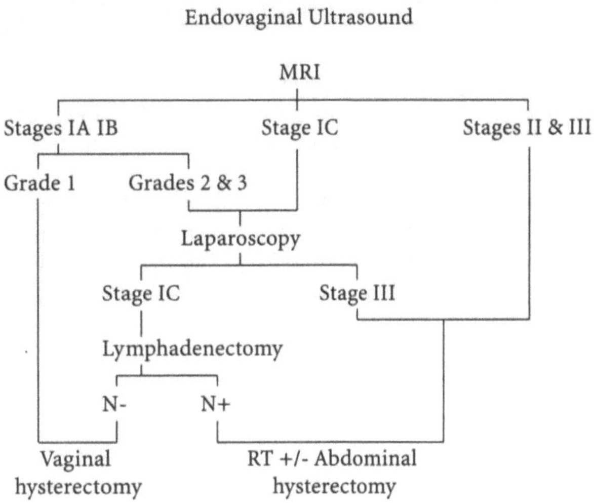

References

1. Al Awani S, Assem M, Belal A, Adel-Hamid H (1991) Magnetic resonance imaging (MRI) of abnormal uterine masses. J Belge Radiol 74: 19-24
2. Belloni C, Vigano R, Del Maschio A, Sironi S, Taccagni GL, Vignali M (1990) Magnetic resonance imaging in endometrial carcinoma staging. Gynecol Oncol 37: 172-177
3. Brown JJ, Thurnher S, Hricak H (1990) MR imaging of the uterus: low-signal-intensity abnormalities of the endometrium and endometrial cavity. Magn Reson Imaging 8: 309-313
4. Buthiau D, et coll (1992) TDM et IRM en gynécologie pelvienne. In: Buthiau D, Piette JC, Khayat D, Nizri D (eds) TDM et IRM cliniques: Abdomen-pelvis. Frison Roche, Paris, pp 266-291
5. Chen SS, Rumancik WN, Spiegel G (1990) Magnetic resonance imaging in stage I endometrial carcinoma. Obstet Gynecol 75: 274-277

6. Dargent D, et al (1993) Cancer de l'Endomètre. In: Buthiau D, Dargent D (eds) Imagerie clinique en gynécologie. Vigot, Paris, pp 219-234
7. Dargent D (nov 1993) Cancers utérins, I'extension en image. 21èmes journées de fertilité et orthogénie (Cohen J) Paris
8. Harrill CD, Kopecky KK, Weaver SR, Sutton GP (1990) Magnetic resonance imaging in the preoperative assessment of clinical stage I endometrial carcinoma. Comput Med Imaging Graph 14: 191-195
9. Hirai Y, Kaku S, Teshima H, Chen JT, Hamada T, Fujimoto I, Yamauchi K, Mine H, Hasumi K, Masubuchi K (1989? Use of angio computed tomography to evaluate extent of endometrial carcinoma. Gynocol Oncol 33: 372-375
10. Hricak H (1991) Cancer of the uterus: the value of MRI pre- and post-irradiation. Int J Radiat Oncol Biol Phys 21: 1089-1094
11. Hricak H, Hamm B, Semelka RC, Cann CE, Nauert T, Secaf E, Stern JL, Wolf KJ (1991) Carcinoma of the uterus: use of gadopentetate dimeglumine in MR imaging. Radiology 181: 95-106
12. Hricak H, Rubinstein LV, Gherman GM, Karstaedt N (1991) MR imaging evaluation of endometrial carcinoma: results of an NCI cooperative study. Radiology 179: 829-832
13. Lien HH, Blomlie V, Trope C, Kaern J, Abeler VM (1991) Cancer of the endometrium: value of MR imaging in determining depth of invasion into the myometrium. Am J Roentgenol 157: 1221-1223
14. La Fianza A, Dore R, Di Giulio G, Alerci M, Di Maggio EM, Franchi M, Donadello N, Campani R (1990) Lymph node metastasis of carcinoma of the cervix uteri. Role of Iymphography and computerized tomography. Radiol Med (Torino) 80: 486-491
15. Mittl RL Jr, Yeh IT, Kressel HY (1991) High-signal intensity rim surrounding uterine leiomyomas on MR images: pathologic correlation. Radiology 180: 81-83
16. Posniak HV, Olson MC, Dudiak CM, Castelli MJ, Dolan J, Wisniewski RA, Isaacs JH, Sharma SK, Bychkov V (1990) MR imaging of uterine carcinoma: correlation with clinical and pathologic findings. Radiographics 10: 15-27
17. Sironi S, Colombo E, Villa G, Taccagni G, Belloni C, Garancini P, Del Maschio A (1992) Myometrial invasion by endometrial carcinoma: assessment with plain and gadolinium - enhanced MR imaging. Radiol 185: 207-212
18. Sironi S, Taccagni G, Garancini P, Belloni C, Del Maschio A (1992) Myometrial invasion by endometrial carcinoma: assessment by MR imaging. Arn J Roentgenol 158: 565-569
19. Taxt T, Lundervold A, Fuglaas B, Lien H, Abeler V (1992) Analysis of uterine corpus tumors in magnetic resonance imaging. Magn Reson Med 23: 55-76
20. Trerotola SO, Fishman EK, Kuhlman J (1989) Computed tomography of uterine sarcomas. Clin Imaging 13: 208-211
21. Varpula M, Komu M, Klemi P (1992) Magnetic resonance imaging of the uterus at an ultra low (0.02 T) magnetic field. Magnon Res Imaging 10: 195-205
22. Weinrerb JC, Barkoff ND, Megibow A, Demopoulos R (1990) The value of MR imaging in distinguishing leiomyomas from other solid pelvic masses when sonography is indeterminate. Am J Roentgenol 154: 295-299
23. Yamashita Y, Harada M, Sawada T, Takahashi M, Miyazaki K, Okamura H (1993) Normal uterus and FIGO stage I endometrial carcinoma: dynamic gadolinium-enhanced MR imaging. Radiology 186: 495-501

CHAPTER 35

Cancer of the ovary

Clinicians
M. Marty, E.-Ch. Antoine, O. Rixe, J. Dauplat, A. Zamora, D. Nizri, J.-V. Chantelard, E. Vuillemin, M. Weil, C. Courtieu, D. Khayat

Radiologists
D. Buthiau, J.-P. Rouanet, A. Maubon, L. Lemaître

Diagnosis of ovarian cancers [13]

Applications of CT and MRI [13]

Despite the significant progress in imaging, particularly endoluminal ultrasound for the examination of the pelvis, and CT for the examination of the abdomen, the diagnosis of cancer of the ovary is still usually made at a late stage with a resultant poor prognosis. However, some improvements in treatments have recently been accomplished. These include the introduction of the platinum derivatives and even more recently several other promising drugs (Taxanes...). There have also been advances in surgery which is essentially the first stage of the treatment.

Early detection of cancers poses different problems depending on the age of the patient. In young women, the differential diagnosis with a possible benign tumor (functional cyst, dermoid cyst...) emphasizes the role of imaging. In post-menopausal women, any cystic or soft tissue density adnexal lesion must be considered as suspicious malignancy and requires laparotomy.

The low incidence and prevalence rates of malignant epithelial tumors of the ovary (frequency: 14/100,000 population; 5% of cancer deaths in women) rules out the possibility of any mass screening program in the absence of a definite target population and reliable screening method. The average age is 60 years, the frequency on the increase.

The value of early diagnosis is best illustrated by the 5 year survival rates: 70% for stage I, 4 to 5% for stages III and IV.

Ovarian adenocarcinomas are characterized by a frequently long doubling time and a low proportion of cells in phase S. The duration of the cell cycle and the coefficient of cellular loss are normal. One would therefore assume that it would take at least 2 to 4 years for a tumor to reach a size of 1 cm diameter. The correlation between the size of the ovarian tumor and the prognosis is much less clear than that for other tumors, and this is probably due to the fact of direct "shedding" of cells. However, although the doubling time is not particularly short, the spread to the pelvic viscera (stage II) and peritoneum (stage III) can occur at an early stage due to the release of viable cells from the surface of the ovary. The diagnosis of these lesions is often made late.

It is certain that the possibility of an early diagnosis will depend on the therapeutic aims.

Despite the ever increasing improvements in imaging, it remains an illusion to hope that it will be able to determine the histological nature of ovarian lesions. This is predominantly due to the huge anatomoclinical and histological variety of ovarian tumors. Imaging can only be more specific for the dermoid cyst or fibroma. Although discussion centers on the attempts at the tissue characterization of ovarian tumors, imaging should perhaps restrict itself to much more fundamental questions and in particular the determination of the organ of origin of a large pelvic mass, especially distinguishing between an ovarian or uterine mass.

It also seems to be more realistic and useful to try and improve image interpretation to obtain a greater specificity in the discrimination between a benign and

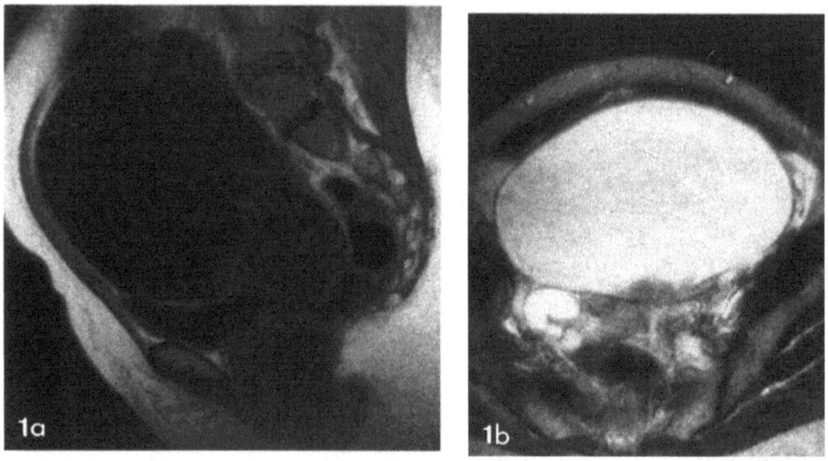

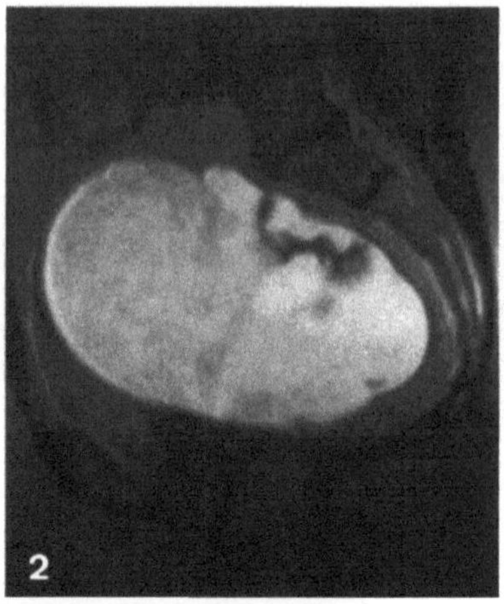

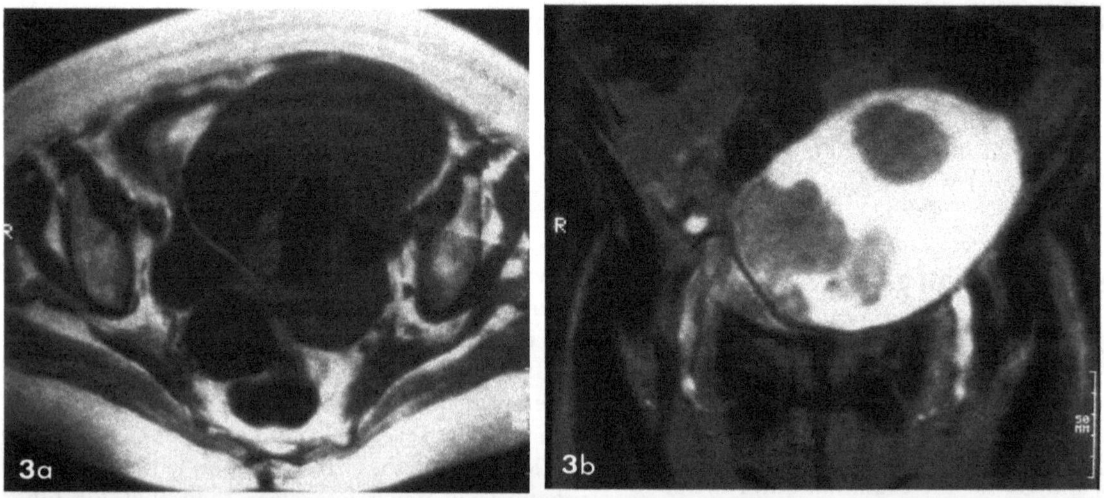

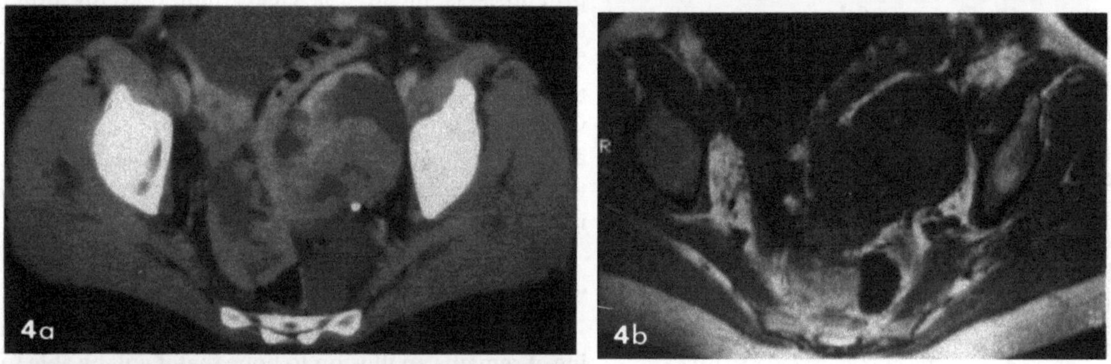

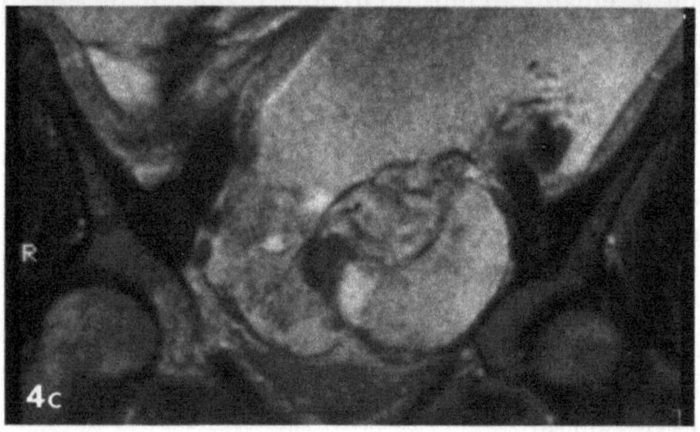

Fig. 35.1. Pelvic MRI: **a** sagittal T1-weighted sequence; **b** transverse axial T2-weighted sequence. Borderline serous tumor of the left ovary. The cyst content is homogeneous fluid with vegetations in its inferior portion

Fig. 35.2. Pelvic MRI, sagittal T2-weighted image. Serous cystadenocarcinoma of the left ovary with marked heterogeneous soft tissue proliferation of the wall

Fig. 35.3. Pelvic MRI: **a** transverse axial T1-weighted image; **b** coronal T2-weighted image. Large bilateral heterogeneous serous cystadenocarcinoma with a very marked soft tissue component

Fig. 35.4. **a** Post-contrast transverse axial CT; **b** T1-weighted pelvic MRI in the transverse axial plane; **c** T2-weighted pelvic MRI in the coronal plane. Bilateral papillary serous cystadenocarcinoma of the ovaries with invasion of the sigmoid colon, peritoneal carcinomatosis and fluid in the pouch of Douglas malignant tumor. In fact, this is the only diagnostic feature that has a critical impact on the choice of surgery and subsequent therapeutic approach.

Ultrasound (especially endovaginal ultrasound) and MRI currently seem to represent the most accurate imaging techniques for analyzing the macroscopic anatomy, as we will describe below.

Specific CT and MRI features of the different types of ovarian tumors [13]

The histopathological classification of ovarian tumors (table 35.1) is based on the histo-embryonic structure of the ovary which comprises of:
- the germinal cells,
- the sex cords and mesenchymal stroma,
- the celomic epithelium.

The normal adult ovary is composed of a cellular medulla (analogous to the Leydig cells) and glandular elements of indeterminate origin ("rete ovari"). The cortical cellular zone includes the theca granulosa.

The term borderline tumor (fig. 35.1) is a response to the concept of attenuated malignancy and is associated with a generally favorable prognosis even in the presence of advanced anatomo-clinical spread. It includes tumors presenting with histological characteristics identical to adenocarcinomas but differentiated from them by the absence of stromal invasion. Conversely, the presence of mitotic activity (although low), and nuclear atypia (also few in number) differentiate borderline tumors from the benign tumors. Serous and mucinous forms are by far the commonest.

Table 35.1. OMS classification of ovarian tumors

1) Epithelial tumors
(derived from coelomic epithelium)
Serous tumors
Mucinous tumors
Endometrioid tumors
Clear cell tumors
Brenner tumors
Any tumor can be benign, malignant or "borderline" to a variable degree
2) Mesenchymal tumors (and sex cord)
Granulosa tumors
Fibrothecal group of tumors
Sertoli-Leyding tumors
Tumors of the sex cords with annular tubules
3) Germinal tumors
Teratomas
Dysgerminomas
Seminomas
Tumors of the endodermal sinus
Yolk sac tumor
Choriocarcinoma
Embryonic carcinoma

Epithelial tumors [13] (figs 35.1-35.6)

These constitute 85% of ovarian tumors (the serous papillary cystadenocarcinoma being the most typical form of ovarian carcinoma). Serous and mucinous tumors may be malignant, borderline (fig. 35.1) or benign. Clear cell and endometroid tumors are almost always malignant whereas the Brenner tumors are almost always benign. The undifferentiated lesions are rare (15% of cases).

Serous tumors (40% of epithelial tumors) (figs 35.1-35.4)

The age of occurrence is very variable. The histopathological diagnostic criteria are indicated in table 35.2. One third of these tumors are malignant.

In view of the fact that these tumors are usually initially cystic, ultrasound seems to be the examination of choice for the early diagnosis. The problems arise when there is an ovarian cyst with ultrasonic signs requiring further investigation, particularly a laparoscopic surgical exploration.

Many authors have been interested in the ultrasonic characterization of lesions. Granberg achieved an 82% sensitivity and 92% specificity in the differentiation of a benign and malignant lesion by endovaginal ultrasound. He attributes great significance to the multilocular nature of the cyst, its size and particularly to the endocystic vegetations (85% of tumors having more

Table 35.2. Serous tumors; 10 macroscopic signs (reproduced from Rouanet JP, et al (1994) In: Buthiau D, Dargent D (eds) Imagerie clinique en gynécologie. Vigot, Paris [13])

Benign	Malignant
Unilocular	Multilocular
Unilateral	Bilateral
Thin wall	Thick wall
Fine, mobile, linear septa	Thick, rigid septa
Harmonious orientation	Acute angulation
Liquid/solid ratio close to 1	Liquid/solid ratio low
Few or no vegetations	External or internal vegetations
Absent or linear calcifications	Large and irregular calcifications
Absence of necrosis	Necrosis within the solid zone
	Ascites

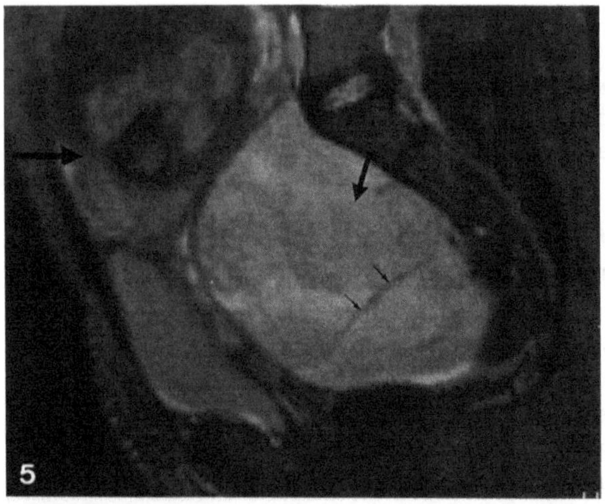

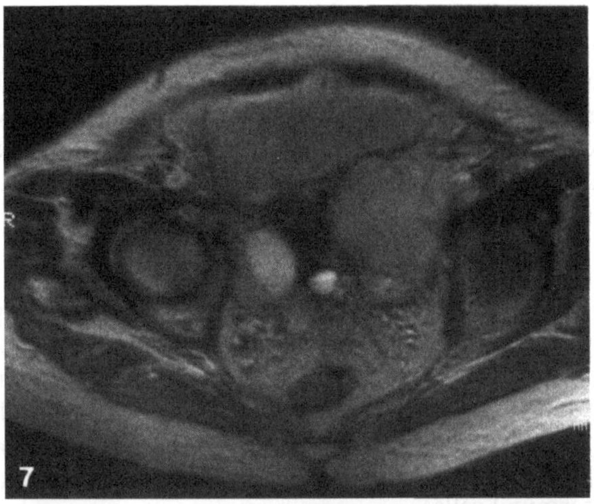

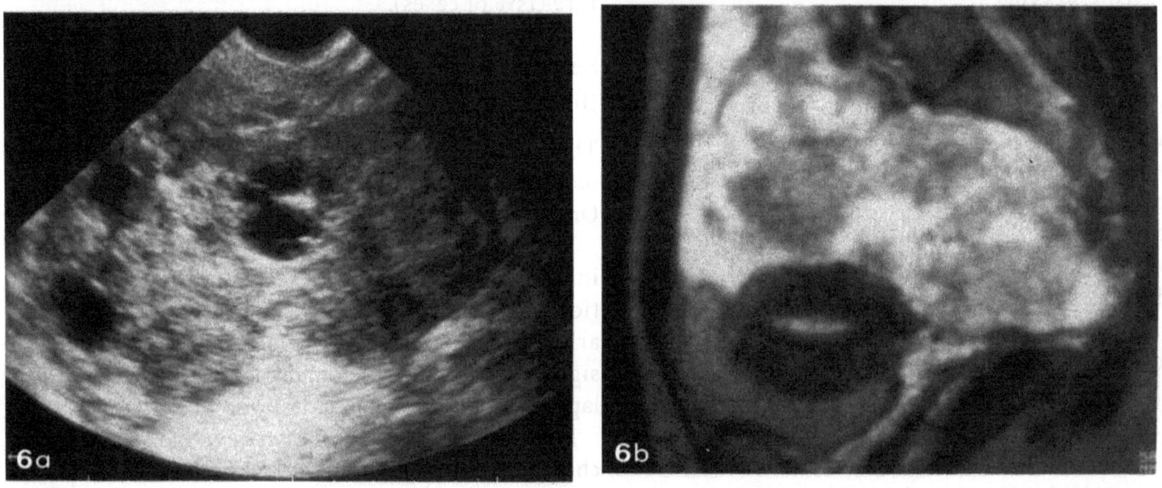

Fig. 35.5. T2-weighted sagittal MRI: mucinous cystadenocarcinoma diagnosed during pregnancy: the fetus *(large arrow)* is displaced by a centropelvic mass *(medium arrow)* containing multiple septa *(small arrows)* more or less grouped together and in the form of a honeycomb

Fig. 35.6. a Suprapubic ultrasound in the transverse axial plane; **b** T2-weighted pelvic MRI in the sagittal plane. Bilateral anaplastic cancer of the ovary with invasion of the pelvic bowel loops

Fig. 35.7. T2-weighted pelvic MRI in the transverse axial plane. Kruckenberg tumor: bilateral ovarian metastases from a bowel adenocarcinoma: note the mucoid content of the fluid cyst on the right ovary

than 5 vegetations were found to be malignant). Sassone reports a specificity of 83% and a sensitivity of a 100% for ultrasound by taking into account the internal structure of the cyst, thickness of the cyst wall, the presence or absence of septa, and the echogenicity of the cyst contents. In a study by Rouanet et al [13], ultrasound achieved the best result by taking into account 10 macroscopic signs (table 35.2), with or without endovaginal scanning, followed by MRI and CT. Ultrasound is significantly superior for the demonstration of intracystic septa.

However, attention should be drawn to the results from a study by Meman which indicate that even a cyst demonstrating all the ultrasonic criteria of a benign lesion can represent a true ovarian cancer.

CT clearly demonstrates calcifications, the walls of the tumor, the proportion of cystic and solid content, and the development of endo- or exophytic lesions from the soft tissue compartment (fig. 35.4). With the exception of calcifications, MRI (figs 35.1-35.4) provides identical information to CT but gives a better assessment of the endolesional contents (purely serous, hemorrhagic...). Post-contrast CT and MRI (figs 35.1-35.4) can demonstrate the tumor vessels. This may also be possible using color doppler ultrasound.

Mucinous tumors (fig. 35.5)

These are the least common (20% of primary ovarian tumors), and approximately 20% are malignant. The cyst contents are frequently thicker than in the serous tumors. The lesions are often large, with a multilobulated outline containing areas with a beehive appearance (fig. 35.5). The macroscopic criteria differentiating between benign and malignant lesions are shown in table 35.3.

Endovaginal ultrasound and MRI primarily have the greatest capacity to assess all the differential macroscopic signs and are the investigations of choice in this pathology. The cyst content, however, may be relatively poorly appreciated ultrasonically in hemorrhagic case, but this is also the case for CT (densitometry is not reliable) and MRI. In the latter case, the intralesional signal intensity is often low but can be variable, particularly appearing more intense in the more mature cysts or those with a high glycoprotein or hemorrhagic content. The injection of contrast agent on CT or MRI may be useful for assessing the tumor vascularization.

Endometrioid tumors (see fig. 35.10)

These lesions are relatively rare (slightly less than 10% of ovarian tumors) and partly demonstrate the anatomo-macroscopic appearances of the differentiated endometrial cancers. They are associated with an endometrial cancer in 20% of cases and with endometriosis in more than 33% of cases.

On CT, there is a solid soft tissue lesion with only a limited fluid component apart. The exception is the specific form of adenoacanthoma which has a pseudoserous cystic appearance and a posterior oblique paraovarian localization mimicking an endometriotic cyst.

Table 35.3. Mucinous tumors: macroscopic signs [13]

Benign	Malignant
Unilocular	Multilocular
Thin wall	Thick wall
Septa in pockets	Thicker septa
Arciform relationship	Geometric at variable angles
Few papillae	Numerous papillae
Liquid/solid ratio close to 1	% Liquid/solid ratio low
Homogeneous fluid	Hemorrhagic fluid
Absence of necrosis	Necrosis in the solid areas

On MRI, the signal intensity may be close to that of the normal endometrium, namely hyperintense on T2- and even on T1-weighted imaging in the presence of hemorrhagic changes.

Brenner tumors

These lesions are rare (1% of ovarian tumors) and rarely malignant. In 25% of cases, they are associated with a mucinous or simple serous cyst.

CT demonstrates the small homogenous well defined soft tissue lesions which quite frequently contain fine microcalcifications. There may be a relative heterogeneity on MRI, hypointense on T1-weighted imaging and isointense to muscle on T2-weighted imaging.

"Clear cell" tumors (fig. 35.8)

These relatively rare lesions (slightly less than 5% of ovarian cancers) are presumed to be of Müllerian origin and are associated in a quarter of cases with endometriosis. They are malignant tumors appearing of soft tissue density on CT sometimes with discrete cystic components containing septa and broad based nodular vegetations. MRI also demonstrates these signs. The lesions appear and hypointense on T1-weighted imaging and relatively heterogeneous and hyperintense on T2-weighted imaging.

Tumors of the mesenchyme and sexual cords [13]

These represent little less than 5% of primary ovarian tumors.

Granulosa tumors

These estrogen secreting lesions are associated, in almost 50% of cases, with secondary endometrial hyperplasia.

On CT, these lesions are more or less rounded, bilobulated or reniform in shape with mixed fluid and soft tissue contents. The peripheral part is usually fluid, often containing hemorrhagic pockets, and the central zone is solid. The peripheral capsule can sometimes be demonstrated. Ultrasound also demonstrates well these peripheral pockets.

MRI is more sensitive than CT for the detection of hemorrhagic contents and the endometrial hyperplasia. The signal intensity of the lesion is that of soft tissue and fluid, usually hypointense on T2-weighted imaging but sometimes hyperintense, this being due to possible intracellular lipid content.

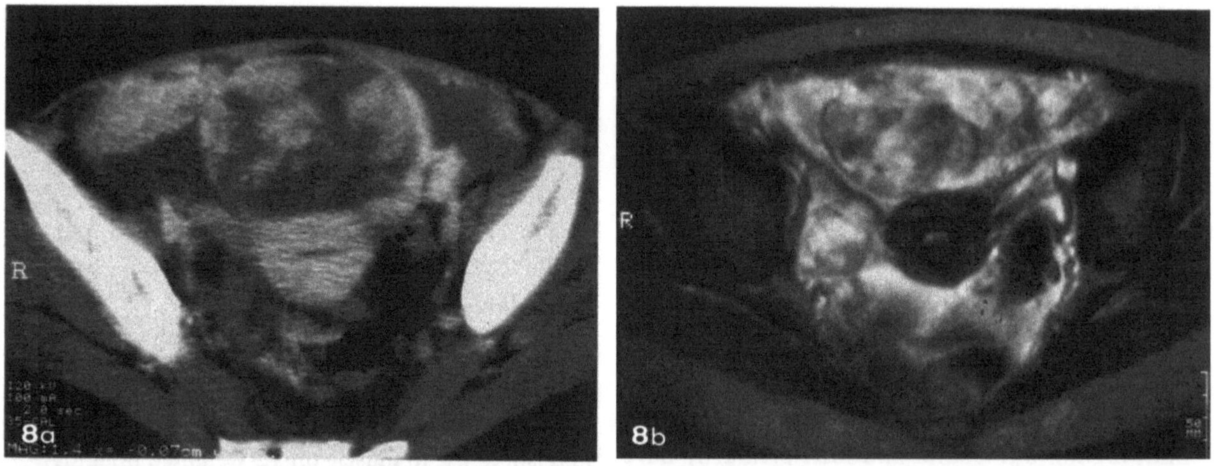

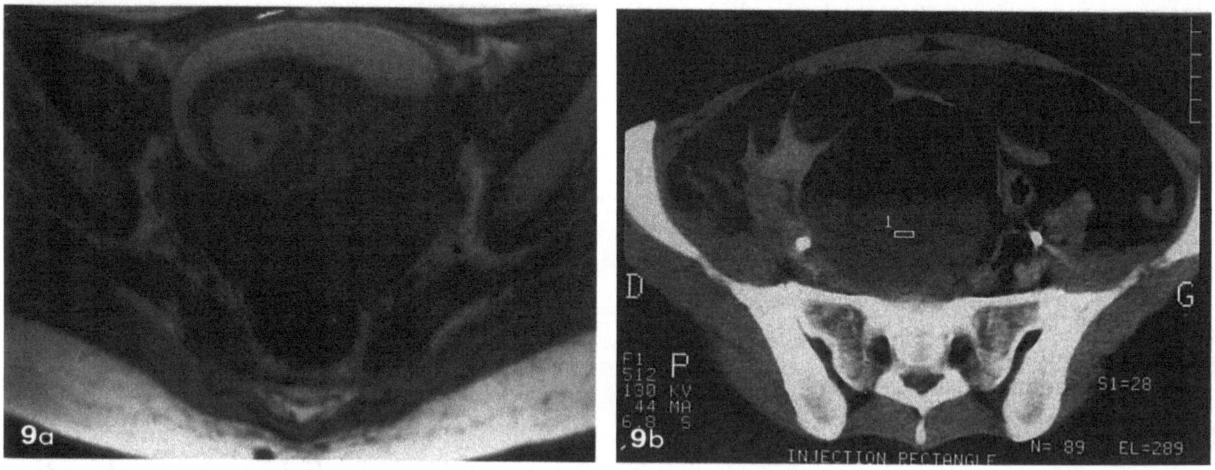

Fig. 35.8. a Pelvic CT, transverse axial section; **b** T2-weighted pelvic MRI, transverse axial sections. Clear cell cancer of the right ovary with pelvic and peritoneal invasion with large intraperitoneal tumor masses

Fig. 35.9. a T2-weighted pelvic MRI in the transverse axial plane. Pleuripotential dermoid cyst of the right ovary with a Rokitansky mass and a fatty component appearing hyperintense (image courtesy of Pr. J Dauplat, Clermont-Ferrand). **b** Ovarian abscess occurring within dermoid cysts with an air-fluid level and displacement of the opacified right ureter

Sertoli-Leydig tumors

These rare lesions (2/1000 of ovarian tumors) are essentially virilizing due to androgen secretion (estrogen secretion is possible but exceptionally rare). These tumors have a slight malignant potential and demonstrate no specific features on imaging, their contents being soft tissue and cystic in equal proportions, sometimes hemorrhagic or necrotic, which are better appreciated by MRI. Bilateral lesions are common.

Tumors of the sexual cords with annular tubules

These lesions have a very favorable outlook, with or without only a slight malignant potential, and are associated with the Peutz-Jeghers syndrome in a third of the cases. There are no characteristic imaging features apart from their large size (greater than 5 cm in 60% of cases) and possible progressive calcification, better demonstrated by CT.

Fibrothecal tumors

These are really benign tumors which may pose problems in the differential diagnosis with malignant ovarian tumors, particularly in the pre- and perimenopausal period. These tumors are often mixed with the ovarian fibrothecoma type and represent approximately 2% of all ovarian lesions. There is the possibility of confusion with a subserosal pedunculated uterine fibroid in the large forms of the tumor. MRI provides the best assessment of the lesions.

Germinal tumors [13]

Usually benign (dermoid cyst), these common lesions (more than 20% of ovarian tumors) are malignant in about 5% of cases. They are usually detected in young adults.

Mature pluripotential cystic teratomas or dermoid cysts (fig. 35.9a)

These cysts have very variable contents with fat, fluid, solid, hemorrhagic, sometimes with bony, cartilaginous, dental, muscular elements, as well as elements of the exoskeleton such as hair, nail and skin. The presence within the cyst wall of a soft tissue mass, so-called Rokitanski mass, is quite characteristic. The size of this prominence is a function of the tissue complexity of the cyst itself.

The plane abdominal radiograph strongly suggests the diagnosis in the presence of pelvic calcification of the bony type or in the form of a tooth. Ultrasound may confirm the polymorphic nature or, alternatively, fail to demonstrate the lesions.

CT of the abdomen and pelvis without bowel preparation has a vital role due to its simplicity and specificity. It is able to discriminate well between the different constituents, particularly the fatty and calcific density.

MRI (fig. 35.9a) is less rewarding than CT because it may lead to confusion with a hemorrhagic serous cystadenoma containing an endocystic vegetation, in the presence of a Rokitanski mass, or the demonstration of the fatty content (value of the fat suppression imaging sequences). Malignant transformation is rare (1%) and has no specific imaging features. Infection is always possible (fig. 35.9b).

Mature monopotential teratomas

This is concerned with either a carcinoid tumor or an ovarian goiter. Their specific imaging features are not known apart from their relatively regular well defined character and the absence of capsular break.

Immature teratomas

These extremely rare lesions (1/10 0000 of primary ovarian tumors) are irregular, disordered and associated with capsular rupture with a tendency to recurrence. These tumors of endodermal tissue (yolk sac tumors) are particularly renowned for their tendency to recur and appear as mixed cystic lesions but with clear solid and hemorrhagic areas. There are no other specific imaging features, as with the very rare gonadoblastomas and choriocarcinomas.

Dysgerminomas

There are no known specific imaging features since the lesions are essentially solid, commonly with microhemorrhagic changes and often associated with ovarian malformations. These lesions are infrequent, in the order of 1% of ovarian tumors.

Secondary tumors of the ovary (fig. 35.7)

These ovarian metastases usually originate from a colonic primary (Kruckenberg syndrome) breast primary or lymphoma, and exhibit non-specific imaging appearances. Bilateral involvement is commonly seen. The lesions comprise of cystic and soft tissues in varying proportions. The clinical context should help in the differential diagnosis.

As for any ovarian tumor, mechanical complications are possible which include rupture or torsion. In this instance, ultrasound demonstrates the peritumoral effusion and alteration in the shape of the cyst with a horizontal fluid level, these signs being taken in conjunction with the clinical findings.

Differential diagnosis [13]

The differential diagnosis of ovarian tumors is essentially with hydrosalpinx, endometriosis and subserosal pedunculated fibromas. Ultrasound is a sensitive technique for diagnosing hydrosalpinx.

The differential diagnosis with endometriosis may be difficult due to the often misleading and variable imaging appearances: the lesion is of oval shape, often with the long axis orientated postero-medially, these signs being entirely non-specific. MRI may be misleading due to the variability of signal intensity encountered in ovarian endometriosis. This is essentially due to the different breakdown products of hemoglobin and the protein content. Ultrasound may also be misleading. In the case of serosal pedunculated uncomplicated fibromas, ultrasound is of value by demonstrating the normal ovary on the ipsilateral side. MRI has some value due to its 3-dimensional capability and by the presence of hypointensity of the lesion on T2-weighted imaging.

Value of the new techniques [13]

Ovarian blood flow studies by color doppler are very promising, although endovaginal scanning still seems to be controversial. A reduction in the resistivity index, less than 4.5 for malignant tumors and remaining greater than 0.5 for benign tumors, constitutes one of the key diagnostic elements even though the sensitivity technique is inadequate, and these findings are yet to be confirmed.

The biochemical analysis by biopsy of the operative specimen provides the best way of understanding the significance of some of the signal intensities on MRI, particularly to explain certain contradictory phenomena which may be linked to the different stages of hemoglobin breakdown and complex protein contents.

CT and MRI imaging also provide information complementary to endoluminal pelvic ultrasound which is particularly helpful in the differentiation between a benign and a malignant tumor. CT is excellent for diagnosing dermoid cysts, demonstrating calcification, and assessing spread but suffers from a lack of specificity. It can sometimes help determine the original organ of large masses. However, it seems that ultrasound, particularly endoluminal ultrasound, is particularly useful in the positive diagnosis of ovarian tumors, complemented by MRI.

Assessment and follow-up of ovarian cancers [27]

Two essential elements must be remembered from the outset:
- first, the critical differences in surgical approach between a benign and malignant tumor, the benign lesions being treated by laparoscopy with or without a suprapubic incision whereas a midline approach is used for malignant tumors;
- second, the initial surgery is indicated regardless of the results of the pretherapeutic imaging findings: the reduction in tumor volume remains a critical element for prognosis (for example in stage III, the prognosis is best if the residual tumor is less than 3 cm)

Cancers of the ovary essentially spread [27] via the serous peritoneum and the pelvic and lumbo-aortic lymphatics. The diagnostic problems of demonstrating this lymphatic spread are identical to those for uterine cancers. Although peritoneal dissemination (30% involve the greater omentum and 60% the peritoneum) remains the critical feature of ovarian cancer, lymphatic dissemination must not be ignored and is present in 10 to 20% of the early stages I and II, 60% of stage III and nearly 100% of stage IV tumors. There is involvement in equal frequency of the external iliac chains by retrograde spread and lumbo-aortic chain, and more rarely the inguinal lymph nodes via the round ligament. Involvement of the retroperitoneal nodes is taken into account in the anatomoclinical classification system of FIGO in 1987 (table 35.4), and

Table 35.4. FIGO classification of ovarian cancer

Stage I	Tumor confined to the ovary
IA	Tumor confined to one ovary, no ascites, no tumor on the surface of the ovary and no capsular break
IB	Tumor confined to both ovaries, no ascites, no tumor on the surface of the ovary and no capsular break
IC	Tumor at stage IA or IB but with vegetations on the surface of one or both ovaries or cytologically malignant ascites or with positive peritoneal cytology or capsular break
Stage II	Tumor involving one or both ovaries with extension into the pelvis
IIA	Extension and/or metastases to the uterus and/or to the fallopian tubes
IIB	Spread to other pelvic tissues
IIC	Capsular tumor IIA or IIB but with tumor on the surface of one or both ovaries, or with capsular break, or with cytologically malignant ascites, or with positive peritoneal cytology
Stage III	Tumor involving one or both ovaries with peritoneal implants beyond the pelvis and/or retroperitoneal or inguinal lymphadenopathy, tumor confined to the pelvis with histologically proven involvement of the small intestine or omentum
IIIA	Tumor completely confined to the pelvis, without regional lymphadenopathy, with micro scopic spread into the abdominal peritoneum
IIIB	Tumor involving one or both ovaries, without regional adenopathy, with macroscopic spread (deposits less than 2 cm) to the abdominal peritoneum
IIIC	Abdominal deposits of greater than 2 cm in diameter and/or inguinal or retroperitoneal lymphadenopathy(ies)
Stage IV	Tumor involving one or both ovaries with distant metastasis In the presence of a pleural effusion, cytological confirmation of malignancy is required to classify a tumor as stage IV Parenchymal hepatic metastases are classified as stage IV, implants on the surface of the liver as stage III

these tumors are staged as IIIc irrespective of the degree of peritoneal involvement.

For spread to the surface of the serous peritoneum [27], the main problem is that of involvement of the ureters, bladder and intestinal wall which determine the necessity for any subsequent intestinal or urinary tract resection. Despite its limitations, classical imaging is still important for the assessment of the latter. Ultrasound and particularly CT are the most useful techniques for detecting distant secondary lesions, notably hepatic, splenic and diaphragmatic ones . CT is particularly useful by its ability to evaluate the viscera and lymph nodes during the same examination.

Surgery remains essential for the staging and initial treatment. It aims to achieve the most complete resection possible of the tumor and its locoregional spread in order to facilitate the results of chemotherapy by prior debulking of the tumor volume. Following treatment, surgery provides a better evaluation of the efficacy of the chemotherapy. However, these follow-up operations are not without risk, and the indications for them have reduced with the advent of other less invasive methods, such as tumor markers (CA125), CT, laparoscopy and even immunoscintigraphy.

These "second-look" operations are often reserved for:

- immediately, following the completion of the course of chemotherapy when this surgery may put the patient into complete remission by the excision of any residual masses;
- at a later stage, at the time of a possible distant recurrence, if remission was already complete at the end of the first laparotomy.

Applications of CT and MRI [27]

For treatment planning [18, 27]

The assessment of the tumor extent is made at the time of the initial routine surgery, and the role of imaging would appear to be less important. Nonetheless, imaging provides information about the presence of retroperitoneal lymphadenopathies, hepatic secondaries, and the relationship of the tumor to ureters and bladder. Infiltration of the omentum, mesentery or the presence of peritoneal carcinomatosis are more difficult to assess.

Ultrasound may demonstrate dilatation of the pelvicalyceal systems, suggestive of ureteric compression. This is facilitated by the detection of secondary hepatic lesions, and large nodular peritoneal deposits, particularly in the presence of ascites. It is, however, of limited value in the evaluation of pelvic spread, especially to the bowel, and also for lymph node and superficial peritoneal spread (in which the lesions are small, less than 1.5 to 2 cm, and spread along the surface of the serous peritoneum).

There are still indications for standard radiography, often guided by CT, to assist surgical intervention. The chest radiograph is essential, mainly for the detection of a pleural effusion. Pulmonary parenchymal metastases are infrequent. Intravenous urography assesses the degree of dilatation of the upper urinary tract due to an obstruction (by compression more often than actual ureteric infiltration). It is rarely performed nowadays and is often replaced by the urographic images which can be obtained at the end of a CT examination (using radio mode) and by the direct assessment of the ureters themselves, both on the axial CT sections and ultrasound. It is still difficult to make the distinction between a simple compression by tumor and subperitoneal pelvic invasion which is more infrequent. Barium enema is still indicated for the detection of colonic involvement, particularly at the rectosigmoid junction, either by direct contiguous spread or by spread along the peritoneum and mesocolon. Lymphography examines the lumbo-aortic and iliac lymph node chains by analyzing both the size and lymph node content. However, some small lacunae are difficult to interpret and not specific, even if there is a good correlation for some of these with the histological findings. This examination is nowadays in the process of being abandoned due to its lack of specificity and has been replaced by routine lymph node sampling at the time of operation.

The short acquisition time of CT, thanks to the angio-CT examination, allows simultaneous examination of the abdomen and pelvis including the supramesocolic, submesocolic, retroperitoneal or pelvic viscera and lymph node chains. Spread to the urinary tract and gut should routinely be looked for. However, CT is of limited value for the detection of peritoneal deposits, especially in difficult areas (diaphragmatic fold or visceral peritoneum), especially when they are of small size (less than 1 cm or 1.5 cm respectively with and without the presence of ascites). The assessment of lymph nodes depends exclusively on size without any evaluation of the content or structure of the node (problems with reactive inflammatory lymph node hyperplasia or neoplastic involvement of a normal size node). Finally, CT is unable to detect the ovarian lesion itself in cases with the preservation of size and morphology of the ovary.

MRI is not well suited to the pretherapeutic assessment of cancer of the ovary. It is inferior to CT in the

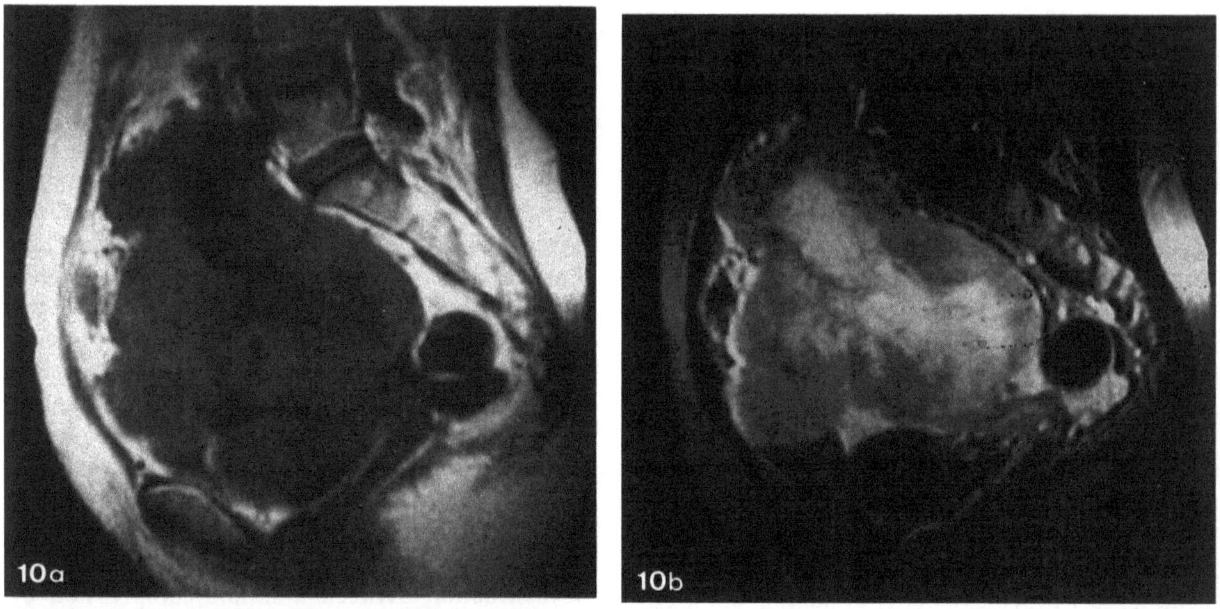

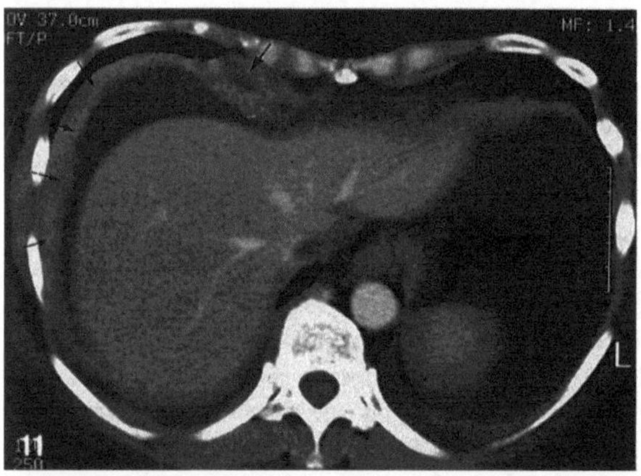

Fig. 35.10 . **a** T1-weighted pelvic in the sagittal plane; **b** T2-weighted MRI sagittal plane. Endometrioid cancer of the ovary: the uterus is displaced inferiorly

Fig. 35.11. Secondary peritoneal implants on post-contrast CT demonstrated in the diaphragmatic recesses *(arrows)* causing an effusion and heterogeneous nodular granulations

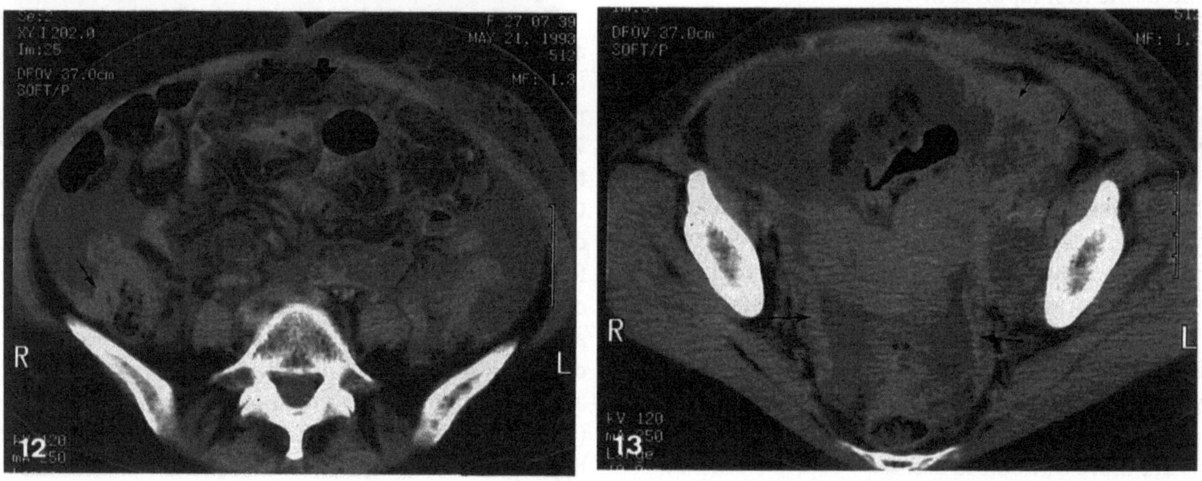

Fig. 35.12. Peritoneal carcinomatosis on post-contrast CT: the carcinomatosis is demonstrated in the form of thickening of the serous peritoneal surfaces without any definite individual mass but with cellulitic infiltration of variable heterogeneity in the peri-intestinal fatty tissue, particularly on the posterior surface of the greater omentum *(short thick arrows)*. There is also involvement of the right parieto-colic gutter *(small arrow)*

Fig. 35.13. Peritoneal carcinomatosis on post-contrast CT: infiltrative thickening of the serous peritoneum of the omentum, mesocolon and fasciae *(arrows)* outlined by ascites assessment of peritoneal involvement and provides no supplementary information compared to CT in the assessment of lymph node spread due to image degradation from respiratory and bowel peristalsis movement artefacts. It may be helpful in the difficult differential diagnosis of hepatic lesions (for example angioma versus metastasis). However, its cost outweighs any benefits.

For follow-up

The follow-up of ovarian cancers treated by surgery and chemotherapy is indicated in two circumstances:
- the monitoring of patients under treatment, in other words analyzing the regression of the tumor elements left behind for which CT has an essential role;
- the detection of local recurrences, for which endoluminal ultrasound and CT have a central role, and distant metastases for which ultrasound and particularly CT again play a crucial role for lymph node and visceral assessment.

CT and MRI signs [27]

CT

CT examination should be performed both with and without the injection of contrast, hepatic angio-CT complemented by an injection at the abdomino-pelvic level, with oral and rectal bowel preparation. Thin sections are useful for a better appreciation of tumor spread and particularly for analyzing a suspicious peritoneal area.

Straight-away, it must be emphasized that ovarian tumors may arise in ovaries of normal size and morphology, from which it must be concluded that the non-visualization of the ovaries or the presence of an ovary of physiological size in no way excludes neoplastic involvement. Such normalities in size are also found at surgery, the invasion being demonstrated histologically. According to the series of Lemaitre [27], the ovarian tumors responsible for peritoneal carcinomatosis were found to be of normal size in a half of the cases. In addition, the tumor itself could not be detected by CT (nor by ultrasound) in one out of two cases. The frequency of bilateral ovarian lesions was in the order of 60% of cases or more for the serosal lesions.

In the late forms of the disease (stages III and IV), peritoneal spread may manifest in the form of a peritoneal carcinomatosis, peritoneal or mesenteric thickening, or nodular peritoneal deposits. CT provides a very useful assessment of peritoneal carcinomatosis with the commonly associated ascites outlines the thickening and infiltration. It should be remembered that an unexplained ascites of recent onset must be considered suspicious in a woman with no significant previous clinical history. Carcinomatosis is demonstrated in the form of thickening, sometimes marked, of the serous peritoneal surfaces which may or may not be associated with micro- or macronodular masses and/or may manifest as a heterogeneous "cellulitic" infiltration of the peri-intestinal and omental fat (particularly in the greater omentum). These infiltrates are generally not parallel, thus distinguishing it from the discretely outlined appearance of the mesentery and omentum by a simple small amount of ascites.

Secondary peritoneal deposits (figs 35.11-35.16 and figs 35.4-35.8 previously) may appear as true soft tissue mass which are more easily demonstrated in the pericolic gutters (fig. 35.12), greater omentum or parietal folds of the peritoneum. Lesions in the pouch of Douglas, Retzius' space, diaphragmatic (fig. 35.11) or visceral folds are, on the other hand, difficult to detect on CT, even on thin sections, which are performed to help distinguish them from the bowel. However, micronodular peritoneal involvement (diffuse semolina grains) may easily be missed on CT.

Thickening and enhancement of the posterior parietal peritoneum are considered as relatively early signs. The nodular granulations must be distinguished from some of the recognized imaging pitfalls (the arcuate ligament of the diaphragm, diaphragmatic incisura, transversalis muscle of the abdominal wall...).

Enhancement of the peritoneal thickening is best seen in the pericolic gutters, subdiaphragmatic region and pelvis (fig. 35.13), particularly if there is abundant intraperitoneal fat and/or ascitic fluid (figs 35.11-35.13).

In the advanced forms of omental involvement at the ultimate stage of thickening and infiltration of the fat of the greater omentum (fig 35.14), there may be a true anterior subparietal tumor cake in the greater omentum (fig. 35.16). Thickening of the mesentery may be simply focal with a linear, stellate or whorled appearance associated at this stage with vascular compression or a neovascular network. During the progression of the disease, true nodules or mesenteric soft tissue masses may appear.

It is certain that stages III and IV disease can exist without ascites, either at the beginning or during the progression of the disease. This absence of ascites considerably limits the detection of peritoneal nodules. In the presence of ascites, apart from the miliary forms

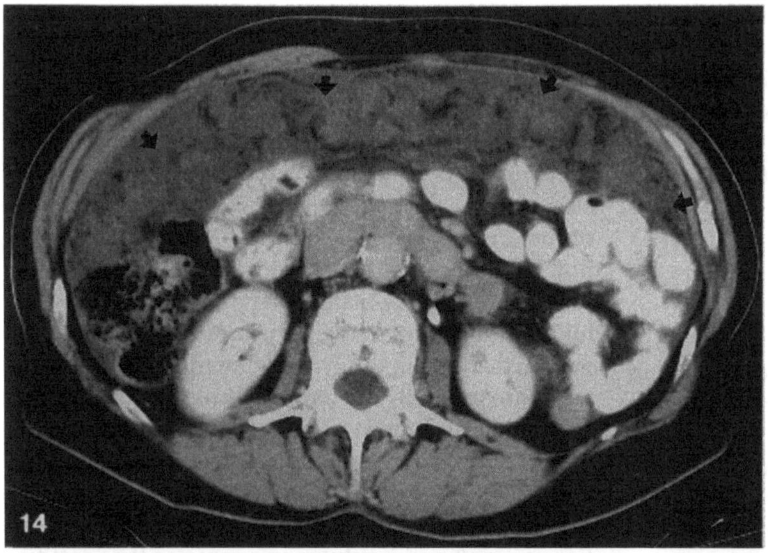

Fig. 35.14. Peritoneal carcinomatosis on post-contrast CT: diffuse involvement of the greater omentum with heterogeneous thickening and infiltration of the fatty tissue located in the greater omentum posteriorly *(arrows)* due to peritoneal spread from a mucinous tumor

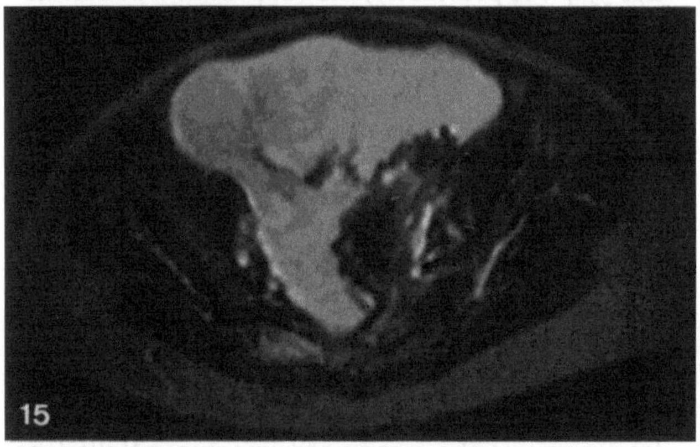

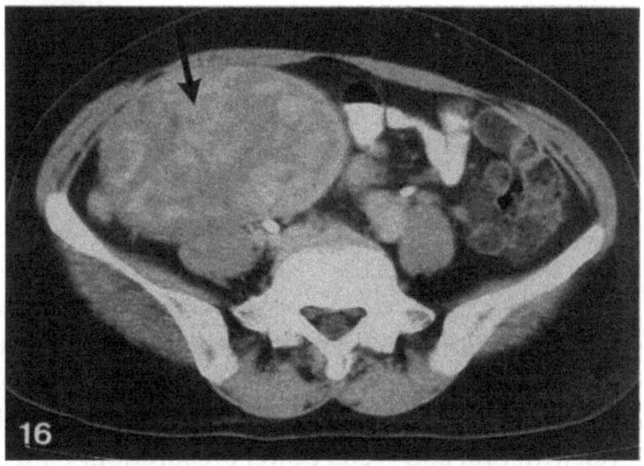

Fig. 35.15. Peritoneal carcinomatosis on axial T2-weighted MRI: there is marked centropelvic ascites outlining the bowel loops, the latter being plastered onto the lateral and postero-lateral pelvic wall; there are only irregularities along the peri-intestinal peritoneal contours; no nodular lesion or direct or indirect sign of granulation has been demonstrated by this technique: there was, however, a micronodular involvement of the peritoneum. MRI, like CT, is unable to demonstrate this miliary pattern of involvement

Fig. 35.16. Peritoneal carcinomatosis on axial CT: advanced form with omental involvement causing a true epiploic tumor cake *(arrow)* located beneath the anterior abdominal wall on the right. Note that this lesion appears well circumscribed and heterogeneous with fluid and soft tissue components corresponding to a peritoneal recurrence away from the treatment sites

which are undetectable by CT, the detection of nodules of greater than 5 or 6 mm is maximal in the subdiaphragmatic regions. Detection rates are less in the pouch of Douglas (80%), greater omentum (60%) and any other sites (50%) [27]. The value of CT for the assessment of locoregional and distant spread depends on the site involved: dilatation of pelvicalyceal systems and ureters is generally due to extrinsic compression proximal to where the internal iliac vessel are crossed by the ureters. Direct infiltration is rarely seen. The urographic image following a CT study can replace conventional intravenous urography. Colonic spread is difficult to demonstrate on axial CT sections. In fact, the distinction between the extrinsic compression and invasion is not easy. A constant and persistent stenosis can be very suggestive of infiltration by contiguous spread in a well prepared patient. Colonic retraction, particularly of the sigmoid colon, or a pericolic infiltrate in the region of the tumor are suggestive but non-specific signs.

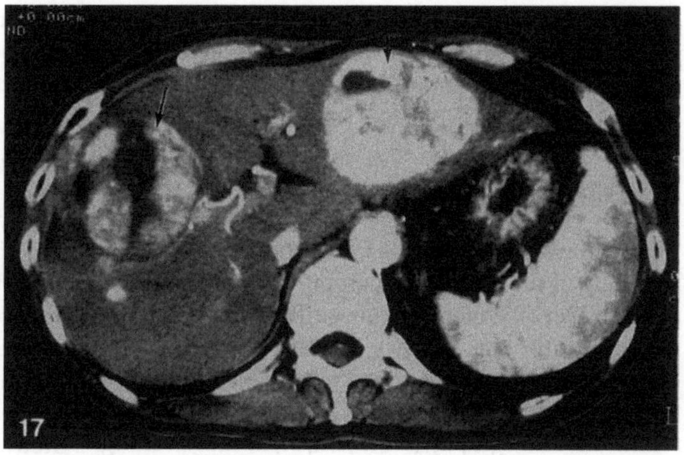

Fig. 35.17. Hepatic metastases from ovarian cancer on angio-CT: two principal macronodular lesions *(arrows)* involving segments 2 and 3 and the junction of the lateral and paramedian sectors of the right lobe of the liver, exhibiting early pseudo-angiomatous vascular kinetics on helical angio-CT

Secondary hepatic lesions are well shown by CT (fig. 35.17) which is complementary to ultrasound. CT can demonstrate particularly well the two routes of hepatic spread, one is the rare intraparenchymal hematogenous route, and the other being peripheral capsular involvement by peritoneal permeation and subsequent subcapsular hepatic parenchymal involvement by contiguous spread. The assessment of lymph node spread depends on CT despite its limitations which primarily concern the involvement nodes of normal size as previously described.

MRI

This technique does not seem to have any role to play because it gives no further information concerning the contents of lymph nodes and does not improve the detection of lymphatic spread compared to CT. In addition, MRI is inferior to CT for the detection of peritoneal deposits (fig. 35.15).

The value of endocavity ultrasound must be remembered which is particularly sensitive for the preoperative assessment and follow-up of ovarian tumors: the endorectal scan evaluates the rectovaginal septum, while the endovaginal scan assesses the parametria, vagina, and the bladder wall to look for angularity or a mass. The barium enema detects a stenosis, extrinsic compression or, particularly, an asymmetrical angulation, pulling-in of the mucosal folds, or fixation in the sigmoid region or flexures.

Other methods of investigation [27]

The most important of these are the tumor markers and isotope techniques.

Tumor markers

Tumor markers can be monitored in tumors of the ovary. For epithelial tumors, only the CA125 level has been clearly demonstrated to be of value despite its lack of specificity. In fact, levels greater than normal are found in more than 5% of patients with benign pathologies (1% of normal subjects) and more than 15% in the first 3 months of pregnancy. As with testicular cancers, the embryonic tumors of the ovary can secrete α-fetoprotein, chorionic hormone (HCG) and β HCG which are extremely valuable markers for follow-up.

It should be remembered that abnormal levels can be seen in other cancers (lung, pancreas, colon and rectum...) and that, particularly in the presence of ascites or non-neoplastic pleural effusion (hepatitis, cirrhosis...), the CA125 level can be extremely elevated.

In little less than 20% of cases, the CA125 levels are normal in patients with ovarian cancers. Therefore, the presence of normal levels of tumor markers do not exclude the diagnosis of an epithelial cancer. Although not entirely specific, CA125 is an extremely useful marker for the prognosis and follow-up of ovarian cancers [17, 32]. CA125 is also used for following the progress of the patients treated by surgery and chemotherapy. A study comparing the CA125 levels, the baseline CT following treatment and the second look laparotomy showed that the results were concordant in 60% of cases and discordant in 40% of cases. In 5% of cases the CA125 and CT were negative and the surgery positive. Conversely, in 5% of cases the surgery demonstrated inflammatory granulomas in the presence of elevated CA125 levels and a positive CT. In the remaining 30%, the CA125 was normal whereas CT and surgery were abnormal [27].

These results agree with others in the literature which confirm that an abnormal CA125 level returning to normal only corresponds to a complete remission of the disease in 56% of cases [18].

Isotopes technique

These represent a real hope for the future:
- a study of the diffusion of an intraperitoneal radioactive tracer (technetium 99m sulfur colloid marker) to determine the efficacy of the intraperitoneal chemotherapy and to detect possible walled-off lesions which limit the efficacy of treatment;
- immunoscintigraphy (for example, immunoscintigraphy using anti-CA125 antibodies) uses antibody markers which concentrate in areas of disease containing the antigen and result in the detection of these lesions by tomoscintigraphy.

Investigations to be performed [27]

For the assessment of ascites

CT seems to be the most sensitive technique, particularly for demonstrating peritoneal carcinomatosis (sensitivity greater than 80%). However, the appearances of peritoneal carcinomatosis are not specific since they may also be seen in lymphomatous involvement of the peritoneum, any other cause of peritoneal carcinomatosis or peritoneal tuberculosis (obviously very rare).

In all cases of an ambiguous pelvic tumor or ascites of indeterminate origin, laparoscopy may be suggested initially to confirm the diagnosis by possible biopsies, only if there is minimal ascites, and to determine an unprepared examination for, the most appropriate eventual surgery or treatment once definitive histology has been obtained.

This pretherapeutic staging guides the surgeon as to the locoregional extent of the disease, the tumor volume, the possibility of lumbo-aortic or pelvic lymph node involvement, peritoneal carcinomatosis and secondary visceral spread, particularly pelvis. However, this is only of relative value due to the fact of the extent of the disease assessed at the time of the routine initial surgery. CT remains the central preoperative examination in association with a chest radiograph and abdominal especially hepatic ultrasound. These examinations are complemented by a barium enema for stages III and IV if bowel involvement is suspected. In fact, in these cases, rather than performing a multiplicity of examinations, it is of greater value for the patient to be warned by the surgeon of the possibility of a bowel resection to prevent imminent obstruction, especially to optimize the debulking of the tumor.

In the context of pelvic tumor

The role of imaging is to determine the origin and localization of the lesion and attempt to assess its nature. Ultrasound has the principal role in this context by confirming the fluid, solid or mixed nature of the lesion. In the case of a mixed or solid tumor in a premenopausal women, it is important to look for signs of benignity so the patient can benefit from limited surgery: laparoscopic surgery or transverse Pfannenstiel incision. Minimal surgery may still be indicated sometimes in young women wishing to become pregnant, if one remembers however the limitations of imaging in the detection of the 6 to 10% of patients with contralateral lesions in supposedly stage IA disease. Conversely, any suspicious signs should be carefully looked for in case of a cystic fluid-filled tumor, the presence of which would preclude any notion of conservative surgery and make it necessary to warn the patient of possibility of extensive surgery (hysterectomy-bilateral adnexectomy) using a large midline incision.

In doubtful cases, it may be useful to complement ultrasound with CT and particularly MRI for the assessment of large masses where the ultrasound findings may be inadequate. Contrast enhancement on CT, and the signal intensity of the endometrium and normal myometrium on T2-weighted MRI are the essential features for diagnosing the original site of the tumor.

For follow-up

Following the initial surgery, there are two possible clinical scenarios:
- If residual disease has been left behind by surgery, it is necessary to perform CT as a baseline at the outset for the follow-up of chemotherapy treatment even though the residual lesion will not be visible either on CT or ultrasound in a considerable number of cases. After adjuvant chemotherapy, CT examination should be repeated unless the initial scan was normal. In this situation, a second look operation is necessary to assess the tumor response.
- If there is no residual disease, and the surgery was macroscopically complete, there is no indication for an immediate CT but rather for one at the end of the course of adjuvant chemotherapy, possibly comple-

mented by ultrasound, lymphography and routine CA125 levels.

At the end of the treatment program and prior to possible second look surgery, it is often advisable to perform a CT examination:
- if CT is normal, it does not exclude micronodular peritoneal involvement, and it is therefore imperative to operate on the patient; even normal CA125 levels do not avoid this surgical inspection [28, 29, 33, 34];
- if CT is abnormal, the continuation or alteration in the treatment must be considered, particularly the possibility of a autograft, or surgery to confirm the presence of a recurrence and secondarily achieving complete debulking of the tumor in the knowledge that the ultimate prognosis is poor.

For the detection of distant spread

Despite its limitations, CT represents the best compromise for examining the abdomen and pelvis, associated with regular CA125 levels. In addition, CT can guide biopsy or lead to a laparoscopic or celioscopic examination.

In the future it can be envisaged that some techniques, notably the intraperitoneal injection of a contrast agent [20, 24] will improve the detection of peritoneal metastases regardless of their localization or size. Similarly, it is expected that imaging will guide peritoneoscopy of laparoscopy in the follow-up of patients to further evaluate recurrences. Immunoscintigraphy is attractive theoretically but still limited by its poor spatial resolution and the difficulty in obtaining specific monoclonal antibodies.

Conclusion [27]

Ultrasound (particularly endoluminal) is considered to be the best technique for the examination of the pelvis, particularly for making a positive diagnosis. MRI is a complementary technique which provides more detailed information (but still non-specific).

Despite its limitations, CT is currently the only indispensable examination for the assessment and follow-up of advanced cancers of the ovary (stages III and IV) in association with the CA125 levels. A single examination provides an assessment of the abdomen and the pelvis. On the other hand, for the initial preoperative assessment, CT only acts as a guide for the surgeon, and for the follow-up. A normal CT examination does not avoid second look surgery. If this CT examination is positive, this may result in a different therapeutic approach or guide the performance of further surgical debulking of the tumor.

The critical problem is spread to the mesocolon and mesentery occurring at the beginning. Standard radiography still has a role which is complementary to CT despite its well recognized limitations for this. For subsequent follow-up, CT remains the best technique for examining the abdomen and pelvis even if the small lesions are missed.

The combination of ultrasound, CT, immunoscintigraphy (still under study) provide the best hope of reducing or even avoiding a second look operation (less than 5% of second look operations are positive when these three examinations are all negative) [27].

References

Diagnosis

1. Ayalon D, Graif M, Het Man M, Abramovicz J, Eckstein N, Vagman (1988) Diagnosis of small ovarian tumor (androgen secreting) by MR: a new non invasive procedure. Am J Obstet Gynecol 150: 905-907
2. Buy JN, Ghossain JN, Sciot C, Bazot M, Guinet C, Prevot S, Hugol D, Laromiguiere M, Truc JB, Poitout P, Vadrot D, Ecoiffier J (1991) Epithelial tumors of the ovary: CT findings and correlation with US. Radiology 178: 811-819
3. Granberg S, Norstrom A, Wikland M (1990) Tumors in the lower pelvis as imaged by vaginal sonography. Gynecol Oncol 37: 224-229
4. Hamlin DJ, Fitzsimmons JR, Pettersson H, Rigall FC, Morgan L, Wilkinson EJ (1985) MR imaging of the pelvis: evaluation of ovarian masses at 0.15 T. AJR 145: 585-590
5. Kier R, Mc Carthy SM, Scoutt LM, Viscarello RR, Schwartz PE (1990) Pelvis masses in pregnancy. MR imaging. Radiology 176: 709-713
6. Kurjak A, Zalud I, Alfirevic A, Jurkovic D (1990) The assessment of abnormal pelvic blood flow by transvaginal color and pulsed doppler. Ultrasound Med Biol 16: 437-442
7. Maiman M, Seltzer V, Boyce J (1991) Laparoscopy excision of ovarian neoplasms subsequently found to be malignant. Obstet Gynecol 70: 563-565.
8. Matsumoto F, Yoshioka H, Hamada T, Ishida O, Noda K (1990) Struma ovarii - CT and MR finding. J Comput AssistTomogr 14: 310-312
9. Mawhinney RR, Powell MC, Worthington BS, Symonds EM (1988) Magnetic resonance imaging of benign ovarian masses. Br J Radiol 61: 179-186
10. Mitchell DG, Marshall C, Spritzek CE, Gussman D, Arger PH, Kressel HY (1987) Adnexal masses - MR imaging observations at 1,5 T with US and CT correlation. Radiology 162: 319-324
11. Okamura M, Akabori T, Takeuchi S, Yamazaki M, Mochizuki M, Itoh H (1987) A case of young woman

with giant ovarian tumor as the manifestation of leukemic recurrence. Nippon Ganka Gakkai Zasshi 25: 1032-1037
12. Rouanet JP, Maubon A, Mares P (1990) Le liquide intratumoral ovarien. Quel signal pour quelle signification? Journées Nationales de Radiologie, Paris
13. Rouanet JP et al (1993) Cancers de l'ovaire - Diagnostic des tumeurs de l'ovaire. In: Buthiau D, Dargent D (eds) Imagerie Clinique en Gynécologie. Vigot, Paris, pp 236-248
14. Sassone M, Timor-Tritsch IE, Artner A, Westhoff C, Warren WB (1991) Transvaginal sonography characterization of ovarian disease: evaluation of a new scoring system to predict ovarian malignancy. Obstet Gynecol 78: 70-76
15. Shetch S, Fischman EK, Buck JL, Hamper UM, Sanders RC (1988) The variable sonographic appearance of ovarian teratomas. AJR 151: 331-334.
16. Varma DG, Thorneycroft IH, Degafu S, Eberly SM, Smith LG (1990) Magnetic resonance imaging of adult ovarian granulosa cell tumor. Clin Imaging 14: 55-59

Assessment and follow-up

17. Aravantinos D, Michalas S, Papazefkos V, Christoforaki M, Stypsaneli A, Vlachos G, Athanasiadis P (1990) Predictive values of CA 125 antigen levels and CT scan in second-look procedures for ovarian cancer. Eur J Obstet Gynecol Reprod Biol 37: 265-270
18. Buthiau D, Dargent D, Darbois Y et coll. (1992) TDM et IRM cliniques. Abdomen-Pelvis. Buthiau D (ed) Frison-Roche, Paris
19. Buy JN, Moss AA, Ghossain MA, Sciot C, Malbec L, Vadrot D, Paniel BJ, Decroix Y (1988) Peritoneal implants from ovarian tumors: CT findings. Radiology 169: 691-694
20. Dunnick NR, Jones RB, Doppman JL, Speyers J, Myers CE (1979) Intraperitoneal contrast infusion for assessment of intraperitoneal fluid dynamics. AJR 133: 221-223
21. Friedman JB, Weiss NS (1990) Second thoughts about second-look laparotomy in advanced ovarian cancer. N Engl J Med 322: 1079-1082
22. Jeffrey RB (1980) CT demonstration of peritoneal implants. AJR 135: 322-326
23. Guidozzi F, Sonnendecker EWW (1991) Evaluation of preoperative investigations in patients admitted for ovarian primary cytoreductive surgery. Gynecol Oncol 38: 241-247
24. Halvorsen RA, Panushka C, Oakley GJ, Letourneau JG, Adcock LL (1991) Intraperitoneal contrast material improves the CT detection of peritoneal metastases. AJR 157: 37-40
25. Hunter VJ, Weinberg JB, Haney AF, Soper JT, Lavin P, Metsch L, Knapp RC, Bast RC (1990) CA 125 in peritoneal fluid and serum from patients with benign gynecologic conditions and ovarian cancer. Gynecol Oncol 36: 161-165
26. Le Bouedec G, Fondrinier E, Kauffmann Ph, Mansoor A, Dauplat J (1992) La lymphadénectomie pelvienne et lombo-aortique dans le cancer primitif de l'ovaire. Presse Med 21: 745-749
27. Lemaître L, et al (1993) Cancers de l'ovaire. Bilan préthérapeutique et surveillance des cancers de l'ovaire. In: Imagerie Clinique en Gynécologie. Buthiau D, Dargent D (eds) Vigot, Paris, pp 249-260
28. Lund B, Jacobsen K, Rasch L, Jensen F, Olesen K, Feldt-Rasmussen K (1990) Correlation of abdominal ultrasound and computed tomography scans with second- or third-look laparotomy in patients with ovarian carcinoma. Gynecol Oncol 37: 279-283
29. Megibow AJ, Bosniak MA, Ho AG, Beller U, Hulnick DH, Beckman EM (1988) Accuracy of CT in detection of persistent or recurrent ovarian carcinoma: correlation with second-look laparotomy. Radiology 166: 341-345
30. Musumeci R, De Palo G, Kenda R, Tesoro-Tess JD, Di Re F, Petrillo F, Rilke F (1980) Retroperitoneal metastases from ovarian carcinoma reassessment of 365 patients studied with lymphography. AJR 134: 449-452
31. Van Nagell JR, Higgins RV, Donaldson ES, Gallion HH, Powell DE, Pavlik EJ, Woods CH, Thompson EA (1990) Transvaginal sonography as a screening method for ovarian cancer. A report of the first 1000 cases scrcened. Cancer 65: 573-577
32. Patsner B, Orr JW, Mann WJ, Taylor PT, Partridge E, Allmen T (1990) Does serum CA 125 level prior to second-look laparotomy for invasive ovarian adenocarcinoma predict size of residual disease? Gynecol Oncol 36: 373-376
33. Reuter KL, Griffm T, Hunter RE (1989) Comparison of abdomino pelvic computed tomography results and findings at second-look laparotomy in ovarian carcinoma patients. Cancer 63: 1123-1128
34. Silverman PM, Osborne M, Dunnick NR, Bandy LC (1988) CTprior to second-look operation in ovarian cancer. AJR 150: 829-832
35. Squillaci E, Salzani MC, Gradinetti ML, Auffermann W, Marsella A, Maresca G, Colagrande C (1988) Recurrence of ovarian and uterine ncoplasms: diagnosis with transrectal US. Radiology 169: 355-358
36. Taal BG, Steinmetz R, Den Hartog Jager FCA (1990) Rectosigmoid obstruction caused by ovarian cancer. Clin Radiol 41: 170-174
37. Walkey MM, Friedman AC, Sohotra P, Radecki PR (1988) CT manifestations of peritoneal carcinomatosis. AJR 150: 1035-1041
38. Weill FS, Costaz R, Guetarni S, Maltoni I, Rohmer P (1990) Le diagnostic échographique des métastases péritonéales chez les malades ascitiques. J Radiol 71: 365-368
39. Yancik R (1993) Ovarian Cancer. Cancer (Suppl) 71: 517-523
40. Young RC, Fuks Z, Hoskins WJ (1989) Cancer of the ovary. In: DeVita VT, Hellman S, Rosenberg SA (eds) Cancer, principles and practice of oncology, 3rd ed. JB Lippincott, Philadelphia, pp 1166-1168
41. Young RC (1987) Initial therapy for early ovarian cancer. Cancer 60: 2042-2049

CHAPTER 36

Cancer of the prostate

Clinicians
M. Gozy, O. Rixe, D. Nizri, J.-L. Misset,
B. Mégarbane, J.-P. Spano, D. Khayat

Radiologist
D. Buthiau

Cancer of the prostate (tables 36.1-36.3 and 36.6) is a common cancer in the elderly. More than 90% of patients are aged between 60 and 85 years. Year after year the incidence and mortality rate of this cancer increase (122,000 cases per year in the USA in 1991 responsible for 32,000 deaths). The mortality rate is 10% of all cancer deaths, second to cancer of the lung [4, 12].

Dosage of prostate specific antigen (PSA) and routine rectal examination of men over 50 years of age is still the best method for the early diagnosis of localized prostatic cancers. The performance of a screening examination in men with no urological symptoms who are consulting for another reason must take into the account the wishes of the patient. This involves fully informing the patient beforehand, particularly of the advantages and disadvantages of this procedure. The aim of the rectal examination is to screen the individual for prostatic cancer. It is primarily indicated in men between 60 and 70 years, but also before 60 years, and the frequency of the tumor has been increased in these latter years. The level of the prostate specific antigen should be obtained if there is any clinical suspicion. Interpretation of this level must consider the normal variations related to laboratories, age and prostatic volume.

Transrectal ultrasound cannot be justified as an initial procedure but is useful for guided prostatic biopsy. Its role is limited in the assessment of extraprostatic spread.

Indications for CT and MRI

[2, 4, 6, 7, 10, 14] (table 36.4)

CT

This examination is useless for making a positive diagnosis and screening because it does not detect localized tumors.

CT underestimates a tumor spread limited to the capsule or the seminal vesicles and does not demonstrate microscopic invasion of the periprostatic fat. Its accuracy is inferior to transrectal ultrasound for the demonstration of capsular invasion. Some authors have recognized that CT has some value in the demonstration of suspected spread in stage B (15 to 20% of cases), reclassifying the disease as stage C and hence altering the therapeutic approach (table 36.1).

The current indications for CT are as follows:
- the general assessment of visceral and lymphatic spread in a single examination for advanced stage disease when there is a clinical indication. The combination of CT lymphography, with or without guided biopsy, gives a 90% efficacy, lymph node sampling being the most accurate technique;
- pretherapeutic radiotherapy planning;
- the assessment of local recurrences, provided the CT examination is performed 6 months after treatment; its value is clear following radiotherapy treatment alone but less justified following a prostatectomy (table 36.5);

Table 36.1. The Whitemore classification

Stage A	Tumor limited to the prostate, impalpable (detected on prostatectomy specimen)
Stage B1	Intracapsular tumor occupying only one lobe of the prostate
Stage B2	Intracapsular tumor occupying two lobes of the prostate
Stage C	Tumor breaking the prostatic capsule
Stage D1	Lymph node metastasis (es)
Stage D2	Visceral metastasis (es)

Table 36.3. IUCC classification

Stage 0	T1a, N0, M0
Stage I	T1a, N0, M0 T1b, N0, M0 T1c, N0, M0
Stage II	T2, N0, M0
Stage III	T3, N0, M0
Stage IV	T4, N0, M0 Any T, N1, M0 Any T, N2, M0 Any T, N3, M0 Any T, any N, M1

Table 36.2. TNM classification

T0	No tumor	
T1	Undetectable tumor (neither classically nor by imaging)	
	T1a	Less than 5% of tumor cells in the resected tissue
	T1b	More than 5% of tumor cells in the resected tissue
	T1c	Tumor identified by needle biopsy (with elevation of the PSA)
T2	Tumor limited to the prostate	
T3	Tumor having broken the prostatic capsule	
T4	Tumor fixed or infiltrating the adjacent structures	
	T4a	Invasion of the bladder neck, external sphincter of the rectum
	T4b	Invasion of the levator muscles and/or the pelvic wall
N0	Absence of lymph node invasion	
N1	Lymphadenopathy less than 2 cm	
N2	Lymphadenopathy greater than 2 cm but not exceeding 5 cm or the presence of multiple lymphadenopathies of less than 5 cm	
N3	Lymphadenopathy (ies) greater than 5 cm	
M0	Absence of metastases	
M1	Distant metastases	
	M1a	Non-regional adenopathy
	M1b	Bone
	M1c	Other site (s)

– sometimes CT helps in the demonstration of secondary bone lesions and their intracanalicular extent within the spine.

MRI (figs 36.1 & 36.2)

Although there is a difference in the signal intensities between normal and pathological tissues on MRI, there is no absolute difference between cancer, adenoma or even benign hyperplasia. MRI cannot be used for making a positive diagnosis, the question of health costs adding to these problems.

MRI represents an advanced method for staging, particularly with the use of an endorectal surface coil for the assessment of involvement of the periprostatic fat, seminal vesicles and periprostatic venous plexus. On whole body MRI, the fibrous capsule is not visible (fig. 36.1), its demonstration being improved by an endorectal coil. For the positive diagnosis of the lesion, MRI does not compete with other equally accurate techniques such as endorectal ultrasound which are much less expensive. It can, therefore, not be used routinely but is reserved for identifying tumor spread, particularly beyond the prostate into the seminal vesicles, despite the possibility of diagnostic errors.

Table 36.4. Cancer of the prostate (reproduced from Buthiau D (ed) TDM et IRM cliniques. Frison-Roche, Paris)

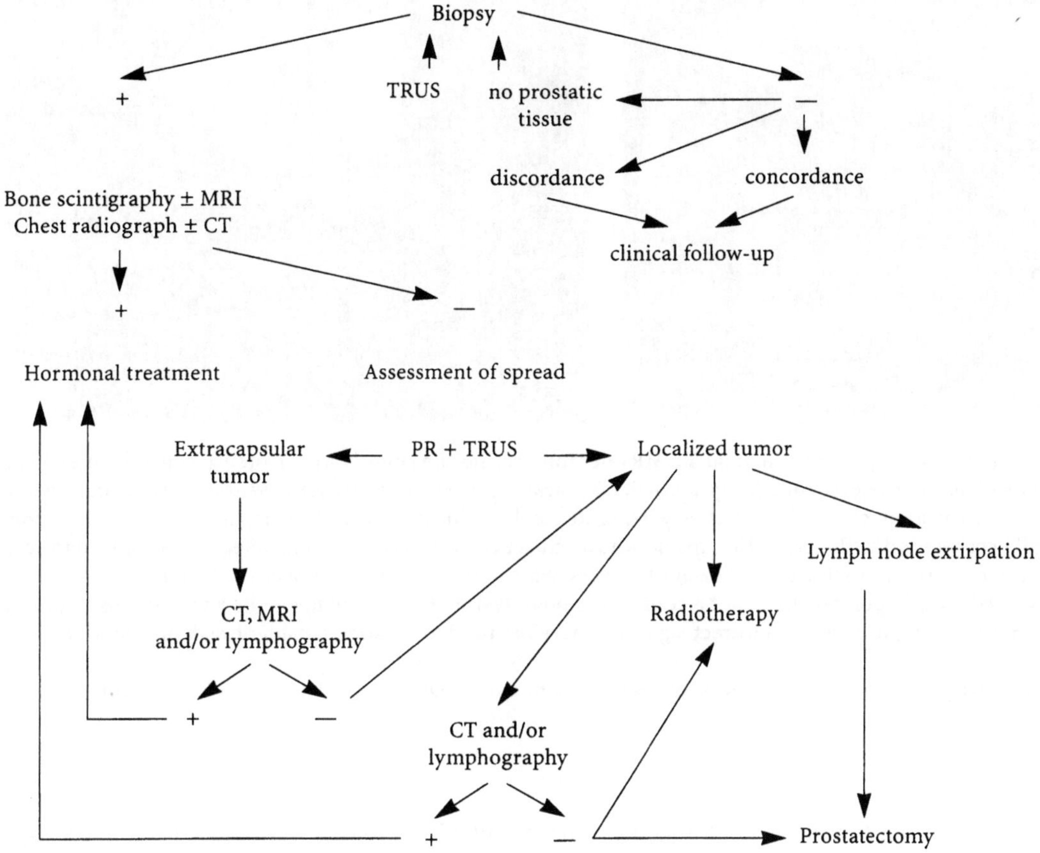

Table 36.5. Follow-up of cancers of the prostate (from D Buthiau et al. Clinical CT and MRI. Frison-Roche, Paris [4])

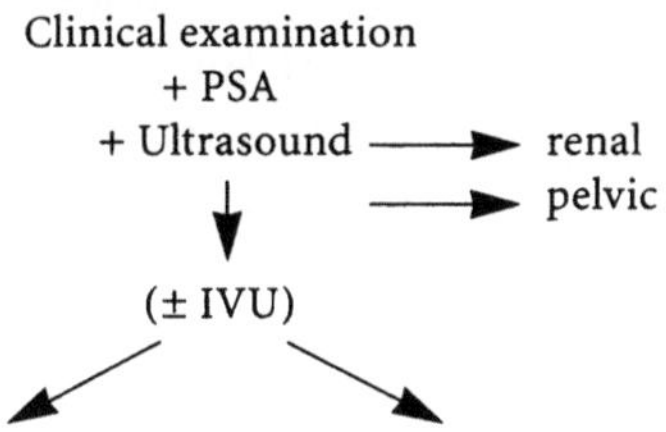

Disseminated disease

- scintigraphy and the value of MRI for bone involvement
- standard chest radiograph + CT if small thoracic

Localized disease

- CT initially (4 to 6 months after treatment), definite role in cases of treatment alone, less of lesions or the least doubt radiotherapy a role for prostatectomy (progress under treatment: different surgical indication)

- MRI as a potential aid in the differentiation of fibrosis and recurrence

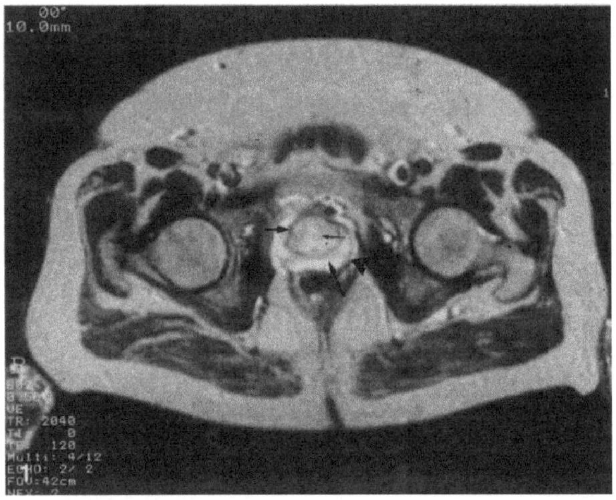

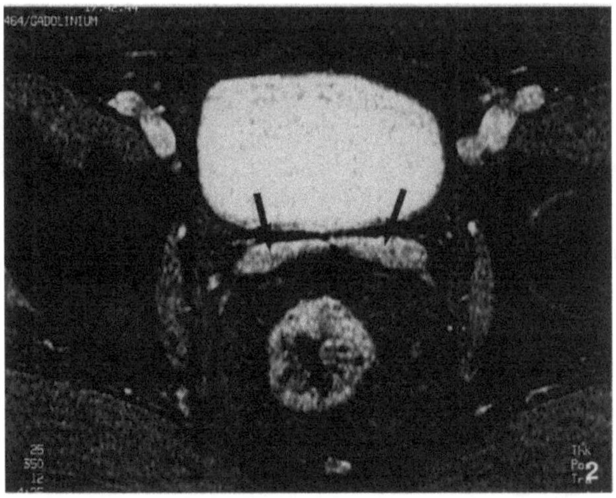

Fig. 36.1. Normal anatomy of the prostate on axial T2 MRI demonstrating the slightly hyperintense central zone *(small arrow)*, clearly hyperintense peripheral zone *(large arrow)*, inseparable from the periprostatic venous plexus, and the low signal intermediate zone *(medium arrow)*. The relatively hypointense thick line located at the periphery of the gland *(arrow head)* does not really correspond to the prostatic capsule whose existence even is controversial. Regardless of its nature, it is an extremely thin structure, approximately a dozen cell layers, which does not in reality seem to be responsible for the hypointensity described. This hypointensity is not a constant enough feature for any change in its single intensity to be a characteristic sign of macroscopic invasion; indirect signs are therefore used to adjudge capsular break or integrity

Fig. 36.2. Normal seminal vesicles on 2D FISP MRI sequence; the seminal vesicles *(arrows)* have a high signal intensity due to their fluid content

MRI has not replaced CT for the assessment of general visceral and lymph node spread, and provides no supplementary information to CT other than the differentiation of lymph nodes and blood vessels without the use of a contrast agent (only of value in patients allergic to iodine).

For follow-up, it has a dual role in differentiating local fibrosis/recurrence and detecting disseminated bone metastases, often nowadays an invaluable complementary technique to scintigraphy (table 36.5).

Signs [4, 7, 12, 14]

CT

There are no differentiating density measurements on CT among hyperplasia, cancer and the normal parenchyma.

For staging purposes:

- the capsule is not visible on CT;
- capsular invasion and spread can only be suspected on indirect signs (see fig. 36.5): asymmetry of the periprostatic fat planes, irregularity of the glandular outline, nodular lesion in the periprostatic fat in contiguity with the gland itself, loss of the fat tissue between the prostate and the pelvic wall, direct spread to the pelvic wall or rectum; these latter signs can be evaluated clinically;
- spread to the seminal vesicles is only suspected in the presence of asymmetrical orientation of the one of the seminal vesicles, focal dilatation, alteration of soft tissue density or filling-in of the retrovesical fat tissue which has no specific value since any increase in the prostatic volume can cause loss of these fat spaces;
- spread to the bladder: this is difficult to appreciate on CT due to the axial plane of the section;
- clearly all these described signs are of any significance only in the absence of any prior locoregional intervention, particularly any prostatic needle biopsy or endoscopic resection: the performance of these interventions nowadays prior to CT makes this examination very difficult to interpret due to the resultant hemorrhagic or local inflammatory changes;
- for lymphatic spread, the sensitivity of CT varies between 70 and 90%; the specificity remains poor, barely more than 50%. This limitation is linked to its

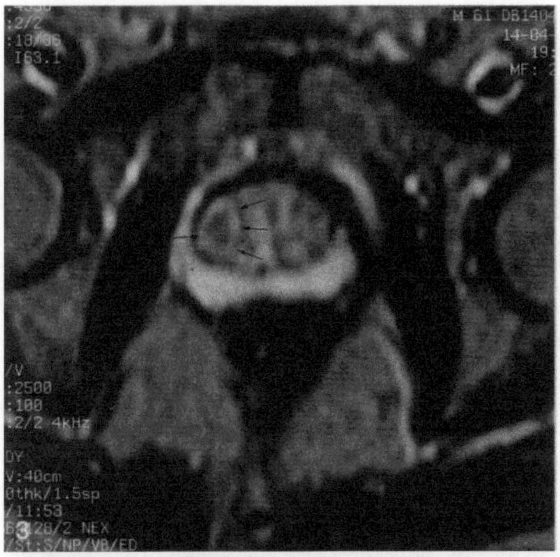

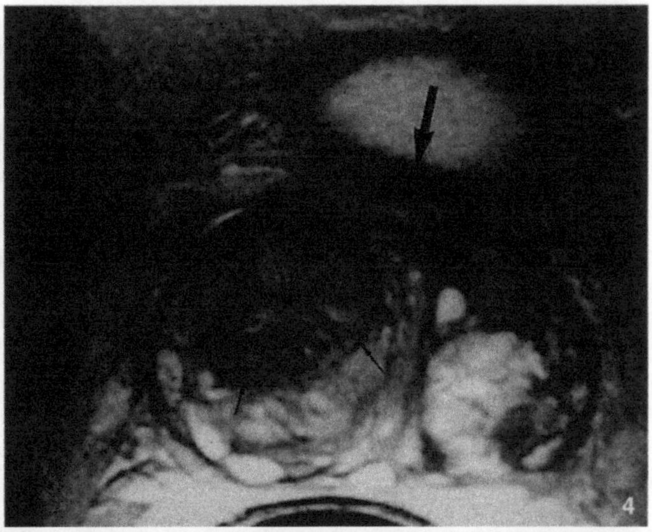

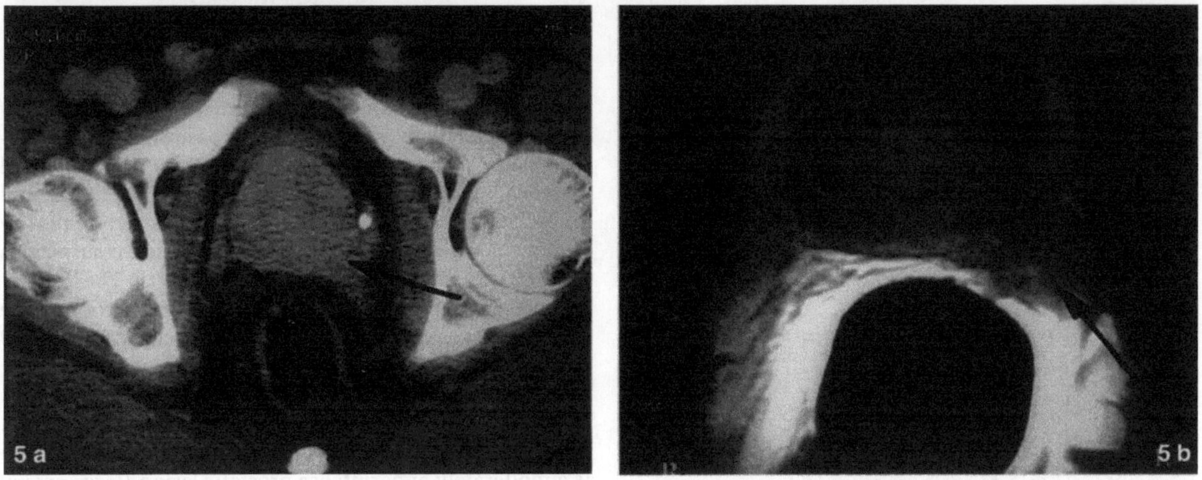

Fig. 36.3. Prostatic cancer on axial T2 MRI: presence of a slightly hyperintense lesion, more or less annular in shape, relatively well defined in the right part of the central zone of the prostate *(small arrows)*, non-specific appearances: in fact, the signal intensity of tumors of the central zone of the prostate raises several controversies, and the criteria of homogeneity are not absolute; the appearances in this patient are indistinguishable from an area of hyperplasia, the diagnosis having been made histologically

Fig. 36.4. Cancer of the prostate on MRI, axial T2 endorectal study: the lesion *(small arrows)* situated in the right part of the prostate is not causing any capsular break nor filling-in of the periprostatic fat and appears to be well differentiated from the prostatic glandular tissue itself. *Large arrow*: anterior fibrous muscular band

Fig. 36.5 a, b. Extracapsular spread from cancer of the prostate. **a** Post-contrast CT demonstrates the left postero-lateral spread, asymmetry of the periprostatic fat plane, irregularity of the posterior and lateral contours, invasion of the periprostatic fat adjacent to the gland itself *(arrow)*; **b** filling-in the left prostato-rectal angle and capsular break *(arrow)* confirmed by MRI using an endorectal surface coil in the same patient

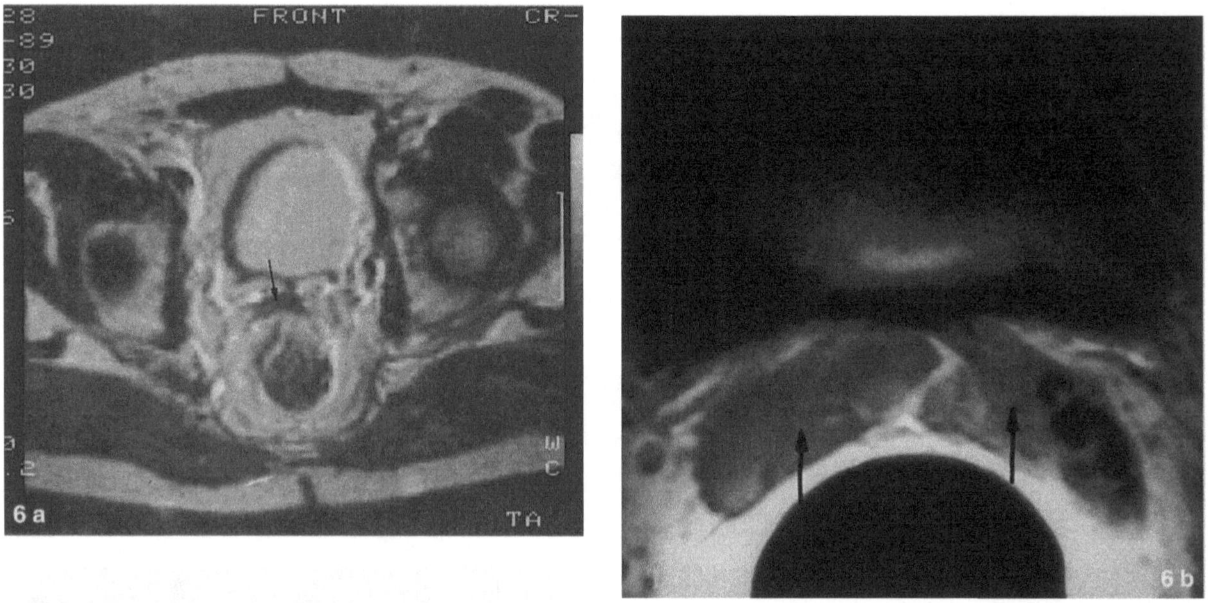

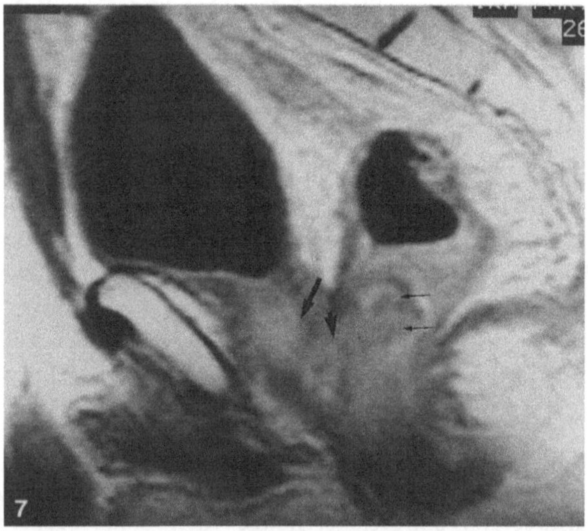

Fig. 36.6 a, b. Spread to the seminal vesicle on MRI. **a** Presence of a well defined asymmetrical hypointensity projecting medially at the level of the base of the right seminal vesicle *(arrow)*. This is not the symmetrical bilateral rounded hypointense appearance related to the deferential ampullae, the asymmetrical nature of this hypointensity within a normally hyperintense seminal vesicle is suspicious of neoplastic invasion (confirmed surgically). **b** The involvement of the right seminal vesicle and medial portion of the left seminal vesicle on T1-weighted endorectal MRI *(arrows)* (image courtesy of Dr A. Dana, Paris)

Fig. 36.7. Rectal spread from cancer of the prostate on MRI. Sagittal T1 MRI image following gadolinium injection. There is a moderately hyperintense prostatic lesion *(large arrow)* with loss of the interprostato-rectal fat planes *(arrow head)* and nodular endoluminal rectal spread *(small arrows)*, confirmed histologically

inability to assess the lymph node content and the relative frequency of lymph node metastases occurring in nodes of normal size. Classically, the physiological upper limit of normal is considered to be 15 mm for the external iliac, iliofemoral and common iliac nodes and 12 mm for the internal and obturator lymph nodes. Increasing this threshold level reduces the sensitivity but increases the specificity, whereas reducing the threshold increases the sensitivity but reduces the specificity. It should be remembered that tumor involvement is found in 90% of nodes over 15 mm, the other 10% being due to inflammatory, fibrotic or hyaline changes. Lymphography is indicated if the CT is normal.

MRI (figs 36.3-36.7)

Around 70% of prostatic cancers arise in the peripheral zone and a little less than 30% in the central or transitional zones although this latter figure is considered to be much less by many authors [7]. The majority of authors agree that the carcinomas arising in the peripheral zone appear as relatively hypointense zones on T2-weighted imaging probably related to a rich cellularity characterized by multiple, relatively compressed glandular elements. The poorly differentiated tumors are of higher signal intensity. This low signal intensity is non-specific and may be seen in glandular hyperplasia, particularly with a muscular predomi-

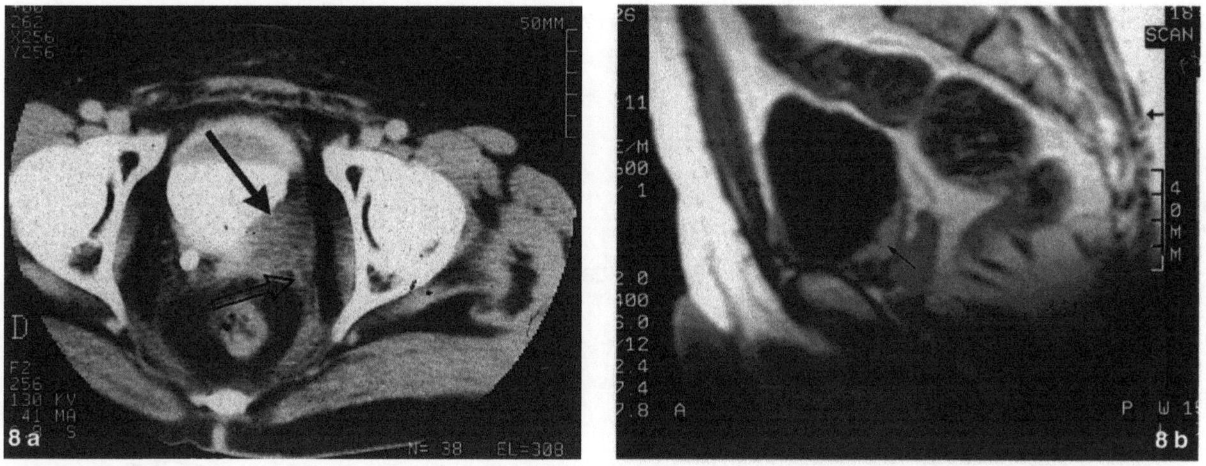

Fig. 36.8 a, b. Recurrent cancer of the prostate. **a** Locoregional recurrence on a post-contrast axial CT section with spread to the left postero-lateral aspect of the bladder *(black arrow)* and left ureteric obstruction *(hollow arrow)*; **b** local recurrence in the bladder wall, 22 months following resection of a prostate cancer: presence of irregular thickening localized to the postero-inferior part of the bladder, enhancing slightly on MRI following gadolinium injection *(arrow)*; sagittal post-contrast T1-weighted image

nance, or sometimes in an area of chronic prostatitis. The low signal intensity does not necessarily correspond to the neoplastic tissue and quite often appears even more extensive than the carcinoma itself resulting in overestimation of the tumor size. It should be recognized that a little less than 60% of lesions greater than 5 mm in diameter are identified by MRI [14]. Also there are other hypointense entities on T2-weighted imaging which can mimic a cancer. These include infarction, focal atrophy, corpora amylacea, recent post-biopsy hemorrhagic changes, post-biopsy fibrosis, or finally simply the smooth muscle around the ejaculatory ducts at the base of the prostate gland itself.

The tumor volume is therefore difficult to assess, often underestimated in extensive cancers and overestimated in small cancers [14].

The tumors of the central zone of the prostate are relatively rare, the signal intensity often varying from one tumor to another. They are always difficult to detect whether they are hyperplastic with an elevated and heterogeneous signal, or not hyperplastic with a low signal intensity (fig. 36.3). Capsular break, defining stage C of Whitemore and classically contraindicating prostatectomy, is also difficult to assess on MRI. Some authors even contest the anatomical existence of the capsule [1]. The capsule is extremely thin, no more than a dozen cell layers, which is indirectly and inconstantly demonstrated on T2-weighted imaging MRI. The hypointense line sometimes seen in the periphery of the gland on T2-weighted imaging is too clear for such a thin layer and therefore does not seem to correspond to it (fig. 36.1). One has to accept indirect signs (fig. 36.5) in order to judge the presence of capsular break. They include asymmetry of the contours, filling of the adjacent surrounding tissue or even extensive asymmetry of the levator muscles. MRI seems to be particularly inaccurate in the detection of microscopic capsular invasion constituting early stage C, but this does not represent a real contraindication to surgical treatment, nor does it constitute such a poor prognostic feature as infiltration of a seminal vesicle or lymph node invasion. The use of an endorectal surface coil (fig. 36.4) improves the demonstration of the fibrous capsule and its early infiltration, although the beneficial effects are still poorly defined, and the studies, as yet, have been too limited to be sufficiently significant. The coronal images obtained with an endorectal coil provide a better delineation of spread from the apical portion of the prostate gland.

Involvement of the seminal vesicles (figs 36.2 & 36.6) is an importantprognostic feature. Neoplastic invasion manifests, according to the majority of authors, as a focal or diffuse hypointensity on T2-weighted imaging, the T1 sequences only giving information on the size, shape and topography of the seminal vesicles. There are, however, a number of false positives, especially in the cases with a diffuse hypointensity of the seminal vesicles since there are other causes for global hypointensity: age of the patient greater than 75 years,

Table 36.6. Diagram showing the spread of prostatic cancers (Whitemore classification)

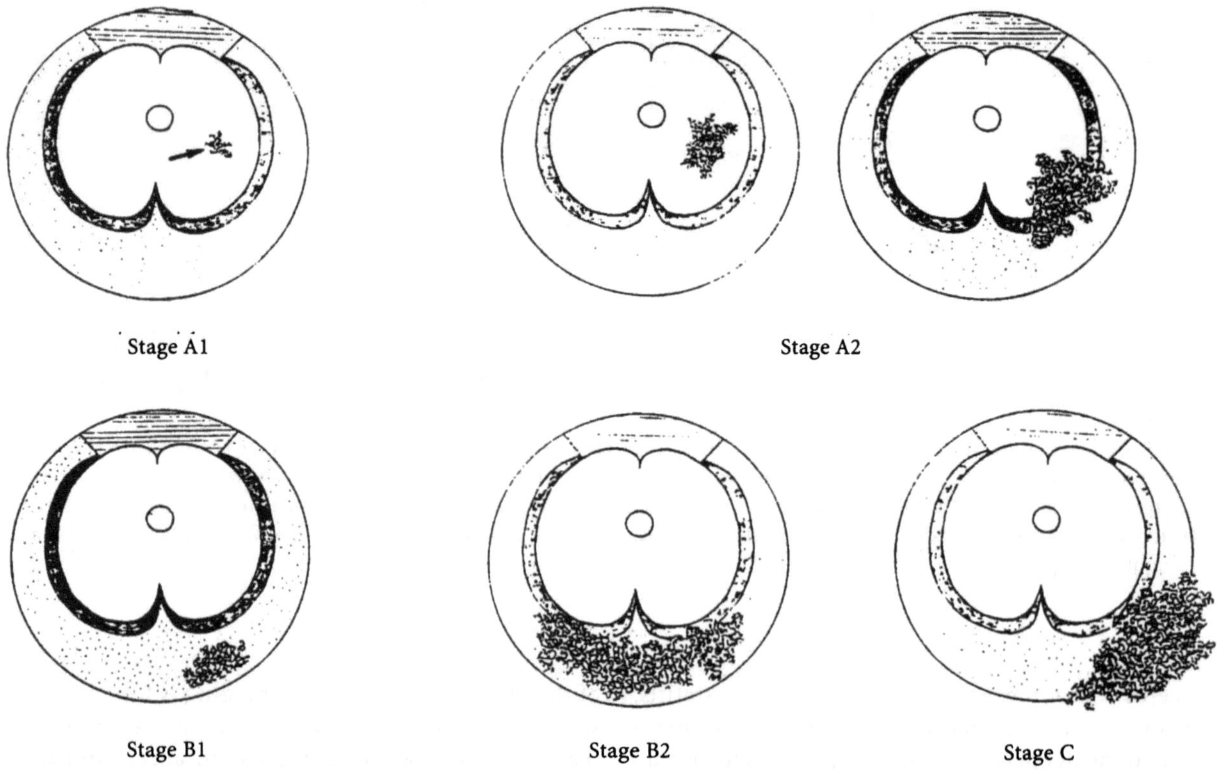

previous radiotherapy or surgical orchiectomy, a history of alcoholism. Many authors [14] consider that any focal hypointensity should be interpreted as being specific of invasion. It must be emphasized [7] that the differential diagnosis with the deferential ampullae (fig. 36.6 a) for hypointensities at the level of the medial part of the base of the seminal vesicle is difficult. The following features of the hypointensity would suggest the latter: well defined, bilateral, rounded symmetrical in a medial projection to the level of the base of the seminal vesicle. On the other hand, intervesico-deferential invasion will be missed by MRI.

Spread to the bladder and rectum is suspected if there is contiguity or loss of the interprostato-vesical or rectal fat, especially if there is an alteration in the signal of the wall or an endoluminal nodularity (fig. 36.7).

Spread along the fascial planes, particularly along the prerectal fascia may be demonstrated on MRI and is much more significant if it involves the frequent route of spread to the presacro-coccygeal planes without involving the rectum.

MRI provides no additional information concerning lymph node spread relative to the combination of CT, lymphography and guided biopsy. The exceptions are the rare cases of allergy to iodine in which MRI can be useful for identifying lymph node lesions without contrast injection. MRI is of limited value for staging following endoscopic resection or simple biopsy due to the inflammatory changes which are undifferentiable from the tumor signal. A recent hematoma or chronic fibrosis can only be recognized on the T1 sequence.

MRI (fig. 36.8) may differentiate fibrosis from recurrence during follow-up, mainly on the sagittal T2 sequence, the active lesions appearing of higher signal intensity than the residual fibrosis provided that there has been delay of at least 6 months following the completion of all treatment.

Conclusion [4, 12]

Following the detection of a lesion suspicious of prostatic cancer by rectal examination, the management approach depends on the clinical findings and a very accurate staging [4]:

- If, quite rarely, the patient is asymptomatic, with a limited B1 or B2 lesion, the tumor size and the life expectancy of the patient can be determined. When the patient is very old or weak, and the tumor volume is moderate, the therapeutic approach will be fairly conservative taking into account the slow evolution of the tumor. Simple clinical follow-up or hormone treatment will suffice.

- In all other cases, biopsy should be performed after PSA estimation and is usually associated with a transrectal ultrasound. The general urological investigation depends on the combination of the urography and ultrasound, provided that the lesion is large and the patient is not symptomatic.

- When the biopsy is positive, chest radiograph and scintigraphy will detect pulmonary and bone metastases, respectively. If these results are positive, further study to look for lymphatic involvement particularly by CT is of no value because this will not influence treatment. Conversely if the results are negative, treatment will depend on the CT examination, and this is indicated unless there is a very large volume prostatic tumor.

- When the biopsy is negative, a repeat ultrasound guided biopsy should be performed. This is also the case when there is discordance with elevated tumor markers prior to the biopsy, again requiring a repeat ultrasound guided biopsy. Alternatively, there is a concordance with the markers which are normal: the presence of a cancer is therefore excluded, and regular clinical follow-up is performed.

In the localized forms, without pulmonary or bone metastases, the choice of assessing lymphatic spread depends on the choice of treatment by the therapist:

If prostatectomy is faced, imaging does not have a role since lymph node sampling will be more accurate.

When radiotherapy is the preferred choice, assessment of lymph node spread would appear to be unnecessary according to the majority of authors when the tumor markers are normal, because the lymphatic chains are irradiated prophylactically; however, the lymph node irradiation is limited in terms of dose and volume.

Imaging is only indicated in the rare cases in whom the tumor markers are elevated or in the search for a contraindication to curative treatment.

In the case of clinically stage C disease, the risk and frequency of clinical and lymph node underevaluation make it essential to perform imaging, particularly CT. Positive CT will be an indication for hormonal treatment. In the presence of visceral metastases, imaging investigations should be kept to a minimum because they are only involved in the diagnosis and follow-up and do not influence the treatment choice.

Conversely, in the forms with significant locoregional spread even without any metastasis, the imaging assessment is indispensable to appreciate the urological sequelae and to guide treatment.

Therefore, CT is reserved for the assessment of spread of the clinically advanced stages (greater or equal to stage C), for the pretherapeutic assessment prior to any radiotherapy, and for the follow-up of patients treated by radiotherapy alone and to monitor recurrences.

The applications of MRI, although still under assessment, concern two areas: staging with follow-up for the detection of recurrences (fig. 36.8), and the differentiation of fibrosis and recurrence. Endorectal surface coils seem to have a significant advantage, with some teams achieving a staging accuracy approaching 90% [14].

The role of MRI remains limited due to the fact that the important elements influencing these surgical choices are directly visualized during the surgery itself and include the periprostatic venous plexus and particularly the periprostatic pelvic aponeuroses. Despite these limitations, MRI seems to be one of the most advanced techniques in the assessment of locoregional spread, particularly with the recent use of endorectal coils (figs 36.4-36.6), but its widespread use has been limited by cost and accessibility.

References

1. Ayala AG, Ro JY, Babaian R, Troncoso P, Grignon DJ (1989) The prostatic capsule: Does it exist? Its importance in the staging and treatment of prostatic carcinoma. Am J Surg Pathol 13; 1: 2
2. Bezzi M et al (1988) Prostatic carcinoma: staging with MR imaging at 1.5 T. Radiology 169: 339-345
3. Bochkish A, et al (1988) Magnetic resonance (MR) imaging of prostatic tumours, a comparison with X-ray CT and transrectal sonography (TRS). Eur J Radiol 8: 54-60
4. Buthiau D, Richard F, Misset JL (1992) Prostate. In: Buthiau D (ed) TDM et IRM Cliniques - Abdomen Pelvis. Frison-Roche, Paris, pp 313-324
5. Hricak H (1988) Imaging prostatic carcinoma. Radiology 169: 569-574
6. Kahn T, et al (1989) Prostatic carcinoma and benign prostatic hyperplasia: MR imaging with histopathologic correlation. Radiology 173: 847-851
7. Le Bastard E, Grenier N, Deminière C, Derws C, Ballager Ph, Le Guillou M, Broussin J (1990) Cancer localisé de la prostate: IRM et correlations histopathologiques. Rev Im Med 2: 523-530
8. Lee JKT, Marx MV (1989) Pelvis. In: Computed body tomography. Raven Press, New York, pp 862-866
9. Mukamel E, et al (1987) Value of computerized tomography scan and magnetic resonance imaging in staging

prostatic carcinoma: comparison with the clinical and histopathologic staging. Radiology 163: 840
10. Platt JF, et al (1987) Accuracy of CT in the staging of carcinoma of the prostate. AJR 149: 315-319
11. Poon PY, et al (1988) MRI of periprostatic venous plexus in staging of early prostatic carcinoma. Canad Assoc Radiol 39: 111-115
12. Richard F, Buthiau D (1990) Cancer de la prostate. Le Généraliste, 11: 4-13
13. Rifkin MD, Dahnert W, Kurtz AV (1990) State of the art: endorectal sonography of the prostate gland. AJR 154: 691-700
14. Rifkin MD, Piccoli CW (1992) Male pelvis and bladder. In: DD Stark, WG Bradley (eds) Magnetic resonance Imaging, 2nd edn. Mosby-Year Book, St Louis, pp 2023-2057
15. Salo JO, et al (1987) Computerized tomography and transrectal ultrasound in the assessment of local extension of prostatic cancer before radical retropubic prostatectomy. Radiology 164: 883-889
16. Schnall MD, et al (1989) Prostate: MR imaging with an endorectal surface coil. Radiology 172: 570-575
17. Vallancien G (1989) Dépistage précoce du cancer de la prostate. Séminaire d'Uro-néphrologie, 15ème série. Masson, Paris, pp 182-185
18. Walsh PC, Epstein JI (1987). Radical prostatectomy with preservation of sexual function. Impact on cancer control. Problem in Urology 1: 42-52

CHAPTER 37

Testicular tumors

Clinicians
E.-Ch. Antoine, J.-P. Droz

Radiologist
D. Buthiau

Tumors of the testicles, although relatively infrequent (less than 1% of cancers in males), are still used as a model for study in oncology, principally as a result of their curability by chemotherapy.

Epidemiologically, the current incidence of malignant testicular tumor seems to be increasing steadily, passing in the USA from 31/100,000 in 1962 to 38/100,000 in 1981 and thus constituting the commonest malignant tumor of the male population aged between 20 and 34 years [39]. In France, the incidence remains low (3 to 5 per 100,000) and essentially occurs between the ages of 20 and 40 years.

Germinal tumors represent more than 95% of malignant tumors of the testicle and can be divided into seminomatous germinal tumors (SGT, 40%) and non-seminomatous germinal tumors (NSGT, 60%): these latter lesions are divided histologically into embryonic carcinoma (15 to 20%), mature and immature teratomas (5%), choriocarcinoma (1.5%) and mixed tumors (40%) [9, 28].

Numerous histological classifications are currently used, according to their authors, with the contradictions and controversy surrounding the histo-oncogenesis of these tumors. These are summarized in table 37.1 remembering that the classification by Puch in 1976 is still the most commonly utilized.

Locoregional spread (principally the abdomino-aortic lymph nodes due to the embryological development of the testicular gland), and distant spread via the hematogenous or lymphatic route (pulmonary, hepatic, more rarely bone or brain) influence the prognosis and treatment strategies. The presence of a tumor mass with multiple metastatic lesions has currently become of foremost importance in determining prognosis and requires a rigorous pretherapeutic assessment by a combination of the biochemical markers and the degree of anatomical spread which is best appreciated by the modern imaging techniques (CT and MRI) [3]. In this respect, the TNM classification contributes little and is only rarely used. Numerous classifications are available based on the prognostic features; the classification of the Royal Marsden Hospital is still the most useful one, along with that from the Indiana University team (tables 37.2 & 37.3) [27].

However, other systems are employed. Many teams are now trying to coordinate their classifications in order to achieve a consensus opinion to allow a common evaluation of the treatment protocols. The Medical Research Council Study of Prognostic Factors in Non-Seminomatous Germ Cell Tumors has recently established a series of prognostic factors which are easily reproducible, the main points of which are summarized in table 37.4 [27].

Indications for CT and MRI

Although imaging testicular tumors is of virtually no help in determining the diagnosis, it has a predominant role for the initial staging (and consequently the choice of treatment), follow-up during and after treatment and ultimately in the appreciation of residual ost-chemotherapy masses.

Table 37.1. Histological classifications

Germinal tumors			
Pure forms			
Dixon and Moon 1932 (USA)	Mustofi and Price 1973 (USA)	WHO 1977	Puch 1976 (GB)
Seminoma	Seminoma: - typical - spermatocytic - anaplastic	Seminoma Spermatocytic seminoma	Seminoma Spermatocytic seminoma
Embryonic carcinoma	Embryonic carcinoma of the adult Polyembryoma	Embryonic carcinoma of the adult Polyembryoma	Undifferentiated malignant teratoma
Adult malignant teratoma	Teratoma: - mature - immature - Malignant degeneration - Juvenile embryonic carcinoma	Teratoma: - mature - immature - with malignant transformation Yolk sac tumor	Differentiated teratoma Yolk sac tumor
Choriocarcinoma	Choriocarcinoma	Choriocarcinoma	Choriocarcinoma
Mixed forms			
Teratocarcinoma	Embryonic carcinoma	Embryonic carcinoma	Teratoma of intermediate malignancy
Teratoma with embryonic carcinoma	with teratoma	with teratoma	
Mixed tumors	Mixed tumor of defined types	Mixed tumor of defined types	Mixed tumor of defined histological type Trophoblastic malignant teratomas (choriocarcinoma & other types)

Other tumors	
Tumors of the sexual cords and gonadal stroma	Leydig cell tumors Sertoli cell tumors Granulosa tumors
Tumors of lymphoid and hemopoietic tissues	Lymphoma Acute leukemia
Secondary tumors	Metastases (prostate++, lung, kidney, colon, stomach...)
Various tumors	Carcinoid tumor
Gonadal like tumors	Gonadoblastoma Other tumors

Initial staging

The anatomical works of Rouvière, as well as the anatomico-surgical correlations of Ray and Donohue have optimized the radiological methods for the evaluation of locoregional spread of testicular tumors [6, 35, 38].

Lymph node spread from germinal tumors of the testicle varies depending on the site of the initial tumor: inter-aortico-caval, precaval, latero-caval, right common iliac (fig. 37.1) and right external iliac nodes for a right testicular tumor; high latero-aortic nodes for a left testicular tumor.

In addition, lymphatic spread via the thoracic duct results in involvement of the left and sometimes right (10%) supraclavicular nodes in cases of anomalies of the lymphatic drainage system.

Table 37.2. Royal Marsden classification and prognostic factors

Stage I		Tumor confined to the testicle
	Stage IM	Elevated tumor markers following orchiectomy
Stage II		Abdominal lymphadenopathy
	Stage IIA	< 2 cm
	Stage IIB	2-5 cm
	Stage IIC	> 5 cm
Stage III		Supradiaphragmatic lymphadenopathy
	Stage III0	Diaphragmatic lymph nodes without abdominal lymph nodes
	Stage IIIA	Diaphragmatic with abdominal nodes < 2 cm
	Stage IIIB	Diaphragmatic with abdominal nodes 2-5 cm
	Stage IIIC	Diaphragmatic with abdominal nodes > 5 cm
Stage IV		Extralymphatic metastases
	L1	Lung less than 3 per field
	L2	Lung more than 3 per field but < 2 cm
	L3	Lung more than 3 per field but > 2 cm
	H+	Liver

Royal Marsden prognostic groups

Good prognosis	Poor prognosis
Stages IM, IIA, IIB, IIIA, IIIB, IV OABL1, IV OABL2 and IIC, IIIC, IVCL1, IVCL2 with markers < 1000 IU/l β HCG < 500 IU/l α FP	IVL3O, A, B, L IV H+ and IIC, IIIC, IVCL1, IVCL2 with elevated tumor markers

Table 37.3. Indiana University classification

Minimal disease	1	Isolated elevation of α FP and/or β HCG markers following orchiectomy
	2	Cervical nodes (with or without impalpable retroperitoneal nodes)
	3	Retroperitoneal nodes (impalpable but uneradicable)
	4	Minimal pulmonary disease: less than 5 metastases per lung field and diameter < 2 cm
Moderate disease	5	Isolated palpable abdominal mass
	6	Moderate pulmonary disease: i.e. 5 to 10 metastases per lung field and diameter < 3 cm or mediastinal mass < 50% ICT or isolated pulmonary nodule > 2 cm with or without impalpable retroperitoneal nodes
Advanced disease	7	Advanced pulmonary disease: mediastinal mass > 50% ICT or metastases > 10 per lung field or metastases > 3 cm and multiple with or without impalpable retroperitoneal nodes
	8	Advanced pulmonary disease + advanced abdominal disease (palpable abdominal mass)
	9	Hepatic, bone metastases or CNS involvement
Poor prognosis	7-8-9	

Hematogenous spread occurs later via the spermatic vein, inferior vena cava and thoracic duct. The organs most commonly involved are the lung, liver, bones, brain and adrenals. Abdomino-pelvic (fig. 37.1) and thoracic CT are routinely performed in practice for the assessment of disease extent.

The distinction between the assessment of the peritoneal region and other levels (thorax, brain) must be recognized.

There are no convincing arguments to suggest that MRI will replace CT at the moment in the assessment of disease extent.

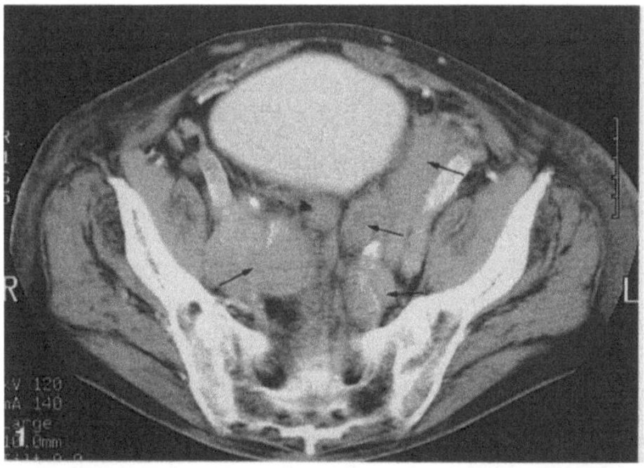

Fig. 37.1. Spread to the pelvic lymph nodes from a testicular germinal tumor on post-contrast CT: the tumor has spread to the right external, common iliac and obturator nodes and also to the contralateral obturator and iliac nodes *(arrows)*

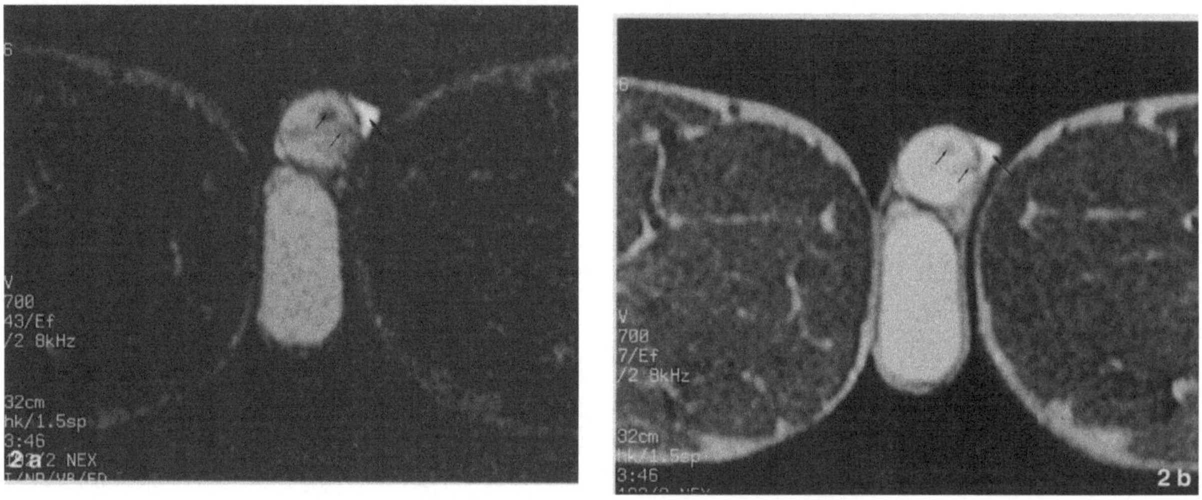

Fig. 37.2 a, b. Testicular seminoma on MRI, axial proton density sequence (**a**) and T2-weighted imaging (**b**). The study demonstrates a biloculated heterogeneous area *(small arrows)* arising in a hypoplastic left testicle. Note the small fluid collection in the serous membrane appearing as a high signal *(large arrow)*

Table 37.4. Poor prognostic factors (Medical Research Council Study)

1. Hepatic, bone, cerebral metastasis (es)	
2. Elevated biochemical markers: AFP>1000 kU/l and β HCG>1000 IU/l	
3. Mediastinal mass > 5 cm	
4. Pulmonary metastases > 20 in number	
5. Absence of embryonic carcinoma or fibrous tissue at initial histology	
No factors (67%)	3 year survival (93%)
Only one factor present (33%)	3 year survival (68%)

For the retroperitoneum

CT is indispensable although its limitations must be remembered.

The problem of assessing the nodes at the upper limit of physiological normality: if the upper limit of normal is taken to be less than or equal to 2 cm, there is a 20 to 30% false negative rate compared to surgery. Conversely, if nodes of less than 2 cm on CT are considered as pathological, there is a 20 to 25% false positive rate relative to surgery.

In the presence of large masses (greater than 5 cm), an ultrasound examination is sufficient, although in practice there is currently a preference for performing CT. This allows later comparisons to be made and helps in the routine search for dilatation of the urinary tract.

It must be mentioned that lymphography seems to have a role in no more than 10% of cases and that it is nowadays only performed in a few centers.

All the results of these complementary examinations are inseparable from the tumor markers following orchiectomy; a doubtful imaging appearance in the presence of elevated tumor markers is considered to be definitely pathological.

The indications for MRI in practice are very limited. Although this imaging modality has a high sensitivity, it is of limited specificity (fig. 37.2) and the main problem is, however, orchiectomy. The detection of infiltrative lymphomatous or leukemic tumor does not seem to be a real problem. It is possible that its role is limited to certain cases for the detection of thrombus in the inferior vena cava.

Assessment of other organs

Thoracic CT must be performed in the presence of clinically stage I or II disease (involvement of the lumbo-aortic lymph nodes). However, in a patient with stage II or the presence of metastatic disease, cranial CT would also seems to be necessary.

MRI only has a role in this context for the pretherapeutic neurosurgical evaluation of cerebral metastases.

Follow-up

Apart from the routine follow-up of treated patients for whom the type, periodicity and duration depends on the initial stage, follow-up using a combination of imaging and tumor markers is suggested as an alternative to routine retroperitoneal lymph adenectomy for stage I disease.

A number of retrospective and more recently prospective studies have been able to demonstrate that following routine lymphadenectomy, 80% of patients with apparent stage I disease (tumor limited to the testis, normal tumor markers and CT following orchiectomy) are true stage I (negative sampling), and 20% have lymph node involvement. Of these 20% false stage I cases initially operated on, a half will relapse, but almost all will be cured by 3 to 4 courses of chemotherapy with cis-platinum. However, of the 80% true initial stage I, 13% will develop hematogenous metastases and will also almost all be cured by subsequent chemotherapy. The remaining 70% will never relapse. Orchiectomy alone therefore is potentially capable of curing 70% of patients with stage I disease [7, 33, 34, 36, 37, 43].

Routine lymphadenectomy (even conservative) is not without morbidity, particularly the considerable risk of retrograde ejaculation (30 to 100% of cases depending on the surgical technique employed) [37]. This is why a number of teams nowadays recommend conservative follow-up only for stage I disease. The recurrence rate varies from 16 to 30%, the majority occurring within the first 6 months in the knowledge that late recurrences (after 3 years) are not uncommon. In terms of survival and because of the almost inevitable success of chemotherapy for recurrences, 98 to 99% of patients who are not operated on for stage I disease are alive and disease free after an average interval of 12 to 121 months depending on the series [36].

Some initial prognostic and particularly histological factors [34] are currently under study to identify the 15 to 30% of patients who will relapse and specifically adapt adjuvant treatment protocols for them. However, the essential elements for this policy of conservative follow-up at the moment depend on imaging and biochemistry (tumor markers) [17].

The periodicity and duration for this follow-up is not yet universally agreed but must take into account the psychological, economic and radiation protection consequences of this type of strategy [36, 43].

Evaluation of residual masses post-chemotherapy

Half of NSGTinitially present with disseminated disease necessitating complementary chemotherapy following initial orchiectomy. The protocols for this are currently adapted to the initial prognostic stage. Although the response rates are high (70 to 90%) [3, 49], the presence of residual masses following induction chemotherapy continues to be a common occurrence, varying between 20 to 89% of cases depending on the series. The treatment strategy relies heavily on the imaging and biochemistry. A progressive tumor mass, as well as persistently elevated markers indicate almost unequivocally a therapeutic failure. Subsequent chemotherapy treatment in the form of second line protocols, treatment intensification or alternating treatment remain the classically accepted treatment strategies [25, 46, 47].

In the more common situation of stable residual masses with normal tumor markers, there is no established consensus opinion. The large series using routine surgery have shown that the residual masses have consisted of necrotic fibrous tissue in 40 to 50% of cases, typically mature teratoma in 30% of cases which is considered as benign, and persistently active tumor tissue in the remaining 20 to 30% (see table 37.6).

The role of imaging in this clinical context is still disputed, and for many cases no specialized examination currently can determine the exact nature of the tissue [2, 8, 20, 21, 31, 40, 45].

Some authors have, however, attempted to establish predictive models based partly on the imaging and partly on the initial histobiological parameters.

Table 37.5. Histology of routine lymphadenectomy specimens following complete biochemical (normal markers) and radiological (normal CT) remission

Team	Protocols	Nbr pts	Necrotic tissue	Mature teratoma (%)	Viable tumor tissue
Fossa [13]	BEP	37	25	11-(30%)	1
Toner [45]	with CDDP	22	17	3-(14%)	2
Gelderman[15, 16]	PVB	5	3	2-(40%)	0
Bracken[4]	with CDDP	22	14	3-(14%)	5

The initial tumor size (greater than or less than 3 cm), the degree of tumor reduction following treatment (less than or greater than 90%), the size of the residual masses (less than 1.5 or 2 cm), as well as the initial histology (presence of a teratomatous component in the testicular tumor) and the initial level of the biochemical markers constitute, for these authors, prognostic indices which are capable of predicting the histological nature of residual masses and particularly the presence or absence of necrotic fibrous tissue or mature teratomas. These probability computation graphs (nomograms) can avoid routine surgical exploration which is known to be of no value in more than 50% of these patients [13, 14, 20, 45].

Therefore, by differentiating seminomas from non-seminomas, the following protocol is suggested:

- for seminomas: follow-up by CT is necessary following chemotherapy, sometimes for many months; if the residual lesion is less than 3 cm, follow-up will be adequate; if the stable lesion is greater than 3 cm, biopsy is also necessary:
- for non-seminomas: if the lesions are greater than or equal to 3 cm before chemotherapy, operation is always necessary following chemotherapy. If the lesion is equal to or less than 3 cm before chemotherapy, operation is only necessary if the tumor regression is less than 90%.

No technique can differentiate with certainty necrosis from active tumor. MRI is undoubtedly the most advanced technique but is not absolutely reliable, even using the strongly T2-weighted sequences or following the injection of gadolinium.

These models have yet to be validated, contested by the majority of teams and appear unreliable compared to the series using surgery from the beginning in patients in complete clinico-biochemical remission with CT scans considered to be normal (table 37.5). In fact, routine lymph node sampling in such patients detected viable tissue, either tumor (5 to 23%) or teratoma (14 to 40%), and no more than a third of these patients had simply necrotic fibrous tissue on histology.

The avoidance of surgery in the presence of residual post- chemotherapy masses with normal tumor markers remains a fundamental dilemma: imaging is currently unable to make the decision.

Signs [26]

The assessment of lymphatic and hematogenous spread by CT (and MRI) is identical to that for any other cancer.

On MRI, the examination of the scrotum in three planes, particularly coronal, demonstrates on T2-weighted imaging any tumor lesion in the form of a hypointense mass relative to the healthy parenchyma. The features suggestive of the tumor type are:

- the large size and heterogeneity, more common in the case of embryonic carcinoma or mixed type;
- the more homogeneous and hypointense appearance of the seminoma;
- generally, one should no longer distinguish various histological forms since in reality all tumors are to some extent mixed.

The assessment of local spread on MRI is of theoretical interest:

- to the rete testis or epididymis, replacement by tissue with the signal intensity of tumor;
- to the albuginea, in the form of interruption or loss of its thin hypointense line;
- to the spermatic cord which appears enlarged, in continuity with the testicular mass, with loss of the physiological fat.

Conclusion (table 37.6)

For diagnostic purposes, testicular CT and MRI have very little value in practice.

CT (and to a variable extent MRI) have a role in routine daily practice for staging of testicular tumors.

Table 37.6. Scrotal enlargement of presumed tumor origin: diagnostic strategy (from B. Martin [26])

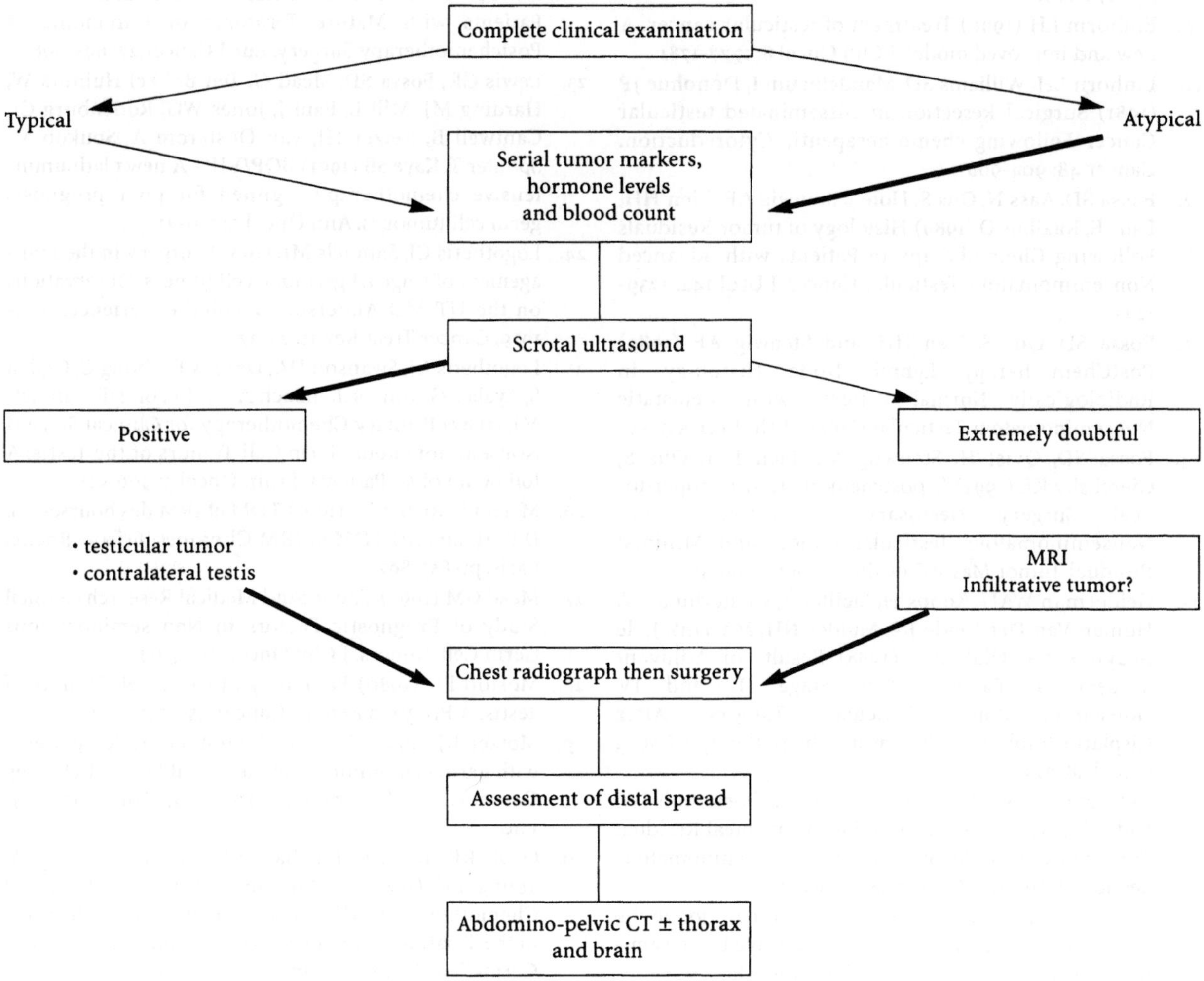

Although it is often indispensable for the assessment, CT (like MRI) is in no way specific (for example the evaluation of lymph node size rather than contents) and is inseparable from the tumor markers and treatment.

References

1. Bajorin DF, Geller NL, Weisen SF, Bosl GJ (1991) Two-drug Therapy in Patients with metastatic Germ Cell Tumors. Cancer 67: 28-32
2. Bassoulet J, Timbal Y, Garretta L (1986) Masses rétropéritonéales résiduelles des tumeurs germinales non seminomateuses du testicule après chimiothérapie. Ann Radiol 29: 607-613
3. Birch R (1986). Prognostic factors for favorable outcome in disseminated germ cell tumors. J Clin Oncol 4: 400-407
4. Bracken BB, Johnson DE, Frazier H (1983) The role of surgery following chemotherapy in stage II germ cell neoplasms. J Urol 129: 39-43
5. Dearnaley DP, Horwich A, A'Hern R, Nicholls J, Jay G, Hendry WF, Peckham MJ (1991) Combination Chemotherapy with Bleomycin, Etoposide and Cisplatin (BEP) for Metastatic Testicular Teratoma: Long-term Follow-up. Eur J Cancer 27: 684-691
6. Donohue JP (1982) Distribution of nodal metastases in non seminomatous testis cancer. J Urol 128: 315-320
7. Donohue JP, Rowland RG (1984). The role of surgery in advanced testicular cancer. Cance, 54: 2716-2721
8. Donohue JP, Rowland RG, Kopecky K (1987) Correlation of computerized tomographic changes and histological findings in 80 patients having radical retroperitoneal lymph node dissection after chemotherapy for testis cancer. J Urol137: 1176-1179
9. Einhorn LH (1989) Classifications of testicular germ cell tumors. In: V De Vita (ed) Cancer Principles and

Practice of Oncology, 3rd edn. Lippincott, Philadelphia, pp 1071-1098
10. Einhorm LH (1990) Treatment of testicular cancer: A new and improved model. J Clin Oncol 8: 1777-1781
11. Einhorn LH, Williams SD, Mandelbaum I, Donohue JP (1981) Surgical Resection in Disseminated testicular Cancer Following chemotherapeutic Cytoreduction. Cancer 48: 904-908
12. Fossa SD, Aass N, Ous S, Hoie J, Stenwig AE, Lien HH, Paus E, Kaalhus O (1989) Histology of tumor Residuals Following Chemotherapy in Patients with advanced Nonseminomatous Testicular Cancer. J Urol 142: 1239-1242
13. Fossa SD, Ous S, Lien HH, and Stenwig AE (1989) PostChemotherapy Lymph Node Histology in Radiologically Normal Patients with Metastatic Nonseminomatous Testicular Cancer. J Urol 141: 557-559
14. Fossa SD, Qvist H, Stenwiig AE, Lien HH, Ous S, Gierchsky KE (1992) Is postchemotherapy retroperitoneal Surgery Necessary in Patients with Nonseminomatous Testicular Cancer and Minimal Residual Tumor Masses? J Clin Oncol 10: 569-573
15. Gelderman WAH, Koops H, Sleijfer T, Oosterhuis JW, Homan Van Der Heide JN, Mulder NH, Marrink J, de Bruyn HWA, Oldhoff J (1988) Results of Adjuvant Surgery in Patients With Stage III and IV Nonseminomatous Testicular Tumors After CisplatinVinblastine-Bleomycin Chemotherapy. J Surg Oncol 38: 227-232
16. Gelderman WAH, Koops HS, Sleijfer DT, Oosterhuis JW, Oldhoff J (1986) Treatment of Retroperitoneal Residual Tumor After PVB Chemotherapy of Non seminomatous Testicular Tumors. Cancer 58: 1418-1421
17. Gressler VH, Levine LA et al (1990) A third option in the management of patients with clinical stage I non seminomatous germ cell tumors? J Clin Oncol 8: 4-8
18. Harstrick A, Schmoll HJ, Kohne-Wompner CH, Bergmann L, Lammers U, Hohnloser J, Dolken G, Reichhardt P, Siegert W, Natt F, Ràth U, Wilke H, Poliwoda H (1991) Cisplatin, Etoposide, ifosfamide, vincristine and bleomycin combination Chemotherapy for Far Advanced Testicular Carcinoma. Ann Oncol 2: 197-202
19. Hendry WF, Goldstraw P, Peckham MJ (1986) Excision of residual masses after chemotherapy for non seminomatous germ cell tumours of the testis. In: NG Jones et al (eds) Advances in the biosciences 55, Germ Cell Tumours. Pergamon Press, Oxford
20. Herr HW. Toner GC, Geller NL, Bosl GJ (1991) Patient Selection for Retroperitoneal Lymph Node Dissection after Chemotherapy for Non seminomatous Germ Cell Tumors. Eur Urol 19: 1-5
21. Husband JE, Howkes DJ, Peckham MJ (1982) CT estimation of mean attenuation values and volume in testicular tumours: a comparison with surgical and histologic findings. Radiology, 144, 553-558
22. Jansen RLH, Sylvester R, Sleyfer DT, Ten Bokkel WW, Kaye SB, Jones WG, Keiser J, Van Oosterom AT, Meyer S, Vendrik CPJ, de Pauw M, Stoter G (1991) Long-term follow-up of Non-Seminomatous Testicular Cancer Patients with Mature Teratoma or Carcinoma at Postchemotherapy Surgery. Eur J Cancer,27: 695-698
23. Lewis CR, Fossa SD, Mead G, Ten Bokkel Huinink W, Harding MJ, Mill L, Paul J, Jones WG, Rodenburg CJ, Cantwell B, Keizer HJ, Van Oosterom A, Soukop M, Splinter T, Kaye SB (1991) BOP/VIP - A new platinumintensive chemotherapy regimen for poor prognosis germ cell tumours. Ann Oncol 2: 203-211
24. Logothetis CJ, Samuels ML (1984) Surgery in the management of stage III germinal cell tumors: Observations on the UT MD Anderson Hospital experience, 1971-1979. Cancer Treat Rev 11: 27-37
25. Logothetis CJ, Swanson DA, Dexcus F, Chong C, Ogden S, Ayala AG, Von Eschenbach AC, Johnson DE, Samuels ML (1987) Primary Chemotherapy for Clinical Stage II Nonseminomatous Germ Cell Tumors of the Testis: A follow-up of 50 Patients. J Clin Oncol 5: 906-911
26. Martin B, Richard F (1991) TDM et IRM des bourses. In: D Buthiau (ed) TDM et IRM Cliniques. Frison-Roche, Paris, pp 853-862
27. Mead GM (1992) The second Medical Research Council Study of Prognostic Factors in Non seminomatous Germ Cell Tumors. J Clin Oncol 10: 85-94
28. Mostofi FK (1980) Pathology of Germ cell Tumors of Testis: A Progress Report. Cancer 45: 1735-1754
29. Motzer RJ (1991) Salvage chemotherapy for patients with germ cell tumors. The Memorial Sloan- Kettering Cancer Center Experience (1979-1989) Cancer 67: 1305-1310
30. Ozols RF, Ihde DC, Lineban WM, Jacob J, Ostchega Y, Young RC (1988) A Randomized Trial of Standard Chemotherapy vs High-Dose Chemotherapy Regimen in the Treatment of poor Prognosis Non seminomatous Germ-Cell Tumors. J Clin Oncol 6: 1031-1040
31. Peckham M (1988) Testicular Cancer. Reviews in Oncology I N°l (in Acta Oncologica Vol.27, Fasc 4): 439-453
32. Pizzocaro G, Salvioni R, Pasi M, Zanoni F, Milani A, Pilotti S, Monfardini S (1985) Early Resection of Residual Tumor following Cisplatin, vinblastine, Bleomycin Combination Chemotherapy In Stage III and Bulky Stage II Non seminomatous testicular Cancer. Cancer 56: 249-255
33. Pizzocaro G, Zanoni F, et al (1986) Orchidectomy alone in clinical stage I non seminomatous testis cancer: A critical appraisal. J Clin Oncol 4: 35-40
34. Pont P, Holtl W, et al (1990) Risk-adapted treatment choice in stage I non-seminomatous testicular germ cell cancer by regarding vascular invasion in the primary tumor: a prospective trial. J Clin Oncol 8: 16-20
35. Ray B, Hadju SI (1974) Distribution of retroperitoneal lymph nodes metastases in testicular germinal tumors. Cancer 33: 340-347
36. Read G, Stenning SP, et al (1992) Medical Research Council Prospective study of Surveillance for Stage I Testicular teratoma. J Clin Oncol 10: 1762-1768

37. Richie JP (1990) Clinical stage I testicular cancer: The role of modifled retroperitoneal lymphadenoctomy. J Urol144: 1160-1163
38. Rouvière H (1932) Anatomie des lymphatiques de l'Homme. Masson, Paris, pp 389-392
39. Senturia YD (1987) The epidemiology of testicular cancer. Br J Urol 70: 285
40. Stomper PC, Jochelson MS, Garnick MB, Richie JP (1985) Residual Abdominal Masses after Chemotherapy for Nonseminomatous Testicular Cancer: Correlation of CT and Histology. AJR 145: 743-746
41. Stoter G, Koopman A, Vendrik CPJ, Struyvenberg A, Sleyfer D, Willemse PHB, Koops HS, Van Oosterom AT, Ten Bokkel Huinink WW, Pinedo HM (1989) Ten year survival and late sequelae in testicular cancer Patients treated with Cisplatin, Vinblastine, and Bleomycin. J Clin Oncol 7: 1099-1104
42. Stoter G, Vendrik CPJ, Struyvenberg A, Sleyfer DT, Vriesendorp R, Koops HS, Van Opsterom AT, TenBokkel Huinink WW, Pinedo HM (1984) Five-year Survival of Patients with Disseminatod Non-seminomatous testicular Cancer Treated with cisplatin, Vinblastine, and Bleomycin. Cancer 54: 1521-1524
43. Sturgeon JFG, Jewett MAS, et al (1992) Surveillance after orchidectomy for patients with clinical stage I non seminomatous testis tumors. J Clin Oncol 10:564-568
44. Tait D, Peckham MJ, Hendry WF, Goldstraw P (1984) Post-chemotherapy surgery in advanced non-seminomatous germ-cell testicular tumours: The significance of histology with particular reference to differentiated (mature) teratoma. Br J Cancer 50: 601-609
45. Toner GC, Panicek DM, Heelan RT, Geller NL, Lin SY, Bajorin D, Motzer RJ, Scher HI, Herr HW, Morse MJ, Fair WR, Sogani PC, Whitmore WF, McCormack PM, Bains MS, Martini N, Bosl GJ (1990) Adjunctive Surgery After Chemotherapy for Non seminomatous Germ Cell Tumors: Recommendations for Patient Selection. J Clin Oncol 8: 1683-1694
46. Vugrin D, Whitmore WF (1985) The Role of Chemotherapy and Surgery in the Treatment of Retroperitoneal Metastases in Advanced nonseminomatous Testis Cancer. Cancer 55: 1874-1878
47. Vugrin D, Whitmore WF, Sogani PC, Bains M, Herr HW, Golbey RB (1981) Combined Chemotherapy and Surgery in Treatment of Advanced Germ-Cell Tumors. Cancer 47: 2228-2231
48. Wettlaufer JN, Feiner AS, Robinson WA (1984) Vincristine, Cisplatin, and Bleomycin with Surgery in the Management of Advanced Metastatic Nonseminomatous Testis Tumors. Cancer 53: 203-209
49. Williams SD, Birch R, Einhorn LH, Irwin L, Greco FA, Loehrer PJ (1987). Treatment of Disseminated Germ-Cell Tumors with Cisplatin, Bleomycin, and either Vinblastine or Etoposide. N Engl J Med316: 1435-1440

CHAPTER 38

Hodgkin's disease and non-Hodgkin's lymphomas

Clinicians
J.-M. Cosset, M. Gil-Delgado, J.-C. Piette, T. Petit, E. Vuillemin

Radiologist
D. Buthiau

The Hodgkin (HD) and non-Hodgkin's lymphomas (NHL) can involve any lymph node chain and any organ. The importance of staging is related to the fact that the prognosis and treatment strategy depend on the extent of the disease and size of the tumor mass.

It is important to perform a selection of complementary examinations for the diagnosis, staging, and follow-up of lymphomas. This applies both to Hodgkin's disease, which theoretically progresses in a predictable fashion with the possibility of locoregional treatment, and non-Hodgkin's lymphomas, which are true systemic diseases.

CT and MRI provide essential information for the assessment of spread, tumor volume, follow-up and the appreciation of regions or organs which are often otherwise difficult to evaluate (brain, retroperitoneum, pelvis).

Lymphoma of lymph nodes and spleen

Assessment of abdominal lymph node involvement

Nowadays the investigation of abdomino-pelvic lymph nodes is achieved using lymphography for Hodgkin's disease, and ultrasound and CT or MRI for Hodgkin's disease and the other lymphomas.

Diagnosis

CT can play an essential role in the diagnosis and allows the performance of guided biopsy of a deep mass, these biopsies also being possible under fluoroscopic or ultrasound control.

Initial staging

CT

CT can simultaneously evaluate the abdominal viscera and all the abdomino-pelvic lymphatic chains. It is also more accurate than lymphography for the internal iliac and celio-mesenteric lymph node chains which are not assessed by the latter examinations; the lymphatic drainage of the foot does not include these lymph nodes in the physiological state, and they are only visible if there is obstruction with reflux.

Although ultrasound can also study all these lymph node chains, it is limited by certain technical constraints: obesity, bowel artefacts.

Like ultrasound, CT is limited in its assessment of the lymph node structure, providing only information on the size (apart from necrosis) unlike lymphography. True lymphatic hyperplasia may turn out to be benign, and 5 to 8% of involved nodes may be of normal size in Hodgkin's disease.

Therefore, lymphography is still indicated in HD and is complementary to CT since the mesenteric nodes are rarely involved. For NHL, CT is the only examination required given the frequency (more than half the cases) of celio-mesenteric involvement (fig. 38.1) which is missed by lymphography.

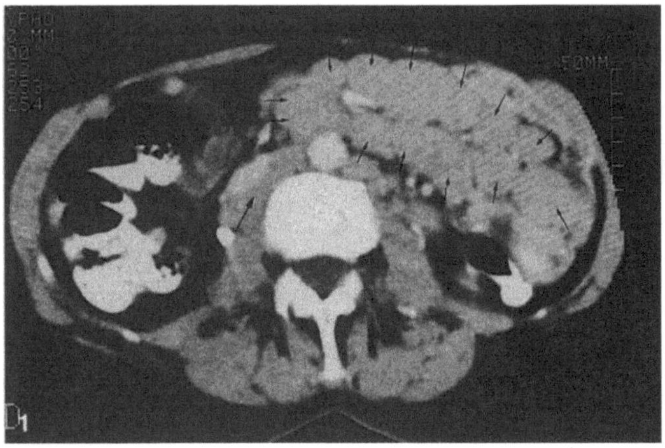

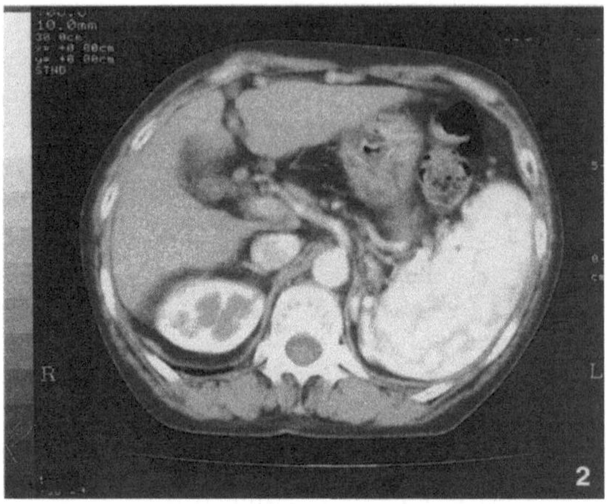

Fig. 38.1. Multiple mesenteric lymphadenopathies in non-Hodgkin lymphoma on post-contrast CT. There are multiple enlarged lymph nodes of variable confluence *(small arrows)* bordering the root of the mesentery. Note the associated retroperitoneal nodes and, in particular, the inter-aortico-caval and retrocaval nodes *(medium arrow)* compressing the inferior vena cava and displacing it away from the spine. There is also compression of the right ureter which is deviated laterally

Fig. 38.2. Lymphomatous splenomegaly with a splenic index of 1.3 on post-contrast CT (helical mode). Note the heterogeneous intrasplenic appearances corresponding to the physiological splenic filling-in at this early stage: these appearances are differentiated from a lymphomatous infiltrate by their transient nature and are concomitant with the injection of contrast

MRI

Generally, the distinction between lymph nodes and vessels, or even parenchymal or muscle structures, is facilitated by MRI. This is particularly true for the iliac and mesenteric lymph node chains. Conversely, like ultrasound and CT, it is limited in the analysis of the internal lymph node structure, the signal intensities on T1- or T2-weighted imaging of a pathological lymph node overlap with those of the normal node. This examination does not provide any added specificity. In addition, certain lymph node chains are difficult to evaluate, for example the vascular pedicle chains (hepatic, but particularly splenic due to the similarity in signal intensity between the node and spleen).

The role of MRI would therefore seem to be limited for the assessment of lymphomas, having no significant advantage over CT.

Assessment of splenic involvement [6, 11]

CT (figs 23.2, 23.17, chap. 23; "Tumors of the liver")

CT is a sensitive but non-specific technique which complements ultrasound and analyzes better the parenchyma and splenic volume (fig. 38.2). The volume is defined by the splenic index which corresponds to the product of the three diameters of the spleen (length, width and thickness); the normal splenic index varies between 150 and 450 cm^3. However, it is of limited value for the demonstration of small subcentimeter lesions. However, micronodules of few millimiters in diameter are not exceptional in Hodgkin's disease and used to be well demonstrated on the routine splenectomy specimens over many years.

MRI

Its specificity is no greater than 50% , with a higher sensitivity of between 80 and 90%, improved by the use of a paramagnetic contrast agent. However, MRI does not appear to have a role in the assessment of splenic involvement in current practice [6].

Assessment of mediastinal lymph node involvement

CT

None of the thoracic lymph node chains escape assessment by CT which demonstrates 30 to 40%

additional lesions relative to classical radiography. It is of particular value for the lymph nodes in the aorto-pulmonary window (left paratracheal), Barety's area (right paratracheal), internal mammary and subcarinal, juxtacardiac, para-aortic or esophageal at the posterior inframediastinal level (also called retrocrural) [12]. This latter point is essential because the demonstration of inferior mediastinal lymph node involvement posterior to the crura of the diaphragm determines the necessity of inferior mediastinal irradiation and therefore includes the heart.

CT assessment is excellent for defining the mediastinal irradiation fields and accurately localizes possible associated lesions: extension by contiguous spread (sternum, anterior thoracic wall, lung, spine), the demonstration of which is important in Hodgkin's disease because it may alter the radiotherapy technique. CT will also look for signs of vascular compression, particularly the superior vena cava, with the presence of a thrombus, or spread to the wall of the vessel. The demonstration of calcification is non-specific but may give information on possible displacement of anatomical structures.

CT should, therefore, be routinely used for the initial assessment of thoracic lymphatic involvement, to define the size of the lymph node masses and degree of compression both in Hodgkin's and non-Hodgkin's lymphoma. This technique has the capability of distinguishing, chain by chain, the lymph node limits and the early microlymphadenopathies.

MRI

See above for abdominal lymphatic assessment.

Assessment of cervical and peripheral lymph node involvement

CT

This evaluation is essentially clinical, CT only having a few indications in very specific circumstances, for example the detection of contiguous involvement.

MRI

This has no recognized role at this time.

Therefore, evaluation of spread to the deep lymph nodes by lymphoma is essentially achieved by CT: both for the therapeutic assessment and follow-up. This technique can also guide percutaneous diagnostic biopsy for lesions which are inaccessible to fluoroscopy or ultrasound.

Extranodal lymphomatous involvement [12]

The demonstration of extranodal disease in Hodgkin's disease determines the treatment, whether this is hepatic, pulmonary, bone marrow, bone involvement (the latter guided by the clinical signs).

The treatment of the non-Hodgkin's lymphomas is less dependent on the degree of spread, the search for extranodal lesions being determined by the clinical and biochemical signs.

The great advantage of CT is its ability to obtain in a single examination an assessment of nodal and extranodal spread in the abdomen and thorax.

Assessment of lesions of the central nervous system

Unlike primary lesions, secondary lymphomas more commonly involve the meninges than the brain.

Intracranial lesions

CT

CT is the key examination for the detection of intracranial lymphomatous lesions in the presence of any neurological signs, or during the course of certain forms of lymphoma (e.g. Burkitt's lymphoma). The frequency of infratentorial lesions is a justification for performing millimetric sections at this level.

MRI

This becomes indispensable when the CT examination is normal in a patient presenting with clinical neurological signs, or for the detection of any complications related to the disease or treatment.

Ocular involvement is considered separately and is detected by clinical examination or orbital ultrasound. These may be complemented by axial and coronal CT for the detection of chiasmatic intracranial lesions. It should be remembered that orbital ultrasound forms part of the routine investigation of primary lymphoma of the CNS and the presence of an ocular lymphoma necessitates regular follow-up of the CNS. MRI, using specific surface coils, can be complementary and replace the ultrasound and CT examinations.

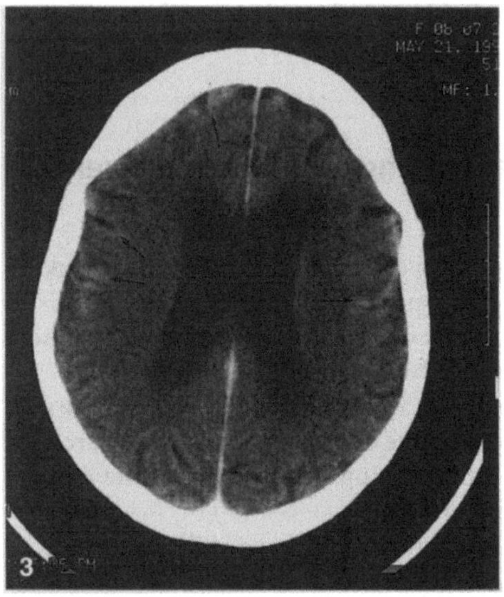

Fig. 38.3. Lymphomatous meningeal spread on post-contrast CT: the examination demonstrates enhancement of the subarachnoid meningeal planes over the convexity *(arrows)*, gyriform appearance and multiple localizations

Meningeal involvement (fig. 38.3)

Meningeal involvement is often only apparent by analysis of the CSF, and the radiological investigation does not, therefore, replace lumbar puncture.

CT is only rarely involved in the search for bone, paraspinal or epidural involvement, MRI having a good specificity (65 to 70% of cases) [6] and an excellent sensitivity (greater than of equal to 90%). As a result, MRI replaces CT, particularly due to its ability to perform sagittal sections, which has obviated the need to perform myelography, and is able to search for possible recurrence following radiotherapy or surgery (on heavily T2-weighted images).

Hepatic involvement

The secondary forms are the commonest, often associated with splenic involvement in HD, the diagnosis being histological. However, biopsies are rarely necessary because hepatic lesions are generally associated with other extranodal tumor localizations, particularly the bone marrow, and documentation of these lesions no longer alters the staging or treatment.

CT

Its specificity is acceptable, in the order of 80%, and is superior to ultrasound [12]. However, its sensitivity is poor and does not exceed 60%. The use of specific contrast agents for the reticulo-endothelial system is rare and not without risk. Despite these limitations, CT is currently routinely used.

MRI

Investigation using T2-weighted sequences would result in a higher sensitivity than CT, but this has still to be confirmed.

Thoracic involvement [1, 9]

CT

In the same single examination, CT evaluates lymph node spread, parenchymal, tracheo-bronchial, contiguous pericardial, chest wall, diaphragmatic and thymic involvement. It helps differentiate the different mechanisms of pulmonary involvement (by contiguous spread or by the hematogenous or lymphatic route). CT also can demonstrate infiltrative or compressive spread to the thymus, trachea, esophagus, and pleural involvement adjacent to an effusion, the pleural localizations and chest wall spread already having been suspected from the routine radiograph. It delineates much more clearly, particularly using fine sections with a millimeter thick, parenchymal nodules or infiltrates, or lesions of the diaphragm, but is limited in the assessment of possible fistulae or breast lesions. Ultrasound remains a key investigation for determining cardiovascular spread, CT being able to appreciate venous compression or even demonstrate iatrogenic lesions such as post-radiation thickening of the aortic wall. Rapid CT (cine CT) is particularly accurate for the visualization of the rare cardiac lesions.

MRI

This is only indicated in certain specific cases, principally for the parietal diaphragmatic spread and the rare cardiac lesion. Some authors [8] advocate performing the examination routinely in the initial staging when there is clinical doubt. MRI can also monitor the progress of these lesions.

Other extranodal sites

See table 38.1 on next page.

Assessment of the therapeutic response, follow-up and detection of recurrence

Follow-up of lymphatic involvement

This can be followed by a plain abdominal radiograph which can monitor previous lymphography, and by ultrasound, which is limited in cases of moderate size and/or deep lesions.

Table 38.2. Decisional algorithm for the investigation of lymphomas (Hodgkin's or non-Hodgkin's lymphoma)

1) Diagnosis
Histological examination of lymph nodes or viscera (-immuno- and possibly histochemical or even molecular genetic studies): role of CT for guiding biopsy of deep lesions.

2) Minimum obligatory investigation for spread and progress
  a) biochemical examinations
    - blood count with platelets
    - assessment of inflammation (sedimentation rate, iron level, C-reactive protein, protein electrophoresis)
    - investigation of liver (transaminase, alkaline phosphatase, bilirubin)
    - LDH
    - HIV serology
  b) radiological examinations
    - chest x-rays (frontal and lateral)
    - CT of the thorax and abdomen
    - lymphography (Hodgkin's disease).
  c) bone marrow biopsy

3) Assessment of spread dependent on the clinical findings: CT indication as a function of each specific regional involvement.

4) Follow-up of residual masses: CT and sometimes MRI

CT is the essential examination for the follow-up of this type of abdominal involvement. It is sometimes used in combination with post-lymphographic plain abdominal radiograph (HD) as it accurately assesses the progress of lymph node masses which can be measured and guide the eventual treatment. Due to its lack of specificity in the differentiation between residual tumor and fibrosis, the only criterion is follow-up by repeated examinations.

MRI is a more advanced technique for making this differentiation, and the majority of authors give an accuracy rate of 80 to 90% [9] for this technique in distinguishing an active hyperintense zone on T2-weighted imaging from a low signal area of fibrosis. Gadolinium is only of less consistent value. MRI is indicated if there is doubt on the CT after a period of time following completion of all treatment.

Thoracic lymphatic involvement: after radiotherapy, CT can demonstrate a recurrence within or on the border of the irradiation field (marginal recurrence) by repeated examination determined by the clinical picture. These investigations, however, are only of value at least 6 months after the completion of all radiotherapy.

Residual mediastinal masses

These masses, generally thymic in the anterior mediastinum [3, 4], are difficult to evaluate on CT since there is no specific density to differentiate an active from a fibrotic lesion. However, the distinction between a mediastinal mass and post-radiotherapy paramediastinal fibrosis is the easiest. Scintigraphy using thallium appears to be of great value for making this distinction. However, MRI is the most accurate method for discriminating between residual tumor and fibrosis, even within an irradiated zone, particularly by demonstrating signal changes on T2-weighted imaging on successive examinations.

Conclusion

CT is indispensable for the diagnosis, pre-treatment staging and follow-up of Hodgkin's and non-Hodgkin's lymphomas. Thoracic CT should be performed routinely, and abdomino-pelvic CT almost routinely apart from those cases in whom ultrasound is adequate. It can assess on the same examination both nodal and extranodal disease, and act as a reference examination by its reproducible nature (table 38.2).

Table 38.1. Other extranodal lesions

CT	MRI
1) Involvement of the sinuses and nasal cavity: ORL (ENT) clinical examination for the detection of the involvement of Waldeyer ring forms part of the routine investigation of any lymphoma.	
CT is an essential complement to standard radiographs of the face and nasal cavities to define lymphatic, bone or even intracranial spread.	Its role is very limited: in theory it would help in the differentiation of a tumor process from simple retained secretions in the sinuses.
2) Involvement of the thyroid and salivary glands: - Thyroid involvement: • CT has no advantage over scintigraphy and ultrasound, • on the other hand: it is necessary for the evaluation of lymph nodes, bone, tracheal, or esophageal spread. - Involvement of the salivary glands: • CT delineates the intraparotid lesion better than sialography but is more limited for the evaluation of the structure of the lesion. Its accuracy is equivalent to ultrasound.	- No known complementary indications currently (see specific chapter)
3) Lymphomatous involvement of bone: It is only used as a complement to scintigraphy and standard radiographs for the investigation of certain localizations, particularly: • the spine, for the evaluation of osteolytic vertebral bone involvement, paravertebral spread and the detection of epidural disease • the sternum, for the evaluation of spread (usually by contiguity with the previsceral mediastinal lymph nodes), • the pelvic girdle, for exact assessment of adjacent pelvic wall involvement (contiguous spread from lymph nodes)	MRI is very sensitive in the investigation of bone marrow (fig. 38.4). The T1 sequences are valuable for demonstrating focal or diffuse lesions in the marrow with reduced signal of the marrow on T1-weighted imaging. MRI is an excellent method for monitoring treatment; it may even avoid repeated bone marrow biopsy in the therapeutic monitoring of some patients. The detection of some lesions in the bone marrow by classical radiology or scintigraphy requires destruction or significant remodeling of the cortical or trabecular bone, generally late in the evolution of lesions of bone marrow origin. Scintigraphy is more sensitive but less specific. The use of marker substances which accumulate in the reticulo-endothelial system reflects fairly poorly the distribution of the hemopoietic marrow but is not currently practiced. The diffuse nature of infiltrative bone marrow lesions and their poor contrast with the normal marrow prevents their detection on CT although this method can demonstrate focal lesions, particularly when there is cortical rupture. The lesions are generally well circumscribed but diffusely distributed in both Hodgkin's and non-Hodgkin's lymphoma. Although MRI is highly sensitive in the detection of focal or diffuse involvement of the bone marrow, it has a poor specificity: in fact, the majority of metastatic lesions also give a reduction in signal. Benign lesions, such as areas of condensation or bone degeneration, traumatic lesions (compression...) or infections, may all give similar appearances. The application of spectroscopy may answer some of the differential diagnostic problems when the history of the patient and character of the lesions cannot suggest the etiology.
4) Lymphomatous involvement of the soft tissues CT represents an important examination for this pathology for the assessment of local and general spread.	Despite its 3-dimensional capability, MRI is only of moderate complementary help compared to CT (better delineation of the tumor contours).
5) Lymphomatous involvement of the gastrointestinal tract: (much commoner in certain forms of NHL) - Gastric involvement: This is the commonest localization in the gastrointestinal tract diagnosed by ToGD and/or endoscopy which should be routine in the search for lymphomatous involvement in the ORL region. • CT is equivalent to ultrasound for the detection of gastric lymphomatous involvement. The major role of endoscopic ultrasound should be remembered. • CT assess the local and distant extent of the disease (visceral and lymph node assessment)	- No indication
- Jejuno-ileal involvement • CT, performed more often than ultrasound (not limited by technical problems) is, however, only of value for the assessment of visceral, lumbo-aortic and mesenteric lymph node involvement; • for local disease, it is only able to visualize those forms arising extraluminally.	- No indication

CT	MRI
- *Colonic and rectal involvement:* • cecal involvement is the commonest, • it is complemented by barium enema in the staging of the disease.	- No known indication
- *Esophageal involvement* (exceptional): - the diagnosis is primarily made endoscopically (or endoscopic ultrasound); - CT helps in guiding biopsy of an intrathoracic mass with difficult access.	- No known indication
6) Other lesions: these are rare, even exceptional. - *Lymphomatous involvement of the bile ducts* (very rare). CT and MRI are not indicated for this (ultrasound).	- No known indication
- *Lymphomatous involvement of the pancreas* • CT provides equivalent information to ultrasound; is only justified in cases of limited ultrasound due to technical problems (bowel artefacts). • It can help guide percutaneous diagnostic biopsy. • ERCP is sometimes necessary to detect the indirect signs of infiltration of the pancreas	
- *Lymphomatous involvement of the adrenal* CT is the best examination suited for the examination of the adrenals and can assess associated spread, particularly renal (in nearly a half of cases) and lymphatic (lumbo-aortic in nearly 85% of cases)	- Studies are under way to look for a possible specificity of the signal intensity on T2-weighted imaging but there is currently no known application for this technique
- *Lymphomatous involvement of the urogenital tract* *a) Renal involvement:* • these lesions are usually secondary, occurring in NHL. - CT is of equal value to ultrasound but can more specifically look for associated abnormalities: - intra- or retroperitoneal lymphadenopathy, - thickening of the perirenal fascial planes, - ureteric obstruction with hydronephrosis (usually lymph node), • alteration in the density of the perirenal fat space. - CT (like ultrasound) can monitor the progress of lymphomatous infiltration following chemotherapy and look for possible iatrogenic complications (subacute or chronic post-radiotherapy nephritis). It also can guide biopsy if this is judged to be technically not possible under ultrasound guidance.	- There is currently no indication for this technique: it can either better demonstrate diffuse involvement (loss of the cortico-medullary differentiation) and unlike CT has no risk in patients in renal failure.
b) Ureteric involvement - Very rarely primary intrinsic disease; ureteric and lymphomatous involvement is usually due to lymph node compression: CT defines the level and can guide possible biopsy. - CT and MRI demonstrate well ureteric infiltration following injection. Regression of the tumor on chemotherapy is a diagnostic sign since the initial appearance is similar to that of the urothelial tumors.	
c) Bladder involvement - Local assessment of the bladder and lymph nodes depends as much on CT as ultrasound, the latter examination demonstrating well the vesical lesions.	- No known indication
d) Lymphomatous involvement of the male genitalia - Prostatic involvement, very rare, can only be diagnosed by suprapubic and particularly endorectal ultrasound: CT has no specific role for this localization (and is only of value for the general assessment of the disease). - The same applies for testicular involvement where ultrasound is very accurate.	- In the presence of prostatic or testicular involvement, MRI is not justified in practice, even if it can demonstrate well the local extensions.
e) Gynecological involvement - CT can detect uterine or ovarian lesions but is entirely nonspecific; ultrasound is adequate; the diagnosis depends on histology.	- This is the most sensitive technique for the detection of gynecological pathology but is not indicated due to its absence of specificity. This technique is of no value for breast lesions.
f) Primary cardiac lymphomatous involvement This is exceptional - CT has no indication	MRI is useful because it is able to demonstrate the infiltrative process even without deformity of the cardiac outline (fig. 38.5).

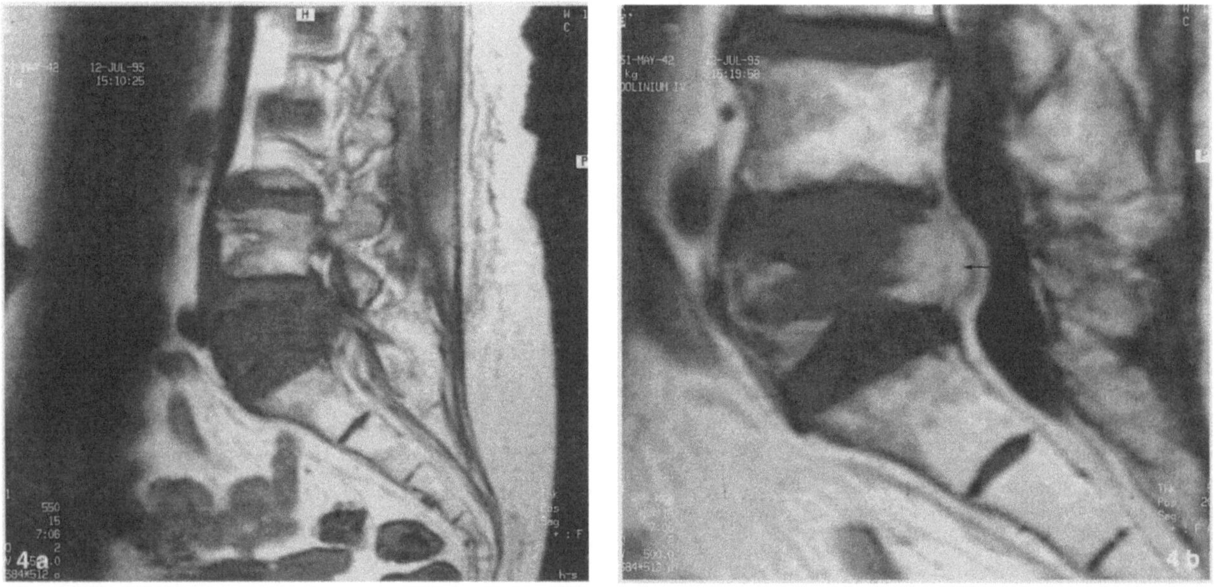

Fig. 38.4 a, b. Lymphomatous involvement of the spine on MRI: examination pre-gadolinium (**a**) and post-gadolinium (**b**) demonstrates infiltration of the bone marrow of L5, breaking the vertebral body and extending into the adjacent intervertebral disc, exhibiting enhancement in the anterior and posterior periphery of the vertebra with centrosomatic destruction. Pathological compression fracture of L5 with bulging of the posterior wall, and adjacent lymphomatous epidural involvement (*arrow* fig. **b**)

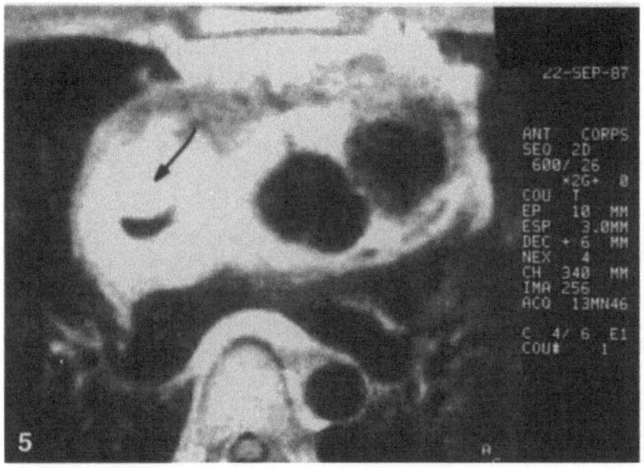

Fig. 38.5. Primary lymphoma of the heart on axial T1 MRI with cardiac gaiting. Infiltration of the right atrial myocardium *(arrow)*, well defined due to the clear inherent contrast between the tumor and healthy tissue, significant thickening of the cardiac muscle without deformity of the contours

MRI is justified in specific circumstances: the assessment of certain lesions, particularly neurological, bony or myocardial; it is also often useful in the distinction between residual tumor and fibrosis in residual masses, and in the diagnosis of recurrence.

It should be noted that CT and MRI are essential to the radiotherapist for planning the radiation fields and enable him to avoid the sensitive organs as much as possible. The new dosimetry softwear for radiotherapy, which projects the isodoses onto the CT images (and soon on to the MRI images), defines the distribution of the irradiation dose. Some softwear can already reconstruct in 3-dimensions the irradiated volume within various organs. The specialty of radiotherapy has greatly profited in the latter stages of the Twentieth Century from the recent advances in imaging, and has become progressively more accurate and less toxic.

References

1. Buthiau D, Jasmin C, Piette JC, Gabarre J, Solal-Céligny P (1991) Indications de la TDM et de l'IRM en Hémato-

logie. In: Buthiau D (ed) TDM et IRM Cliniques. Frison-Roche, Paris, pp 876-882
2. Dooms GS Hricak H, Crooks LE, Higghins CB (1984) Magnetic imaging on the lymph node. Comparison with CT. Radiology 153: 719-728
3. Frija J, Ferme C, Baud L (1988) Radiation-induced lung injuries: a survey by computed tomography and pulmonary function test in 18 cases of Hodgkin's disease. Eur J Radiol 8: 18-23
4. Katz M, Piekarski P, Bayle-Weisberger C, Laval-Jeantet M, Teillet F (1977) Masses médiastinales résiduelles post-radiothérapiques au cours de la maladie de Hodgkin. Ann Radiol 20: 667-672
5. Kœhler PR (1978) Lymphography vs CT of Iymphomas. AJR 131: 1116-1117
6. Kurdziel JC, et al (1988) Magnetic resonance imaging (MRI) of the spleen and bone marrow in hematological disorders. JBR-BTR 71: 211-229
7. Kurdziel JC, Dondelinger RF, Dicato MA, Ries F (1991) IRM de la moelle osseuse en hématologie. In: D Buthiau (ed) TDM et IRM Cliniques. Frison-Roche, Paris, pp 1093-1098
8. Monsuez JJ, Hertz-Pannier L, Frija J, et al (1988) Les localisations cardiaques des Iymphomes non hodgkiniens : suivi thérapeutique par imagerie par résonance magnétique nucléaire. GRAMM, Le Kremlin Bicêtre
9. Nyman R, Rehir S, Glimelins B (1987) Magnetic resonance imaging, chest radiography, computed tomography and ultrasonography in malignant Iymphoma. Acta Radiol 28: 253-262
10. Shuman LS, Libshitz HI (1984) Solid pleural manifestations of Iymphoma. AJR 142: 269-273
11. Strijk SP, Wagener DJT, Bogman MJJT, De Pauw BE, Wobbes T (1985) The spleen in Hodgkin's disease: diagnostic value of CT. Radiology 154: 753-757
12. Thomas F, et al (l988) Thoracic CTscanning follow-up of residual masses after treatment of Hodgkin's disease. Radiother Oncol 11: 119-122
13. Yana C, Frija J, Rain JD (1989) Imagerie fonctionnelle en hématologie. Encycl Med Chir (Sang) Paris, 13000N40, 3, 22 pages

CHAPTER 39

Malignant melanoma

Clinicians
D. Coeffic, E.-Ch. Antoine, A. Benhammouda, M.A. Rocher, C. Soubrane, O. Rixe, A. Eche, E. Vuillemin, P. Banzet, D. Khayat

Radiologist
D. Buthiau

The incidence of malignant melanoma has consistently increased since the beginning of the century: affecting 1 in 1,500 of the population in 1935, the incidence at the end of the 1980's is approximately around 1/130 and will be 1/90 by the year 2,000. There is a great variation between different populations.

The vast majority of patients in whom melanoma is diagnosed have localized disease; at the time of diagnosis, 70% are stage I, 20% stage II, 8-10% are stage III (distant metastases which could be recognized clinically and for whom the primary site is unknown in almost 10%) (table 39.1).

The prognosis is directly correlated with the depth of involvement (Clark's level) and the thickness of the tumor. The 5 year survival rate for stage I disease is between 65 and 80% and reduces to between 27 and 35% for stage II. These figures indicate that at least 20% of patients with stage I and 60% with stage II disease present at the time of diagnosis with occult metastases (table 39.2).

What role could MRI and CT play in the demonstration of these lesions in asymptomatic patients? It is certain that their role is well recognized in current practice (particularly for CT) for the demonstration of secondary lesions at a time when they are asymptomatic, guided sometimes by other investigations. This problem includes the positive diagnosis of visceral (figs 39.1-39.4) and distant lymphatic metastases (see corresponding chapters). This chapter is concerned with the demonstration of asymptomatic lesions and the appropriate investigation at the time of diagnosis.

In a recent study, A.C. Buzaid et al [2] demonstrate that 20% of CT scans performed for stage I disease show abnormalities suspicious of metastases, not revealed by clinical examination. The commonest lesions encountered are solitary hepatic lesions (fig. 39.1), suspicious of secondary involvement, and multiple or, more often, solitary pulmonary nodules . Sometimes subcutaneous nodules, solid renal masses or isolated dilatation of the intra- and extrahepatic bile ducts... are detected. 70% of cases demonstrate a stable appearance or even a reduction or disappearance of the suspicious lesion on the follow-up, either by CT or ultrasound several months after their initial

Table 39.1. Principle metastatic sites

Skin, node	42-59%
Lung	18-36%
Liver (fig. 39.1)	14-20%
Brain (fig. 39.2)	12-20%
Bone	11-17%
Gastro-intestinal tract	1-7%
Others (figs 39.3 & 39.4)	< 1%

Table 39.2. 10 year survival rate as a function of stage (AJCC classification)

Stage I	90%
Stage II	60%
Stage III	30%
Stage IV	10%

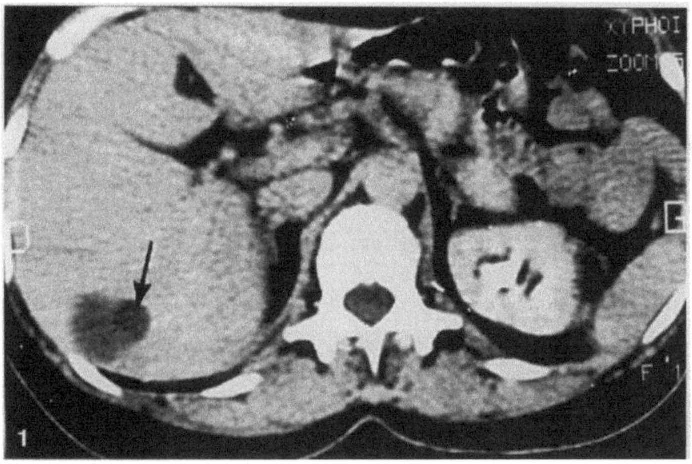

Fig. 39.1. Hepatic metastasis from malignant melanoma on post-contrast CT: note the fatty component *(arrow)* which constitutes an infrequent but peculiar feature of these secondary lesions

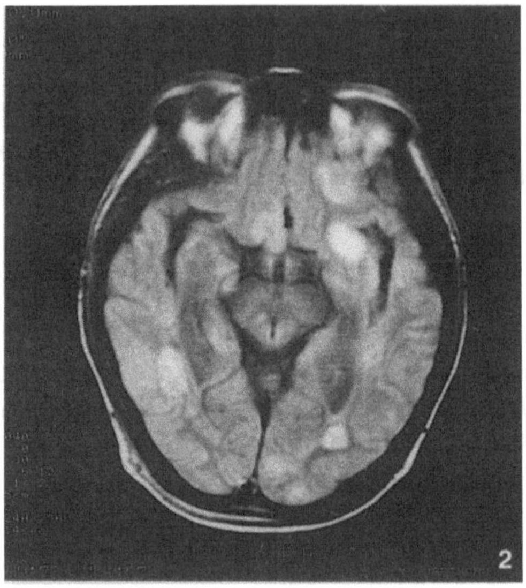

Fig. 39.2. Multiple brain metastases from malignant melanoma on axial proton density MRI: there are multiple diffuse nodular hyperintensities in both hemispheres with edema and relatively limited perilesional gliosis. These lesions involve the same axial level of the brain. A multiplicity of secondary deposits is common in melanoma

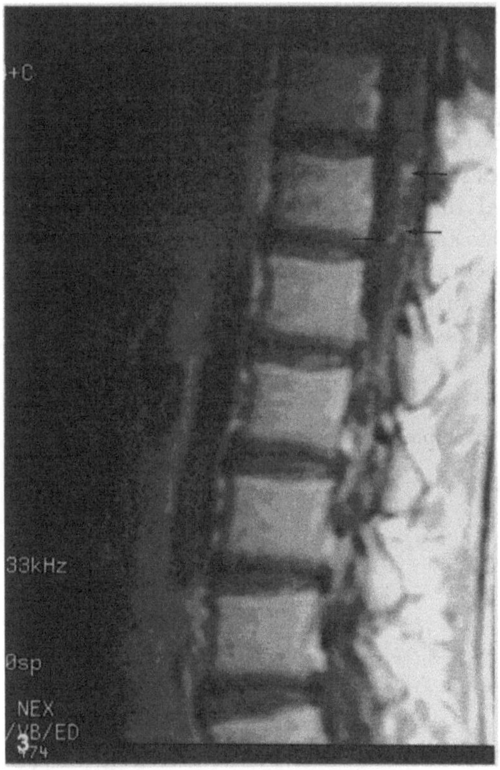

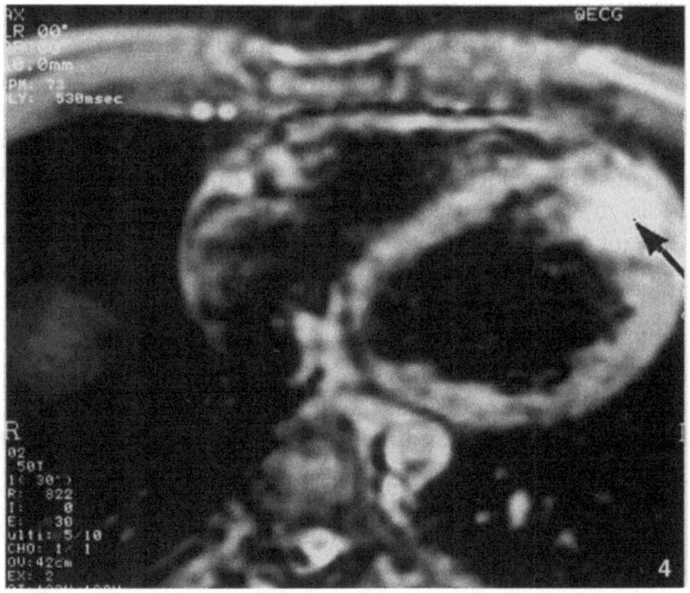

Fig. 39.3. Intradural metastases from melanoma on sagittal post-gadolinium T1-weighted MRI: MRI is the best method for detecting these secondary lesions, even when they are small. There is marked perimedullary enhancement. Note particularly the definite tumor nodules *(arrows)* predominantly in the dependent part of the spine

Fig. 39.4. Cardiac metastasis on MRI, axial T1-weighted section with cardiac gating: there is a hyperintense lesion following contrast injection *(arrow)* at the apex of the left ventricle. Note that cardiac metastases are extremely rare, but melanoma is quite often the responsible primary tumor demonstration. These lesions turn out to be benign on biopsy, or due to artefacts which disappear on the follow-up examination. In 10% of cases there is another primary tumor (for example renal tumor or lymphoma) and in less than 20% of cases the lesions turn out to be secondary deposits (subcutaneous nodules and lymph nodes metastases). Complementary MRI is only justified for the detection of cerebral lesions following an equivocal CT scan (fig. 39.2).

A number of complementary examinations can be proposed in the search for distant metastases at the time of the initial diagnosis of the melanoma. Scintigraphy [4] of the brain, bone or spleen only demonstrates a very few of the metastases (1.5%).

However, several series [5] have shown a relatively high rate of false positives on CT, of the order of 30 to 40% on average. Moreover, the true positives were clearly more numerous than on scintigraphy but less than the presumed figure for secondary involvement at the time of the positive diagnosis. In certain series [3, 5] involving several dozen patients, no CT examination was pathological. This figure becomes higher if there is lymph node involvement, the true positives for CT is exceeding 20% of patients in this instance. Other groups [3] have studied the value of abdomino-pelvic ultrasound: the number of false positives here is also high, and the true positive rate is inferior to that for CT.

CT constitutes the most sensitive method, superior to scintigraphy, ultrasound or plain radiography. Therefore, it would seem reasonable, despite the considerable number of false positives (15 to 20% depending on the series), to perform this examination in the initial assessment of melanomas. When there are no clinical or paraclinical pointers, it is reasonable to perform abdomino-pelvic, thoracic, as well as a brain CT scan, the assessment of bone being poorly adapted to an examination in the axial plane.

Bone scintigraphy is the most appropriate examination for the detection of bone involvement. MRI may occasionally be required as a complementary examination when there is doubt on the CT (particularly brain) and scintigraphy (particularly spine).

When there are localizing clinical signs or guiding paraclinical features, CT is the principle examination for further investigation.

In our experience, the role of CT was not negligible, initially in demonstrating the N+ forms with the risk of false positive or false negative results identical to any lymph node assessment by CT (related to the CT assessment being based solely on size criteria with no evaluation of the internal lymph node content). In our series, the percentage of lesions revealed by abdomino-pelvic, thoracic and brain CT was 11%, increasing to almost 20% when there was lymph node involvement. In these different series, the type of CT scanner must be taken into account, particularly the value of spiral CT (or continuous rotation CT) and helical mode (see fig. 18.4), which can perform very rapid images over a large anatomical region during a single breath hold with angio-CT. This technique is more accurate for the demonstration of lesions because there are no areas "in the shade". The contiguous nature of the sections is guaranteed and there is no variability in the level of section resulting from respiration. The more widespread availability of this type of CT apparatus will increase significantly the sensitivity of CT to allow the earliest possible demonstration of the occult metastases. This seems to be a primary indication of this new technique of continuous rotation CT. Care must be taken not to perform the whole of the investigation in a single study but to fractionate the contrast injection and perform multilevel bolus injections with angio-CT (see chapter 1: Principles and performance of CT and MRI).

References

1. Balch CM, Cascinelli N, DrzewiecLi KT, et al (1992) A comparison of prognostic factors worldwide. In: CM Balch, AN Houghton, GW Milton, Sober, Soong (eds) Cutaneous Melanoma, 2nd edn. Lippincott, Philadelphia, pp 188-199
2. Buzaid AC, Sandler AB, Mani S, Mc Curtis A, Poo W, Bolognia JL, Ariyan S (1993) Role of computed tomography in the staging of primary melanoma. JCO 4: 638-643
3. Khansur T, Sanders J, Das SK (1989) Evaluation of staging work-up in malignant melanoma. Arch Surg 124: 847-849
4. Kirkwood JM, Myers JE, Vlock DR, et al (1982) Tomographic gallium-67 citrate scanning: useful new surveillance for metastatic melanoma. Ann Intern Med 97: 694-699
5. Thomas JH, Panoussopoulous D, Liesmann GE ,et al (1979) Scintiscans in the evaluation of patients with malignant melanomas. Surg Gynecol Obstet 149: 574-576

CHAPTER 40

Investigation of metastases from an unknown primary

Clinicians
E.-Ch. Antoine, F. Guinet, D. Coeffic, M.A. Rocher, C. Borel, D. Paraiso, A.-C. Hardy, E. Vuillemin, D. Khayat

Radiologist
D. Buthiau

This is a relatively common situation since metastases of indeterminate origin represent 5 to 10% of all cancers, depending on the series and the definition adopted. The most restrictive definition only includes metastases whose origin cannot be determined even at autopsy [7]. A more useful definition includes all patients in whom a primary tumor is not demonstrated despite clinical and intensive radiological investigation at the time when the therapeutic decision had to be taken [3]. This latter definition is more commonly used.

These metastases typically pose the problem of the search for the primary lesion and hence the level of investigation to be contemplated. This search is rarely rewarding but most useful in identifying the clinico-histological associations which may benefit from treatment.

Diagnosis of metastatic disease

The commonest clinical presentations are:
- cervical lymphadenopathy in third of cases;
- signs of respiratory problems or a pleural effusion;
- right hypochondrial pain, hepatomegaly or ascites;
- one or several symptomatic bone lesions.

In the case of lymphadenopathy, simple cytology from fine needle aspiration will provide the diagnosis of what is, by definition, a secondary disease, unless the histology demonstrates a lymphoma in which case the lesion may be primary.

Although the plain radiograph can be sometimes be sufficient in the case of thoracic lesion, thoracic CT represents the most sensitive method of detecting pulmonary nodules and mediastinal lymphadenopathy. The distinction between primary and secondary diseases is sometimes difficult. However, there are a certain number of features which are suggestive of metastatic disease: the peripheral location, the presence of several nodules, the absence of mediastinal lymphadenopathy. If no primary is found, the possibility of a carcinoma presenting as a solitary pulmonary nodule (such as a primary bronchial carcinoma) should be considered.

If the presenting signs are abdominal, CT provides a good assessment of hepatic metastases, ascites, peritoneal carcinomatosis, lumbo-aortic or celio-mesenteric lymphadenopathy. Ultrasound is more sensitive for small volume hepatic lesions. However, the distinction between secondary hepatic lesions and a hepatocellular carcinoma may be difficult.

In the case of a bone lesion, scintigraphy is the most sensitive examination but lacks specificity. The plain radiographs centered on the areas of increased uptake may be sufficient, but if these areas appear normal, CT and specially MRI are indicated. As a general rule, multiple bony lesions are due to secondary deposits.

In every case, the diagnosis can only be made histologically. This is the key feature for determining the diagnostic and therapeutic approach. Plain radiography, ultrasound or CT may be able to guide a needle biopsy. However, in the case of a difficult histological diagnosis or for certain specific localizations, a surgical biopsy may be deemed necessary.

Adenocarcinoma is the commonest diagnosis and represents approximately 50% of metastases from an unknown primary [4]. This presents in the form of an abdominal mass in 44% of cases, peripheral lymphadenopathy in 17%, a thoracic mass in 12% and a bone lesion in 10%.

Epidermoid or squamous carcinomas manifest in the form of cervical lymphadenopathy in 50% of cases, a bone lesion in 20% of cases and an enlarged supraclavicular node in 14% of cases.

The very undifferentiated tumors must be particularly carefully assessed because some of these may be highly chemosensitive. In cases of doubt, immunohistochemistry and possible electron microscopy help to provide a more accurate classification. It is important not to ignore a potentially lymphoma (immunotracer to leukocyte common antigen), a germinal tumor (α fetoprotein, HCG and β HCG levels), or a neuroendocrine tumor. These undifferentiated tumors present in the form of abdominal mass in 25% of cases, cervical lymphadenopathy in 23%, bone lesion in 20% and supraclavicular lymph node enlargement in 14%.

Search for the primary tumor

Once the diagnosis of metastatic disease has been established, it would seem logical to search for a primary tumor. Such an investigation which would include routinely a thoracic, abdomino-pelvic CT, pelvic MRI, bronchoscopy, esophagogastroscopy, colonoscopy, is invasive, time consuming, expensive and rarely rewarding in terms of detection of the primary.

It would seem more logical to extend the investigation depending on the clinical presentation and histological results with a view to separate out those disease entities for which there is sometimes a curative treatment.

Cervical lymph node involvement (excluding the supraclavicular nodes)

Half of these tumors are epidermoid or squamous carcinomas which points towards a primary head and neck tumor, particularly in a patient with a history of heavy alcohol and tobacco consumption. It is useful, therefore, to perform a panendoscopy of the ORL (ENT) region, and CT of the neck and facial complex. If these examinations are negative, it is justifiable to look for a bronchial cancer by bronchoscopy and thoracic CT.

Twenty-five per cent of these tumors are undifferentiated. Lymphoma, germinal tumor (α-fetoprotein and β-HCG levels) and neuro-endocrine tumors must therefore be excluded. CT and EBV serology are performed to look for a tumor of the nasal cavity (cavum) particularly in a young subject from North Africa.

Ten per cent of cases with this presentation are due to adenocarcinoma, and a tumor of particularly thyroid origin must be excluded since this is amenable to treatment: level of tumor markers, thyroid ultrasound, immunolabeling by thyroglobulin.

Axillary lymph node involvement

The most commonly encountered histologies are lymphoma, adenocarcinoma, melanoma, and, more rarely, epidermoid (squamous) carcinoma and undifferentiated tumors.

An adenocarcinoma in a women is suggestive of a primary breast tumor. In fact, a subclinical breast cancer is confirmed following mastectomy in 30 to 50% of cases in whom the mammogram is negative [6]. One should obtain the CA15.3 levels and a mammogram to anticipate before the biopsy the level of hormonal receptors whose presence confirms the diagnosis even in the absence of breast lesion.

An adenocarcinoma in a man or an epidermoid (squamous) carcinoma is suggestive of a bronchial origin and justifies a bronchoscopy and thoracic CT.

Undifferentiated tumors require the performance of immunolabeling to LCA to look for lymphoma, and to the neuron specific enolase (NSE) pointing towards a small cell bronchial carcinoma. In both cases, bronchoscopy and thoracic CT are justified.

Malignant melanoma from an unknown primary, revealed by lymph node disease is an interesting example of diagnostic and therapeutic strategies. First of all, it is important not to fail to recognize the histological diagnosis of malignant melanoma which can occur in cases of an achromatic tumor. Secondly, the problem is not so much to find the primary (any suspicious nevus will obviously need biopsy) but more to confirm the strictly locoregional nature of the disease. The axillary lymph node group is the most commonly involved, followed by cervical and inguinal node involvement. Lymph node sampling is only indicated if there is no involvement of any other lymph node group (mediastinal in the case of axillary involvement, iliac or lumbo-aortic in the case of inguinal involvement) and no evidence of visceral spread or cutaneous secondaries. Pulmonary and hepatic metastases, together or separately, and cerebral metastases are particularly common. Bone metastases are rare, and lesions of the gastro-intestinal tract are possible, particularly the stomach and small bowel.

Inguinal lymph node involvement

In cases of inguinal presentation, it is rare for the primary tumor not to be found [12]. In all cases, abdomino-pelvic CT is useful (fig. 40.1). In effect:
- an epidermoid (squamous) tumor suggests a tumor of the cervix or vulva in a female (a tumor of the anus in either sex). A gynecological examination is essential, proctoscopy should always be performed;
- an adenocarcinoma in a female should always suggest a lesion of a ovarian origin and requires the performance of a pelvic ultrasound and a CA125 level;
- in cases of a transitional cell histology but also squamous or adenocarcinoma, a tumor of the bladder should be suspected and requires the performance of cystoscopy, as well as the TPA level. Also, in the case of a poorly differentiated histology, a malignant melanoma and lymphoma (fig. 40.1) must be excluded, the latter becoming more likely when no other primary can be identified [2].

Supraclavicular lymph node involvement

This is usually from an epidermoid (squamous) carcinoma, adenocarcinoma or undifferentiated tumor.

In the case of an epidermoid carcinoma, a bronchial origin is the most likely and requires bronchoscopy and thoracic CT.

For an adenocarcinoma, the two hormone sensitive cancers must be looked for: cancer of the breast in a woman and cancer of the prostate in man. The commonest primary tumors are, however, pulmonary and gastrointestinal. A CA15-3 level and mammography should therefore be performed in a woman, the prostate specific antigen level and endorectal ultrasound in a man, and a thoracic CT, gastroscopy and colonoscopy in both sexes.

The management of undifferentiated tumors is the same for that of a cervical lymphadenopathy.

Involvement of the midline lymph nodes (mediastinal and/or retroperitoneal)

This represents advanced disease with a poor prognosis in cases of differentiated histology. The commonest primary extrathoracic tumors of origin are from the head and neck, urogenital tract and breast. Malignant melanoma is also a possibility.

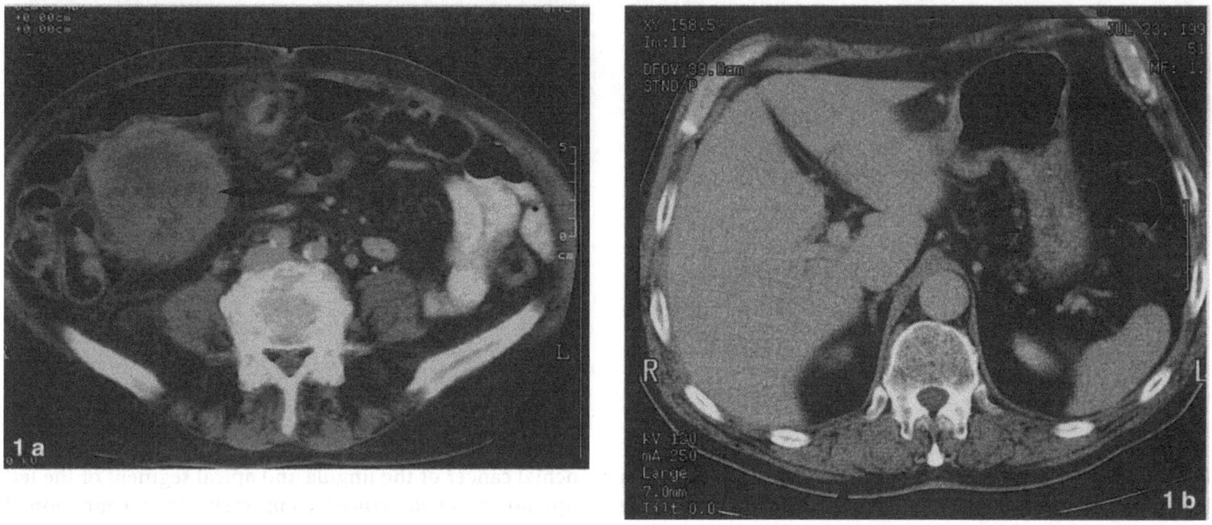

Fig. 40.1 a, b. Sixty-six year old man presenting initially with inguinal lymph node involvement: abdomino-pelvic CT demonstrates a pericolic and right colonic wall mass (*arrow* fig. **a**) corresponding at histology to lymphoma of the bowel and lymph node. There is, in addition, a collection of lymph nodes, limited in size and number, in the lesser omentum in the celiac region (*arrow* fig. **b**)

In cases of poorly differentiated histology, apart from lymphoma which must always be excluded in the presence of a solitary node, several other chemosensitive disease entities merit identification:

- extragonadal germinal tumors with the production of HCG and/or α fetoprotein;
- poorly differentiated neuro-endocrine tumors identified by positive immunobinding to NSE, chromogranin and the presence of neurosecretory granules on electron microscopy;
- poorly differentiated carcinoma which cannot be differentiated from the germ cell tumors or neuro-endocrine tumors.

In all cases, the detection of the primary does not alter the therapeutic management and investigations should therefore be limited.

Intrathoracic metastases

Solitary pulmonary nodule

It may be difficult to say whether this represents a primary tumor or a metastasis. In the case of an epidermoid (squamous) carcinoma or small cell cancer, the tumor of origin is pulmonary. If it is an adenocarcinoma, it is likely to be of gastrointestinal or pancreatic origin.

Multiple pulmonary nodules

All the primary lesions described in the cases of a solitary nodule are equally possible. In a young man, a testicular primary should be looked for and the level of the β HCG and α fetoprotein levels are therefore essential. In a young woman, a trophoblastic tumor should be considered and the HCG and β HCG levels will confirm the diagnosis.

Lymphangitis carcinomatosa

This suggests tumor of breast, gastric or pancreatic origin. However, given the terrible prognosis and the rapid progression of this form of disease, any investigations should be limited and non-invasive.

Pleural effusion (fig. 40.2)

In a man, this is usually from a bronchial carcinoma (fig. 40.2); thoracic CT and bronchoscopy are then justified. In a woman, a breast or ovarian origin is common, requiring the performance of mammography

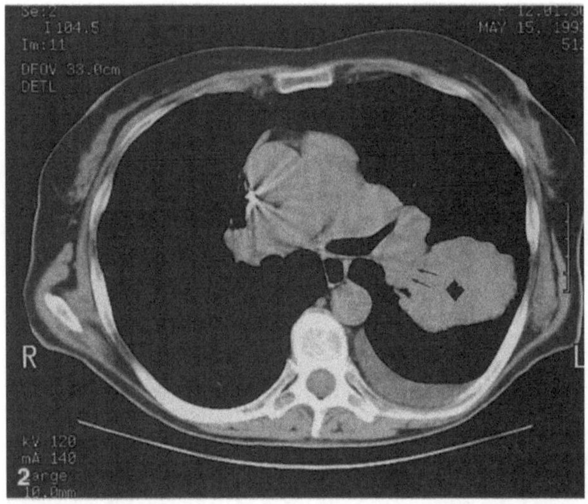

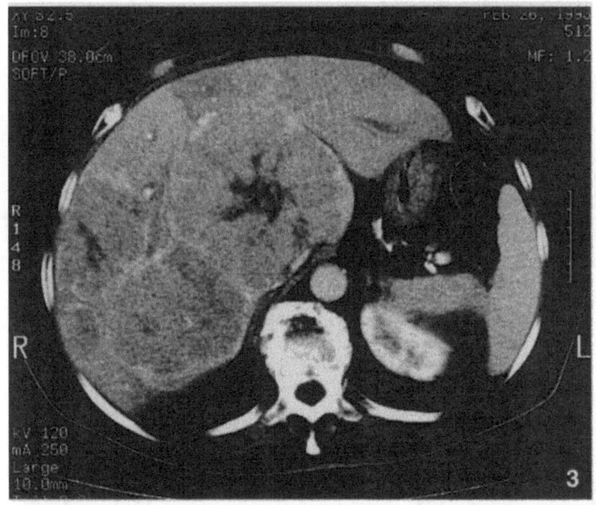

Fig. 40.2. Left pleural effusion as the presenting feature of a bronchial cancer of the lingula and apical segment of the left lower lobe *(diamond)* with enlargement of the principal hilar lymph nodes *(small arrows)*, compressing the termination of the left main bronchus, with encasement of the lingular bronchus and displacement and encasement of the left lower lobe bronchus

Fig. 40.3. Multiple and diffuse hepatic metastases without a known primary in a woman of 70. Colonoscopy did not demonstrate any lesion, the primary remaining unknown and pelvic ultrasound. Mesothelioma is rare but must not, however, be misdiagnosed.

Abdominal metastases

Hepatic metastases (fig. 40.3)

The liver is the commonest organ involved. It is the most frequent site of visceral involvement and is usually due to an adenocarcinoma. The differential diagnosis between a hepatocellular carcinoma and secondary lesions can be difficult. The α fetoprotein level should be routinely obtained. Although a subdiaphragmatic tumor of origin is the commonest, particularly gastrointestinal but sometimes gynecological, a supradiaphragmatic origin is also possible. In addition to routine abdomino-pelvic CT, the investigation should include a chest radiograph and mammography. If the primary is still not identified, colonoscopy is justified given the frequency of primary colonic lesions and the value of surgical intervention in preventing bowel obstruction.

Peritoneal carcinomatosis (fig. 40.4)

This suggests a tumor of ovarian origin in a female, and a lesion of the digestive tract in both sexes (pancreas, stomach, colon). The level of the tumor markers CA125, ACE and CA19-9, as well as an abdomino-pelvic CT should routinely be obtained.

In a woman, peritoneal carcinomatosis with an occult primary should be considered to be of ovarian origin (fig. 40.4) [11].

Bone metastases

Five tumors of origin should be carefully looked for because they may benefit from treatment specific to each tumor:
- breast: the lesions are usually multiple and lytic;
- prostate: the sclerotic nature of the lesions is very suggestive;
- thyroid;
- myeloma: necessitating the routine performance of protein electrophoresis;
- renal: abdominal CT and IVU are justified because this tumor may respond to immunotherapy (interleukin 2 and/or interferon).

Finally, a pulmonary tumor of origin is common justifying the performance of a chest radiograph, thoracic CT, and even bronchoscopy if there is any doubt.

Cerebral metastases (fig. 40.5)

In 60% of cases, the primary tumor remains undiagnosed despite exhaustive investigations. When a pri-

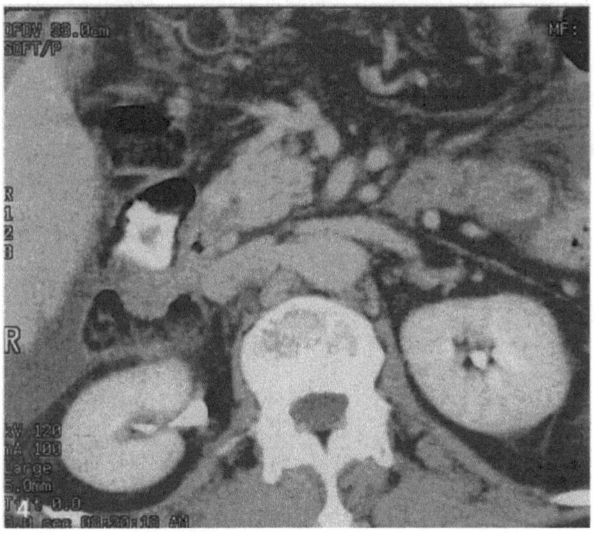

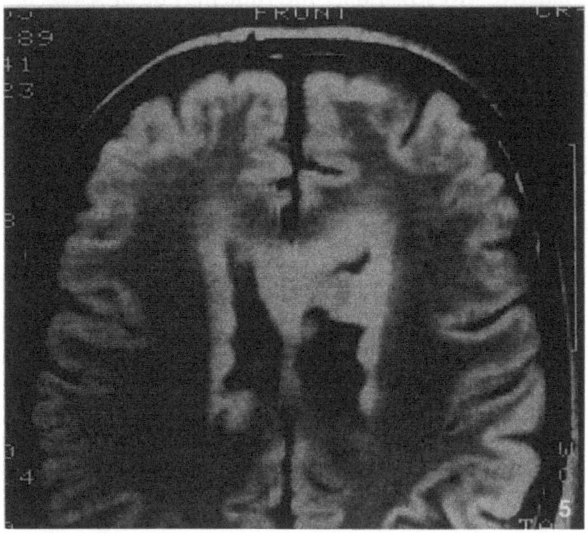

Fig. 40.4. Peritoneal carcinomatosis on CT in a 62 year old woman with no known primary: an ovarian origin was the most likely cause, and this was confirmed subsequently

Fig. 40.5. Cerebral metastasis as a presenting feature on MRI; the study demonstrates subependymal spread from a secondary lesion located in the genu of the corpus callosum mary is found, it is a bronchial carcinoma in 90% of cases [2] (fig. 40.5). This is a justification for the performance of a thoracic CT and bronchoscopy. The other principal tumors of origin are renal and malignant melanoma (which is not an unusual cause).

Cutaneous metastases

This is a relatively rare presentation. The primary tumor is most commonly found in the bronchus, although cancer of the kidney and malignant melanoma are also not uncommon causes. Cutaneous metastases have also been described in the breast, ORL cancers, and peritoneal carcinomatosis in the form of umbilical nodules [9].

Conclusion

It is of prime importance to identify a clinico-histological association in the presence of metastatic disease from an unknown primary. The primary tumor can often be suspected using a knowledge of these associations, and this may help to target the investigations appropriately.

It is important not to perform any invasive investigation if the result is not going to alter the treatment. Moreover, it often takes a long time to perform exhaustive investigations, and time may be precious in this type of patient who may benefit from the rapid administration of a treatment, whatever its nature may be.

In the final analysis, investigation must be governed by their contribution clinically:
- demonstration of an anatomo-clinical entity which is likely to benefit from a specific efficient treatment (thyroid...);
- early treatment of lesions which are likely to progress into medico-surgical emergencies.

The value of demonstrating the primary for an adenocarcinoma from a previously occult primary following very extensive investigation must be questioned since this has very little impact on the treatment and prognosis [1].

References

1. Altman E., Gadman E. (1986) An analysis of 1.539 patients with cancer of unknown primary site. Cancer 57: 120-124
2. Casciato DA, Tabbarah HJ, Rice DH (1985) Metastases of unknown origin. In: Haskell CM (ed) Cancer Treatment, 2nd edn. WB Saunders, Philadelphia, pp 225-243
3. Fisher DS (1975) Management of cancer of unknown primary. Conn Med 39: 205-208
4. Greager JA, Wood D, Dasgueta TK (1983) Metastatic cancer from an undetermined primary site. J Surg Oncol 23: 73-76
5. Greco FA, Vaughn WK, Hainsworth JD (1986) Advanced poorly differentiated carcinoma of unknown primary site: recognition of a traitable syndrom. Ann Intern Med 104: 547-556
6. Haskell CM, Cochran AJ, Barsky SH, et al (1988) Metastasis of unknown origin. Curr Probl Cancer 1: l-50
7. Holmes FF, Fouts TL (1970) Metastatic cancer of unknown primary site. Cancer 26: 816-820
8. Mc Cunnif AJ, Raben M. (1986) Metastatic carcinoma of the neck from an unknown primary. Int J Oncol Biol Phys12: 1849-1852
9. Scarpa FJ, Dincen JP, Boltax RS (1979) Visceral neoplasia presenting at the umbilicus. J Surg Oncol 11:351-359
10. Steckel RJ, Kagan AR (1980) Diagnostic persistence in working up metastatic cancer with an unknown primary site. Radiology 134: 367-369
11. Strnad CM, Grosh WW, Baxter J, et al (1989) Peritoneal carcinomatosis of unknown primary site in women. Ann Intern Med 111: 213-217
12. Zaren HA, Copelan EM (1978) Inguinal pode metastases. Cancer 41: 919-923

CHAPTER 41

CT and MRI in radiotherapy

Clinicians
O. Bernard, D. Nizri, R. Dendale, P.-Y. Pagan, E.-Ch. Antoine, L. Zelek

Radiologist
D. Buthiau

In radiotherapy, the use of cross sectional imaging for planning the treatment planes has the advantage of combining precise anatomical details (tumor volume, critical organs) with the differences in tissue density necessary for dose calculations. A diagnostically targeted CT is used to choose the number and position of sections necessary for calculating the distributions of the dose.

CT and radiotherapy (figs 41.1 & 41.2)

Techniques used

Treatment assessment

The therapeutic decision is determined by the clinical and radiological findings in terms of the degree of locoregional and distant spread of the tumor. This assessment nowadays should include at least a CT or even an MRI examination.

Radiotherapy represents a therapeutic stage targeted to locoregional disease (curative or palliative) and should comply with certain rules with regards to its indications, administration, control and follow-up.

The irradiation fields are determined clinically and by the imaging findings from which simulation can be performed as the first stage of treatment in radiotherapy.

Simulation

The simulation techniques and retention methods depend on the individual preferences, the aim being to determine the volume to be irradiated, the ports of access of the beams, the limits of irradiation field. All this information can be obtained from the radiographs and cutaneous landmarks. As a matter of routine, the following must be apparent; the points of entry of the radiation beams, the limits of the field, their size, the D.S.P, the position of the stand, the rotation of the collimators, position of the masks, position of the patient, and their characteristics (mode of retention).

Once the simulation has been completed, it is important to check it and determine the distribution of the dose to the tumor volume and to the rest of the irradiated volume, specifying the dose to the I.C.R.U. point. It is during this vital stage of the treatment and radiotherapy that CT has a role called "CT planning".

CT planning

The value of CT in radiotherapy concerns on one hand, the precise anatomy of the regions of the interest and the tumor, and on the other hand, a knowledge of tissue density whose heterogeneity must be taken into account for the dose calculations.

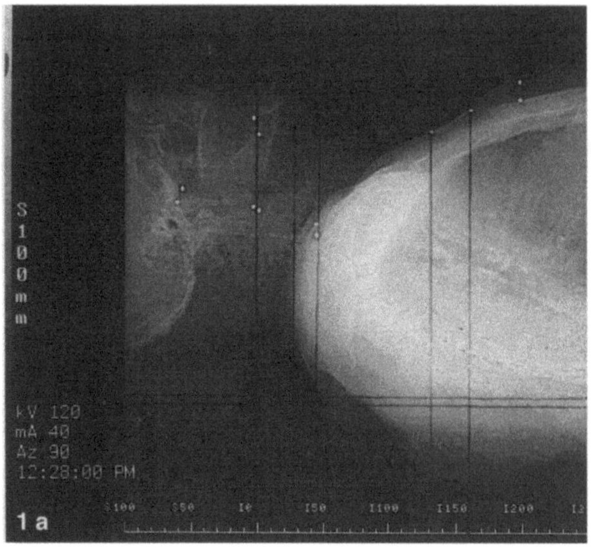

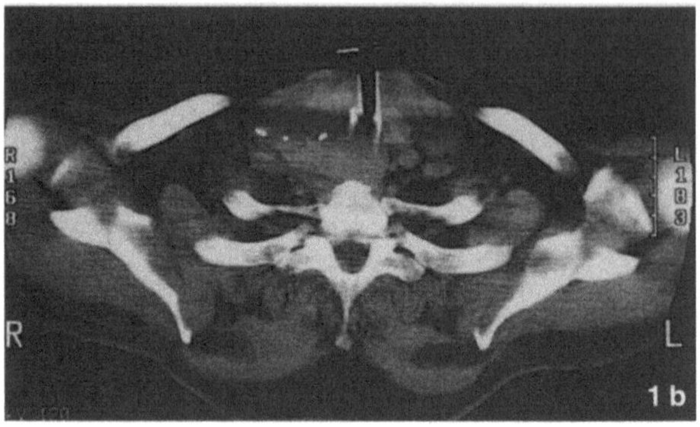

Fig. 41.1 a-d. Dosimetry, cancer of the larynx: an example of dosimetry in the transverse axial and sagittal planes with acquisition of the data by CT

It is possible to obtain all the necessary anatomical information on a single examination of the treatment area and, by direct computer linkage, to have a simultaneous representation of the different irradiation fields in the various planes in space and also the distribution of the dose in the volume of interest. Nonetheless, it is still important to take precautions, as much in the acquisition of the CT data as in their subsequent use for the dosimetric calculations [12, 14, 16].

Data acquisition

A different procedure is required to that for the diagnostic examination.

Flat and rigid CT table top: adequate aperture of the tunnel. Patient in the treatment position, immobile, normal respiration (condition of treatment). The acquisition of the section takes on average 10 seconds. This balances the differences, in the order of 15 to 20%, which exist both for the area and lung density between the two respiratory phases.

Marking with ball bearings and/or plumb lines the entry points of the centers of the beams, possibly the limits of the fields, sometimes the important anatomical points.

Frontal and lateral scan in radio-mode.

The acquisition area should include all the external contours of the patient, even a minimal representation of the support.

Work using a conversion window (grey scale/ Hounsfield units) wide enough to reduce the distortion of these structures.

Transfer of data

a) Direct: all the matrices, whose number is related to the CT sections, are transferred to a computer used to calculate the dose distributions. The contours are calculated automatically, and the treatment can be planned directly on the computer.
b) Indirect: by photography of the image on the screen of the scanner, this is subject to errors in determining the dimensions of the organs, the tumor volume and the restoration of the contours. The density values are not accessible, and the dosimetry work requires the use of theoretical values.

Restoration to a life-size scale can be helped by a pantograph or any other appropriate apparatus.

However, during the performance of the examination and on certain scanners, it is possible to obtain some values from the console; the dimensions and/or densities can be measured and extracted one by one, enabling corrections to be made.

Number and position of slices

The choice of the number of sections depends on the localization and information required. Certain treatments necessitate the performance of a large number of contiguous sections (from 20 to 40), allowing a 3-dimensional representation required for more precise targeting of ballistic irradiation (stereotactic treatment). Generally, however, the majority of treatments only require a limited number of axial sections, in the order of 3 or 4, of 10 mm thickness and, depending on the localization, with or without contrast agent. Their

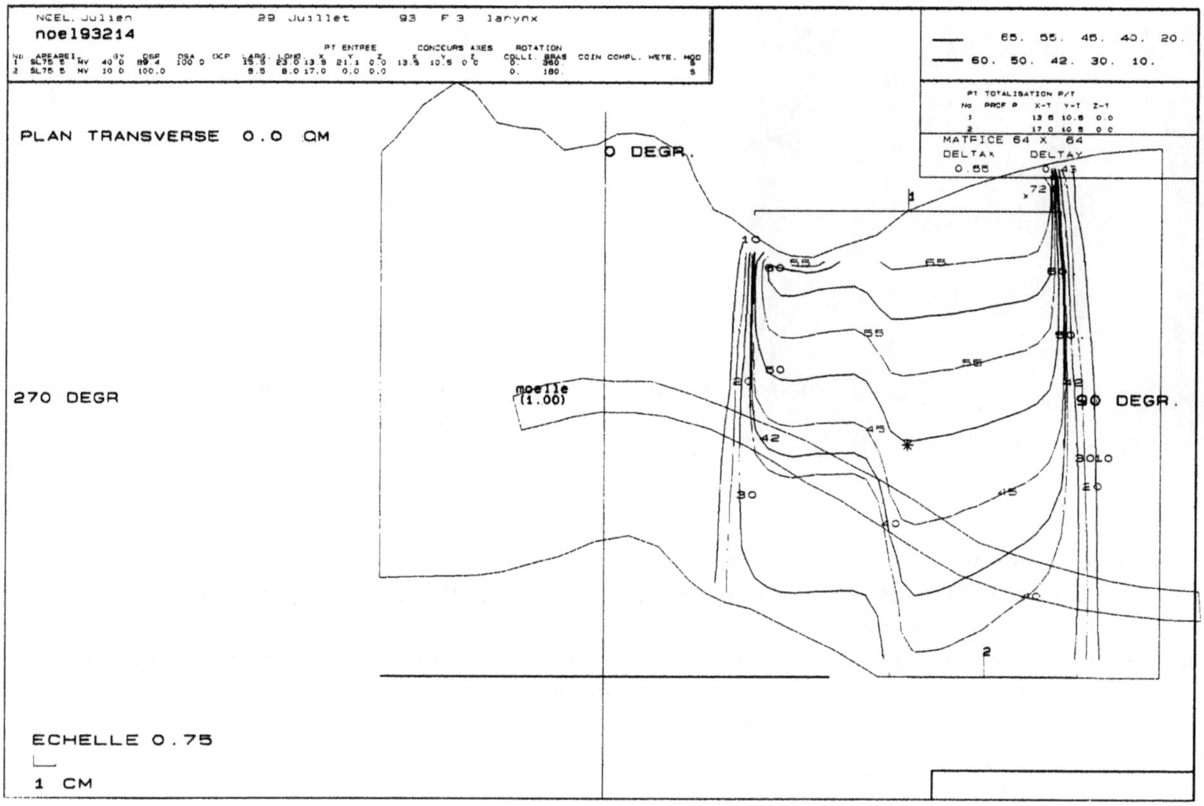
NOEL Julien 29 Juillet 93 F 3 larynx
noe193214
PLAN TRANSVERSE 0.0 CM
0 DEGR.
270 DEGR
90 DEGR.
moelle (1.00)
65. 55. 45. 40. 20.
60. 50. 42. 30. 10.
MATRICE 64 X 64
DELTAX DELTAY
ECHELLE 0.75
1 CM

1 c

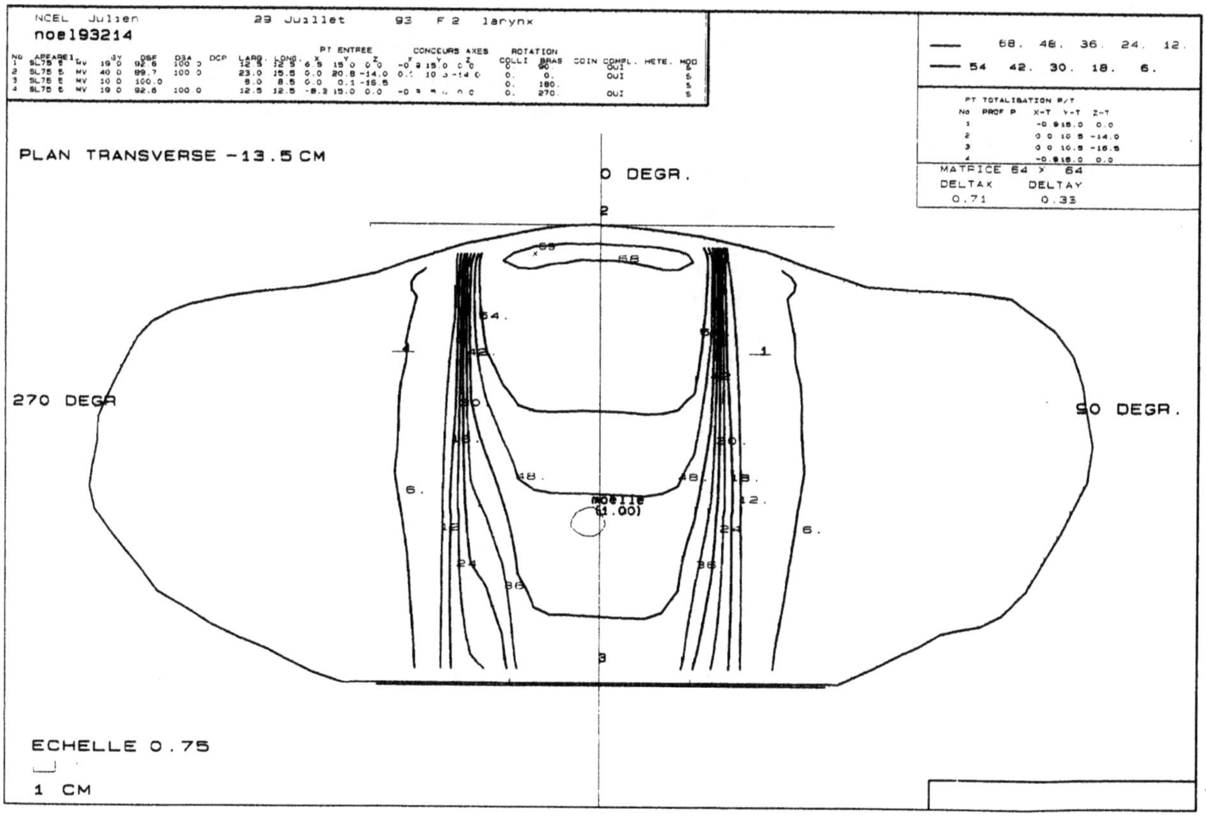
NOEL Julien 29 Juillet 93 F 2 larynx
noe193214
PLAN TRANSVERSE -13.5 CM
0 DEGR.
270 DEGR
90 DEGR.
moelle (1.00)
58. 48. 36. 24. 12.
54 42. 30. 18. 6.
MATRICE 64 X 64
DELTAX DELTAY
0.71 0.33
ECHELLE 0.75
1 CM

1 d

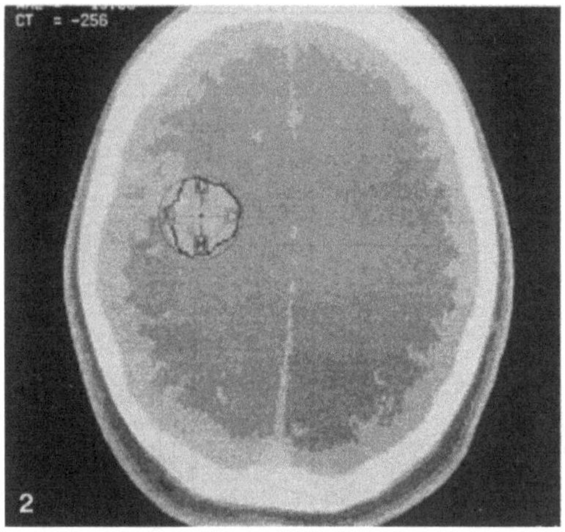

Fig. 41.2. Treatment of an arteriovenous malformation. Acquisition in stereotactic mode of the hemographic anatomical sections with markers. Automatic contouring

position and validity limits are determined by the shape of the patient and the differences in thickness over the irradiation volume. The plane of section should routinely pass through the axis of the beams, and this reference section determines the calculation of the treatment time and hence the value of the dose really delivered.

A too limited number of sections in some anatomical regions with a significant thickness gradient (ORL) may result in distortions of the isodoses and an overestimation of the amount and extent of the areas of over- and underdosage. As a result, it is important for the radiotherapist at the time of CT planning to oversee the examination and determine the number and thickness of the sections in order to optimize the representation of the dose distribution. According to a study at the Gustave Roussy Institute, a correct representation of the dose distribution can be obtained using a limited number of regularly spaced sections, every 3 cm for lesions of the ORL region, every 5 cm for lymphomas and every 4 cm for tumors of the liver [2].

It may be necessary during the course of the treatment to perform a new series of CT sections due to any significant anatomical change which needs to be taken into account in order to modify the treatment and optimize the dose. This is the case particularly in the ORL tumors with markedly enlarged lymph nodes.

Calculation of density [14]

The corrections for heterogeneity are subject to some difficulties, related to the fact that the energies used by the CT (Sc) and the treatment apparatus (Rx) are very different (not forgetting the hardening of the CT x-ray beam by the effects of tissue filtration).

This may explain why there is not always a linear relationship between the CT units and the electron densities.

However, it seems that by referring to the average density of each organ (if it approaches that of water ≤ 100 Hounsfield units), it is possible to establish a linear relationship.

For those tissues with a higher density, this linearity no longer exists; the electron densities are dependent on the atomic number (which must be known). This is the case for prosthetic materials (cardiac, orthopedic).

MRI and radiotherapy

This examination which is under full development and at the heart of modern imaging does not yet have a well defined role in radiotherapy treatment. It does have some advantages over CT:

- an improved detection sensitivity and remarkable topographic definition due to a higher soft tissue contrast;
- the potential of obtaining sections in 3-dimensions, as well as 3-dimensional reconstructions (very useful for stereotactic treatments);
- the disadvantages currently preventing direct use of these images are:
  - geometric distortion, particularly in the periphery (attributable to the machine, the patient and/or the examination time);
  - the absence of any information on electron density;
  - the acquisition times for the images are still long.

MRI remains therefore, for the moment, a complementary examination to CT for establishing the treatment plane with a particular role in the CNS, for the detection of skip lesions and monitoring the tumor response.

Conclusion

The CT examination in conjunction with the development of computer systems make it possible to obtain accurately targeted irradiation for radiotherapy. The acquisition and handling of the data must, above all, be done methodically, using a rigorous technique and with certain precautions. This aims to reduce the causes for errors. The improvement in the accuracy of treatment planning depends primarily on the position of the patient, the number of sections, as well as taking into consideration the anatomical changes which occur during treatment. The role of MRI in radiotherapy is still under study.

References

1. Austin-Seymour MM, Chen GTY, Castro JR, Saunders WM, Pitluck S, Woodraff KH, Kessler M (1986) Dose volume histogram analysis of liver radiation tolerance. Int J Radiat Oncol Biol Phys 12: 31-35
2. Beaudre A, Bridier A, Chavaudra J, Houlard JP, Eschwege F, Cosset JM (1991) Données scanographiques minimales pour l'établissement des plans de traitement en radiothérapie externe en vue de leur application a un grand nombre de patients. XXX Congrès de la SFPH Rennes
3. Becker G, et al (1989) Presentation and evaluation of 3D dose distributions in radiotherapy planning. In: Lemke HU, Rhodes ML, Jaffe CC, Felix R (eds) Computer assisted radiology. Springer-Verlag, Berlin
4. Bridier A and Dutreix A (1981) The interest of CT scanning for tumour dose determination in radiotherapy. In: Computerized Tomographic Scanners in Radiotherapy in Europe. Br J Radiol (Suppl) 15: 106-108
5. Bridier A, Wibault P, Chavaudra J, Houlard JP, Eschwege F (1991) Amélioration de la méthode utilisée à l'IGR pour l'établissement des plans de traitement en radiothérapie ORL. Bull. Cancer Radiother 78: 55-58
6. Brown AP, Urie MM, Barest G, Cheng E, Coia L, Emami BN, Galvin J, Kutcher J, Manolis J, Wong JW, Yahalom J (1991) Three-dimensional treatment planning for hodgkints disease. Int J Radiar Oncol Biol Phys 21: 205-215
7. Buthiau D, Gardeur D (1987) Protocoles d'examen TDM. Shering
8. Chavaudra J (1992) Acquisition des données anatomiques : avec quelle méthode ? Bull Cancer Radiother 79: 515-521
9. Dahlin H, Ekstrom P, Schneider W (1989). Computer based workstations in radiation oncology. In: Lemke HU, Rhodes ML, Jaffe CC, Felix R (eds)Computer assisted radiology. Springer-Verlag, Berlin
10. Day MJ, Harrison RM (1983) Cross-sectionnal information and treatment simulation in radiation therapy planning. In: NM Bleehen, E Glastein, JL Haybittle (eds) Chap. 4, pp 87-132
11. Drzymala RE, Moban R, Brewster L, Chu J, Goitein M, Harms W, Urie M (1991) Dose-volume histograms. Int J Radiat Oncol Biol Phys 21: 71-78
12. Dutreix A (1980) Use of computerized tomography in photon and electron treatment planning. In: RH Thomas,V Perez-Mendez (eds) Advances in Radiation Protection and Dosimetry in Medicine. Plenum Press, New York, pp 557-577
13. Dutreix A (1984) When and how can we improve precision in radiotherapy? Radiother Oncol 2: 275-292
14. Dutreix A, Bridier A (1986). Peut-on améliorer la précision en radiothérapie grâce à l'utilisation des coupes scanographiques pour le calcul des doses ? XXV~ Congrès SFPH, Toulouse
15. Eschwege F, Bridier A, Gabrielle P, Pichon C, Dutreix A, Piekarski JD (1981) The role of CT scanners in treatment planning of head and neck tumours. In: Computerized tomographic scanners in radiotherapy in Europe". Br J Radiol (suppl) 15: 18-21
16. Glatstein E, Lichter AS, Fraass BA, Kelly BA, Van de Geijn J (1985) The imaging revolution and radiation oncology: use of CT, ultrasound, and NMR for localization, treatment planning and treatment delivery. Int J Radiat Oncol Biol Phys 11: 299-314
17. Kett H, et al (1989) The value of 3D MRI in the treatment planning in radiation therapy. Society of Magnetic Resonance in Medicine. Book of Abstracts, 2: 991
18. Kutcher GJ, Fuks Z, Brenner H, Brown AP, Burman C, Cheng E, Coia L, Krippner K, Manolis JM, Mohan R, Simpson JR, Urie M, Vikram B, Wallace R (1991) Three-dimensional photon treatment planning for carcinoma of the nasopharynx. Int J Radiat Oncol Biol Phys 21: 164-182
19. Ling CC, Rogers CC, Morton RJ, eds (1983) Computer tomography in radiation therapy. Raven Press, New York
20. Lukas P, Heuck A (1989) MR challenges CT for therapy management. Diag Im International: 4-48
21. Lyman JT (1985). Complication probability as assesed from dose-volume histograms. Radiat Res 104: S13-19
22. Lyman JT (1989) Optimisation of radiation therapy: a dose volume histogram reduction algorithm. Int J Radiat Oncol Biol Phys 17: 433-436

23. Rosenwald JC (1992) Acquisition des données anatomiques. Dans quel but ? Bull Cancer Radiother 79: 511-513
24. Vermillard D, Lafforgue B, Regal R, Lauche H (1992). Dosimétrie TDM et IRM par numérisation des images au moyen d'un scanner XRS Omnidemia 3 CX. Bull Cancer Radiother 79: 523-524
25. Toonkel LM, et al (1988). MRI assisted treatment planning for radiation therapy of head and neck. Magn Reson Imaging 6: 315-319
26. Fraass A, Moshan DL, Diaz RF, Ten Haken RK, Aisen A, Gebarski S, Glazer G, Lichter AS (1987) Integration of magnetic resonance imaging into radiation therapy treatment planning. I. Technical consideration. Int J Radiat Oncol Biol Phys 13: 1897-1906
27. Battista JJ, William D, Rider D, VanDyk J (1980) Computed tomography for radiotherapy planning. Int J Radiat Oncol Biol Phys 6: 99-107

CHAPTER 42

Interventional CT in oncology

Radiologist
R.F. Dondelinger

CT guided percutaneous biopsies

The performance of percutaneous biopsies of circumscribed lesions guided by imaging represents a fundamental technique. This adds diagnostic specificity to the high sensitivity of lesion detection attributable to cross-sectional imaging. The anatomical precision of CT lends itself readily to the guidance of percutaneous biopsies. The modern scanners offer the necessary conditions for a reliable and rapid technique. The large aperture and flaring of the gantry allow easy access to the patient. The laser marker systems on the inside and outside of the gantry determine the site of needle entry on the skin surface and the millimetric control of the table top movements helps to find the desired plane of section. The rapid review of the images and volumetric acquisitions reduces the time of the procedure. The availability of a television screen inside the examination room allows the operator to remain close to the patient all the time [18]. Clinical colleagues must give the radiologist the freedom to decide whether a percutaneous biopsy is indicated. This decision is made with a full knowledge of the patient's history. The biopsy is usually performed during the course of the diagnostic examination. This approach minimizes the delay in reaching a definitive diagnosis and reduces health costs.

Indications

Any imaging appearance which is suggestive but not pathognomonic of a tumor requires confirmation of its nature by percutaneous biopsy. The general indications can be summarized in the following fashion, without considering the specific particular indications of the different organs:

- Appearance suggestive of a primary malignant tumor (fig. 42.1): confirmation of the diagnosis is essential if radiotherapy or chemotherapy are planned prior to surgical resection, or in the case of an advanced tumor when the treatment can only be palliative. The confirmation of the diagnosis of malignancy may also help some previously resistant patients to accept the need for surgical exploration.
- Metastasis(es) in the lung, liver, lymph nodes, bone or other sites (fig. 42.2). There are three possible outcomes:
  - the primary tumor is known, but the metastasis(es) are in an unusual site for this type of cancer;
  - the patient presents with several concomitant primary tumors, or a cancer and a lymphoma, or a malignant hematological tumor;
  - the patient is in clinical remission.
- Appearance suggestive of a tumor which persists following the initial regression of the lesion under the effects of chemotherapy or radiotherapy. Is the lesion sterile or does it still contain tumor cells? Pulmonary metastases from germinal tumors represent a typical example.
- The differential diagnosis between post-radiation fibrotic scarring and residual tumor. The typical example is the situation following amputation of the rectum.
- The differential diagnosis between a benign tumor and metastasis in an organ which is commonly the site

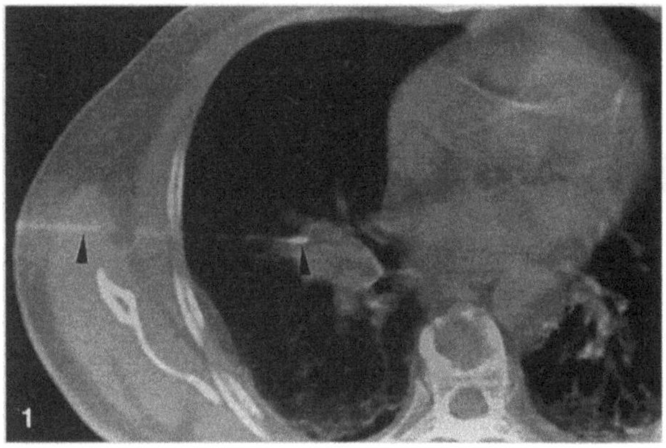

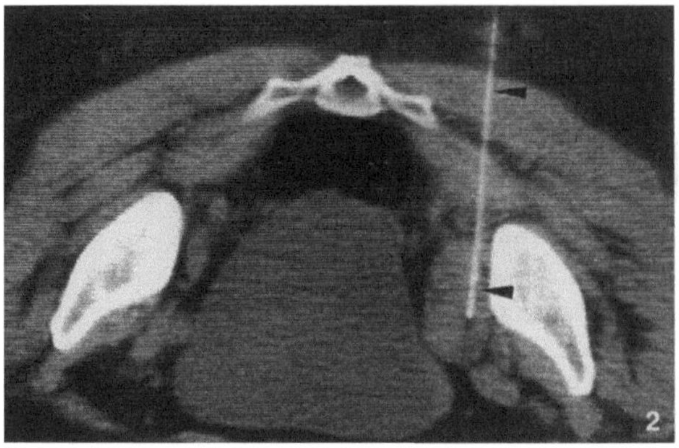

Fig. 42.1. Pulmonary tumor of 3 cm in diameter in the right hilum. Negative transbronchial fibroscopic biopsy. Percutaneous biopsy *(arrow)* under CT guidance via the right axillary approach: undifferentiated or anaplastic bronchial epithelioma

Fig. 42.2. Lymphadenopathy in the right iliac chain causing vesical indentation. Percutaneous biopsy under CT control via the transgluteal approach *(arrows)*. Lymph node metastasis from a previously resected cancer of the uterine cervix

of solid benign tumors. The adrenal glands are frequently involved by metastases from bronchial cancer but are the also the site for non-functioning adenomas in 7% of the population.

- Appearances atypical of a benign tumor: necrotic pseudocystic metastases, biliary or pancreatic cystadenocarcinomas, or pseudocystic renal carcinomas (hypernephromas) are examples of tumors which may suggest a benign cyst. Another example is the differential diagnosis between hepatocellular carcinoma and a dysplastic or regenerative nodule.
- Sampling for the level of the hormone markers, for DNA cytometry, or for in vitro treatment sensitivity tests.
- Preoperative needle localization of pulmonary nodules under fluoroscopic control prior to resection [20].

Contraindications

These are of a general nature for abdomino-pelvic percutaneous biopsies, provided that the diameter of the needle is less than 1 mm. Needling through bowel is acceptable for an anterior approach to deep lesions, but the risk of infection is increased by transection of a distal bowel loop. When a hypervascular hepatic tumor is biopsied, some healthy tissue should remain interposed between the liver capsule and the lesion in order to avoid hemorrhagic complications. The majority of the relative contraindications concern pulmonary biopsies: solitary lung, recent myocardial infarction, diffuse pulmonary emphysema or emphysematous bullae along the needle tract, pulmonary arterial hypertension, cardiac failure, artificial ventilation, etc. Prior to performing any biopsy, a hydatid cyst or normal and abnormal vascular structure must be identified. Any clotting abnormality, intrinsic or induced by medication, should be corrected prior to the biopsy. The patient must be fully cooperative. Dyspnea, hiccups, pain and distress can be limiting factors for performing a percutaneous biopsy. A concise explanation of the aim and performance of the procedure is the best guarantee for obtaining the cooperation of the patient.

Technique

The performance of a CT examination, both with and without contrast, is essential before percutaneous biopsy of any circumscribed lesion.

The aim of the enhancement is:

- to recognize a normal vascular structure, aneurysm, pseudoaneurysm or arteriovenous fistula;
- to establish the diagnosis of a typical angioma on the basis of the characteristic dynamic pattern of contrast uptake, thus making percutaneous biopsy unnecessary;
- to demonstrate the septa and wall thickening in a cyst-like tumor, recognizing that ultrasound is superior to CT;
- to appreciate the degree of vascularity of the lesion which determines the choice of the biopsy needle;

- to identify areas of central tumor necrosis which should be avoided by the needle;
- to recognize the anatomical tissue adjacent to the target structure, and the vessels, nerves or viscera to be avoided.

CT guided percutaneous biopsies are preferably performed in the transverse axial plane using a perpendicular approach or one parallel to the plane of the examination table. This makes the use of goniometric devices or any other system of angulation measurement unnecessary and makes it possible to perform all visceral biopsies by hand. The site of the skin puncture is determined so that the internal trajectory of the needle is as short as possible and crosses the least number of anatomical compartments or different organs before reaching its target.

If the tumor is suspected to be of a high grade malignancy, the needle track is planned in fashion that will include it within an eventual surgical resection block of tissue. The laser guidance system indicates on the patient's skin the level of the CT section which contains the needle tract. The site of the injection on the skin is marked by a needle which is placed perpendicular to the plane of section and traced on the surface of the skin. The intersection between the needle and plane of section determines the entry point on the skin. The cutaneous and subcutaneous tissue planes are anesthetized. The intraparenchymal progression of the flexible needle is almost painless. Only the diaphragm, neurinomas or certain tumors with an associated inflammatory reaction are painful to biopsy. A needle inserted into the intercostal nerves, presacral plexus or sciatic nerve is recognized by the distribution of the pain. The needle tip is recognized by distal hypodensity (needle tip artefact).

The choice of the biopsy needle is determined by the radiologist, cytologist or the histopathologist. The same applies to the choice of technique for mounting the material on slides and the fixation process of the histological fragments. It is not worth frequently changing the type of needle used because the efficiency of the different fine needles available is equivalent [10]. The simplest needles give excellent results [5]. On the other hand, the radiologist should have several different needles at his disposal for visceral biopsies, for lesions with a high cellular consistency, such as sarcomas, or marked stromal reaction, and for bone biopsies. When an automatic biopsy gun is used, the length of advancement of the needle should be less than the diameter of the lesion. These devices have the advantage of obtaining biopsies of a consistent quality [2]. In practice, needles whose diameter is around 18 gauge tend to be used. The configuration of the needle tip allows simultaneous acquisition of histological and cytological material, multiple passes of the needle (of the order of 3 to 4) and the performance of biopsies as a day case. It is only necessary to monitor the patient for 1 to 4 hours afterwards. As well as multiple passages using a free hand technique, coaxial or tandem techniques can also be used.

- The tandem technique consists of inserting several identical needles of the same length in close proximity by following a parallel course to the first needle whose position inside the lesion has been previously verified on CT. This technique is particularly useful for performing multiple biopsies rapidly in a small lesion which is difficult to localize, such as within the pancreas for example [16].
- The coaxial technique consists of inserting a smaller diameter needle through a first needle which is already in place. This facilitates repeat biopsies within the target lesion without repeating the guidance [17]. This technique is useful for pulmonary biopsies, the external coaxial needle being inserted just into contact with the pleura. It is then sufficient to introduce a small caliber needle in the required direction into the pulmonary lesion by using the previously correctly placed coaxial needle.

Results

Hepatic, pulmonary, adrenal and bone biopsies are the most commonly performed in oncology. These have a diagnostic accuracy of 90 to 95% for the demonstration of a malignant tumor. The yield is 85% for pancreatic lesions [18]. The positive predicative value of a percutaneous biopsy is in the order 98%, and false positive diagnoses are rare. The yield from percutaneous biopsies is greatly influenced by the size of the lesion. Fine needle biopsies of hepatocellular carcinomas of between 1 and 2 cm in diameter are falsely negative in 50% of cases. The confirmation of recurrent lymphoma is relatively easy. However, it is difficult to confirm the diagnosis of lymphoma or determine whether the lesion is of the Hodgkin or non-Hodgkin variety on the basis of a percutaneous biopsy [8, 17]. Lymphomas with a marked stromal reaction, as well as the cellular depleted Hodgkin varieties require large specimen for accurate typing.

Complications

Clinically significant complications resulting from percutaneous fine needle biopsy are rare. Two reviews of nearly 65,000 patients have documented an overall complication rate of 0.1-0.5%, a major complication rate of 0.05%, and a mortality rate of 0.008% [13, 22]. The most worrying complications are acute hemorrhagic pancreatitis, intraperitoneal hemorrhage, biliary peritonitis and sepsis. The observation of a meticulous technique is essential for the prevention of these complications. The seeding of metastases along the biopsy track or into the skin results from a high number of biopsies (>10) and the use of a large caliber needle (16 or 14 G).

Percutaneous neurolysis of the celiac plexus and splanchnic nerves

The high resolution of CT is useful to guide the injection of neurolytic substances into the structures which conduct the sensory thoraco-abdominal nerve fibers. Neurolysis of the celiac plexus and splanchnic nerves, stellate ganglion block, infiltration of the thoracic and lumbar sympathetic chain, as well as the sacral plexus, are preferably performed under CT control. We will limit ourselves to a description of percutaneous neurolysis of the celiac plexus under CT guidance [9, 12].

Indications

The semilunar ganglia receive sensory fibers from the upper abdominal organs (pancreas, liver, biliary tract, spleen, stomach). Neurolysis of these ganglia or those of the splanchnic nerves is indicated in the treatment of pain emanating from tumors lying within these organs or which directly infiltrate the nerves. Cancer of the body of the pancreas is the best descriptive model. Direct tumor invasion of the median preaortic retroperitoneal space or the desmoplastic reaction around the nerve structures are responsible for the so-called celiac pains which are deeply localized within the abdomen with classical radiation posteriorly.

Technique

This is based on the radio-anatomical observations [6]. The ganglia of the celiac plexus are situated either side of the line between the origin of the celiac trunk and superior mesenteric artery and remain in constant contact with these arteries. The splanchnic nerves form a common trunk which results from the convergence of the nerve fibers at the T11 level. They are situated in the fatty space either side of the aorta, posterior to the diaphragmatic crura. For percutaneous neurolysis of the celiac plexus, the patient is fasted and placed supine. The T12 level is determined by a digital radiograph of the abdomen. The aortic origins of the celiac trunk and superior mesenteric artery are recognized following an intravenous injection of contrast agent. A 22 gauge needle is introduced by an anterior transabdominal approach at the level of the plane of section which contains the root of the celiac trunk. The needle tip is advanced to the anterior surface of the abdominal aorta (fig. 42.3). The needle track should avoid crossing the healthy pancreatic parenchyma. Passage through the gastric wall should be performed with a true biopsy needle because the Chiba type of needle is easily deviated by the stomach walls. One to 3 ml of dilute contrast are injected through the needle. Stasis of the contrast agent around the needle tip is confirmed by control sections. If the procedure is performed in a pain free period, or if the patient is still on analgesic medication at the time of the procedure, 1 to 3 ml of absolute ethanol are injected through the needle. This injection provokes the usual pains and confirms the correct position of the needle tip. Then, 10 ml of 1% Xylocaine are injected down the needle. The pain should be instantly alleviated. 25 ml of ethanol are also injected through the needle. The injection is repeated after repositioning the needle on the other side of the celiac trunk, only if the contralateral diffusion of ethanol from the first injection has not been satisfactory. Before any injection of ethanol, a prolonged aspiration into the syringe is necessary to confirm that the needle tip is not within the lumen of a vessel. Control sections demonstrate the local diffusion of ethanol by the negative densities anterior to the aorta either side of the midline. The postero-lateral percutaneous route of access is much less comfortable for the patient who has to be placed in the prone position. However, neurolysis of the splanchnic nerves should be performed using a posterior latero-spinal approach at the T11 level. 15 to 20 ml of ethanol are injected on each side.

Results

Neurolysis of the celiac plexus results in a subjective analgesic effect and a reduction in the intake of medication in 87% of cases [9]. The causes for failure of the procedure are linked to the incorrect positioning of the needle too far from the celiac ganglia, a too lateral, retroperitoneal and anterior diffusion of the eth-

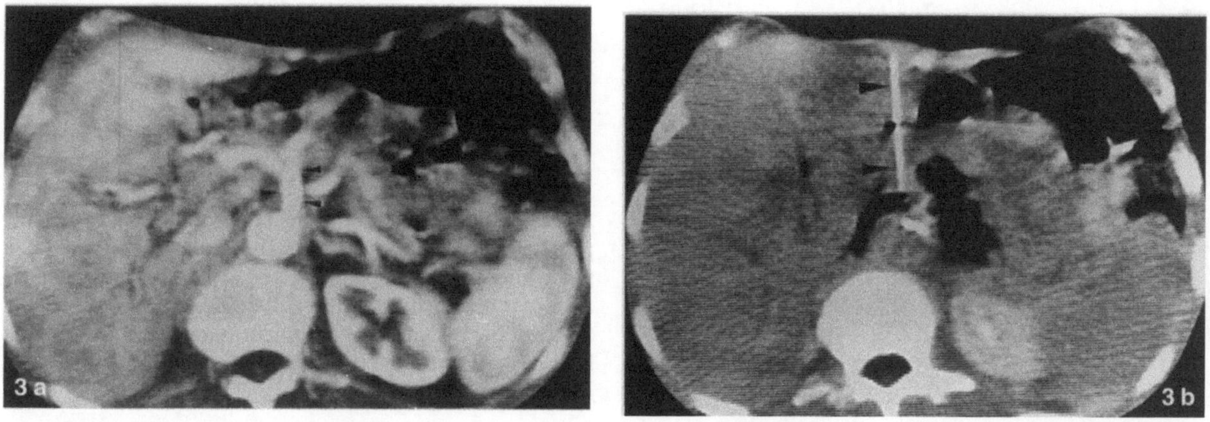

Fig. 42.3. a. Cancer of the pancreas responsible for celiac pain resistant to analgesic medication. CT examination following an intravenous bolus injection of contrast is at the level of the origin of the celiac trunk *(arrow)*; **b** pre-aortic diffusion of 40 ml of absolute ethanol injected at the root of the origin of the celiac trunk (the ethanol is apparent by the negative densities). Note the anterior transvisceral percutaneous approach *(arrow)* and the diffusion of ethanol either side of the origin of the celiac trunk

anol, an insufficient quantity of ethanol injected, regeneration of the demyelinated nerve fibers, progression of the subjacent tumor and the development of other sensory pathways.

Complications

The complications are usually minor and do not require any specific treatment. Rapid venous absorption of the ethanol may cause an alcoholemia and various clinical manifestations. The overactive vasomotor response in the splanchnic circulation may cause a transient systemic hypotension due to pooling of blood in the mesenteric region, and therefore the patient should be kept for several hours under observation following the procedure. We have observed a persistent diarrhea in several patients for up to 2 to 3 months. Diffusion of the ethanol too anteriorly may irritate the posterior parietal peritoneum and result in a moderate transitory chemical peritonitis manifesting as an ileus. The other complications related to the percutaneous approach are avoided by a meticulous technique under CT guidance. Pancreatitis, pneumothorax, hemothorax or perforation of the bowel are exceptionally rare occurrences.

Other interventional procedures

- CT is occasionally used as a method for guiding percutaneous implantation of radioactive sources in the treatment of local tumor recurrence or a residual lesion from a breast or bronchial cancer within the chest wall, CT can also assess the results, including the liver changes [14]. It is also used to direct the transperitoneal insertion of radioactive implants for the local treatment of cancer of the prostate (fig. 42.4).
- The therapeutic monitoring of other procedures which are currently performed either by arterial catheterization or under ultrasound control is achieved using CT. This involves the percutaneous treatment of hepatic carcinomas by the injection of absolute alcohol, or the application of cryotherapy probes, laser probes or thermal ablation, high energy ultrasound or electrocoagulation waves in the treatment of hepatic tumors [1, 4, 11, 21, 23].

CT demonstrates the devascularization or necrosis of tumors following local treatment. In the case of tumor reactivation, there is enhancement at the periphery of the nodule following the injection of contrast agent or the development of satellite tumor lesions in the immediate vicinity of treated lesions (fig. 42.5).

- CT is useful to make a map of the distribution for intra-arterial chemotherapy [3]. Before any therapeutic infusion into the pelvic viscera for example, it is advisable to perform an arterial CT examination by the injection of contrast through infusion catheters placed in the two internal iliac arteries. This examination identifies the dominant vessel in the vascularization of a tumor located in the midline and confirms the total or partial treatment of the tumor by infusion into the catheterized vessels (fig. 42.6).

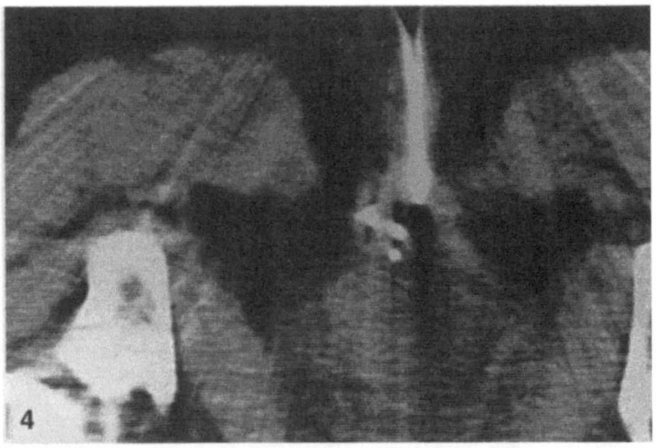

Fig. 42.4. Implantation of radioactive iodine sources via the posterior percutaneous approach, the patient having been placed in the prone position, in an area of local recurrence from cancer of the rectum following surgical resection. Study of the pelvic cavity demonstrating the midline distribution of the radioactive sources in the posterior pelvic region

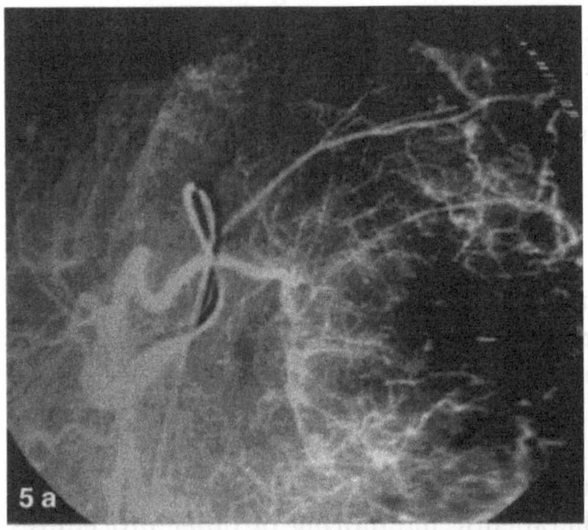

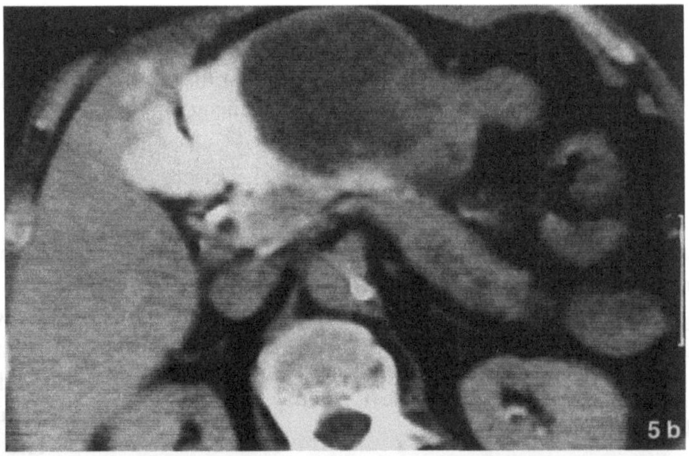

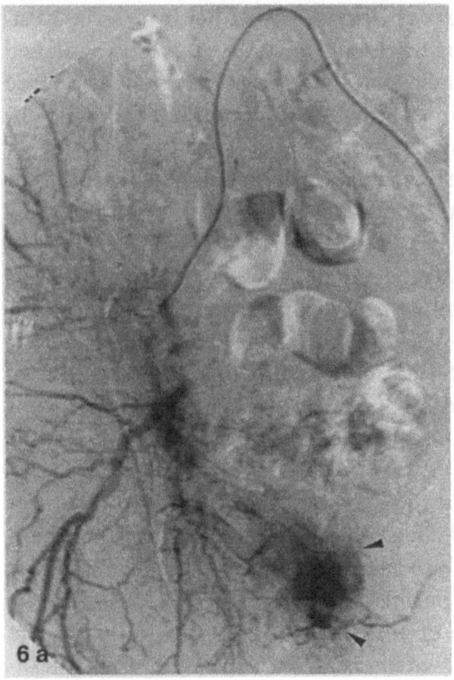

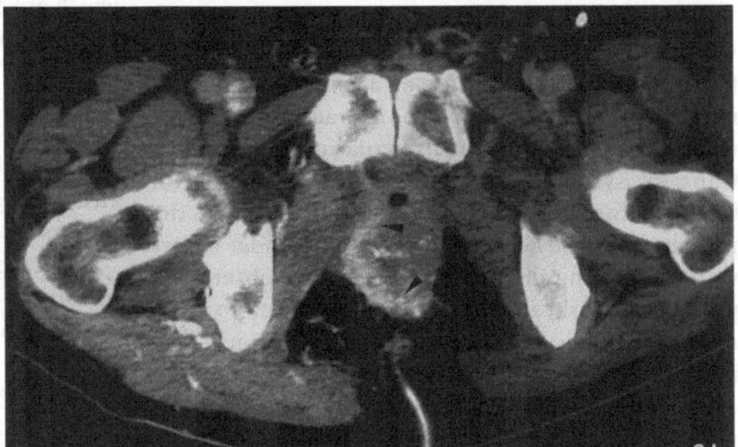

Fig. 42.5. a Chemo-embolization of a hepatocarcinoma in the left lobe of the liver: hypervascular tumor arising from the left hepatic artery in segment 3; **b** devascularization and subtotal necrosis of the tumor on an arterial CT examination performed by injecting contrast into the hepatic artery following the 5th treatment, one year after the commencement of treatment

Fig. 42.6. a Infusion of local chemotherapy for palliative and analgesic treatment of a recurrent cancer of the rectum. Catheterization of the right internal iliac artery. Right perirectal hypervascular tumor *(arrow)*; **b** CT examination performed during the intra-arterial injection of contrast, confirming the intratumoral diffusion of the contrast agent prior to the infusion of the therapeutic agent *(arrow)*

- Finally, CT is usefully employed, in combination with arteriography, for the assessment of hepatic cancers by performing arterial CT examinations or CT portography to demonstrate the extent of hepatic metastases [19, 15].

Spiral acquisition, combined with the possibility of 3-dimensional reconstructions and the volumetric visualization of the organ, provide an accurate segmental localization of all lesions relative to the reference vascular structures.

These 3-dimensional representations are equally useful for certain interventional radiological treatments, such as portal embolization, which is performed percutaneously and induces contralateral hypertrophy of the embolized lobe [7].

References

1. Amin Z, Bown SG, Lees WR (1993) Liver tumor ablation by interstitial laser photocoagulation: review of experimental and clinical studies. Seminars Intervent Radiology 10: 88-100
2. Bernardino ME (1990) Automated biopsy devices: significance and safety. Radiology 176: 615-616
3. Chuang VP, Wallace S (1980) Hepatic arterial redistribution for intraarterial infusion of hepatic neoplasms. Radiology 135: 295-299
4. Dachman AH, Smith MJ, Burris JA, Vandemerwe W (1993) Interstitial laser ablation in experimental models and in clinical use. Seminars Intervent Radiol 10: 101-112
5. Dahnert WF, Heller Hoagland MH, Hamper UM, Erozan YS, Peirce JC (1992) Fine-needle aspiration biopsy of abdominal lesions: diagnostic yield for different needle tip configurations. Radiology 185: 263-268
6. Dal Pozzo G, Bozza A, Fargnoli R, Brizzi E (1985) CT identification of coeliac ganglia. Eur J Radiol 11: 24-26
7. De Baere T, Roche A, Vavasseur D, Therasse E, Indushekar S, Elias D, Bognel C (1993) Portal vein embolization: utility for inducing left hepatic lobe hypertrophy before surgery. Radiology 188: 73-78
8. Erwin BC, Brynes RK, Chan WC (1986) Percutaneous needle biopsy in the diagnosis and classification of lymphoma.Cancer57: 1074-1078
9. Herpels V, Kurdziel JC, Dondelinger RF (1988) Percutaneous CT guided nerve block of the coeliac plexus and splanchnic nerves. Ann Radiol 31: 291-296
10. Hopper KD, Abendroth CS, Sturtz KW, Matthews YL, Shirk SJ (1992) Fine-needle aspiration biopsy for cytopathologic analysis: utility of syringe handles, automated guns, and the nonsuction method. Radiology 185: 819-824
11. Joseph FB, Baumgarten DA, Bernardino ME (1993) Hepatocellular carcinoma: CT appearance after percutaneous ethanol ablation therapy. Work in progress. Radiology 186: 553-556
12. Kurdziel JC, Dondelinger RF (1990) Celiac Plexus. In: Dondelinger RF, Rossi P, Kurdziel JC, Wallace S (eds) Interventional Radiology. Thieme, Stuttgart, PP 768-772
13. Livraghil R, Damascelli B, Lombardi C, Spagnoli I (1983) Risk in fine needle abdominal biopsy. J Clin Ultransound 11: 77-81
14. Marn CS, Andrews JC, Francis IR, Hollet MD, Walker SC, Ensminger WD (1993) Hepatic parenchymal changes after intra-arterial Y-90 therapy: CT findings. Radiology 187: 125-128
15. Matsui O, Fadoya M, Susuki M (1983) Work in progress: dynamic sequential computed tomography during arterial portography in the detection of hepatic neoplasm. Radiology 146: 721-727
16. Morettin LB, Brown RW, Amparo EG, Matteson R (1987) Multiple simultaneous percutaneous needle biopsy technique for masses of the abdomen and peritoneum. Eur J Radiol 7: 98-101
17. Moulton JS, Moore PT (1993) Coaxial percutaneous biopsy technique with automated biopsy devices: value in improving accuracy and negative predictive value. Radiology 186: 515-522
18. Otto RC, Dondelinger RF, Kurdziel JC (1990) Abdominal biopsy. In: Dondelinger RF, Rossi P, Kurdziel JC, Wallace S (eds) Interventional Radiology. Thieme, Stuttgart, pp 33-52
19. Oudkerk M, Van Ooijen B, Mali SPM, Tjiam SL, Schmitz PIM, Wiggers T (1992) Liver metastases from colorectal carcinoma: detection with continuous CT angiography. Radiology 185: 157-161
20. Plunkett MB, Peterson MS, Landreneau RJ, Ferson PF, Posner MC (1992) Peripheral pulmonary nodules: preoperative percutaneous needle localization with CT guidance. Radiology 185: 274-276
21. Sironi S, Delmaschio A (1993) Follow-up imaging of hepatocellular carcinoma treated with percutaneous ethanol injection. Seminars Intervent Radiol 10: 78-79
22. Smith EH (1984) The hazards of fine needle aspiration biopsy. Ultrasound Med Biol 10: 629-634
23. Tanaka K, Okazaki H, Nakamura S (1991) Hepatocellular carcinoma: treatment with a combination therapy of transcatheter arterial embolization and percutaneous ethanol injection. Radiology 179: 713-717

CHAPTER 43

Primary malignant tumors of bone and soft tissues

Clinicians
G. Delépine, N. Delépine, J.-M. Ziza,
J.-C. Desbois, J.-L. Misset

Radiologist
D. Lardé

Primary malignant bone tumors

Before the advent of the new treatment protocols, immediate high amputation used to represent the only treatment for sarcomas of the limbs. Unfortunately, this did not prevent the development of metastatic disease in more than 90% of cases of Ewing's sarcoma, 80% of osteosarcomas and nearly a half of the chondrosarcoma cases.

Two advances have transformed the life expectancy and functional prognosis for bone sarcomas, particularly those arising in the limbs:
- the advent of digital medical imaging (CT and MRI) has provided a very accurate assessment of the tumor extent, enabling an almost complete excision of the tumor in a single block, as well as preserving the function of the limb [13];
- the appearance of chemotherapy protocols [43, 44] has resulted in more and more patients surviving.

Since 1989, osteosarcoma has become a curable disease with a survival rate in primary complete remission close to 100% [18]. This figure is also more than 90% for Ewing's sarcoma [14].

However, the prognosis for bone sarcomas of low grade malignancy depends, above all, on the quality of the surgical treatment which is guided by an accurate staging.

The therapeutic advances and development of protocols depend on an international classification system, initially proposed by Ennecking. This distinguishes:
- sarcomas of low grade malignancy (degree I);
- sarcomas which have a risk of metastasis (degree II);
- sarcomas whose general malignancy has already been expressed by macroscopic metastasis (degree III).

Locally, it distinguishes:
- tumors which only involve bone (intracompartmental tumors or group A);
- bone tumors which invade the adjacent soft tissue (extracompartmental tumors or group B).

The detection of a bone tumor, sometimes in a deceptive clinical context, depends on the radiographic examination.

The comparison of the radiological and clinical findings can provide, in a limited number of cases, a definitive diagnosis and represents the only acceptable exception to biopsy (table 43.1).

Table 43.1. Permissible exceptions to biopsy

1. Monostotic lesion - benign metaphyseal lacuna (cortical defect, non-ossifying fibroma) - asymptomatic osteogenic exostosis - non-fractured solitary cyst - vertebral angioma
2. Polyostotic lesions - fibrous dysplasia, - enchondromatosis - exostotic disease - bone involvement from histiocytosis X - bone metastasis from a known primary

A complementary CT and/or MRI examination may improve the diagnostic certainty in a few cases by:
- morphological analysis (study of the cortex and soft tissues);
- analysis of the density or signal intensity to establish the fatty, cystic, soft tissue and/or calcific nature of the lesion (e.g. intraosseous lipoma).

In the majority of cases, this comparison of the clinical features with these complementary examinations can only provide a presumptive diagnosis. When the possibility of a progressive lesion cannot be excluded or malignancy seems probable, the principal aim of the morphological examination (CT and/or MRI) is to determine accurately the extent of the lesion prior to histological assessment by biopsy.

CT

The assessment of local spread depends on the following simple principals:
- definition of a reference anatomical plane (e.g. the femoro-tibial line for the lower limb);
- evaluation within a centimeter of the longitudinal extent of the osteomedullary lesion;
- measurement in 3 planes of the soft tissue mass (with evaluation, if necessary, of the tumor volume);
- definition of the relationships of the vascular structures and determining the vascularity of the lesion by systemic injection of an iodinated contrast agent using the bolus method.

Osteomedullary involvement

This is the usual site of origin of a tumor process [19, 20].

In the physiological state, the medullary compartment has a negative density value due to its fatty content (density usually between -40 and -110 HU). The presence of a soft tissue process increases the density value (positive).

The associated inflammatory phenomena or the aseptic necrobiosis do not cause significant alterations in the accuracy of the assessment of medullary spread.

The assessment of spread tends to be a little more precise in the metaphyso-epiphyseal region due to the presence of spongy bone. The inadequacy of this method in this region is reduced by the improved spatial resolution of the latest generation scanners.

Corticospongy involvement is generally more lim-ited than that of the medullary spread. The appearance of the periosteal reaction indicates the progressive nature of the tumor and its osteogenic capabilities. Its description remains of secondary interest.

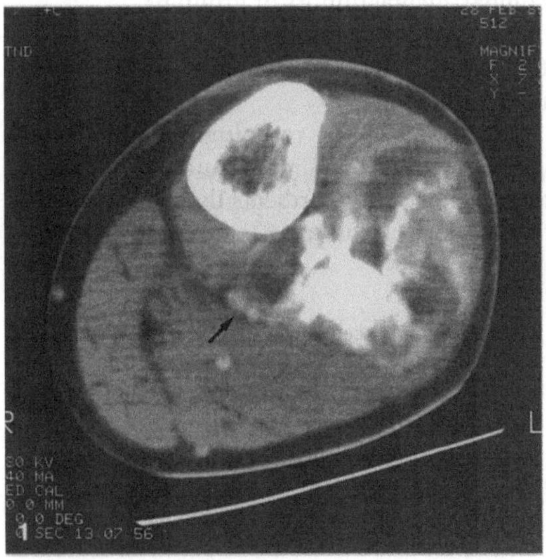

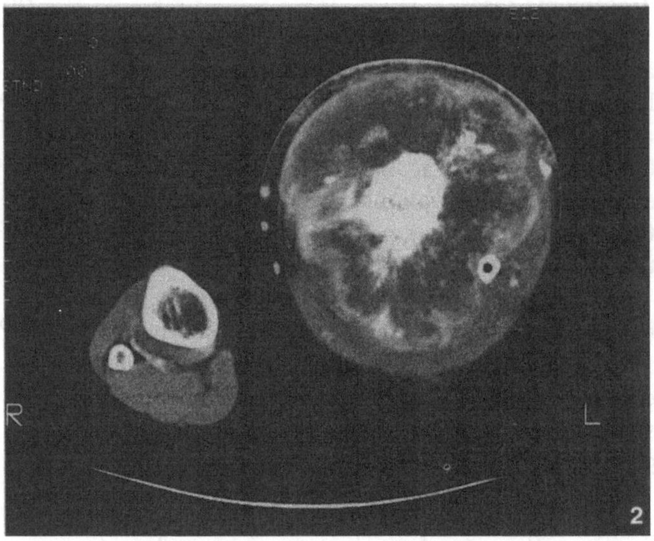

Fig. 43.1. Osteosarcoma of the fibula on CT. Spread into the adjacent soft tissues is well demonstrated following injection of intravenous iodinated contrast. It is predominantly in the anterior and perineal compartments, and displaces posteriorly the posterior tibial neurovascular bundle *(arrow)*

Fig. 43.2. Osteosarcoma of the tibia on CT. Extensive spread into the peripheral soft tissues, the limits of the lesion are highlighted by the peripheral enhancement. The mass is predominantly necrotic

Soft tissue lesions

Prior to injection of contrast agent, the mass is hypodense and may contain calcified elements.

In current practice, the contrast injection is performed straight away (repeated boluses). This allows appreciation of the hypervascular composition of the tumor (with better definition of the limits of the lesion) and evaluates the degree of necrosis (figs 43.1 & 43.2) [35]. The position of the principal neurovascular axis is usually visualized.

The detection of possible intra-articular spread is still difficult.

Pitfalls and limitations [9, 27]

The nutrient vessels of the bone cause a punctiform intramedullary hyperdensity. This pitfall can usually be avoided.

Diaphyseal skip lesion may be missed by CT if the whole of the bone is not examined in contiguous sections.

Small corticoperiosteal abnormalities are better seen on conventional radiographs (of secondary interest in practice). The contrast between the fat and tumor tissue is reduced in the metaphyso-epiphyseal region by the presence of spongy bone.

The assessment of the tumor extent in the small bones (humerus, fibula) is adequate although the assessment of the more distal regions is less accurate.

The assessment of tumor spread into the soft tissues may be distorted by the presence of a post-biopsy hematoma.

MRI

The assessment of locoregional spread must nowadays follow a well established protocol [32]:
- this requires an examination of the whole length of the bone (using the body coil in the majority of cases);
- the examination is performed:
  . in at least 3 planes on T1-weighted imaging, and in one of the 3 planes on T2-weighted imaging:
  . in at least the longitudinal plane on T1-weighted imaging (medullary lesion) and in the axial plane on T2-weighted imaging (soft tissue lesion);
- the injection of a gadolinium compound (always performed after an initial examination) is contributory [52]. It is especially valuable for assessing the degree of necrosis.

The tumor is usually hypointense on the T1 sequences and hyperintense on T2 sequences [41]. No precise diagnostic information can be obtained by a study of the signal intensities or their distribution within the lesion [3].

Osteomedullary tumor spread

This is best assessed on the T1-weighted sequences in the longitudinal plane including the whole length of the involved bone.

The lesion is exquisitely demonstrated in the form of a low signal intensity replacing the high signal intensity of the normal bone marrow (fig. 43.3).

The skip metastasis are easily recognized (fig. 43.4).

In a child, the epiphyseal cartilage is clearly identified as a hypointense line.

The evaluation of tumor spread in the metaphyso-epiphyseal region can be complemented, if necessary, by the T2 sequences, the hyperintense tumor contrasting with the hypointense trabeculae of the spongy bone.

Intra-articular extension is assessed, if necessary, by the use of specifically adapted surface coils which can analyze the capsulo-ligamentous structures.

Soft tissue lesions (fig. 43.5)

These are better appreciated on the T2 sequences, the hyperintense tumor contrasting with the normal low signal intensity of the muscle structures.

The degree of necrosis can be measured by the injection of gadolinium, the active vascularized parts of the tumor enhanced on T1-weighted imaging. However, gadolinium is of little use for defining the limits of the tumor [46].

The anatomical position of the principal vascular axes (displacement, encasement) is well assessed on the longitudinal sequences.

Pitfalls and limitations

- The assessment of the cortical bone is inaccurate [4] (absence of signal and the frequency of chemical shift artefacts);
- small calcifications are not visible (loss of diagnostic information for tumors of a cartilaginous nature);
- the limited spatial resolution makes it difficult to detect small lesions of the soft tissue [54];
- enhancement of the signal of the osteomedullary lesion by gadolinium may efface the boundaries which become isointense with the adjacent fatty marrow (hence the importance of an initial pre-gadolinium scan);

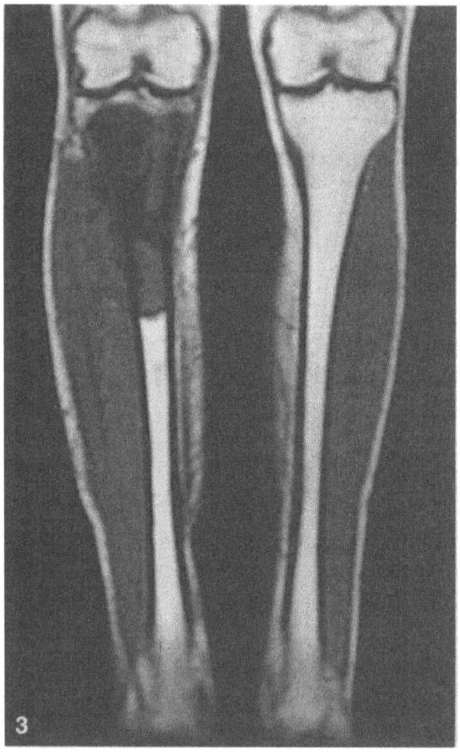

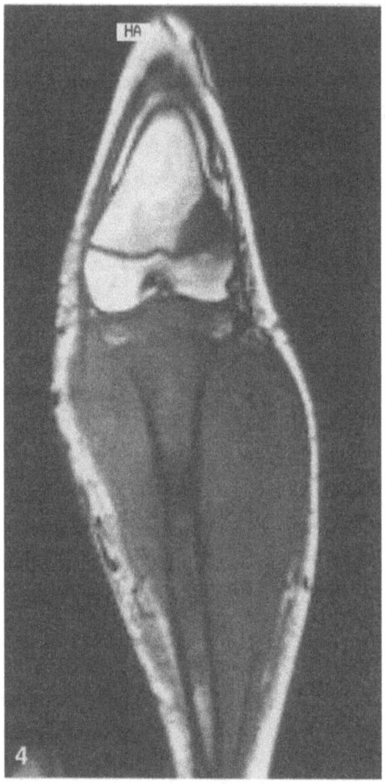

Fig. 43.3. Bone sarcoma of the superior end of the right tibia on MRI. Spin echo T1 sequence. The longitudinal medullary spread of the tumor is well appreciated, appearing hypointense

Fig. 43.4. Large sarcoma of the tibia on MRI. T1 spin echo sequence. Skip lesion in the inferior metaphyseal region of the femur (hypointense)

– the assessment of spread in an active cellular bone marrow (particularly in children and around the pelvic lesion) may be very difficult whatever the sequence is used (T1 or T2);
– the degree of tumor necrosis may be overestimated in cases where the cells secrete mucus with a signal intensity identical to that of necrosis [54];
– the principle risk is an overestimation of the extent of the tumor on the T2 sequence due to the high sensitivity of the method, and the limits of the lesional hyperintensity may be increased by the associated inflammatory reaction or aseptic necrosis (table 43.2).

Table 43.2. Advantages and disadvantages of CT and MRI

Advantages	Disadvantages
CT	
- simple rapid examination - reliable - cheap	- examination of the extremities - skip metastasis
MRI	
- multiplanar examination - study of the whole length of bone (skip metastasis) - better analysis of the metaphyso-epiphyseal and articular regions -relationship to the vascular structures	- poorer spatial resolution - poor demonstration of calcification - tendency to overestimate the extent of the lesion (inflammatory phenomena)

Histological types

It is vital to establish the histology of the lesion.

Osteosarcoma

This is the commonest malignant primary bone tumor.

Recognition of the different classifications is of little practical value. It is, however, particularly useful to distinguish the bone sarcomas of low grade malignancy, for whom the treatment is essentially local, from the sarcomas of high grade malignancy requiring pre- and post-operative polychemotherapy.
– the primary osteosarcoma of high grade malignancy involves mainly the active metaphyses of the adolescent during the growth period.

There is a clear male preponderance with a peak incidence in the second decade of life.
– The juxtacortical osteosarcoma is the most classical form of the osteosarcomas of the low grade malignancy. It particularly occurs in the fifth decade of life with perhaps a female predominance. It arises on the surface of the bone and has a slow evolution encircling

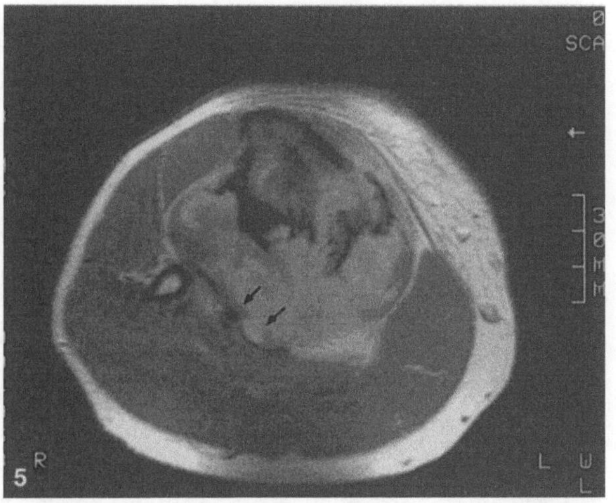

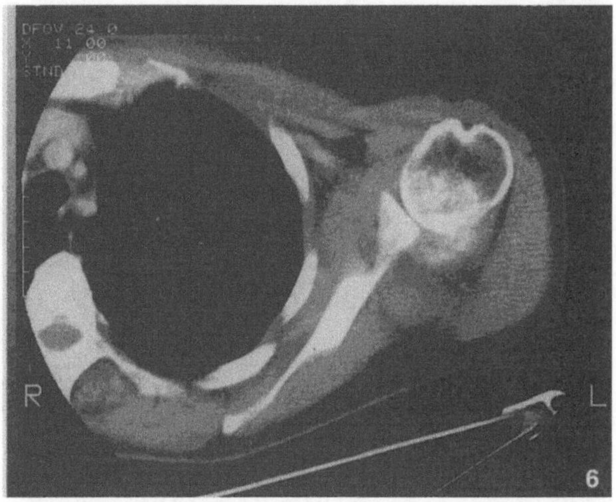

Fig. 43.5. Bone sarcoma of the tibia on MRI. On post-gadolinium T1-weighted imaging, the lesion is hyperintense with well defined limits. The posterior tibial vascular axis is displaced posteriorly and laterally *(arrow)*

Fig. 43.6. Juxtacortical osteosarcoma of the humerus on CT. Spread into the medulla of the humeral diaphysis with partial replacement of the fatty marrow hypodensity by a calcified structure (posterior part)

the bone. There is a predominant osteoblastic activity with homogeneous bone thickening and well defined borders in the adjacent soft tissues. The connection to the cortex is usually limited.

It occurs particularly on the posterior surface of the lower femur. The principle role of imaging is to exclude any associated medullary involvement (completely changing the therapeutic protocol) (fig. 43.6).

Ewing's sarcoma

This is the commonest bone sarcoma of children of less than 12 years with a male predominance.

It probably belongs to the group of primary neuroectodermal tumors [45].

The microscopic appearance is that of a tumor containing sheets of small round cells containing glycogen granules without any connective tissue matrix. The radiological appearances are variable, particularly dependent on the position, with a more lytic evolution in the flat bones and sclerotic progression in the long bones. There is usually a significant extension into the peripheral soft tissues [22, 51].

It is, in fact, a diffuse disease and is treated as such by chemotherapy.

Chondrosarcoma

Three forms can be distinguished:

- The enchondrosarcoma (primary) is mainly encountered in adults between the ages of 30 and 60 years. The tumor usually evolves slowly, expanding the bone and slowly invading the soft tissues, with secondary deposition of calcific materials. There are numerous deceptive forms;
- the ecchondrosarcoma (secondary) often develops in the cartilaginous cap of an exostosis, rapidly invading the soft tissue. However, spread to the bony base of the exostosis occurs much later (fig. 43.7);
- the differentiated form of the chondrosarcoma has a peak incidence in the seventh decade of life (predominantly male). It is essentially a lytic lesion with spread into the soft tissues (usually without calcific deposits). There is a significant metastatic potential [11].

Miscellaneous forms: fibrosarcoma, malignant fibrous histiocytoma, giant cell sarcoma

The diagnosis depends essentially on the histological findings.

Chordoma

A rare malignant tumor, the chordoma has a mainly locally progressive potential with invasion of the soft tissues.

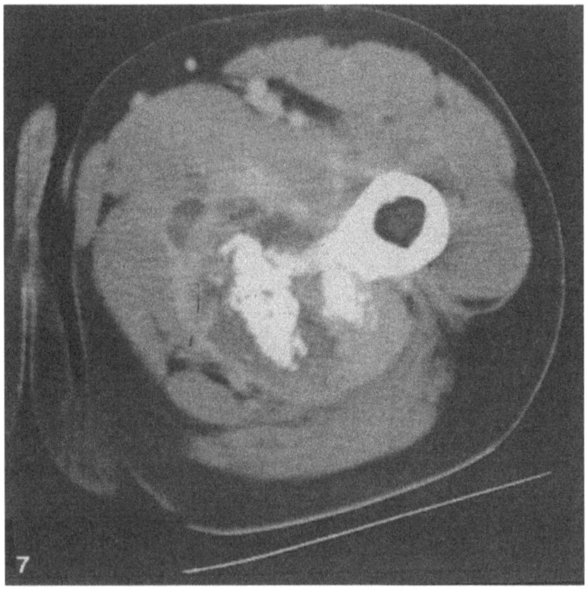

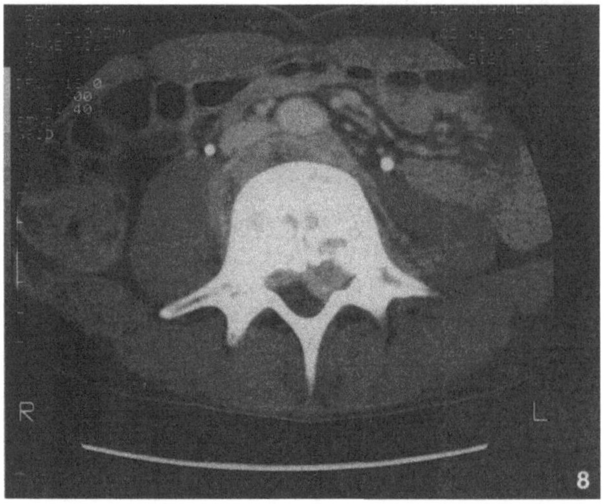

Fig. 43.7. Chondrosarcoma arising in an exostosis (medial surface of the left femur) on CT. The cartilaginous cap is clearly thickened greater than 2 cm (it is considered to be suspicious if greater than 1 cm), with a partially vascularized soft tissue structure. The superficial femoral vascular bundle is away from the lesion. The medulla of the femur is unaffected

Fig. 43.8. Osteosarcoma of the lower limb. Post-contrast CT. Increased uptake in L3 on scintigraphy. Secondary deposit with tumor spread into the prevertebral soft tissues (displacing the aorta and inferior vena cava anteriorly), and intraspinal spread (causing a significant indentation of the anterior of the surface of the dural sac)

The tumor arises from the embryonic remnants of the notochord and consequently is located in the axial skeleton. The sacrococcygeal region is the commonest localization (more than 50% of cases) followed by the skull base.

It usually effects middle aged adults with a male predominance. The evolution is usually slow and insidious. There is often a large associated soft tissue mass at the time of detection of the tumor.

In the classical sacral localization, the osteolysis is poorly defined. CT and/or MRI define the degree of extension into the soft tissues and the relationships of the tumor. The lesion is usually hypovascular, sometimes with a fairly characteristic loculated appearance. Calcium deposition is common but minimal.

The primary differential diagnosis of a sacral chordoma is a chondrosarcoma. Plasmocytoma, bone metastasis and nerve tumors (ependymomas, Schwannomas) are other possibilities [55]. There is usually only limited extension into the soft tissues in the case of giant cell tumors. Complete surgical excision is difficult, resulting in the frequent recurrences, even following combined radiotherapy. Metastasis may be seen late in the evolution of the disease.

Adamantinoma

This is an exceptionally rare bone tumor with a slow growth rate which is located in the diaphysis of the tibia in almost 9 out of 10 cases.

The etiology and pathology are still disputed. A history of previous trauma is present in two thirds of cases. The lesion may occur at any age, the peak incidence being in the third decade. It causes cortical osteolysis, usually without break, and a rather multiloculated appearance surrounded by reactive osteosclerosis. Metastases are possible (lungs). Wide surgical excision is the only hope of cure.

Preoperative management

There must be a rigorous approach when the diagnosis of malignancy has not been excluded:
- assessment of local extent by CT or MRI, which makes it possible to plan the surgical excision in a single block and to choose the most suitable approach for biopsy [12];
- anatomopathological examination performed on the surgical biopsy material (allowing an adequate quan-

tity of pathological tissue to be examined) with preoperative histological and cytological examination.

In bone sarcomas of high grade malignancy

Neoadjuvant chemotherapy (preoperative) is commenced on the same day as the biopsy.

The general assessment is performed during the days following the induction chemotherapy and must include at least bone scintigraphy (fig. 43.8) and pulmonary CT to look for secondary deposits

The efficacy of the chemotherapy can be evaluated by:
- angiography (digital), this requires the performance of 2 examinations separated by an interval of 3 weeks to 1 month with an assessment of the tumor vascularity;
- CT (evaluation of the tumor volume, vascularity and the progression of the necrosis);
- or MRI, with assessment of the extraosseous component of the tumor [24]. Although the signal changes on T2-weighted imaging can give some indication of the efficacy of chemotherapy [21, 34], there are, in fact, no sufficiently reliable criteria to predict a good response [25]. The reduction in tumor volume and the increase in the hypointense zones can be present and independent of a good histopathological response in more than a half of the cases. The dynamic injection of gadolinium provides a better evaluation [5, 21], particularly with the help of subtraction techniques, allowing distinction between neoplastic and inflammatory enhancement (the latter being more progressive) (D. Vanel);
- phlebography is indicated preoperatively, especially when the tumor is large and compressing the principal vascular axes, in order to look for possible intravenous thrombi (thus modifying the operative technique).

In bone sarcomas of low grade malignancy

For sarcomas of low grade malignancy (juxtacortical osteosarcoma, grade 1 and grade 2 chondrosarcoma...), the treatment is essentially surgical and is dependent on an accurate assessment of local extent.

Follow-up

CT

The quality of the local CT follow-up is largely dependent on the surgical technique employed. The use of reconstruction prostheses made of titanium (surrounded by allograph from the bank) reduces the resultant metal artefacts sufficiently to allow a fairly reliable analysis of the periprosthetic soft tissues. The techniques used for the CT examination are the same as those for the initial scan.

In the majority of cases, the recurrent tumor appears as a mass in the soft tissues (with variable neovascularization). It must be distinguished from the post-operative changes;
- hematomas often form well defined and avascular cavities:
- enhancement of the fibrosis following contrast injection is generally homogeneous, moderately intense, stable or diminishing on successive examinations;
- the presence of corticospongy material which is often used in abundance for consolidating the bone at the junction of the banked allograft and the remaining bone of the patient must be recognized and distinguished from possible tumor recurrence with an osteoid matrix.

Follow-up for distant spread is particularly concentrated on the lungs in the search for possible secondary lesions.

MRI

MRI remains feasible in patients with titanium metallic prosthetic implants.

The signal of a tumor recurrence does not differ from that of the initial lesion (hypointense on T1-weighted imaging: hyperintense on T2-weighted imaging).

Yet again, the high sensitivity of the technique is offset by its relatively poor specificity.. Therefore, the presence of an abnormal high signal intensity on the T2 sequences does not necessarily correspond to a tumor recurrence. It can equally well represent any other lesion with a high water content: infective lesions (osteitis or abscess), necrotic tissue (notably following radiotherapy alone), fluid cavity.

The use of a gadolinium contrast agent can usually distinguish the cavity lesions (not altered by the gadolinium) and vascularized soft tissue (which enhance on the T1-weighted sequences).

The dynamic injection of gadolinium with subtraction techniques may make it possible to differentiate young active fibrosis (particularly caused by chemotherapy or radiotherapy) from tumor recurrence, the enhancement of the tumor appearing more rapidly of that of the fibrosis (D. Vanel).

Strategy

It is essential to obtain a reference baseline examination following the stabilization of the post-operative changes (after the sixth week). For sarcomas of high grade malignancy, the local (CT and MRI) and general monitoring is performed every 3 months for the first 2 years, and every 6 months for the following 3 years. The frequency of these follow-up examinations can obviously be modified depending on the clinical findings. For sarcomas of low grade malignancy, the local surveillance must continue for 10 years because late recurrences are possible. 3D volumetric CT imaging seems promising (see later fig. 43.14).

Malignant tumors of the soft tissues

The tumors of the soft tissues have benefited from the same diagnostic and therapeutic advances as those for bone sarcomas [15].

The clinical picture is dominated by the discovery of a generally painless soft tissue mass. Its often well defined character on clinical examination is a poor and sometimes misleading indicator of the benign or malignant nature of the lesion. The routine assessment of the drainage lymph nodes may help point to the diagnosis.

Ultrasound is usually the first examination requested. This confirms the organic nature of the lesion and defines its cystic or soft tissue nature.

If the diagnosis is in doubt and histological confirmation is planned, particularly in the presence of an echogenic or "soft tissue" lesion, complementary investigation by CT and/or MRI is necessary.

CT

The performance of the examination does not differ from that described for bone tumors (definition of a reference anatomical plane, measurement in centimeters in all 3 planes).

The injection of an intravenous iodinated contrast using the bolus method is particularly important. It often improves the delineation of lesion, defines the degree of vascularization and necrosis, and demonstrates the vascular relationships (and confirms the patency of the principle vessels) (fig. 43.9).

CT may also be of diagnostic value for:
- verifying the cystic nature of a lesion, some synovial cysts having an echogenic content (viscosity of the fluid);
- confirming lipomas (negative density of the fat);
- recognizing some liposarcomas;
- suggesting the vascular nature of angiomas and angiopericytomas.

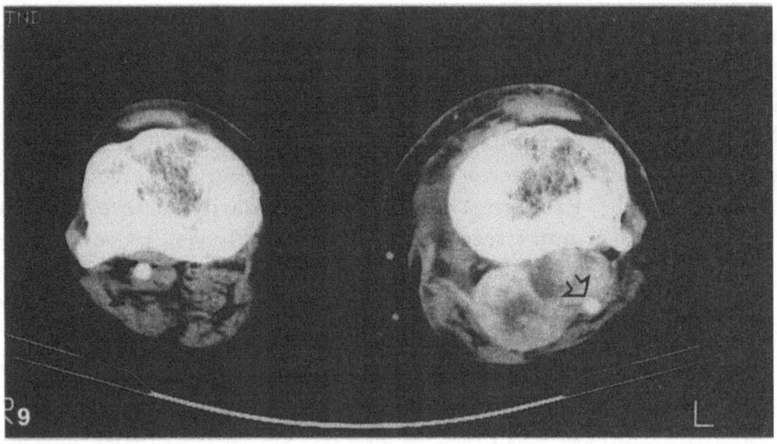

Fig. 43.9. Liposarcoma of the left popliteal fossa on CT. Injection of iodinated contrast agent using the bolus method. The mass is hypervascular (with a small central hypodense component due to necrosis). The popliteal artery is displaced postero-laterally in contact with the lesion *(arrow)*

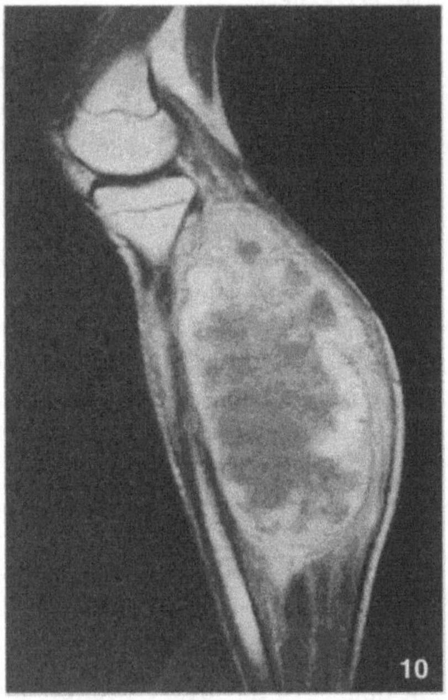

Fig. 43.10. Synovial sarcoma of the calf. Post-gadolinium sagittal T1 MRI section defining the predominantly necrotic nature of the lesion

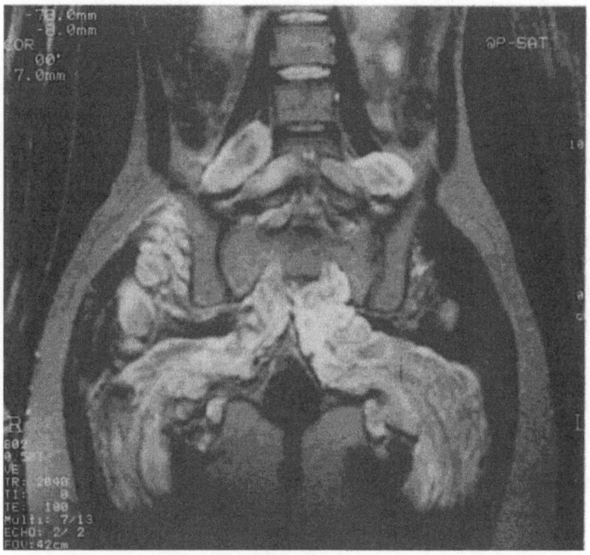

Fig. 43.11. von Recklinghausen's neurofibromatosis on MRI. Coronal T2 sequence (second echo). The neurofibroma (hyperintense) extend along the different nerve axes from the L3 level, with involvement of the predominantly nerve root of the cauda equina

This examination is especially important in assessing the extent of the lesion, guiding the biopsy approach, and modifying the therapeutic management.

The finding differs little from that described for bone tumors which spread into the soft tissues. The lesion may arise exclusively in the soft tissues or extend into bone (a rare situation).

MRI

The reference plane for the examination of soft tissue tumors is the axial plane with the performance of T1- and T2-weighted spin echo sequences. These are complemented, if necessary, by coronal or sagittal sequences, particularly around the joints [17, 49] (fig. 43.10).

The injection of gadolinium is not necessary. It may efface the spontaneous contrast between the hypointense tumor and hyperintense adjacent fatty tissue (T1-weighted spin echo sequences). The evaluation of the necrotic composition is of no practical value, chemotherapy being an adjuvant treatment following surgery. However, the use of gadolinium should be considered when the various sequences (T1 and T2) suggest the presence of a cystic formation, since intramuscular myxomas may have identical characteristics on the sequences without contrast injection [39].

The benign or malignant nature of a soft tissue lesion may be suspected in a number of cases [2], based on the morphological criteria and distribution of the signal. The benign lesion is well defined, and its signal is homogeneous. There is neither encasement of the neurovascular bundle nor osteolysis. The distinction between a benign and malignant lesion remains difficult, however, for the desmoid fibromas (infiltrative lesion), the tumoral form of villonodular synovitis, and a benign tumor progressing to become necrotic (neurofibroma). However, in the majority of cases, the analysis of the signal provides little information on the histological nature of the soft tissue mass, the exceptions being a lipoma, subacute hemorrhage, hemangioma and certain well differentiated liposarcomas [6, 30, 42, 50]. Regardless of the site of the tumor and its histological type, the lesion is usually hypointense on T1-weighted imaging and hyperintense on T2-weighted imaging.

The principal role of MRI is definitely still in the assessment of tumor extent prior to surgical biopsy (fig. 43.11).

Respective roles of the two examinations

Although the capabilities of the two examinations are very similar [1, 8, 26, 38, 40], MRI has today tended to be the method of choice due to the precise assessment of muscle spread and the aponeurotic relationships. MRI is the easiest method of analyzing the neurovascular structures [17, 49] but remains poor for the detection of calcifications or ossifications (which may possibly guide towards the diagnosis).

Both methods are equally inadequate in predicting the integrity of the periosteum or the possible tumor adherence to the adjacent neurovascular structures.

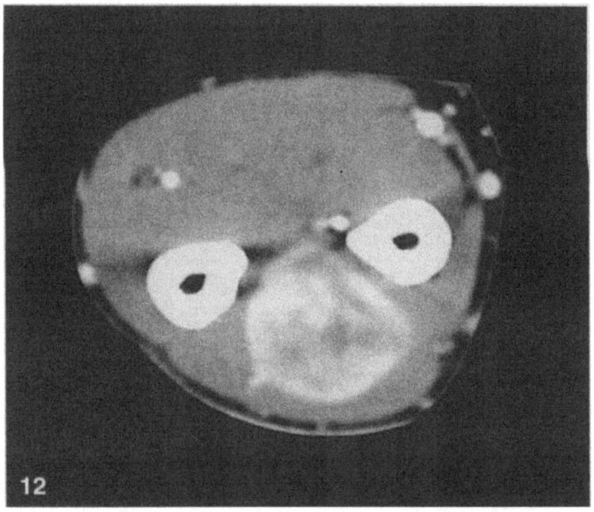

Fig. 43.12. Malignant fibrous histiocytoma of the posterior compartment of the forearm. Angiographic CT defines the hypervascular nature of the lesion (almost 3 cm in diameter) and the position of the principal vascular axes

Findings specific to histological type

Malignant fibrous histiocytoma (fig. 43.12)

This is one of the commonest tumors encountered and is more commonly observed between the ages of 50 and 70 years. It arises in the muscle or fascia and often has indistinct boundaries [29, 37].

The tumor usually becomes necrotic, bone extension is rare. The tumor is lymphophilic.

The CT and MRI appearances cannot differentiate it from the other soft tissue tumors. The presence of a low signal intensity on the spin echo T2-weighted sequences has been reported in several cases [48].

Liposarcoma

This may occur at any age (more common in middle aged adults) and anywhere in the body (predisposition for the thigh and sites close to the neurovascular bundles).

The myxoid form is the commonest with an identical appearance on imaging to other tumors. The presence of fatty tissue may suggest the diagnosis. There are rarely well organized areas of fat, but rather deposits arranged in a linear fashion, or in small pockets, which should be carefully looked for [49].

The fatty composition may predominate (lipomatous liposarcoma).

The presence of irregular contours and heterogeneity excludes the diagnosis of a simple lipoma (rare form).

The liposarcoma is generally well defined, pseudoencapsulated, and usually with the presence of septa [49]. Metastatic spread is rare and usually occurs to the lungs and liver.

Synovial sarcoma (malignant synovioma)

This is a mesenchymal tumor affecting particularly the young adult, often in the vicinity of joints (bursae and tendon sheaths), but usually without any connection to the articular synovium. It is, in fact, a lesion whose histological appearance is close to that of the synovial tissue although its development within the joint synovium is extremely rare [7, 16].

The tumor is often hypervascular [47]. The presence of calcific structures is observed in approximately 30% of cases.

On MRI, the multilocular configuration of lesion with the presence of septa is fairly suggestive [36]. Its boundaries tend to be poorly defined (infiltrative lesion). Fluid levels may be seen within the mass, related to the hemorrhagic or necrotic abnormalities (fig. 43.10). The tumor is lymphophilic.

Fibrosarcoma

This has no specific characteristic pathological features. It may occur in children, particularly at birth (congenital fibrosarcoma), or in the first 2 years of life in the limb extremities with a better prognosis. The risk of metastasis depends on the degree of malignancy histologically. Pulmonary lesions are the commonest.

Rhabdomyosarcoma

This arises in striated muscle and is the commonest soft tissue tumor in children (pelvis and neck) in whom it is usually the highly chemosensitive embryonic form. It may also occur in the young adult (limbs) in whom the alveolar and pleomorphic variants are the rule and chemotherapy is much less efficacious.

The lesion is usually hypervascular with poorly defined boundaries. It may contain calcifications. Spread to bone is quite common. The tumor is highly lymphophilic.

Leiomyosarcoma

This arises from the white muscle fibers with a predilection for the thigh and along the vascular pathways (venous wall).

The lesion occurs in the adult and is usually pseudo-encapsulated and poorly vascularized. It has a significant metastatic potential via venous spread (lungs, lymph nodes, bone) and often presents with an isolated phlebitis.

The presence of endovenous spread (routinely looked for by phlebography) is a feature of a poor prognosis.

Two lesions of the soft tissue merit special mention due to the resultant diagnostic problems (myositis ossificans) or therapeutic problems (desmoid fibroma) which they may cause.

Myositis ossificans circumscripta

This does not always arise in the context of trauma. It is spontaneous in approximately a third of cases, posing the problem of a possible progressive tumor.

The radiological and, if necessary, CT appearances are sufficiently characteristic to avoid surgical biopsy (the histological study is often very difficult and sometimes can be confused with osteosarcoma).

Desmoid fibroma

This is a benign tumor histologically, developing from the musculo-aponeurotic structures. However, it has the tendency to recur frequently, and wide surgical excision of the lesion is often difficult, mainly due to its infiltrative and often multifocal nature (fibromatosis).

On CT, it usually appears as a hypervascular mass of homogeneous density which may be observed anywhere in the body and at any age [28]

On MRI, the signal intensity depends on the cellularity of the lesion and the abundance of collagen which tends to be more distributed in the periphery [23]. Several appearances can be observed:

- either non-specific (hypointense on T1- and hyperintense on T2-weighted imaging);
- or hypointense on both the T1- and the T2-weighted spin echo sequences due to the acellularity of the tumor and the abundance of collagen [48];
- the presence of hypointense linear or curvilinear opacities on both sequences within a lesion which appears hyperintense on T2-weighted imaging is also suggestive of the diagnosis of fibromatosis [31].

Tumor recurrence may be difficult to differentiate from fibrotic scarring with enhancement fairly close to soft tissue density or signal intensity following the injection of contrast [53].

Management strategy

The diagnostic and therapeutic management is nowadays well rationalized.

Small volume tumors

In the case of a small superficial tumor for which a wide excision is without any obvious problem: excision biopsy in a single procedure.

Large subaponeurotic tumors

Standard radiology is still essential (study of the density of the lesion and adjacent bony structures).

Ultrasound may be performed at the same time as radiography to confirm the organic nature of the tumor and to define its cystic or soft tissue character;

The assessment of spread is undertaken by CT or ideally by MRI (method of choice), these two examinations allow planning of the surgical excision of the tumor in a single block [10];

"Planned" biopsy, taking into account the excision of the biopsy track at the time of surgical intervention [12];

The indication for angiography depends on the tumor localization, its size and associated clinical signs;

Assessment of distant spread:
- if the tumor is lymphophilic, the search for lymphadenopathy will usually be performed by CT,
- confirmation of the normality of the pulmonary parenchyma (and pleura) by CT;
- in the majority of cases, the treatment is surgical straight-away, apart from the following exceptions:
- chemosensitive tumors (e.g. embryonic rhabdomyosarcoma of children);

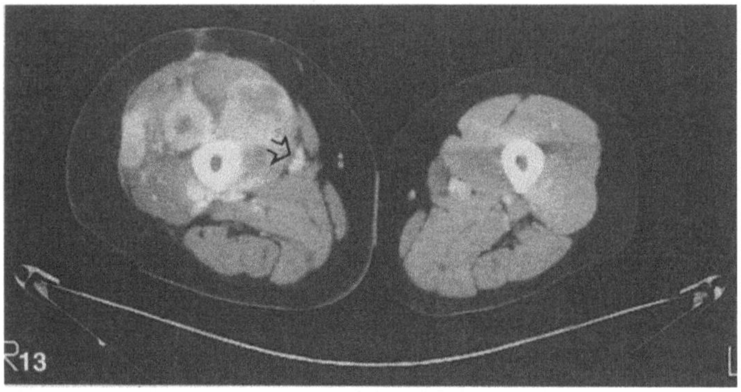

Fig. 43.13. Recurrence of a rhabdomyosarcoma in the anterior compartment of the right thigh on CT. The tumor recurrence is multifocal and clearly enhanced following contrast. Close relationship with the superficial femoral vascular pedicle *(arrow)*

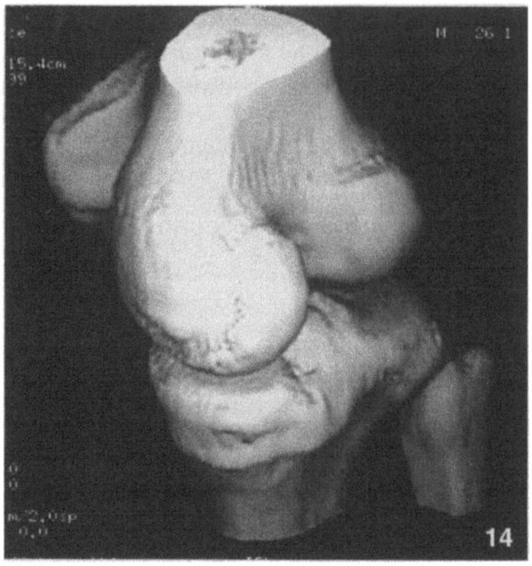

Fig. 43.14. 3-D volumetric study on helical CT of a normal left knee (image courtesy of Dr D Buthiau, scanner Paris 14)

- or those which cannot be excised in a single block without significant mutilation;

Monoblock surgical excision may require reconstructive surgery for bone and vascular resection, or musculocutaneous plastic surgery to achieve skin coverage. When the surgery is radical (total ablation of the invaded muscle compartment), no complementary local treatment is necessary. When surgery has not been able to remove the invaded muscle in its entirety, it is complemented by post-operative radiotherapy (45 grays over a large field and 20 grays to the tumor bed);

Adjuvant chemotherapy for soft tissue sarcomaswith a tendency to metastasize (histological degrees 2 or 3 and tumor size greater than 5 cm).

A locoregional assessment at three months (CT-MRI) will act as a baseline for further follow-up: performed every 3 months for 2 years, then every 6 months for a minimum of 5 years, associated with a search for pulmonary metastasis by CT.

The CT and MRI findings for recurrence is the same as that described for bone sarcomas (fig. 43.13).

Finally, helical CT seems to be promising (fig. 43.14) but is still under evaluation.

References

1. Aisen AM, Martel W, Braunstein EM, et al (1986) MRI and CT evaluation of primary bone and soft-tissue tumors. AJR 146: 749-756
2. Berquist TH, Ehman RL, King BF, et al (1990) Value of MR imaging in differentiating benign from malignant soft tissue masses: Study of 95 lesions. AJR 155: 1251-1255
3. Bloem JL, Bluemm RG, Taminiau AH (1987) MRI of primary malignant bone tumors. Radiology 7: 425-445
4. Bokyo OB, Cory DA, Cohen MD, et al (1987) MR Imaging of osteogenic and Ewing's sarcoma. AJR 148: 317-322
5. Bonnerot V, Charpentier A, Frouin F, et al (1992) The use of factor analysis of dynamic MR Imaging in predicting the response of osteosarcoma to chemotherapy. Investigative Radiology (to be published)
6. Burk DL, Dalinka MK, Shiebler ML, et al (1988) Strategies for musculoskeletal magnetic resonance imaging. Radiology 26: 653-672
7. Cadman NL, Soule EH, Kelly PJ (1965) Synovial sarcoma: an analysis of 134 tumors. Cancer 18: 613-627
8. Chang AE, Matory YL, Dwyer AJ (1987) Magnetic resonance imaging versus computed tomography in the evaluation of soft-tissue tumors of the extremities. Ann Surg 205: 340-348
9. Coffre Ch, Vanel D, Contesso G, et al (1985) Problems and pitfalls in the use of computed tomography for the local evaluation of long bone osteosarcoma: report on 30 cases. Skeletal Radiol 13: 147-153
10. Cohen MD, Weetman RM, Provisor AJ (1986) Efficacy of magnetic resonance imaging in 139 children with tumors. Arch Surg 121: 522-529
11. De Lange EE, Pope TL, Fechner RE (1986) Dedifferentiated chondrosarcoma: radiographic features. Radiology 160: 489-492
12. Delepine G, Goutallier D (1986) La biopsie dans les sarcomes des membres. Réflexions à propos d'une série homogène de 135 cas. Presse Med 15: 1145-1147
13. Delepine G, Delepine N, Desbois JC, et al (1989) Sarcome ostéogène des membres en 1989. Une maladie curabie sans mutilation. La Médecine Infantile 7: 539-545
14. Delepine G, Delepine N, Deshois JC (1989) Sarcome d'Ewing; tendances thérapeutiques actuelles. La Médecine Infantile 7: 529-536

15. Delepine G, Delepine N, Jasmin Cl, et al (1989) Results of multidisciplinary limb salvage in 272 sarcomas. 4th International Symposium on Limb salvage
16. Delepine G, Delepine N, Desbois JC (1989) Synovialosarcome. La Médecine Infantile 7: 564-574
17. Demas BE, Heelan RT, Lane J, et al (1988) Soft-tissue sarcomas of the extremities: comparison of MR and CT in determining the extent of disease. AJR 150: 615-620
18. Desbois JC, Delepine N, Delepine G (1988) L'ostéosarcome ostéogénique, un modèle de maladie devenue curable grâce à l'approche multidisciplinaire de son traitement. CR Soc Biol 182: 523-537
19. Enneking WF, Dagan A (1975) Skip metastases in osteosarcoma. Cancer 132: 2192
20. EnneLing WF, Dagan A (1978) Transepiphysed extension of osteosarcoma: incidence, mechanism and implications. Cancer 41: 1526
21. Erleman R, Sciuk J, Bosse A, et al (1990) Response of osteosarcoma and Ewing sarcoma to preoperative chemotherapy: assessment with dynamic and static MR Imaging and skeletal scintigraphy. Radiology 175: 791-796
22. Ginaldi S, De Santos LA (1980) CT in the evaluation of small round cell tumors of bone. Radiology 134 : 441-446
23. Hauwnaur JM, Jenkins JPR, Isherwood I (1990) Magnetic resonance imaging of musculoaponevrotic fibromatosis. Skeletal Radiol 19: 509-514
24. Holscher HC, B loem JC, Nooy MA, ct al (1990) Thc value of MR imaging in monitoring the effect of chemotherapy on bone sarcomas. AJR 154: 763-769
25. Holsher HC, Bloem JC, Vanel D, et al (1992) Osteosarcoma: chemotherapy induced changes at MR imaging. Radiology 182: 839-844
26. Hudson TM, Hamlin DJ, Enneking WF, et al (1985) MRI of bone and soft-tissue tumors: early experience in 31 patients compared with CT. Skeletal Radiol 13: 134-146
27. Jones ET, Kuhns LR, Arbor A (1981) Pitfalls in the use of computed tomography for musculoskeletal tumors in children. J Bone and Joint Surg 63: 1297
28. Kalifa G, Lalande G, Larde D, et al (1982) Les fibromes desmoides chez l'enfant. Ann Radiol 25: 25-33
29. Kearney MM, Sole EH, Ivins JC (1980) Malignant fibrous histiocytoma: a retrospective study of 167 cases. Cancer 45: 167-178
30. Kransdorf MJ, Jelinek JS, Moser RP, et al (1989) Soft- tissue masses: diagnosis using MR imaging. AJR 153: 541-547
31. Kransdorf MJ, Jelinek JS, Moser RP, et al (1990) Magnetic resonance appearance of fibromatosis. Skeletal Radiol 19: 495-499
32. Larde D, Coffre C, Delepine G (1991) Tumeurs des os et des parties molles. In: D Buthiau (ed) TDM et IRM cliniques. Frison-Roche, Paris, pp 1069-1092
33. Levine E, Wetzel LH, Neff JR (1986) MR imaging and CT of extrahepatic cavernous hemangiomas. AJR 147: 1299-1304
34. Mc Vicar AD, Ollif JFC, Pringle J, et al (1992) Ewing sarcoma: MR imaging of chemotherapy induced changes with histologic correlation. Radiology 184: 859-864
35. Mail JT, Cohen MD, Mirkin LD, et al (1985) Response of osteosarcoma to preoperative intravenous high dose methotrexate chemotherapy: CT Evaluation. AJR 167: 783-785
36. Morton MJ, Berquist TH, Mc Leod RA, et al (1991) MR imaging of synovial sarcoma. AJR 156: 337-340
37. Paling MR, Hyams DM (1982) Computed tomography in malignant fibrous histiocytoma. J Comput Assist Tomogr 6: 785-788
38. Petasnick JP, Turner DA, Charters JR, et al (1986) Soft tissue masses of the locomotor system: comparison of MRI with CT. Radiology 160: 125-133
39. Peterson KK, Renfrew DL, Feddersen RM, et al (1991) Magnetic resonance imaging of mixoïd containing tumors. Skeletal Radiol 20: 245-250
40. Petterson H, Gillespy T, Hamlin DJ (1987) Primary musculoskeletal tumors: examination with MR imaging compared with conventional modalities. Radiology 164: 237-241
41. Petterson H, Slone R, Spanier S (1988) Muskuloskeletal tumors: Tl and T2 relaxation times. Radiology 167: 783-785
42. Reiser M, Rupp N, Heller HS (1984) MRI in the diagnosis of malignant soft tissue tumors. Eur J Radiol 4: 288-293
43. Rosen G, Caparros B, Huvos AG (1982) Preoperative chemotherapy for osteogenic sarcoma: selection of post-operative adjuvant chemotherapy based on thc response of the primary tumor to preoperative therapy. Cancer 49: 1221
44. Rosen G, Caparros B, Groshen S, et al (1984) Primary osteogenic sarcoma of the femur: a model for the use of preoperative chemotherapy in high risk malignant tumors. Cancer Invest 2: 181-192
45. Rousselin B, Vanel D, Terrier-Lacombe MJ, et al (1989) Clinical and radiologic analysis of 13 cases of primary neuroectodermal tumors of bone. Skeletal Radiol 18: 115-120
46. Sieger LL, Widoff BE, Bassett LW, et al (1991) Preoperative evaluation of osteosarcoma: value of gadopentetate dimeglumine-enhanced MR imaging. AJR 157: 347-351
47. Sundaram M, Mc Guire MH, Fletcher J, et al (1986) Magnetic resonance imaging of lesions of synovial origin. Skeletal Radiol 15: 110-116
48. Sundaram M, Mc Guire MH, Schajowicz F (1987) Soft-tissue masses: histologic basis for decreased signal (short T2) on T2 weight MR images. AJR 148: 1247-1250
49. Sundaram M, Mc Leod RA (1990) MR imaging of tumor and tumorlike lesions of bone and soft tissue. AJR 155: 817-824
50. Sundaram M, Baran G, Merenda G, et al (1990) Myxoid liposarcoma: magnetic resonance imaging appearances with clinical and histological correlation. Skeletal Radiol 9: 359-362
51. Vanel D, Contesso G, Couanet D, et al (1982): CT in the evaluation of 41 cases of Ewing's sarcoma. Skeletal Radiol 9 : 8-13

52. Vanel D, Coffre Ch, Contesso G, et al (1988) Apport du gadolinium DOTA dans 20 tumeurs primitives des os et des parties molles. J Radiol 69: 735-739
53. Vanel D, Ubaldino V, Coffre Ch, et al (1989) Intérêt de l'imagerie par résonance magnétique dans la surveillance des fibromatoses. J Radiol 70: 33-36
54. Vanel D, Coffre Ch, Couanet D, et al (1990) Limites et erreurs dans l'interprétation de l'imagerie par résonance magnétique dans les tumeurs primitives des os et des parties molles. Rev Im Med 2: 89-93
55. Wetzel LH, Levine E (1990) MR Imaging of sacral and presacral lesions. AJR 154: 771-775s

CHAPTER 44

Progress in helical CT in oncology

Clinicians
E.-Ch. Antoine, M. Gozy, D. Coeffic, D. Khayat

Radiologist
D. Buthiau

Virtual endoscopy in oncology

Virtual endoscopy (or internal navigation) in oncology may have a role in the evaluation of the tracheobronchial, ENT, digestive and urological systems.

The advent of helical CT has enabled the performance of single volumetric breathold acquisitions of the thorax by a combination of continuous table movement at a constant velocity during the data collection and concomitant rotation of the tube and detectors at a constant speed and direction [11, 14, 21]. Further calculation, called interpolation, reduces artifacts caused by patient movement during the acquisition [12,16]. Similarly, respiratory motion artifacts are eliminated. High quality 3D reconstruction can be obtained as a result of the contiguous anatomical slices [20]. These reconstructions can be volumetric by using a slice thickness formed by the summation of several adjacent sections (Multi Projection Volume Reconstruction, MPVR). It is also possible to select minimal intensity (mIP) [12, 13] or maximum intensity (MIP) algorithms to obtain image projections of the tracheobronchial tree viewed from the outside. So-called surface reconstructions give an appearance in relief [9, 15, 18, 19].

Methods

This technique has been developed from virtual endoscopic reconstruction modalities [7] performed on a CT scanner (Highspeed Advantage: General Electric Medical Systems, Milwaukee, USA) with an image processing console (Research Center GEMS, Buc, France). The slices were acquired using helical mode, 1:1 pitch, with a 360° tube rotation/s, covering a 10-15 cm segment and effective slice thickness of 1.5 to 3 mm. The data was processed on an Advantage Windows Workstation (GEMS). 3D reconstruction was performed from the axial sections by rejecting all voxels with a density greater than 50 Hounsfield units and then generating an endoluminal view (software still under development) which gives an in relief effect using a light and shade technique dependent on the calculated position relative to the lens of the endoscope.

Potential clinical applications

Pulmonary disease [1-5, 16, 17]

Virtual tracheobronchial endoscopy (figs 44.1-44.4)

This type of 3D endo-tracheobronchial reconstruction can produce images very similar to those seen at fiberoptic endoscopy (fig. 44.1). It is even possible to pass down the tracheobronchial lumen in real time and perform a virtual endoscopy by adjusting the position of the virtual endoscope on a 2D multiplanar section. In this way, the carina, the main bronchi and the bronchial tree can be assessed, as well as allowing a concomitant study of the bronchial endolumen from

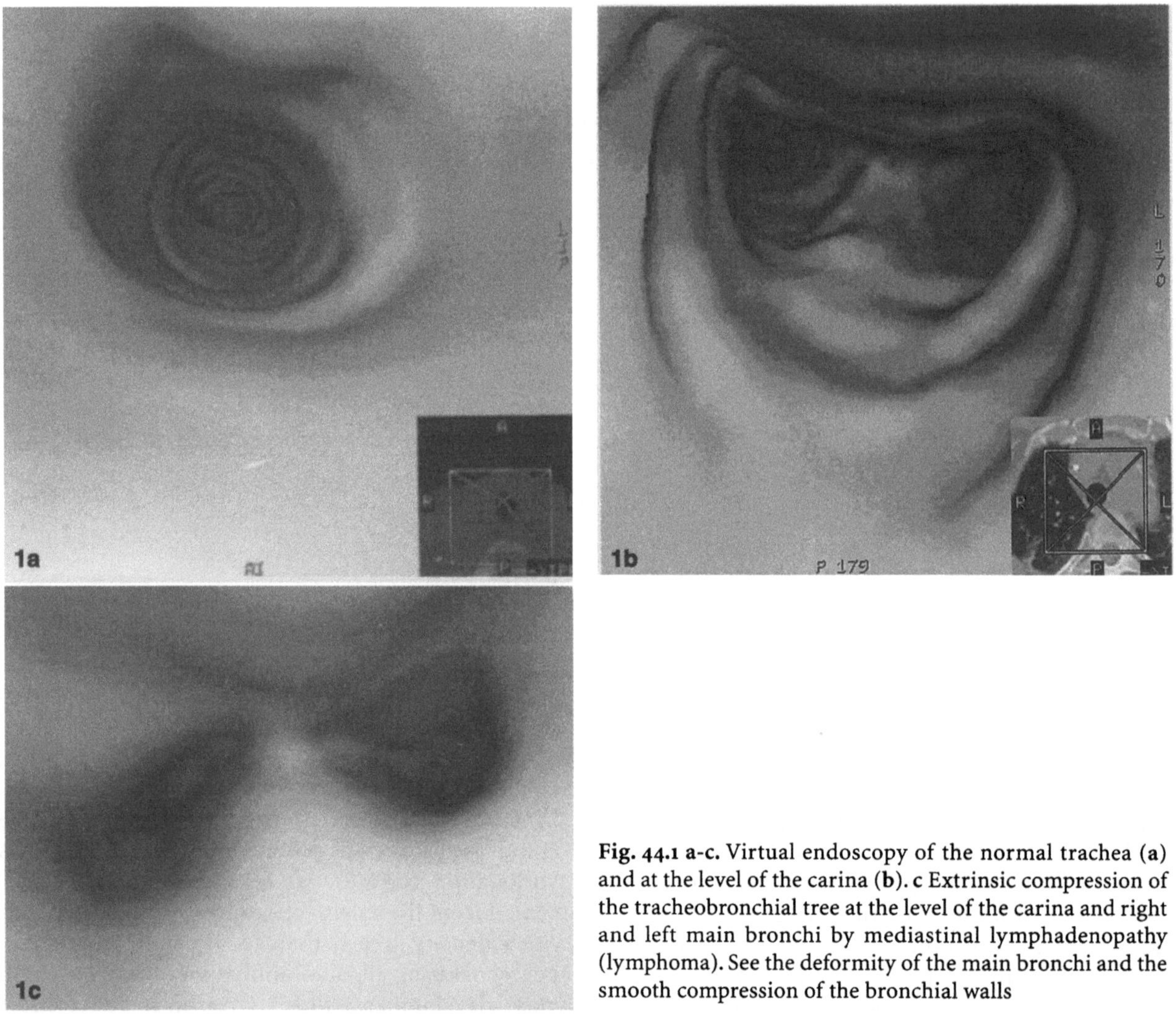

Fig. 44.1 a-c. Virtual endoscopy of the normal trachea (**a**) and at the level of the carina (**b**). **c** Extrinsic compression of the tracheobronchial tree at the level of the carina and right and left main bronchi by mediastinal lymphadenopathy (lymphoma). See the deformity of the main bronchi and the smooth compression of the bronchial walls

direct axial and reconstructed coronal and sagittal sections (figs 44.2 & 44.3).

It is also possible to evaluate the bronchial wall, its thickness, caliber and submucosal or peribronchial structures, essentially lymphatics and blood vessels. Thus, a multiplanar analysis of both the extra- and endobronchial structures can be made on the same study. A multidirectional study can be performed using virtual endoscopy allowing retrograde visualization and demonstration of segmental bronchi distal to a stenosis. The possible diagnostic applications of this new technique are still under evaluation [1-5, 8, 17]. It is not the aim of this reconstruction technique to replace bronchoscopy which remains indispensable for obtaining a biopsy for histology. Initial comparisons suggest that the traditional fibroscopic images and the data from virtual endoscopy are superimposable. However, CT gives additional information on the extrabronchial structures (figs. 44.2 & 44.3).

Possible clinical applications [10, 15, 16] include a more complete representation of certain complex pathologies, such as post-therapeutic tracheobronchial changes (e.g. post-radiotherapy) and malformations of the tracheobronchial tree. This atraumatic technique could be useful in the post-treatment follow-up of bronchopulmonary carcinomas, particularly to assess the reduction in the endoluminal extension and extrinsic compression (fig. 44.1), bronchial obstruction and more tangible appreciation of response to treatment which may even be accurately quantifiable. In fact, the absence of an endoscopy probe allows repeated studies. The follow-up of other

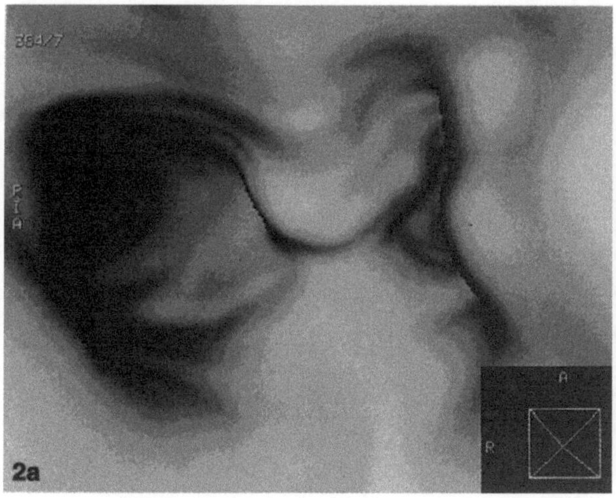

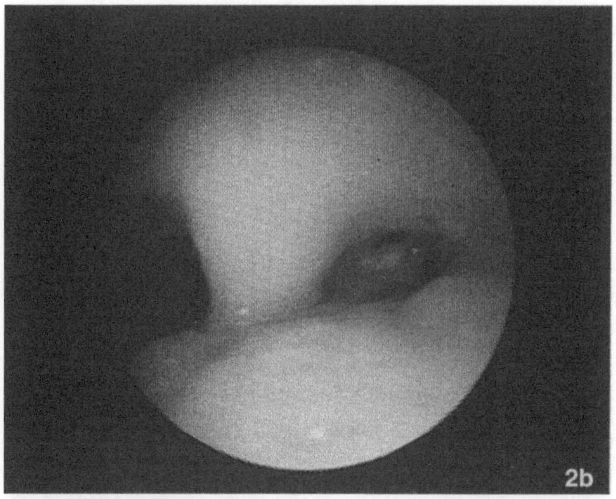

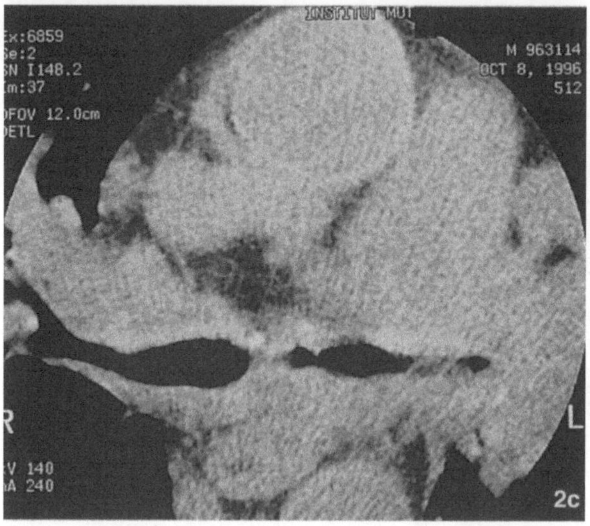

Fig. 44.2 a-c. Lung carcinoma invading the posterior wall of the carina and the main left bronchus. **a** Virtual endoscopy. **b** Standard endoscopy. **c** Axial view (courtesy of Dr. Baldeyrou, Paris)

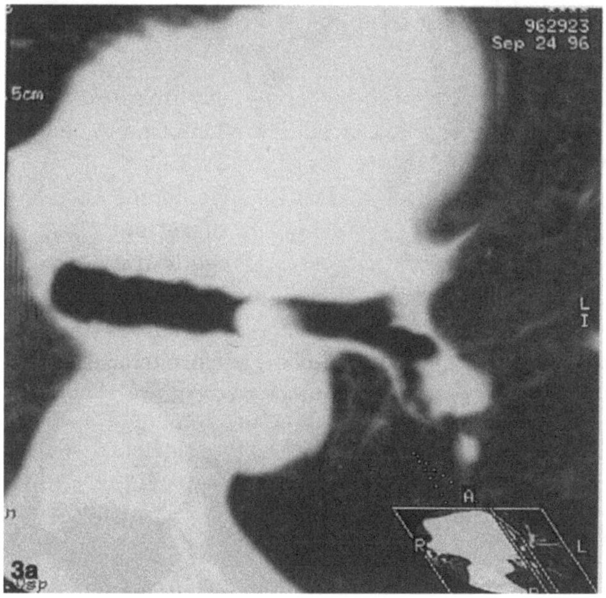

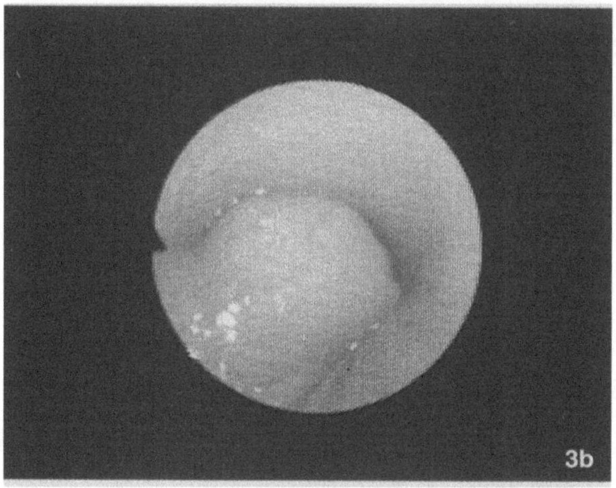

Fig. 44.3 a, b. Lung carcinoma invading the main left bronchus. **a** Demonstration of the bulging tumor of the main left bronchus on axial view; **b** the equivalent aspect with standard endoscopy (courtesy of Dr. Baldeyrou, Paris)

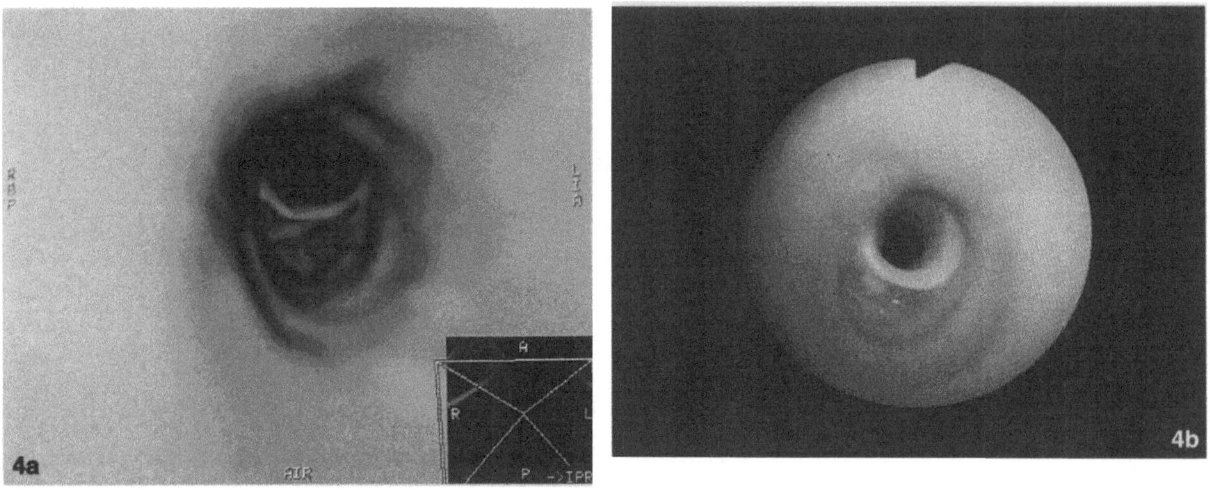

Fig. 44.4 a, b. Follow-up of prosthesis. Normal aspect of a Dumont prosthesis, by virtual endoscopy (**a**) and standard endoscopy (**b**)

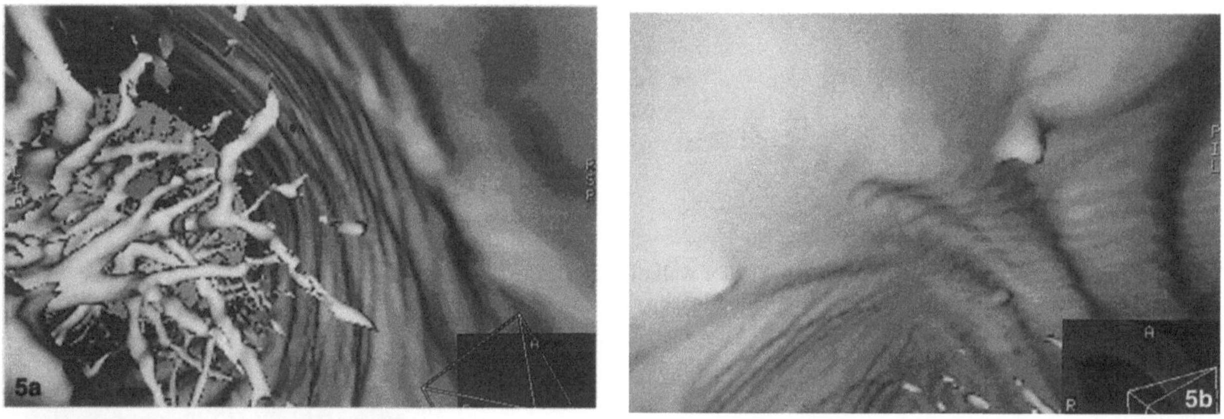

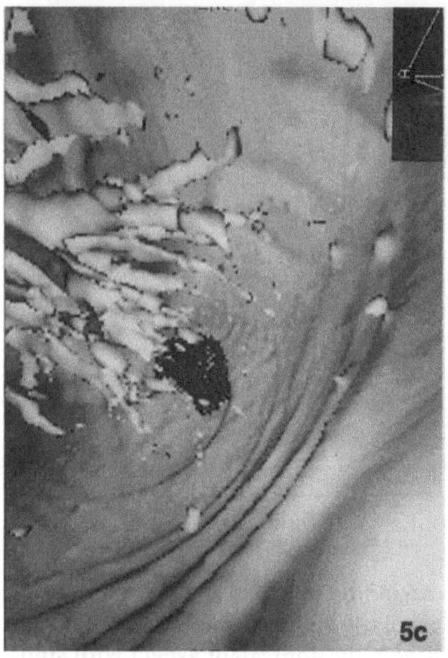

Fig. 44.5. a Normal endothoracic virtual view of the left hemithorax. See the pleural surface and bronchovascular peripheral tree. **b** Peripheral nodular metastasis from kidney cancer, invading pleural wall. Intrathoracic endoscopic view by helical CT shows directly the visceral pleural nodes. **c** Hematogenous secondary peripheral nodes from breast cancer; intrathoracic virtual endoscopy. Pleural and parenchymal metastases are directly demonstrated on this picture

types of known bronchial lesions can be considered, notably, bronchial stenosis of any etiology (particularly following lung transplant). The differentiation between extrinsic compression (fig. 44.1) and infiltration of the bronchial wall is still under study. However, nodular endobronchial (figs 44.2 & 44.3) or tracheal extension has already been well visualized by this technique in patients with bronchopulmonary carcinomas or infiltrative mediastinal pathology, particularly lymphatic lesion (lymphoma or metastatic lymphadenopathy).

This technique [7] may be of value in other situations, for example, the pre-radiotherapy calculation of the target volume (brachy-radiotherapy), or laser treatment of bronchial stenosis and preliminary evaluation of bronchial endoprosthesis insertion (fig. 44.4).

Furthermore, this technique may prove to be ideal in the assessment of tracheobronchial abnormalities due to polychondritis, Wegener's granulomatosis or any cause of tracheomalacia where standard endoscopy is not advisable or even contraindicated (due to the fragility of the tracheobronchial wall or the risk of worsening of respiratory failure). In addition, the degree of stenosis and the caliber of the tracheobronchial lumen can be evaluated in inspiration and expiration in order to identify the degree of weakness of the tracheobronchial rings and walls. Nonetheless, many questions such as the effect of slice thickness and the distal limit for bronchial exploration still remain unanswered. Moreover, this technique must be fully understood before utilization, since it can produce false positive or negative images or make the contours of tracheobronchial walls artificially disappear. This problem is greatly reduced by verifying on the axial sections or simple multiplanar reconstruction that the structures of interest have not been effaced.

In summary, the following applications may be envisioned:

- in the investigation and the guidance of semi-distal lesions which cannot be seen at standard endoscopy but only with a thinner endoscope;
- in the follow-up of bronchial carcinomas, allowing retrograde visualization and evaluation distal to a stenosis;
- in the follow-up of bronchial endoprostheses;
- as an aid in performing brachytherapy;
- in the follow-up of the stability of sutures after surgery for benign as well as malignant pathologies (transplants, grafts, resection and anastomoses);
- in monitoring the clinical progression of polychondritis.

Endothoracic virtual imaging [5] (fig. 44.5)

Our preliminary studies were aimed at investigating perspective volume rendering as a means to "fly through" CT imaging data sets to perform "virtual endoscopy". Although the experience is short, we believe that these techniques can have implications in diagnostic imaging and provide an effective new means of communication. This technique could be of value in directly visualizing the peripheral anatomy, subpleural space, the apex and base of the lung and the costo-phrenic angles. The visceral pleura, mediastinal pleura, distal vessels, diaphragm, mediastinal great vessels and cardiac walls can be clearly demonstrated. Although this technique leads to a contour image, it can provide complementary information on pleural extension or pleural nodes, parenchymal nodes (fig. 44.5) and diaphragmatic involvement with a good correlation with surgery and without any gray areas or any technical limitation, except for navigation of the hilum and perihilar space where the vasculature and bronchi are dense and artifacts are possible. Applications could include the evaluation of the local extent of peripheral and subsegmental lung carcinoma, the direct demonstration of hematogenous secondary pulmonary nodes, of primary or secondary pleural disease and of the extent of diaphragmatic involvement. This technique could also allow these lesions to be followed atraumatically after treatment and could be applied to any distal and semi-distal pleuro-parenchymatous diseases (e.g. pleuro-pneumopathies, pulmonary embolism...) and could include planning of transthoracic biopsies and guided procedures.

In conclusion, perspective volume rendering is a new way to view CT imaging data that may expand the clinical use of these techniques by reaching spaces that cannot be visualized with mechanical endoscopy. With considerable investigation and refinement, perspective volume rendering may become an alternative to the current review of tomographic sections for the primary interpretation of CT imaging data. Before that time comes, perspective volume rendering will most likely need to become a real-time examination, and extensive comparisons between perspective volume rendering, review of tomographic sections, and pathologic results must be made to optimize and validate this technique.

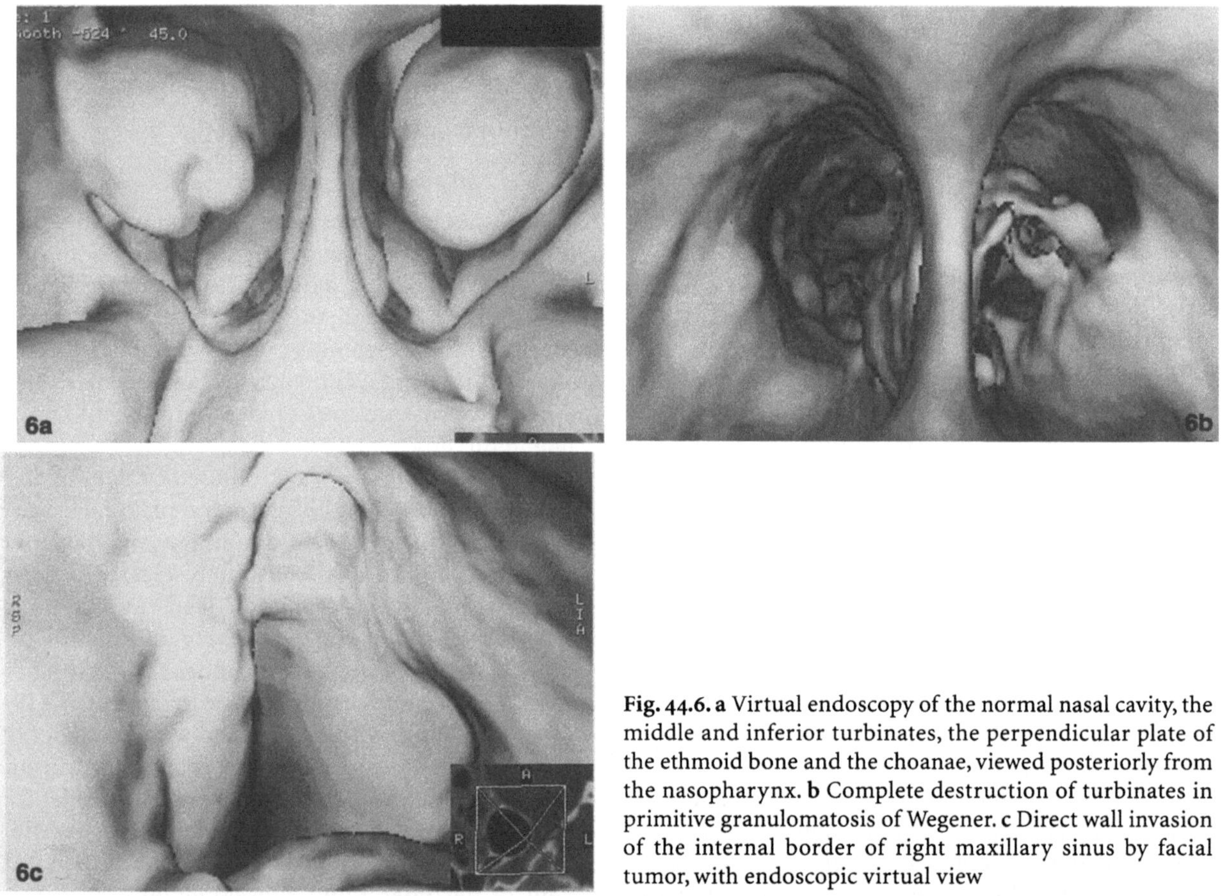

Fig. 44.6. a Virtual endoscopy of the normal nasal cavity, the middle and inferior turbinates, the perpendicular plate of the ethmoid bone and the choanae, viewed posteriorly from the nasopharynx. b Complete destruction of turbinates in primitive granulomatosis of Wegener. c Direct wall invasion of the internal border of right maxillary sinus by facial tumor, with endoscopic virtual view

ENT virtual endoscopy [1-5] (fig. 44.6)

In the investigation of ENT carcinomas, the value of this technique would be its ability to allow an evaluation of all of the sinuses and pharyngo-laryngeal cavities in association with standard axial CT scanning. Thus, from one and the same scanning session, additional information could be gathered:
- on the type and degree of the tumoral extension (fig. 44.6),
- on the distinction between compression and tumor invasion (being evaluated),
- on the severity of a stenosis, of an extrinsic compression or of destruction by contiguity (for example, it is very difficult differentiate between inflammatory and infiltrative pathology).

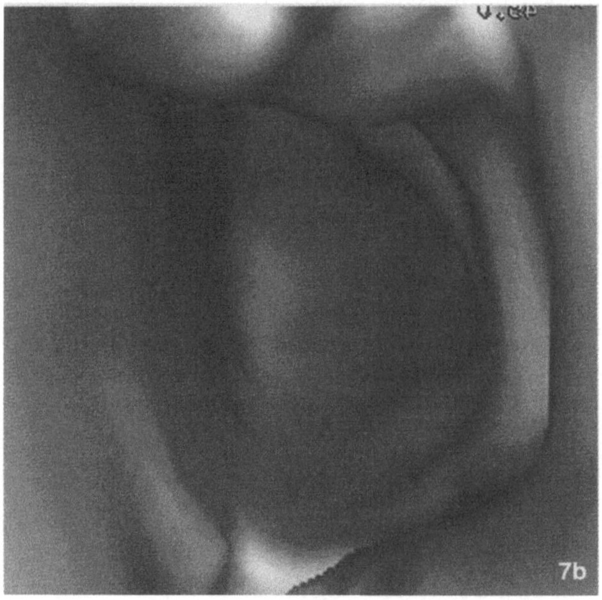

Fig. 44.7. Normal ileocolic valvula in virtual endoscopy

Digestive virtual endoscopy [3] (figs. 44.7-44.10)

This is a non-invasive examination which does not involve the injection of any contrast material or anesthetic agent and which can be carried out during a

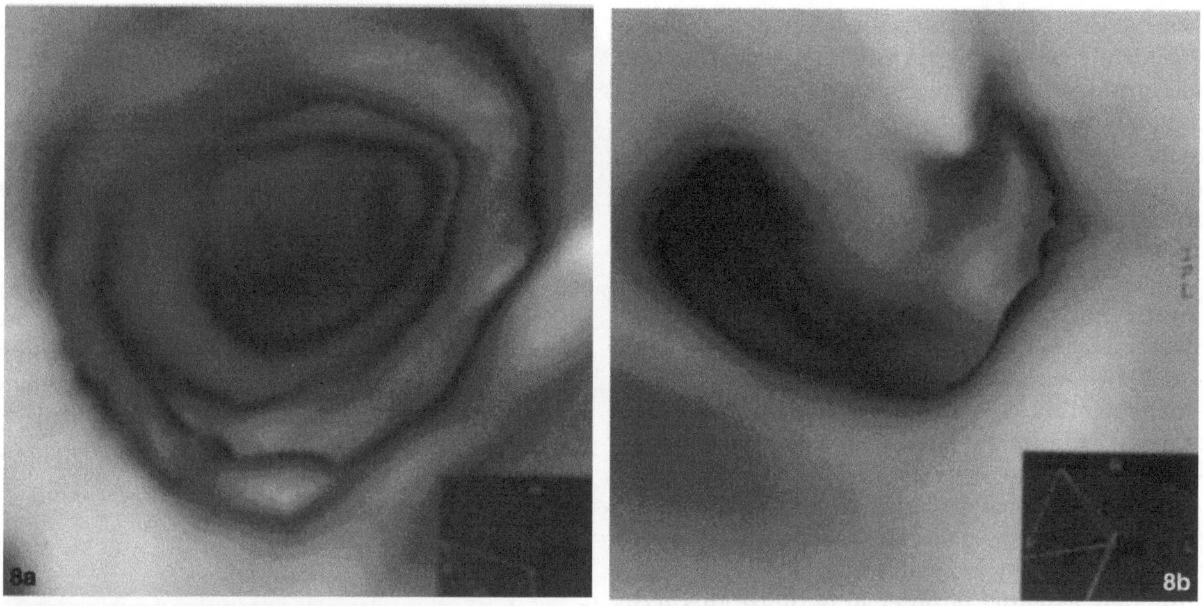

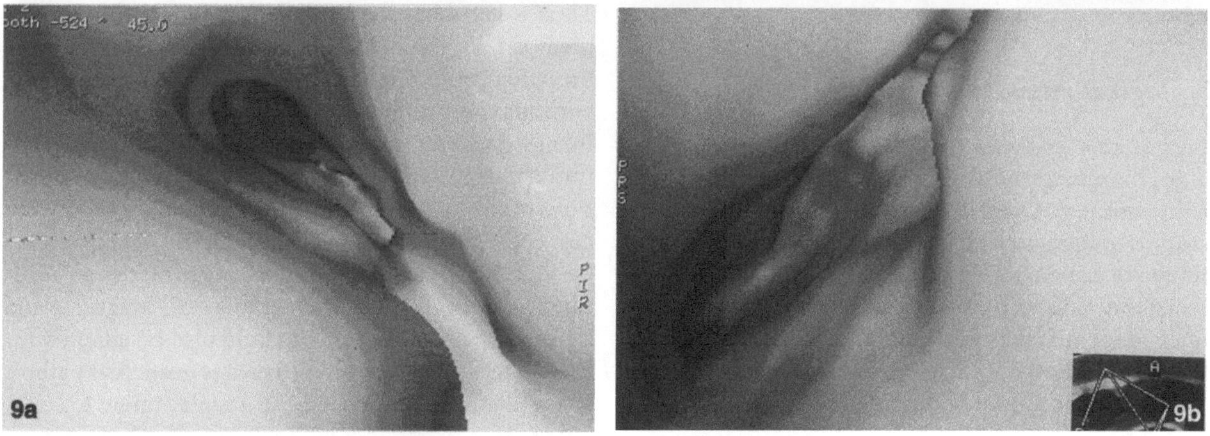

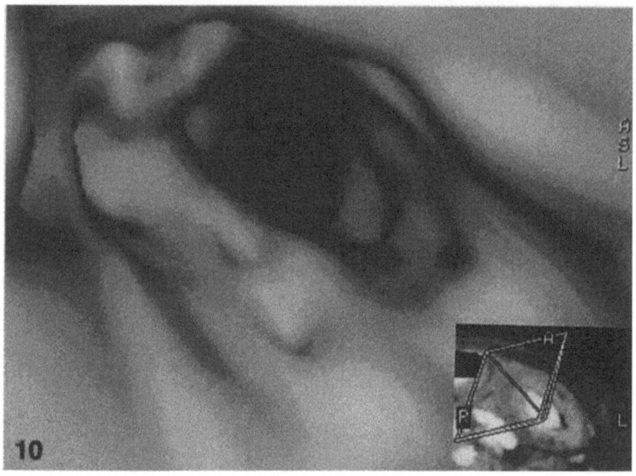

Fig. 44.8. a Tumoral stenosis from left colic cancer on endoscopic virtual view. **b** Colic cancer by helical CT and endoscopic view, bulging inside the colic lumen

Fig. 44.9 a, b. Gastric antrum carcinoma in virtual endoscopy: see the important narrowing of the antrum, especially the pre-pyloric region (**a**), with straight anterior and posterior walls

Fig. 44.10. Antral carcinoma by endoscopic virtual view: see the important thickening of the gastric wall on the axial view *(down left of the picture)* and the important irregularities of the gastric outlines routine scan. However, it does necessitate a preparation identical to that performed for colonoscopy and with insufflation (using a Pouliquen cannula). This is currently being evaluated. In theory, it could be of value in the decision to operate a polyp based on the volume measurement; it could be used for the non-invasive follow-up of known pathologies and even, one day, have a role in the diagnosis of digestive pathology before colonoscopy. This technique could, nevertheless, be an alternative to a barium enema. Its main limitations are:

- the lack of a tissue sample for histology,
- the inability to provide an etiologic diagnosis because the technique generates contour images,
- the lack of reproducibility.

It should be pointed out that, in the management of digestive tract pathologies, close cooperation between the specialist physician, endoscopist and radiologist is absolutely essential in order to optimize this technique.

Urological virtual endoscopy [3] (fig. 44.11)

It is possible to obtain virtual cystoscopic images (fig. 44.8), thanks to the ability to set precise thresholds, using iodine contrast material to fill the bladder with a radio-opaque product. The applications of this technique are not currently known. In fact, this technique is just starting to be evaluated. It may be of importance in identifying and, in particular, in investigating relapses of known infiltrative and especially bulging lesions (fig. 44.8b), in evaluating the anatomical relationship between the tumor and the ureteric orifices and in ureteroscopic studies (fig. 44.11). It may also be potentially useful in the evaluation of the vesical extension of prostatic tumors. This technique is potentially of value in the exploration of tumors of the bladder, prostate and renal pelvis and calyces, although its applications have not so far been evaluated. With respect to the kidney, two applications may be envisaged: firstly, the study of renal cysts and especially their walls (when the cyst is large) in order to more accurately identify the type of cyst and to distinguish between benign and malignant cyst. Secondly, it may be possible to detect vascular pathology, particularly thrombosis due to neoplasia in the renal veins and inferior vena cava.

Conclusion

Thus, we now have at our disposal a new non-invasive method for the endoluminal assessment of the tracheobronchial tree. The virtual endoscopy is performed, without the use of any endoscopic probe, from the image data obtained by helical CT scanning. It is important to remember that the diagnostic applications of this technique, both pre- and post-therapy, are currently being evaluated. Nevertheless, it can already be stated that the virtual endoscopy provides an accurate anatomical image. Even at this early stage, it could be used as a teaching aid. It could also be adapted for the clinical investigation of tracheobronchial pathology, even though it is no sense a replacement for clas-

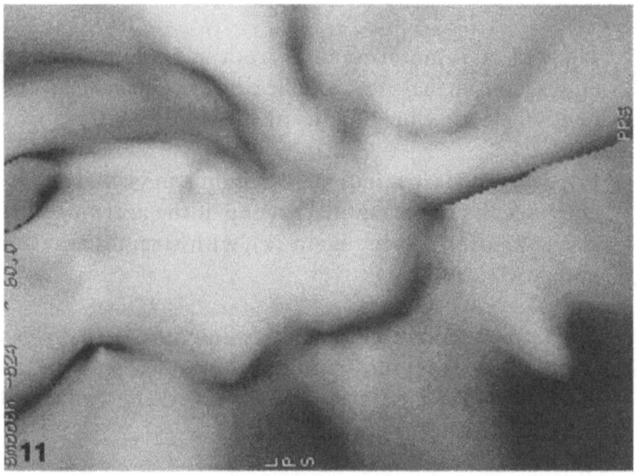

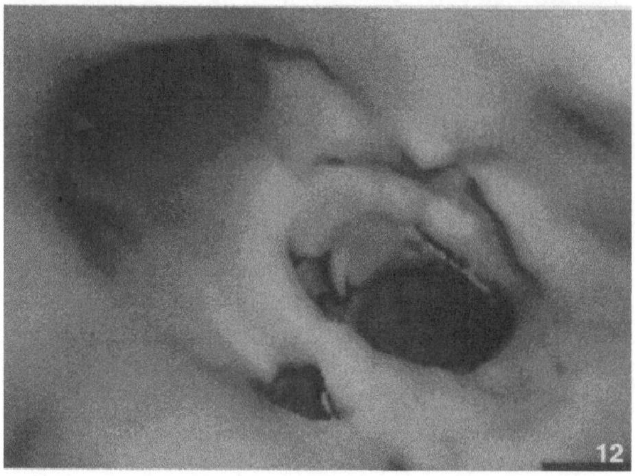

Fig. 44.11. Bladder carcinoma invading the basis, with bulging outlines, near the ureteral aperture (*left on the picture*)

Fig. 44.12. Irregular shaped neoplasic thrombus within the inferior vena cava in endoscopic view, from kidney carcinoma extension sical fiberscopy which allows a tissue sample to be taken. Its non-invasive nature and its reproducibility make it of potential value in the monitoring of known malignant lesions and the evaluation of tracheobronchial lesions in situations where fiberscopy would be difficult or contraindicated. Moreover, this technique may have applications in other areas which are still being studied: ENT, the digestive tract, urology and vascular lesions (fig. 44.12). With respect to the digestive tract, it is possible to consider morphological assessment in health as well as disease given that the patient is prepared in the same manner as for colonoscopy with the use of a moderate degree of insufflation. It is important to remember that this is not a supplementary, but rather a complementary technique which can be performed at the time of a standard CT scan and provides additional information. It does not, therefore, constitute an increased burden on the public health budget [1-5].

Clinical measurement of volumes with the helical scanner [6]

Acquisition techniques [6]

Spiral CT allows a single breath-hold acquisition of a liver volume (usually the entire liver volume); this eliminates respiratory artifacts but ensures the acquisition of perfectly continuous sections [1-5]. The CT sections were acquired on a CT scanner (Highspeed Advantage; General Electric Medical Systems, Milwaukee, USA), using the following parameters:
- acquisition parameters: 7 mm sections, pitch 1 to 1.5 in relation to the patient's ability to hold his breath, tube rotation through 360° in one second, 120 kV, 250 mA on average, level of acquisition related to level of liver or any organ in patient;
- reconstruction parameters: 7 mm section every 5 or 6 mm; reconstruction filter selection for maximum density resolution.

The complete series of images acquired after injection of iodinated contrast was transferred to an Advantage Windows Workstation (General Electric Medical Systems, Buc, France) for image processing.

Reconstruction technique [6]

Using the software for 3-dimensional visualization (3D) in Advantage Windows (Voxtool) it is possible to create a volume of data derived from the planar acquisitions. This 3-dimensional reconstruction is based on two stages:
- volume reconstruction from the axial sections;
- segmentation of the volume of interest allowing elimination of the data for densities less than 500 HU (Hounsfield Units).

The quality of this 3D reconstruction, as well as the accuracy of the measurements of surface and volume are correlated with the size of the voxel (acquisition field, reconstruction matrix, slice thickness, reconstruction gap).

The software offers different methods for extraction of the volumes of interest. In view of the heterogeneity of the structures studied, the most suitable method is manual contouring section by section. To facilitate the tracing, the software is able to detect interfaces corresponding to an abrupt change in density. The volumes so defined may be previewed in order to verify the contouring before applying the segmentation.

The corresponding volume is then calculated by counting the voxels. Thus, this is a computerized method for measurement of volumes; the software establishes the volumetric estimation of the object which has been selected by summation of the total number of voxels (smallest unit of volume) composing this object. This very powerful software takes into account all the data of the internal composition of this volume (the interior of the volume is digitally reconstructed, and may be visualized in any plane of section passing through this volume).

This is therefore very different from 3D morphologic "surface" reconstruction, which show only the exterior of the volume (it is a virtual reconstruction in the interior of the volume not being taken into account and being "hollow"). These are, from the computer aspect, easier to produce. It is possible to construct an histogram of the segmented volume to extract different statistics on the distribution of the components.

Results [6] (fig. 44.13)

The aim of this preliminary study was to assess the feasibility and reliability of volume measurements by helical CT, correlating the results obtained with the macroscopic findings (at surgery or autopsy). This macroscopic correlation has been obtained for four main groups of disorders: retroperitoneal lymphadenopathies, mediastinal lymphadenopathies, liver metastases, and primary cerebral tumors.

In comparing the macroscopic and CT assessments of lesional volumes, a certain percentage of error

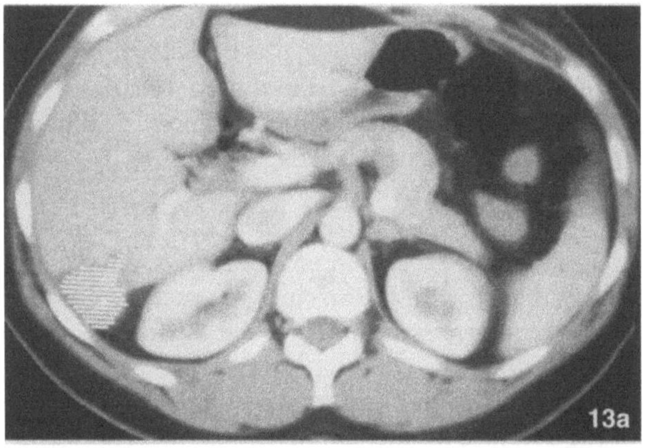

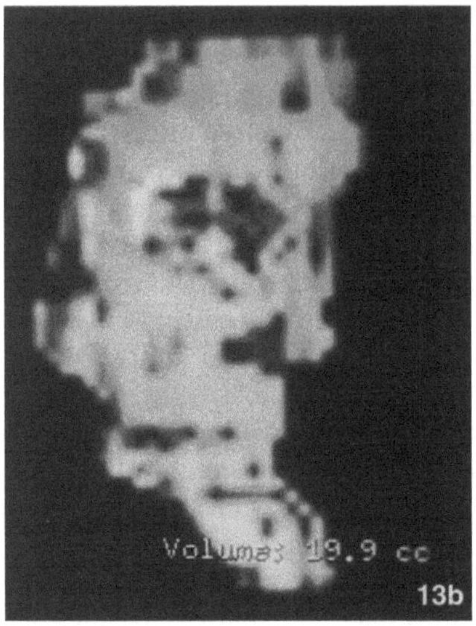

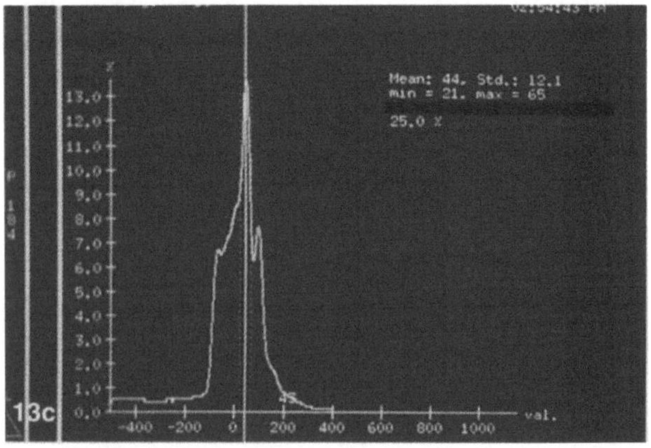

Fig. 44.13 a-c. Clinical measurement of volume with helical scanner. **a** Contouring of whole right hepatic lesion, in projection on an axial transverse section. **b** Measurement of volume of the lesion: 19.9 cm^3. **c** Statistics of densitometric distribution within the examined volume. Mean density is situated at 30 Hounsfield Units, with tissue components and also lipomatous components (metastasis form melanoma)

appeared: 4.5% for retroperitoneal lymphadenopathies, 5% for mediastinal lymphadenopathies, 6% for hepatic metastases and 9.5% for primary cerebral tumors. The overall mean percentage error in the volumetric calculation was 6.25%.

Several factors should be noted: the more limited the volume of the lesion, the higher the percentage of error may prove; errors of over-estimation are more common than errors of underestimation; the percentage of error is less when the structure measured is surrounded by structures of very different densities, thus facilitating the contouring of the lesions (retroperitoneal lymphadenopathies, mediastinal lymphadenopathies). The slightly higher figure for discordance of volume evaluation of primary cerebral tumors may be explained by the greater difficulty of assessing the precise boundaries of the lesion, edema and adjacent gliosis.

Discussion [6]

It would seem from this preliminary study that there is a satisfactory correlation between the measurements of volumes established by helical CT and that obtained by direct macroscopic study (surgery or autopsy). This correlation shows a scatter of 6.25% between the measured and true values so that this may be considered as one of the best techniques currently available, both in the evaluation of visceral anatomic volume in terms of macroscopic anatomy in vivo and in assessment of lesional volume in clinical and surgical practice. However, the study continues and may have recourse to larger series to define better the sites where this correlation is maximal (a priori, greater sensitivity for lesions surrounded by very different densities, e.g. lymphadenopathies, pulmonary or hepatic masses rather than for breast lesions). The next stage is to correlate this technique with the classical techniques of two-dimensional tumor measurement in the framework of a phase II study in clinical oncology. If this study of volumes by helical CT proves satisfactory, reproducible and reliable, we should have at our disposal a technique of great value in the assessment of tumor volume both as a factor of prognosis, in predicting therapeutic response, in assessing surgical accessibility and evaluation before radiotherapy, and as a factor in the actual assessment of therapeutic response (the most precise evaluation of tumoral regression under cytotoxic treatment). The current two-dimensional surface study has obvious theoretic limitations and may prove inadequate for these purposes.

Parallel to volumetric evaluation, the study of the distribution of the components within the volume may permit estimation of the nature of the mass syndrome and its course under treatment (assessment of the nature of residual masses after chemotherapy in the context of non-seminomatous germinal tumors, necro-tic course in lymphomas, etc.). Thanks to histograms of density, it is possible to differentiate the fluid, tissue, calcified, adipose, necrotic or hematological components, and to assess their percentage distribution within the volume investigated (fig. 44.13). This evaluation is still under study but may be promising.

Thus, after this preliminary study, the establishment of satisfactory correlation and concordance between volume assessment by helical CT and by macroscopic anatomy may be able to validate this technique, subject to subsequent multicenter confirmation. In that case, this could lead to direct measurement of the volume of organs in vivo or of any structure (provided it is sufficiently different in density from adjacent structures). In the context of clinical application, especially in oncology, it may result in a reevaluation of the measurement of tumor masses in terms of volume, in the context of the WHO criteria for assessing cytotoxic treatments.

References

1. Buthiau D, Antoine EC, Piette JC, Nizri D, Baldeyrou P, Khayat D (1996) Virtual tracheobronchical endoscopy: educational and diagnostic value. Surg Radiol Anat 18: 125-131
2. Buthiau D, Antoine EC, Gozy M, et al. (1996) Endoscopie trachéobronchique virtuelle. Cahiers d'Oncologie 5: 114-118
3. Buthiau D, Antoine EC, Khayat D (1996) Endoscopie virtuelle en cancérologie. La Lettre du Cancérologue V, 6: 261-267
4. Buthiau D, Blum A, Régent D (1996) Scanner hélicoïdal: principes et perspectives cliniques. Rev Med Interne 17: 243-254
5. Buthiau D, Soyer P, Blum A, et al (1994) Scanner hélicoidal de l'abdomen. In: Buthiau D (ed) Progrès en scanner et IRM. Vigot, Paris, pp 58-75
6. Buthiau D, Antoine EC, Stefani E, et al (1996) Clinical measurement of volumes using helical CT. Surg Radiol Anat 18: 227-231
7. Ferretti G, Knoplioch J, Coulomb M, Brambilla C, Cinquin P (1995) Reconstruction 3D endoluminale de l'arbre trachéobronchique (bronchoscopie virtuelle). J Radiol 76: 531-534
8. Heiken JP, Brink JA, Vannier MW (1993) Spiral (helical) CT. Radiology 189: 647-656
9. Kitaoka H, Yumoto T (1990) Three-dimensional CT of the bronchial tree. Invest Radiol 25: 813-817
10. Mc Guinness G, Naidich DP, Garay SM, Davis AL, Boyd AD, Mizrachi HH (1993) Accessory cardiac bronchus: CT features and clinical significance. Radiology 189: 563-566
11. Naidich DP (1994) Helical computed tomography of the thorax. Radiol Clin North Am 32: 759-774
12. Napel S, Rubin GD, Jeffrey RB (1993) STS-MIP: a new reconstruction technique for CT of the chest. J Comput Assist Tomogr 17: 832-838
13. Napel SA, Bergin CJ, Paranjpe DV, Rubin GD (1992) Maximum and minimum intensity projection of spiral CT data for simultaneous 3dimensional imaging of the pulmonary vasculature and airways. Radiology 185: 132
14. Newmark GM, Conces DJ, Kopecky KK (1994) Spiral CT evaluation of the trachea and bronchi. J Comput Assist Tomogr 18: 552-554
15. Ney DR, Kuhlman JE, Hruban RH, Ren H, Hutchins GM, Fishman EK (1990) Three-dimensional CT-volumetric reconstruction and display of the bronchial tree. Invest Radiol 25: 736-742
16. Rémy J, Rémy-Jardin M, Giraud F, Wannebroucq J (1994) Le balayage spiralé volumique et ses applications en pathologie thoracique. Rev Mal Resp 11: 13-27
17. Rémy J, Rémy-Jardin M, Petyt L, Wannebroucq J (1994) La trachéobronchoscannographie sans contraste par reconstructions multiplanaires et tridimentionnelles surfaciques (RMP-3D) et volumiques (MIP). Rev Im Med 6: S210
18. Rubin GD, Dake MD, Napel S, et al (1994) Spiral CT of renal artery stenosis: comparison of three-dimensional rendering techniques. Radiology 190: 181-189
19. Stern RL, Cline HE, Johnson JA, Ravin CE (1989) Three dimensional imaging of the thoracic cavity. Invest Radiol 24: 282-288
20. Vahlensieck M, Lang Ph, Chan WP, Grampp S, Genant HK (1992) Three-dimensional reconstruction. Part I: applications and techniques . Eur Radiol 2: 503-507
21. Vock P, Soucek M, Daepp M, Kalender WA (1990) Lung: spiral volumetric CT with single breath-hold technique. Radiology 176: 864-867

CHAPTER 45

Progress in MR imaging in oncology

Clinicians
E.-Ch. Antoine, M. Gozy, E. Malaurie, M. Gil-Delgado, D. Nizri, C. Durier, J.V. Chantelard, D. Khayat

Radiologists
J.P. Laissy, D. Buthiau, D. Régent

MR angiography in oncologic patients: clinical uses

MR imaging is usually sufficient to display vessel involvement within or close to tumors. One example concerns the liver where hepatic vessel involvement is well identified, by the hepatocellular carcinoma or metastases [1]. In addition to the clinical diagnostic properties of MR imaging, MR angiography (fig. 45.1) and dynamic MR imaging studies have potential clinical applications in oncologic patients. However, a small number of studies limited their conclusions to the feasibility of the technique. Moreover, none of these described in the following pages concluded that MR angiography should substitute for other techniques (i.e. ultrasound and/or CT).

Neoplasm of the central nervous system

Extradural tumors - Dural sinus involvement and meningiomas

Preoperative assessment of meningiomas includes study of dural venous involvement. This has long been performed with either conventional or digital intraarterial cerebral angiography. MR venography has already demonstrated a high level accuracy in dural venous thrombophlebitis. Hence, it should be used in the preoperative assessment of venous involvement in meningiomas, but further studies would be necessary to demonstrate its real usefulness in this disease [2].

Pituitary tumors should also been examined with keeping in mind that hyperprolactinemia can be due to endosellar kinking of the internal carotid artery [2].

Brain tumors [12, 14]

MR imaging of the venous system of the brain already plays an important role in the diagnosis and follow-up of intracranial venous vascular diseases [4]. However, MR angiography (fig. 45.1 a)s not yet able to help characterization of brain tumors. In vascular tumors, only one study to date demonstrated the usefulness of spin-echo MR imaging and MR angiography. This study consisted of 17 patients with venous angiomas, 4 of whom had associated cavernous angiomas. All underwent MRI with spin-echo T1- and T2- and T1-weighted sequence post-gadolinium; MR angiography (MRA) was also performed with 3D and 2D time-of-flight technique. 3D and 2D MRA, as well as contrast-enhanced MRI demonstrated all the lesions, but cavernous angiomas (24% in our study) were better identified on T2-weighted images.

At the present time, however, dynamic MR imaging provides data to differentiate neoplasms from infectious conditions, in particular lymphoma from brain infections in HIV patients.

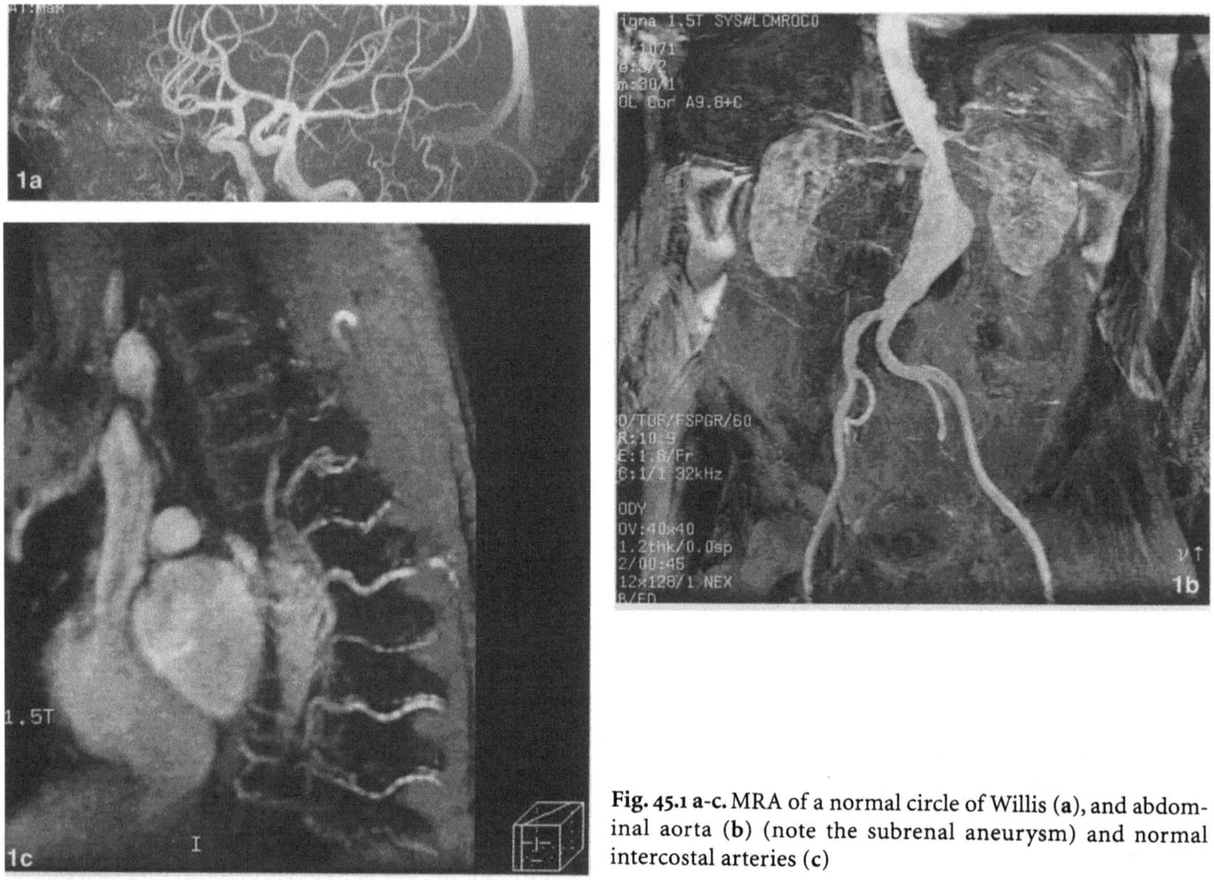

Fig. 45.1 a-c. MRA of a normal circle of Willis (**a**), and abdominal aorta (**b**) (note the subrenal aneurysm) and normal intercostal arteries (**c**)

An important diagnostic problem is indeed to differentiate between toxoplasmosis, CNS primary lymphoma and other causes of CNS mass lesions in AIDS patients. The particular concern of distinguishing between toxoplasmosis and lymphoma relies on the need of early specific treatment in both diseases, and on different prognosis. Several studies have described the typical imaging patterns of each of these diseases. Unfortunately, most of the authors admit that these two diseases often exhibit similar features.

The current approach is to treat focal enhancing lesions empirically with antitoxoplasma therapy without prior biopsy and follow-up the disease by MR imaging. However, the rapid doubling time of lymphoma compared with the slow growth of toxoplasmosis abscess could shorten the time of follow-up and lead to a stereotaxic biopsy despite a non-negligible morbidity and mortality, allowing an earlier effective management of lymphoma.

One recent study showed that measuring the relative signal enhancement of lesions could help differentiate toxoplasmosis from lymphoma. Toxoplasmosis lesions peaked at 39% six minutes after injection of gadolinium-DOTA, while lymphoma peaked at 56% at 8 minutes [14].

Thus, in the evaluation of space occupying lesions of the brain complicating the course of AIDS, dynamic enhanced rapid MR imaging might help to quickly select patients highly suspected of CNS lymphoma, and to lead to immediate stereotaxic biopsy and radiation treatment.

Glomus tumors

Patients with suspected glomus tumors undergo at the present time CT and angiography. Preoperative assessment of glomus tumors requires angiography to characterize and locate tumor and arterial feeders. In a recent study [21], arterial MR angiography and MR venography were evaluated for tumor detection in 40 patients with suspected glomus tumors (fig. 45.2). Sixteen of 18 proved tumors were detected with spin-echo (SE) images alone. Although four high-lying jugular bulbs were misinterpreted as tumors due to similar signal intensity, combined evaluation allowed differentiation between tumor and sinusal blood flow

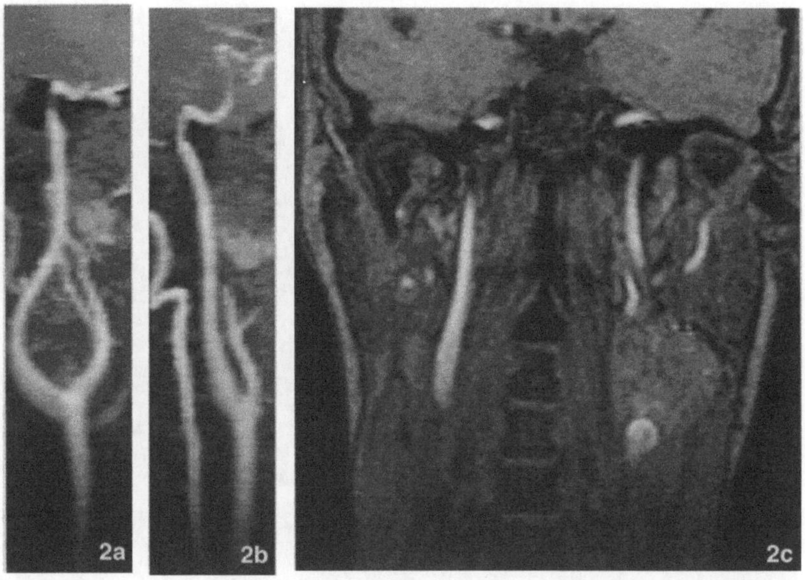

Fig. 45.2. MRA in a young female patient with suspected left carotid artery dissection. MIP reconstruction from a 3D GRE acquisition shows enlargement of the left carotid bifurcation (**a**) when compared with the right (**b**). Source image shows a glomus tumor developed between the left internal and left external carotid arteries

in all cases. It was concluded that combined SE imaging and MR angiography are recommended for ruling out tumors in patients with pulsatile tinnitus.

Lung neoplasms

Vascular involvement

In thoracic diseases, MRA has not been extensively evaluated, particularly because MRA of the thorax is difficult to perform due to cardiac and thoracic motion. Infiltration of mediastinal vessels is crucial to thoracic surgeon when sleeve or double-sleeve resection and vascular reconstructions are planned. MRA can provide information upon vessel displacement, stenosis and perfusion defects due to space occupying lesions. However, it is only a complementary technique to MR imaging as its indications are not yet well defined. A recent paper has demonstrated the value of MRA in the assessment of the patency of mediastinal vessels before thoracic surgery in patients with various thoracic neoplasms, in particular lung carcinoma [11].

Superior sulcus tumors are a rare bronchogenic carcinoma. The pretherapeutic assessment relies on imaging, before considering surgery or combination chemotherapy-radiotherapy . The selection of appropriate candidates for surgery requires a precise preoperative assessment of tumor resectability. Brachial plexus invasion does not influence prognosis. Vertebral body and vessel invasion have been demonstrated to be bad prognosis factors, although it is not a contraindication to tumor resections. Vascular involvement is an important problem in the preoperative staging, as it leads to a more radical resection. It has recently been demonstrated that MRA might be a valuable noninvasive diagnostic complementary method to MR imaging for detecting vascular involvement in the preoperative work-up of superior sulcus tumors with Pancoast syndrome. The use of selective presaturation allows separate studies of arteries and veins, without superimposition of both structures.

Dynamic MR assessment of mediastinal lymph node involvement

Pretherapeutic local and regional spread of bronchogenic carcinoma is usually evaluated with CT. Some reports have compared the accuracy of MR imaging with CT in mediastinal tumor invasion and mediastinal node involvement. The major problem of CT and MR imaging is their lack of accuracy in preoperative evaluation of bronchogenic carcinoma, due to poor specificity in the diagnosis of enlarged mediastinal lymph nodes. Therefore, a false-positive diagnosis of mediastinal involvement deprives patients of a potentially curative surgical procedure, whereas false-negative diagnosis may results in unnecessary surgery.

The lack of specific imaging features is primarily due to an inability to distinguish between enlarged anthracotic or inflammatory lymph nodes from metastatic lymph nodes on the basis of density or signal intensity node size. Given that enlarged anthracotic

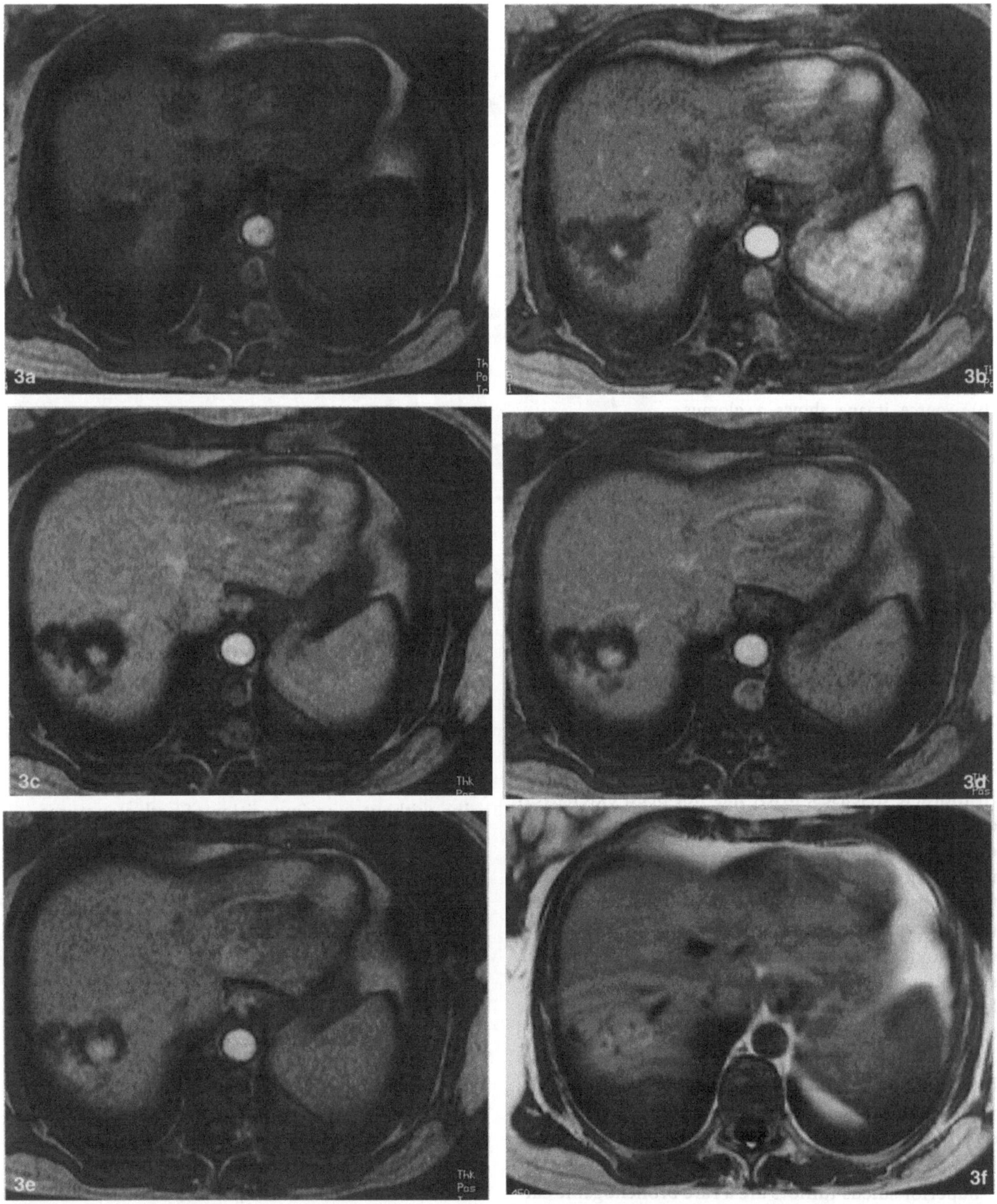

Fig. 45.3. Dynamically enhanced MRI of the liver in a patient diagnosed as having two focal hepatic masses during the follow-up of breast cancer. **a** Unenhanced axial T1-weighted GRE image demonstrating two hypointense masses located in segments 7 and 8. **b** 30 seconds post-injection, the mass in segment 8 has enhanced homogeneously, whereas the large lesion in segment 7 is incompletely filled-in by the contrast. **c, d, e** Later images showing progressive filling-in of the lesion in segment 7. **f** SE T1-weighted image obtained 5 minutes later shows completely homogeneous enhancement of the segment 7 lesion, a pattern highly suggestive of a hemangioma

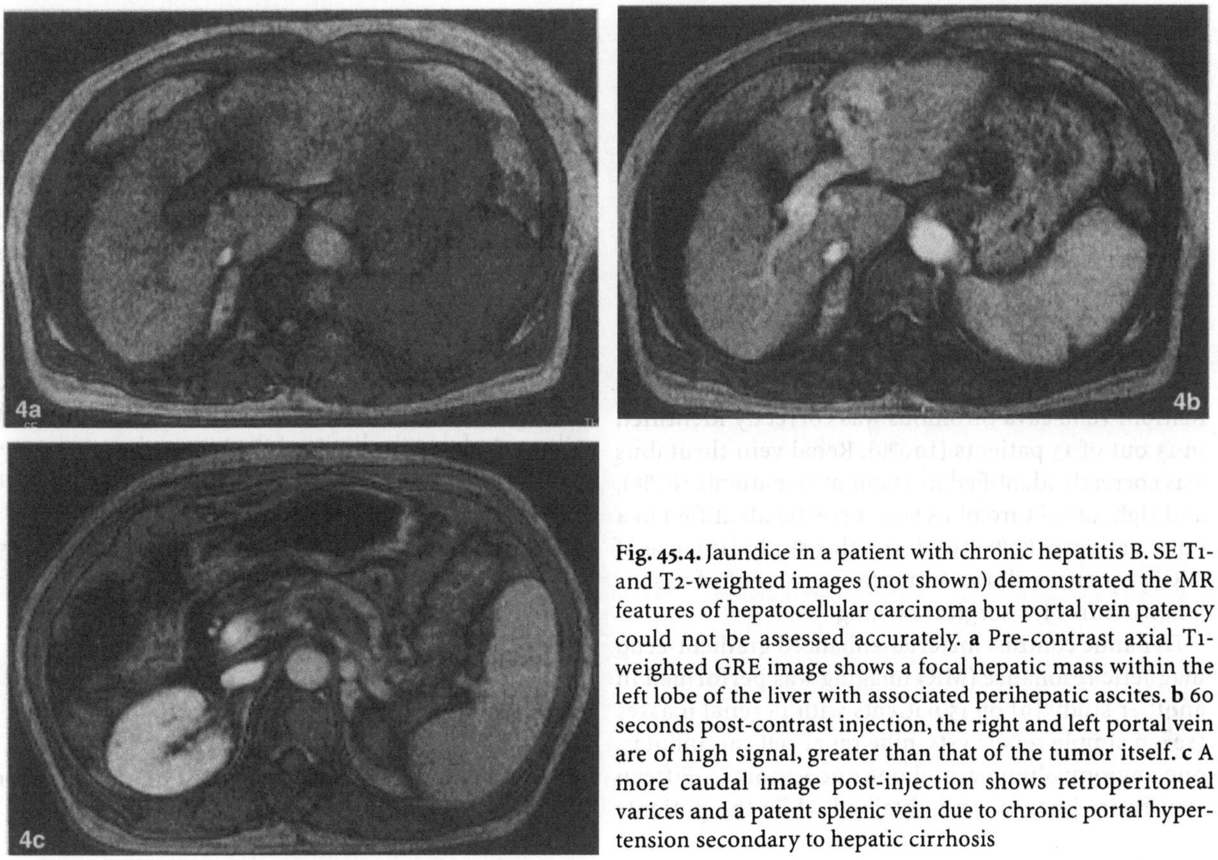

Fig. 45.4. Jaundice in a patient with chronic hepatitis B. SE T1- and T2-weighted images (not shown) demonstrated the MR features of hepatocellular carcinoma but portal vein patency could not be assessed accurately. **a** Pre-contrast axial T1-weighted GRE image shows a focal hepatic mass within the left lobe of the liver with associated perihepatic ascites. **b** 60 seconds post-contrast injection, the right and left portal vein are of high signal, greater than that of the tumor itself. **c** A more caudal image post-injection shows retroperitoneal varices and a patent splenic vein due to chronic portal hypertension secondary to hepatic cirrhosis

and metastatic nodes should display different enhancing patterns, a prospective study [13] showed that enhancement kinetics offered reliable data upon lymph node characterization. Metastatic nodes displayed enhancement curves similar to those of lung tumor, while anthracotic and granulomatous nodes did not enhance significantly.

Moreover, this study identified a high frequency of enlarged nodes that were not metastatic compared with the number of metastatic mediastinal lymph nodes reported in previous studies.

Hepatic neoplasm

Characterization of hepatic lesions [5, 7, 8, 15] (figs 45.3 & 45.4)

MR imaging is taking an important place in clinical practice for the evaluation of patients with focal hepatic masses. Newly developed fast MR sequences have been tested with the two major goals of decreasing motion artefacts and increasing intrinsic liver to lesion contrast. Dynamic gradient-echo (GRE) MR sequences have been recently developed to obtain fast acquisition of images and have been used to improve identification of focal hepatic masses.

Encouraging results have been reported using this technique.

CT vs MR arterial portography (CTAP vs MRAP) [3, 4, 16, 19]

By using a multisection GRE technique, several authors have demonstrated the superiority of MR arterial portography over CT arterial portography and unenhanced MR imaging.

MR arterial portography is a highly accurate preoperative imaging technique to detect focal hepatic masses, displaying a sensitivity up to 93% and a specificity of 100%. Nevertheless, because no significant difference have been reported in sensitivity between MR and CT arterial portography, MR arterial portography should not be performed on the basis of cost-effectiveness in assessment of patients with focal hepatic masses.

Venous involvement in kidney neoplasms

(fig. 45.5)

MR imaging has been suggested as a noninvasive alternative method to vena cavography and computed tomography for the detection of venous extension of renal adenocarcinoma. Several study designs have been used for the imaging of vascular structures. Complementary to spin-echo (SE) MR imaging, the preoperative gradient-recalled echo (GRE) MR images of 26 patients with renal adenocarcinoma were compared with findings at surgery and pathologic examination. Vena cava thrombus was correctly identified in 13 out of 13 patients (100%). Renal vein thrombus was correctly identified in 23 out of 26 patients (88%), and right atrial thrombus was correctly identified in 4 out 5 patients (80%) [6]. From this study [18], use of GRE sequences allows accurate assessment of vascular structures for surgical planing.

Dynamic contrast material-enhanced gradient-echo magnetic resonance (MR) imaging was performed in another study [9] on 15 patients with 18 renal masses (seven simple renal cysts, nine renal cell carcinomas, one angiomyolipoma, and one oncocytoma). Fifteen sequential images were obtained while the patients held their breath during a 2.5-3.5-minute interval during and immediately after intravenous administration of gadolinium-DTPA; delayed images were also obtained for 15 minutes. None of the simple renal cysts showed enhancement. All renal cell carcinomas were isointense with the renal cortex and demonstrated variable enhancement. Both the angiomyolopoma and the oncocytoma showed brisk, homogeneous enhancement. This dynamic MR imaging technique appeared to be useful in the detection and characterization of simple renal cysts and solid neoplasms.

In conclusion, CT remains the best technique to assess regional extension of kidney neoplasms, as it allows studying the limits of the tumor, the renal compartment and its walls, the renal vein and the inferior vena cava, the neighboring organs and the contralateral kidney all together. Its findings allow defining the indications of MRI which can be sometimes complementary to assess venous invasion.

Uterine masses

Dynamic MR imaging has been used in one study for the staging of uterine tumors. Usefulness of paramag-

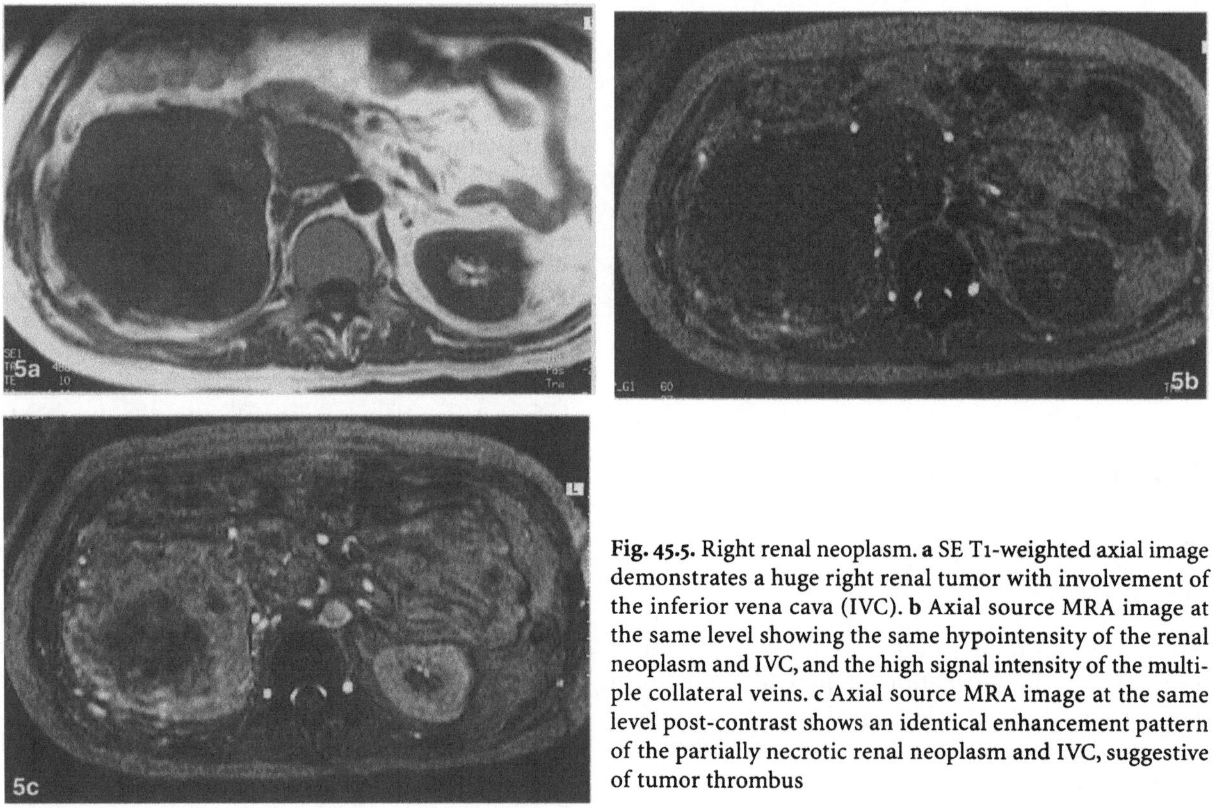

Fig. 45.5. Right renal neoplasm. **a** SE T1-weighted axial image demonstrates a huge right renal tumor with involvement of the inferior vena cava (IVC). **b** Axial source MRA image at the same level showing the same hypointensity of the renal neoplasm and IVC, and the high signal intensity of the multiple collateral veins. **c** Axial source MRA image at the same level post-contrast shows an identical enhancement pattern of the partially necrotic renal neoplasm and IVC, suggestive of tumor thrombus

netic contrast agents with MR imaging in uterine neoplasms was evaluated in 53 patients with endometrial carcinoma and 15 patients with cervical carcinoma. T1- and T2- weighted MR images were obtained before the contrast material was administered. After a bolus injection of gadopentetate dimeglumine, dynamic MR images were acquired, followed by static T1-weighted images. Gadolinium-enhanced MR images revealed relatively small endometrial carcinomas in the uterine cavity as high signal intensity in four cases and invasion of the myometrium as low signal intensity in 20 cases. In eight cases, endometrial tumors showed irregular, early enhancement compared with that of the myometrium on dynamic images; these cases were associated with poor prognosis. Tumor extension into the lower part of the uterus, parametrium, and paracervical fat was well seen on enhanced images in cases of cervical carcinoma. The authors believe that gadolinium-enhanced MR imaging will prove helpful in the staging of uterine neoplasms [10].

Musculoskeletal neoplasms

(fig. 45.6)

Magnetic resonance (MR) angiography has also been tested to preoperatively depict vascularity of musculoskeletal neoplasms in 23 prospective examinations [20]. 92% of vessels in proximity to tumor were noted by blinded readers. The post-contrast technique provided supplemental data in 47% of cases, usually related to better delineation of in-plane feeder vessels and areas with pulsatile blood flow. Of the 28 branch feeder vessels, 23 were noted on both conventional arteriograms and MR angiograms in a nonblinded review, but 16 were difficult to distinguish as feeders because of lack of associated tumor blush. From the results, MR angiography promised to replace conventional arteriography for orthopedic preoperative planing.

Other applications

(figs 45.7 & 45.8)

New MR angiographic applications can also be applied to oncologic patients. These can include diagnosis and assessment of extension of lower limb thrombophlebitis which is often present in these patients. Compression of iliac veins by pelvic neoplasms can also be easily demonstrated. Cervical and mediastinal veins can also be examined with MR angiography to assess thrombus extent, in particular in patients with indwelling catheters. However in these cases, MR angiography does not compare favorably with Duplex-Doppler study in terms of cost-effectiveness.

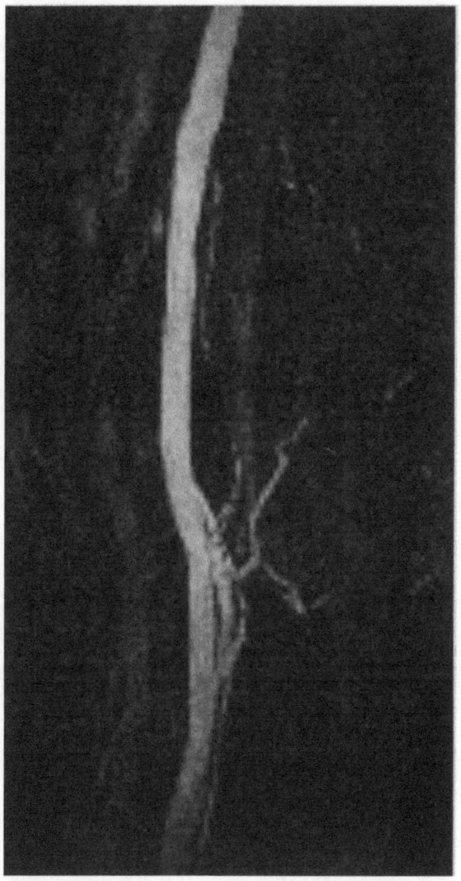

Fig. 45.6. Soft tissue sarcoma arising in the distal femur. A MIP reconstruction angiogram shows arterial feeding vessels running around the tumor

Conclusion

MR angiography is a technology undergoing rapid development, but is facing serious competition of spiral CT. Despite the intrinsic advantages of MR angiography in portraying, the whole vasculature,noninvasively measuring blood flow and regional perfusion, and with dynamic MR imaging to study the specific enhancement of tissues, the main limitation of this technique is its high cost, when compared with the other available techniques.

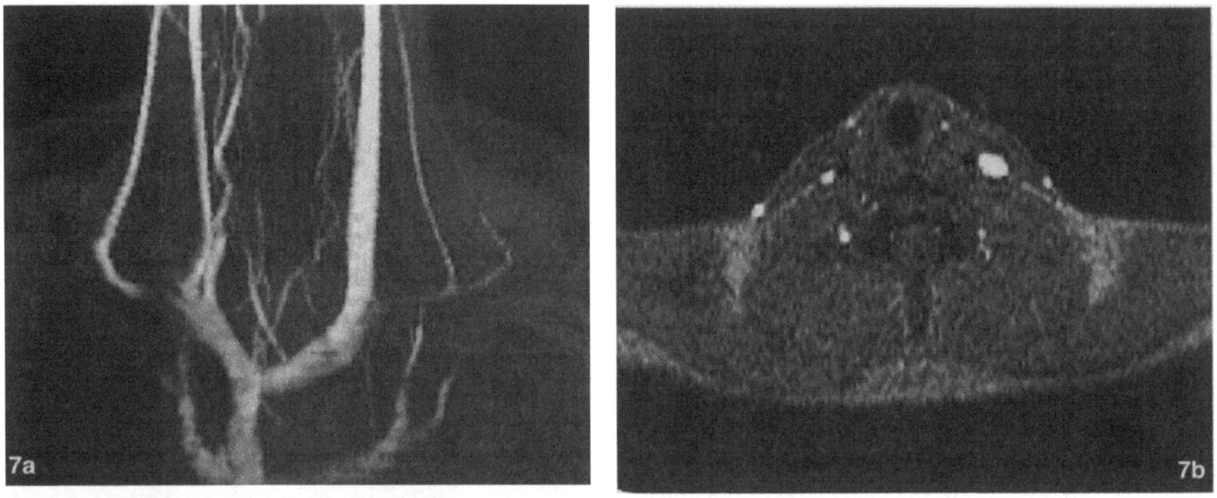

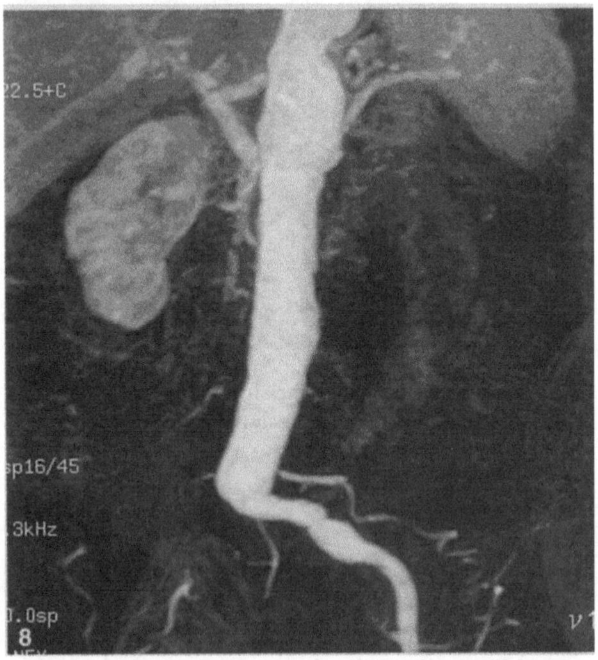

Fig. 45.7. MR venography of the cervico-mediastinal veins following retrieval of an infected internal jugular catheter. **a** The MIP reconstruction hardly displays the right internal jugular vein. Note the hypertrophied right external jugular vein. **b** Axial source image shows a small but patent right internal jugular vein

Fig. 45.8. Right iliac vein obstructed by enlarged lymphomatous lymph nodes

MR cholangio-pancreatography

Stationary or slightly mobile fluid (physiologic CSF-containing cysts, endolymph, aqueous humors of the eye, as well as fluid within bowel loops, the urinary tract and especially the hepato-biliary-pancreatic ducts) is ideally suited for MR imaging using heavily T2-weighted sequences.

This is due to the very high contrast obtained between the homogeneous high signal of the endoluminal fluid and the low signal of the surrounding parenchyma and vascular structures (irrespective of blood flow).

MR cholangiography [17]

(fig. 45.9)

MR cholangiography can be performed on current machines at mid-field strength (0.5T), but the acquisition times are generally long (several minutes).

The acquisition times on the high field strength systems (1T and particularly 1.5T) are reduced to the order of 1.5 to 2 seconds per slice, especially by using strong phase encoding gradients ("hypergradients" > 20mT/m/s). The image quality also depends on the data collection system and is markedly improved by the use of phased array surface coils.

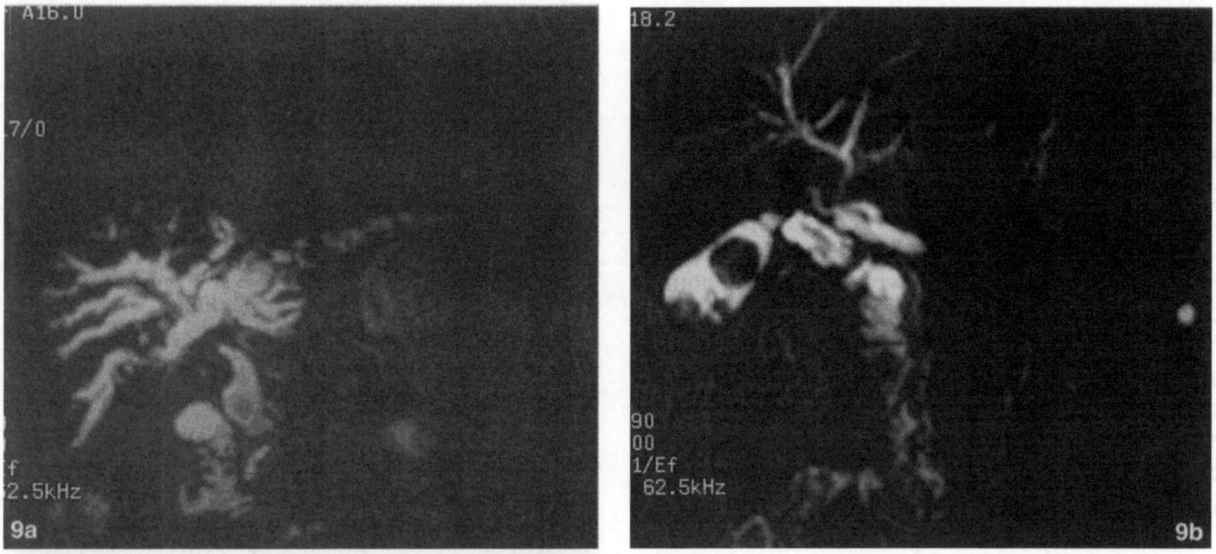

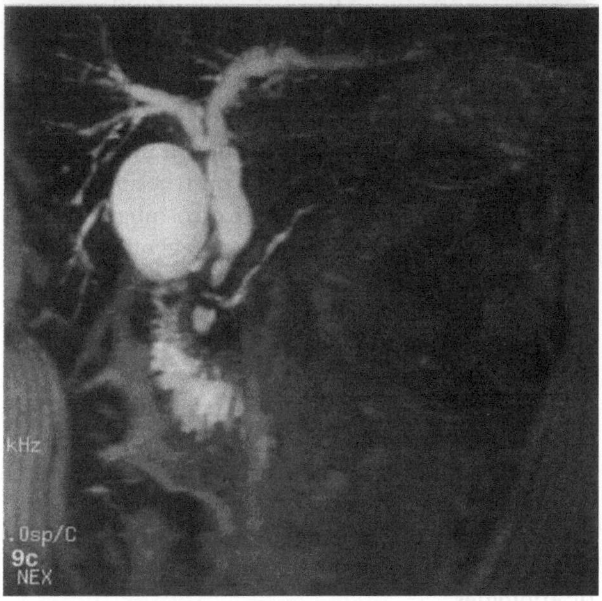

Fig 45.9. **a** MR cholangiography showing generalized biliary tract dilatation due to a carcinoma of the pancreatic head. **b** Acrolithiasis of the gallbladder shown on MR cholangiography. **c** Ampulloma with a stenotic main retropancreatic bile duct and proximal dilatation

The software controls the acquisition sequences which are conducted by the application of successive ultrafast magnetic field gradients allowing the required signal to be obtained in the study slice from the structures under examination (using T2-weighting in the case of MR cholangio-pancreatography).

It is in this area that the major advances have been witnessed, thus enabling MR cholangio-pancreatography to become a routine technique which provides very high quality anatomical and diagnostic information.

Single breath hold acquisitions can be achieved using current techniques:
- either 10-20 sections acquired in one or two breath holds of 15-20 seconds each
- or single successive sections (of the "incremental" type using the CT analogy) of a variable thickness (3-50 mm, with an average of 20 mm for "thick" sections and 5-7 mm for "thin" sections) with an acquisition time of only 2 seconds per section.

These very rapid sequences in a single "excitation" (single shot) utilize a very long echo train (68-128 echoes) allowing a complete readout of the section (in fact only a half readout is performed in the Fourier plane, the rest of the image being calculated due to the symmetry in this plane).

There are two types of sequence currently available which are based on this principle:

• HASTE (Half Fourier Acquisition Single Shot Turbo Spin Echo) has been used for two years in clinical practice and has produced well recognized results in MR cholangiography by the acquisition of series of sections in apnea which are then reconstructed into images by a process of "summation" of the MIP (Maximum Intensity Projection) type .

• SS-FSE (Single Shot Fast Spin Echo from GE) has just become available to users, and its strong point is the ability to acquire thick sections (nominal optimal thickness 20 mm) which allow visualization of almost the entire biliary and pancreatic ductal system in 2 seconds on a single image. This is achieved without the necessity of long image processing which tends to be of variable quality due to its empirical nature.

Unfortunately, it is not possible to transform an "average" MRI scanner into one which is ideally suited to the performance of MR cholangio-pancreatography without changing the hardware (especially the "hyper-gradients"). Although this is technically feasible, it necessitates a costly upgrade. However, this is perfectly justifiable when one considers the resultant complete transformation in the possible MRI applications (particularly in body imaging).

The aim of imaging both for the clinician and the radiologist is to obtain a macroscopic representation of an often complex anatomical structure as accurate as possible by constructing an impression from a global view. Subsequently this will be complemented by analytical images with improved definition using thinner superimposed sections.

In this respect, it is directly the "esthetic" quality of the images, particularly the absence of flow artefacts, which leads to the diagnosis with a complete representation of the whole of the hepato-biliary-pancreatic ductal system.

Artefacts and limitations [17]

Endoluminal areas of low signal (pseudolacunae) are seen within dilated bile ducts using the breath-hold MR cholangiography sequences (HASTE and SS-FSE) both on the coronal and axial sections. These artefacts, which have yet to be clearly explained, can be very misleading by simulating intraductal stones. They should, however, be recognized by their central location and the progressive nature of the endoluminal signal loss. The same phenomena can be seen in any dilated tubular structure (e.g. Wirsung's duct or ureters).

Value of MR cholangiography in cases of neoplastic pancreatico-biliary obstruction

It is in the investigation of pancreatico-biliary obstructions that the thick sections of MR cholangio-pancreatography using the SS-FSE sequence can provide crucial information as to the etiology and possible operability by clearly demonstrating the degree and precise level of obstruction of the dilated ducts.

Wirsung's duct is visible in 100% of cases in the region of the pancreatic head and isthmus. Thus, it becomes very easy to decide whether the responsible tumor is situated at/or in the immediate vicinity of the ampulla of Vater, or alternatively if the obstruction is purely choledochal (adenocarcinoma of the bile duct), or if there is an infiltrating carcinoma of the pancreatic isthmus causing cut off of Wirsung's duct in this region. A simple and accurate analysis of the ancillary signs, namely dilatation of the biliary and pancreatic ducts, in every case precludes the necessity for an invasive contrast ERCP examination which can be dangerous due to the introduction of infection into the stagnant bile proximal to the obstruction.

The precise map of the pancreatico-biliary system which can be obtained in all cases (even in the aged since a breath-hold of only 2 seconds is required) optimizes the treatment options: surgery, insertion of an endoprosthesis or stent via the endoscopic or transhepatic route.

In a series of 29 cases comparing ERCP with MR pancreatico-cholangiography [17], good concordance was seen with a k = 0.68. Discordance was mainly encountered in cases of post-cholecystectomy bile duct dilatation and diagnostic oddities. The concordance was excellent (9 out of 10 cases) for the neoplastic etiologies.

Assessment of tumor size and operability is better with MR pancreatico-cholangiography compared to ERCP due to the reliable visualization of the tissues around the dilated pancreatico-biliary ducts.

Size is the limiting feature for lesion detectability by MR cholangiography which is probably superior in this respect to endoscopic ultrasound. This latter technique provides more accurate information for the assessment of vascular invasion and local lymph node involvement by the tumor, as well as the precise localization of the lesion (adenocarcinoma of the lower end of the CBD vs adenocarcinoma of the pancreatic head or ampulla).

MR pancreatico-cholangiography is superior to endoscopic ultrasound in the evaluation of the extent of infiltrating tumors of the pancreatic head or isthmus because it gives an unequivocal and very precise representation of the dilated ducts proximal to the tumor.

ERCP should no longer be performed in a purely diagnostic role but be reserved as an interventional procedure. The image quality obtained from ERCP is greatly inferior to that from MR cholangio-pancreatography both for the extrahepatic bile ducts (with the exception of the lower biliary confluence) and the intrahepatic bile ducts.

As with all organ imaging techniques, significant further improvements in image quality of MR cholangio-pancreatography can be expected with thanks to several possible already open avenues of progress:

• The reduction in acquisition times to less than 1 second, an essential factor for limiting flow movement, an improvement in spatial resolution by performing thin sections, increased signal to noise ratio and increase in the number of phase encoding steps, optimization of the volumetric acquisitions either by using thick sections or by the summation of thin sections, the development of techniques for obtaining three dimensional models of the whole of the parenchyma, excretory ducts and blood vessels. These "models" can subsequently be used to guide surgery and interventional procedures, possibly even to automate them.

References

1. Apicella PL, Mirowitz SA, Weinreb JC (1994) Extension of vessels through hepatic neoplasms: MR and CT findings. Radiology 191: 135-6
2. Atzor KR, Stolz H, Kauczor HU, Urban V, Tintera J, Perneczky A, Stoeter P (1995) 3D-high resolution imaging of tumors and aneurysms at the cranial base-comparison of CT and MR. Comput Biol Med 25: 277-91
3. Bluemke DA, Fishman EK (1993) Spiral CT arterial portography of the liver. Radiology 186: 576-579
4. Dravid VS, Shapiro MJ, Mithcell DG, Outwater Ek, Piccoli CW, Feld RO, Wechsler RJ, Rosato FE (1994) MR portography: preliminary comparison with CT portography and conventional MR imaging. J Magn Reson Imaging 4: 767-71
5. Edelman RR, Siegel JB, Singer A, Dupuis K, Longmaid HE (1989) Dynamic MR imaging of the liver with Gd-DTPA: initial clinical results. AJR 153: 1213-1219
6. Eilenberg SS, Lee JKT, Brown JJ, Mirowitz SA, Tartar VM (1990) Renal masses: evaluation with gradient-echo Gd-DTPA-enhanced dynamic MR imaging. Radiology 176: 333-338
7. Goldberg MA, SainiS, Hahn PF, Egglin TK, Mueller PR (1991) Differentiation between hemangiomas and metastases of the liver with ultrafast MR imaging: preliminary results with T2 calculations. AJR 157: 727-30
8. Hamm B, Fischer E, Taupitz M (1989) Differentiation of hepatic haemangiomas from metastases by dynamic contrast-enhanced MR imaging. J Comput Assist Tomogr 14: 205-216
9. Helenon O, Denys A, Chretien Y, Souissi M, Melki P, Cornud F, Dufour B, Moreau JF (1992) Role of MRI in the diagnosis of cancer of the kidney. J Urol (Paris) 98: 3-13
10. Hirano Y, Kubo K, Hirai Y, Okada S, Yamada K, Sawano S, Yamashita T, Hiramatsu Y (1992) Preliminary experience with gadolinium-enhanced dynamic MR imaging for uterine neoplasms. Radiographics 12: 243-56
11. Kauczor HU, Gamroth AH, Tuengerthal SJ, et al (1992) MR angiography: clinical applications in thoracic surgery. Eur Radiol 2: 214-222
12. Knopp EA. Venous disease and tumors. Magn Reson Imaging 1995; 3: 509-28
13. Laissy JP, Soyer Ph, Sekkal SR, Tebboune D, Servois V, Sibert A, Menu Y (1995) Assessment of vascular involvement with Magnetic resonance angiography (MRA) in Pancoast syndrome. Magn Reson Imaging 13: 523-530
14. Laissy JP, Soyer Ph, Tebboune D, Gay-Depassier Ph, Casalino E, Lariven S, Sibert A, Menu Y (1994) Value of dynamic contrast-enhanced fast MR imaging in differentiating brain toxoplasmosis and lymphoma in AIDS patients. J Comput Assist Tomogr 18: 714-718
15. Mirowitz SA, Lee JKT, Gutierrez E, Brown JJ, Heiken JP, Eilenberg SS (1991) Dynamic gadolinium-DTPA-enhanced rapid acquisition spin-echo MR imaging of the liver. Radiology 179: 371-376
16. Pavone P, Giuliani S, Cardone G, et al (1991) Intraarterial portography with gadopentetate dimeglumine: improved liver-to-lesion contrast in MR imaging. Radiology 179: 693-697
17. Régent D, Bigard MA (1997) Cholangiopancréatographie IRM en séquence SS-FSE. Dialogues Gastro-Entérologie. Nicholas diffusion-édition
18. Roubidoux MA, Dunnick NR, Sostman HD, Leder RA (1992) Renal carcinoma: detection of venous extension with gradient-echo MR imaging. Radiology 182: 269-72
19. Soyer Ph, Laissy JP, Sibert A, Blanc F, Belghiti J, Marmuse JP, Zeitoun G, Levesque M, Menu Y (1994) Focal Hepatic Masses: Comparison of Detection during Arterial Portography with MR Imaging and CT. Radiology 190: 737-740
20. Swan JS, Grist TM, Sproat IA, Heiner JP, Wiersma SR, Heisey DM (1995) Musculoskeletal neoplasms: preoperative evaluation with MR angiography. Radiology 194: 519-524
21. Vogl TJ, Juergens M, Balzer JO, Mack MG, Bergman C, Grevers G, Lissner J, Felix R (1994) Glomus tumors of the skull base: combined use of MR angiography and spin-echo imaging. Radiology 192: 103-110

Index

Impressions DUMAS
42100 SAINT-ÉTIENNE
Dépôt légal : Avril 1998
N° d'imprimeur : 34308
Imprimé en France

MIX
Papier aus verantwortungsvollen Quellen
Paper from responsible sources
FSC® C105338

If you have any concerns about our products,
you can contact us on
ProductSafety@springernature.com

In case Publisher is established outside the EU,
the EU authorized representative is:
Springer Nature Customer Service Center GmbH
Europaplatz 3, 69115 Heidelberg, Germany

Printed by Libri Plureos GmbH
in Hamburg, Germany